SPORT AND THE BODY:

A Philosophical Symposium

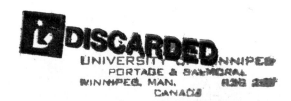

SPORT AND THE BODY:

A Philosophical Symposium

Edited and with Introductions and Bibliographies by

ELLEN W. GERBER, Ph.D., J.D.
formerly Associate Professor
University of Massachusetts, Amherst
now Staff Attorney
Legal Aid Society of Northwest North Carolina
Winston-Salem, North Carolina

and

WILLIAM J. MORGAN, Ph.D.
Assistant Professor of Physical Education
Adjunct Assistant Professor of Philosophy
The University of Tennessee
Knoxville, Tennessee

Second Edition

LEA & FEBIGER   Philadelphia · 1979

Ruth Abernathy, Ph.D., Editorial Adviser,
Professor Emeritus, School of Physical and Health Education,
University of Washington, Seattle, Washington 98105

First edition, 1972
  Reprinted 1974

Library of Congress Cataloging in Publication Data

Gerber, Ellen W.   comp.
  Sport and the body.
  Includes bibliographies.
  1. Sports—Philosophy—Addresses, essays, lectures.
I. Morgan, William John, 1948–   II. Title
GV706.G47   1979   796'.01   79–16599
ISBN 0–8121–0679–9

Published in Great Britain by Henry Kimpton Publishers, London

Printed in the United States of America

Print Number 3 2 1

Preface

It has been only six years since the preface to the first edition was written. Rereading those words one senses the excitement of something new, an awakening interest in studying the phenomenon of sport, an incipient focus on the experience of the body in sport. The sparcity of historical attention to the study of the sport phenomenon from a philosophical viewpoint was evident in the selections and the bibliographies for each section of that first symposium. The editor of the first edition remembers clearly the luxury of being able to include among the selections everything written that she deemed to be of appropriate quality. Moreover, she was extremely grateful to Lea & Febiger for their willingness to chance the commercial success of a book for which there seemed to be at best only an extremely limited market of a dedicated band of scholars.

The situation in 1979 is markedly different. The philosophic study of sport and the body is now a vigorous, well-developed and recognized field of study. Students, scholars, sports participants, and the merely curious have come together in a joint effort to gain more understanding and insight into this interesting phenomenon. Thus it was understandable that soon after the publication of the first edition, the Philosophic Society for the Study of Sport was organized. Its founding meeting was held on December 28, 1972 in conjunction with the meetings of the eastern division of the American Philosophical Association, ratifying in some formal sense the alliance between sport and philosophy.

The Society began publishing the *Journal of the Philosophy of Sport* in 1974. It soon became a fine source for increasingly sophisticated analyses of sport, as testified to by the articles reprinted in this volume. Moreover, a glance through its table of contents reveals that scholars in this field have creatively expanded their approaches to the study of sport, finding rich and interesting avenues to consider.

Of course, a field of study requires more than writing and organizations to give it life. It needs active, ongoing dialogue of the kind that goes on in classes, seminars and scholarly meetings. At the time of the first edition, a small band of people interested in the philosophic study of sport and the body met from time to time at the State University of New York, College at Brockport. There a faculty remarkable in its devotion to this subject played host to the faithful providing a forum for presentation of papers and free-wheeling discussion. From those informal meetings came the annual meetings of the Philosophical Society for the Study of Sport and special symposia such as the recent R. Tait McKenzie Symposium on Sport sponsored by the University of Tennessee.

Perhaps most important has been the growth of the philosophic study of sport and the body as a curricular subject. Undergraduate and graduate classes throughout the country have focused their attention on this approach to sport. Some classes are held under the auspices of departments of physical education; others by departments of philosophy or by new, specialized units that focus on American culture. The courses of study have enabled innumerable people to begin to understand the dimensions of their personal sport experience, to plan for the future when as teachers, coaches or sport leaders they will guide the sport experiences of others and perhaps to glimpse the meaning of the phenomenon to the individuals of the world at large—for sport clearly is an international phenomenon, present in virtually every culture throughout all of human history.

The second edition of *Sport and the Body* reflects the growth and development of these past six years. To the best and most representative of the articles in the first edition have been added a richly diversified and sometimes more sophisticated compilation of recent analyses. In their quality and insight into contemporary concerns, we believe that each selection offers to the interested individual an opportunity to better understand sport and the experience of it. Happily (and in contrast to the first edition), we found ourselves presented with a plethora of riches from which to choose. Inevitably, many persons will disagree with our selections. Clearly they represent the editors' tastes, critical acumen and classroom experience; we accept full responsibility for our choices.

We sought to bring to the reader, to the student of sport, an anthology that would provide a broad range of approaches to the phenomenon of sport and the body, while keeping narrowly within the definition of sport as it was defined in the first edition:

> Sport is a human activity that involves specific administrative organization and a historical background of rules which define the objective and limit the pattern of human behavior; it involves competition or challenge and a definite outcome primarily determined by physical skill.

As in the first edition, we tried to introduce students to the spectrum of scholars writing on sport from a philosophic viewpoint. Although we particularly preserved the works of classical philosophers, inevitably the thrust of this edition is the presentation of ideas engendered within the last five years. In this way we have been able to take advantage of the product of

the growth of the field as described in this preface.

Because of the academic interest in sport philosophy on both the graduate and undergraduate levels, and in society at large, we also have attempted to meet a variety of needs within this one anthology. There is a sufficient quantity of articles to permit teachers (and casual readers) to choose selections from those offered according to the level of sophistication of their students and with attention to the unique interests and focus of a particular course.

The organization of the first edition has been repeated in the second edition. It proved to be useful both as a means of organizing the collection of articles into meaningful theoretical groups of concepts and also for providing units of manageable size for curricular purposes. Moreover, it permits the reader interested in a particular aspect of the study of sport to have an opportunity to focus on it with some depth of material available within this one volume.

Lastly, we take pleasure in acknowledging those who have provided us with assistance, or inspiration, or just plain emotional support and sustenance during the process of putting together this book. Those who deserve special mention in this regard include Leonard Ehrlich, Don Franks, Robert Osterhoudt, Madge Phillips, Terry Roberts and Clarence Shutte. A special note of thanks is also owed Steve LeMay for his careful and adroit editorial assistance. And finally, our deepest appreciation goes to the original lonely band who formed the collegial nucleus that made possible the growth of this field and ultimately the need for a second edition.

We are grateful for the patience and trust exhibited by Lea & Febiger and in particular its executive editor for Health, Human Movement and Leisure Studies, Edward H. Wickland, Jr. Ed has been unfailingly helpful, generous and prompt in his response to our requests.

It is always difficult to find time to write when the burden of other responsibilities goes on and on; inevitably, the frustration shows. Therefore, it is those women with whom we each live, Pearl Berlin and Linda Morgan, respectively, who deserve the greatest thanks because inevitably they are the ones who bear the burden of offering support and encouragement when we are at our most obnoxious.

Greensboro, North Carolina Ellen W. Gerber
Knoxville, Tennessee   William J. Morgan

Contents

SECTION I

The Nature of Sport

INTRODUCTION

Fundamental to an examination of sport in its diversified and meaningful roles is an understanding of its nature as a phenomenon. There are numerous methods useful for discerning the nature of sport. Operating from the conviction that a given noun (e.g., sport) has a describable essence—an essentialistic philosophical position—a variety of techniques can be employed to analyze the phenomenon. These include definition, characterization, classification, and comparison.

Definition is basically an application of inductive reasoning. To define sport one might begin by listing all activities intuitively accepted as sport. If one rejects the personalism of intuition, convention or social agreement can be substituted as a better basis for constructing such a list. In either case, from this list of specific activities an all-embracing definition can be induced. The definition must be general enough to include all the activities one wishes to accept as sport and specific enough to exclude all activities which one rejects as non-sport. Robert Osterhoudt's article "The Term 'Sport': Some Thoughts on a Proper Name" and Bernard Suits' essay "What is a Game?" are excellent examples of this form of logic.

Characterization, although similarly beginning with an idea of the activities accepted as sport, is an example of deductive logic. From the generalized idea of what is sport (or from an accepted definition of sport), are deduced the characteristics of sport, viz. their common elements. The characteristics decided upon must be present in all activities accepted as sport and that precise combination of characteristics should not be found in activities not considered sport. "The Nature of Play" by Johan Huizinga, and "Sport and Play: Suspension of the Ordinary" by Kenneth Schmitz both represent the application of deductive logic as the process used to ascertain the nature of sport.

At least since Aristotle, classification has been an important technique for delineating the essence of something. It can serve the purpose of clarifying the basic relationships that are inherent in sport activities. In many ways classification is similar to characterization because it groups subjects that have like elements. It may even be considered a secondary form of analysis because it is dependent upon the identification of common characteristics before grouping can be accomplished. Probably the most frequently cited model for classifying games was designed by Roger Caillois; it is presented here in the chapter called "The Classification of Games." John Loy expressed a somewhat different system in his article "The Nature of Sport: A Definitional Effort."

The last two selections in this section exemplify further ways in which the question concerning the definitional status of sport may be approached. In his essay, "Toward a Non-Definition of Sport," McBride argues, using ordinary language as his normative standard, that the concept of sport is a vague, imprecise one, and thus, one that cannot be defined. The final essay in this section, Morgan's "Some Aristotelian Notes on the Attempt to Define Sport," takes an entirely different stance towards this definitional question and in so doing initiates a critical response to McBride's work. Adopting what might be termed a critical-essentialist position, Morgan argues that the concept sport can indeed be defined provided that the conceptual model brought to the definitional venture includes Aristotle's theory of "focal meaning," or something akin to it.

In general, attempts to apply the technique of philosophical analysis to the nature of sport have been sparse. Most of the important writings on the subject are included in this book. There are, however, other important essays dealing with this topic that the reader might be interested in pursuing. Champlin's recent essay (1977) discusses the need for developing a critical definition of sport and sets out the notion of "universe of discourse" as a pivotal criterion for constructing such a definition. Thomas (1976) approaches the definitional issue by examining concepts closely tied to the conceptual ken of sport (games, rules, competition and the like). Paddick (1975) provides an insightful analysis of physical activity, arguing that what makes an activity a physical activity is not its lack of mental involvement, nor its simple dependence on gross movement, but rather its express valuation of certain bodily movements. Suits' essay (1973) extends his definitional account of a game in terms of the kindred concept of sport which he defines as a specific type of game involving physical skill, a wide following, and a certain measure of institutional stability. Weiss (1969) develops a comparative analysis of play, sport and game, noting their similarities. Metheny (1969) formulates a definition of sport using the deductive method. Fogelin (1968) presents another variation of the analytic approach to this issue. Approaching play as a behavior, Avedon and Sutton-Smith (1971) proffer a critical analysis of the theories of Huizinga and Caillois. In their anthropological study on "Games in Culture," Roberts, Arth and Bush (1969) provide an interesting classification of games somewhat different from Caillois' version. Melvin (1960) does a good comparison between play, work, and leisure. Sutton-Smith (1959) offers an excellent analysis of game characteristics in an article on "game meaning." Stone in his two articles (1957, 1969) presents the results of a sociological study which shows the varied meanings inherent in the symbolic term sport, to groups

with different social characteristics. And going back to the turn of the twentieth century, Graves' work (1900) set the stage for much of the work in this area by raising the problematic conceptual status of the term sport. There is also a body of literature on game theory which includes analyses of game characteristics, but the writings are too tangential to this book to be noted here.

It seems safe to say that we have yet to achieve reasonable closure in our efforts to concisely characterize the concept sport. A cursory perusal of the readings and bibliographical citations included herein indicates as much. Yet at least two possible lines of interpretation, which reflect to a greater or lesser extent the prevailing philosophic tenor of our age, offer themselves for inspection here. On the one hand, we could simply beg off from answering the question altogether, arguing that in fact the question cannot be answered. And it seems that we would have a good prima facie case for doing so; for the definitional ventures that have been proffered thus far reflect a great diversity of thought, much of it of a conflicting nature. On this view, we are persuaded to resist our definitional impulse, to, as it were, simply get used to the idea that sport is an inherently ambiguous concept. For getting used to this idea forestalls, so the argument goes, the pseudo-problems that inevitably occasion the stubborn insistence on pursuing such impulses.

However, as indicated above, another possible interpretation is forthcoming here. On this latter view, the welter of thought concerning this definitional issue is viewed from a synoptic vantage point. As such, one is pressed not so much to simply look for differences (these are certainly important but only in a preliminary way) but rather to look for a progressive development of thought, one that winds itself at times through apparent contradictions and widely divergent philosophic perspectives. Hegel provides the general heuristic clue in this regard: ". . . opinion . . . does not comprehend the diversity of philosophic systems as the progressive unfolding of truth, but rather sees in it simple disagreements. The bud disappears in the bursting-forth of the blossom, and one might say that the former is refuted by the latter . . . These forms are not just distinguished from one another, they also supplant one another as mutually incompatible. Yet at the same time their fluid nature makes them moments of an organic unity in which they not only do not conflict, but in which each is as necessary as the other; and this mutual necessity alone constitutes the life of the whole." ("Preface" to Hegel's *Phenomenology of Spirit*, p. 3, Miller Translation). With respect to the issue of the definability of sport then, the latter position commits us to regard each definitional endeavor as an integral moment or step on the path to a fully "systematic" rendering of the "nature of sport."

Now it is quite clear that in the latter case the definability of sport remains a viable philosophic topic. Yet even the former case sanctions the relevance of this question in at least this one sense: namely, that in order to establish the philosophic insignificance of the definitional question one must first pose the question itself. In this case, one is prompted to consider the question as but a necessary step in the process of refuting its importance. To do anything less is to trade philosophy for vulgar dogmatism.

Thus, on both fronts, their disparate character notwithstanding, the definitional question about sport retains its philosophic vitality, if for no other reason than to make clear the referent of our discussions of this phenomenon. And as hopefully has been shown, what is required in this context is an unbiased examination of the possible answers to this question as well as the conceptual models that undergird them. But beyond this, the practical implications of these theoretical deliberations must also come under our critical purview. That is to say, the relevance of the question concerning the definitional status of sport takes on further significance when viewed from the more concrete vantage point of the sport practitioner (included by the latter are all those charged in one way or another with the actual conduct of sport: teachers, coaches, trainers and the like). Here decisions about what is or is not sport manifest themselves in quite determinate ways. For instance, if our definition of sport is sufficiently broad to include such activities as dog shows, cock fighting, bull fighting, demolition derby, and the like, and assuming we possess the requisite resources, then it seems quite reasonable to insist that we make curricular provision for such in our respective sport programs (e.g., physical education classes and recreation programs). Similarly, if our definition of sport is compatible with the notion of professional sport, then, perhaps, a thorough re-examination of the role and place of sport in our educational institutions is in order. The possible list of pertinent issues that could be generated in this context are, no doubt, legion, but the upshot of it all is simply this: such questions as what is the "nature of sport," what are its fundamental characteristics, how can it be distinguished from other kindred human movement phenomena, have great practical import, and for this further reason, deserve our careful scrutiny.

The Term 'Sport':
Some Thoughts on a Proper Name*

ROBERT G. OSTERHOUDT

At bottom, the subject of this essay is sport. Few phenomena are so veiled in ambiguity as this one, however. It is fashionably conceived either as in some sense excluding, in some sense including, or in some sense serving as the basis for distinguishing such as dance, exercise, movement, physical education, play, and recreation. But it is not altogether clear as to in precisely what sense this is so in any of these cases. This essay will attempt to lay away some of this ambiguity by concisely saying what sport is. First it will be necessary to give an account of what is expected of terms, or linguistic expressions in general. Then it will be possible to demonstrate in what the term 'sport' consists, and in this demonstration to show as well what constitutes the basic nature of dance, exercise, movement, physical education, play, and recreation. The distinctions between sport and these others, and in significant measure the basic character of sport itself will thereby be made explicit.

A term, or linguistic expression which names a spatio-temporal particular (a person, place, thing, quality, idea, or activity) signifies that particular. That is to say, it utters a conventionally (or esoterically) accepted phrase which represents that particular. Such expressions thereby symbolize a mutually and continuously held, as well as informed, understanding with respect to the particulars to

*From *International Journal of Physical Education*, xiv (Summer, 1977), 11–16.

which they refer. In this way, these expressions fulfill their general communicative function, and recognize as well their aesthetic obligations. The search here is for a linguistic expression (or logico-linguistic characterization) which adequately signifies the phenomenon fashionably known as sport. This expression must be sufficiently general so as to refer to all of the sorts of activity properly included by the term 'sport', yet sufficiently specific so as to avoid mention of all the sorts of activity properly excluded by it. It must include explicit or tacit mention—it must recognize—all of the major forms of activity designated by the term, and only these forms. The attempt here is to determine the expression or characterization which is most aptly descriptive/prescriptive of this phenomenon, not for the purpose of arbitrarily reforming or revising it, but for the purpose of promoting a more fully and carefully developed understanding of, and appreciation for it—for the purpose of unveiling its basic character. Moreover, this discussion will confine itself to talk about the logico-linguistic bases of these determinations; thereby avoiding comment on the status of even prominent historical developments, and on the socio-politico-economic exigency, or administrative implications of such determinations.

The difficulty in successfully completing such a treatment is substantial, for the precise meaning of the phenomena and terms considered is elusive. This is so largely because the stipulations which distinguish each of these phenomena and terms themselves wait significantly on yet more basic presuppositions about reality in general—elaborate presuppositions which it is neither the purpose nor the capability of this essay to uncover, and presuppositions to which not even every rational, informed, and insightful person will agree. The "provocations" which follow thereby represent what, within the limits of a few pages and moments, can be plausibly said about the most preferred alternatives on the subject from among all of the many others.

Perhaps the most basic phenomenon prominently talked about in discussions concerning the fundamental character of sport is movement. The notion of movement implies a sense of mobility, as distinct from a sense of immobility; a sense of the dynamic, as distinct from the static; a sense of activity, as distinct from inactivity. Further implied by this is the view that movement entails an interpenetration or interaction, whereby "something" comes to displace or succeed "something else." In spatial terms, then, movement is apparently tantamount to displacement; in temporal ones, it is equivalent to succession. And, the yet more basic presupposition of these two notions is *change* itself. All of this comes to saying that, spatially, change, as the ground of movement, expresses itself as a "something" coming-to-occupy-the-place-of a "something else"; temporally, it takes the form of a "something" preceding or following a "something else."[1] It may also profit to observe that the spatial characterization is closely related to the temporal in that displacement and succession entail one another. That is to say, displacement carries with it the notion of preceding or following, and succession carries with it the idea of coming-to-occupy-the-place-of. Because "everything" is in this sense changing,[2-4] movement needs to be considered the motive force inherent in the entire fabric of things. It is the universal principle of change, or history. According to this account, then, the notions of displacement and succession together make up change, and change in turn reveals itself as the constitutive basis of movement.

When prominently expressed in the form of self-conscious "bodily" or "physical" displacement-succession of a particular intentional and objective sort, movement evidently provides such as dance, exercise, physical education, and sport with a definitive medium. But movement, as the general principle of change in the world, refers in some sense to all phenomena, and not merely or distinctively to an animating presence in dance, exercise, physical education, and sport. Movement as such consequently excludes little and is therefore insufficiently discriminating to conclusively secure the sorts of distinctions here sought.

Among the other basic phenomena considered in discussions of this type, play is perhaps the most notable. Play is not itself a concrete activity in the sense in which such as gymnastics, boxing, and baseball are concrete activities, for play does variously "attach" itself[5] to these and other concrete activities, and provides such activities with an axiologic guide (a guide as to value or purpose). Play is therefore of a different order than concrete activities as such; it is effectively a way of regarding these activities. It is the quality of concrete activity by which the activity(ies) to which it is "attached" (or in which it inheres) is intrinsically valued, or valued in-and-for-itself, and so voluntarily engaged, of an extraordinary or supra-mundane and disinterested character, and aesthetically ordered. Play is consequently a function of our purposeful, our self-conscious regard for activities, as distinct from a function of the objective mosaic of characteristic which distinguishes activities themselves. And its conceptual opposite, work, or the instrumental mode of valuing, is the result of saying what not-play is, and is as such secondary to play. The notion of intrinsicality is needed prior to, and as a basis for the notion of instrumentality, for the latter is effectively a flying away from the former. Play is positive, independent, and primary; work is negative, dependent, and derivative.

Insofar, then, as dance, physical education, and sport assume a genuinely human posture, they are primarily played. But this is what may and must be said of all types of human activity authentically disposed; that is, disposed to a fulfillment of human beings, as distinguished from being disposed to an instrumental regard for, and use of them. The notion of play, like that of movement, is nonetheless helpful here in its carrying out some fundamental distinctions; but it is not decisive in the end of this carrying out, because it, as such, fails to discriminate between the phenomena that it is our charge to discriminate between, and that it is in the character of our experience to distinguish.

The basic character of recreation is closely associated with the notion of play. It is commonly conceived as that collection of activities, voluntarily undertaken in the time unobligated to work—in leisure time—and primarily for the "enjoyment" it evokes. This is tantamount to characterizing recreation as the category of concrete activities conducted at play, or intrinsically valued. Though this characterization implies an inversion of the play-work relation earlier discussed, it does not, on further inspection, actually carry out such an inversion. The negative reference to recreation as occurring in the time unobligated to work merely succeeds in reinforcing the previously adduced insight that play and work are mutually exclusive. This reference does not penetrate to the basic constitutions of play and work themselves except to observe that the two are qualitatively distinct. This needs to be so because the contrary results in a confusion (in the form of an inversion) with respect to what is meant by positivity and negativity. In any case, recreation conceived in this way is virtually as inconclusive in making the distinctions tacit in our experience which it is the objective of this essay to make evident, as play itself. For it is nothing other than the concrete substance in which the play spirit resides. And insofar as recreation is thought a category of concrete activities which is not distinguished by the terms of its concretion, but by a mode of valuing this concretion, recreation may be understood as including any sort of concrete activity—dance, physical education, and sport being perhaps among the most prominent of these—which has the intrinsic mode of valuing at its axiologic center. And this is in prospect the case for any and all concrete activities.

Unlike recreation, exercise is by its nature instrumental. In general terms, it entails an organization of concrete events fashioned so as to produce an improvement of some sort in one's disposition or ability to perform designated activities. As applied to the phenomena here under examination, the notion typically refers to an organization of "bodily" or "physical" movements performed primarily for the purpose of enhancing the structuro-functional disposition of the self. As such, the principal interest in these movements is in their external effects, as distinct from in the movements themselves and in their possibilities for human fulfillment. Exercise is thereby conducted in the spirit of work, as opposed to that of play. And though it is of concern to such as dance, physical education, and sport, in the form of its producing effects which are useful in these, it is of such concern largely as a preliminary or preparatory tool, and not as a part, let alone the whole of these per se.

With the lot of prior discussion now in hand, adequate foundation has been laid for a productive conversation about sport itself. All sporting activity is governed by an elaborate mosaic of constitutive rules[6] which stipulate the material goals aimed at, and the means permitted in attempting to achieve these goals. These rules individually define particular sporting activities, and collectively they contribute much to saying what sport in general is. For one, pertaining to this latter, the goals they posit serve no utilitarian purpose.[7] These goals, together with the means to them, merely make possible an experience of a certain, compelling sort, and in this they serve the spirit of play. For another, the experience made possible by these rules entails a standing in viable relation to the performance of another (or others), and/or a stipulated standard of performance. This is the agonistic or competitive motif in sport. It is that by which one is constrained to achieve difficult-to-achieve goals. The goals of sport are thereby neither impossible (else they could not be seen as viable, and sought after) nor are they gratuitous (else there be nothing but cavalier emptiness to achieve). And for yet another, these rules embody an emphasis on the "physical" which makes the way in which movements are performed highly significant. The final outcome of these movements does not exhaust their significance, as is so in the movement of chess pieces and in other board and in card games as well. In these games, the terms of movement themselves are incidental, in any constitutive or genuinely interesting sense, as compared to the importance of the position (or state) moved from and to. In sport, however, the movements themselves are idealized and become an engaging part of the activity. This is so on two principal counts. Firstly, these movements require great skill to perform well. One's success in sport thereby depends primarily on the skillful execution of these movements, as distinct from any chance occurrence of them (which counts most in such as dice). And secondly, these movements (together with their connections to final outcomes, and their connections to competitive strife) constitute the concrete substance of sport's aesthetic appeal. They are the basis of sport's well known sense of beauty.

Even at this, however, we come upon activities which apparently meet these conditions, but which it is nonetheless our inclination to exclude from any strict and full notion of sport. Such activities as barrel jumping, hurling, jai alai, hula hooping, and jousting, among similar others, have an insufficiently wide basis in our geographico-historical experience to be included. They have not affected the human circumstance in sufficient measure to have gained anything other than a geographically or historically isolated practice—to have had anything other than a highly limited cultural or temporal experience. And activities involving self-propelled mechanical contrivances (e.g., automobile, motorcycle, and hydroplane racing) and animate non-humans (e.g., bull fighting, rodeo, horse racing, polo, hunting, and fishing) do not fully meet the voluntary and self-conscious requirements of playful and peculiarly human endeavor. So-termed "conquest" or "nature" sports (e.g., mountain climbing, parachuting, and surfing) apparently persist on the edge of these distinctions and must be considered sport insofar as they obtain sufficient geographico-historical, or institutional grounding.

The activities which most unequivocally satisfy these conditions are the individual, dual, and team sports[8] which follow:

individual sports:
  classical forms of individual sport:[9]
    gymnastics: classical forms of aerial movement.
    swimming and diving: classical forms of aquatic movement.
    track and field athletics (including cross country): classical forms of grounded movement.
  individual winter sports: alpine skiing, biathlon, bobsledding, cross country skiing, figure skating, luge, ski jumping, and speed skating.
  other individual sports: archery, bowling, canoeing, cycling, golf, modern pentathlon, rowing, shooting,[10] weightlifting, and yachting.
dual sports:
  dual combative sports: boxing, fencing, and wrestling.
  dual court sports: badminton, court tennis, handball, squash, and table tennis.
  other dual sports: billiards, croquet (or roque), and curling.
team sports: basketball, cricket-baseball, field hockey, ice hockey, lacrosse, rugby-football, soccer, volleyball, and water polo.

The problems with this conception are not yet at an end, however. For dance too apparently satisfies all of the conditions here laid out for sport, and yet it is not consonant with our experience of either sport or dance to consider dance a sport.[11] The two bases on which dance and sport are most commonly distinguished have to do with the alleged competitive emphases of sport (and the apparent absence of such emphases in dance), and the typically more numerous, elaborate, and inflexible rules of sport (than those which "gov-

ern" dance). What is usually made of the first basis is that the intention of dance is fundamentally expressive, and the intention of sport is fundamentally competitive. But this characteristic (the competitive characteristic) was reduced in our prior discussion of it to a being constrained by standards of variously expressed (by the performances of other participants or by other "independently" stipulated standards of performance) excellence, and in this basic constraint dance shares, though perhaps in different degree than sport.[12] The cogency of this reduction is further demonstrated by the earlier argued conclusion which has sport a peculiarly human undertaking (a purposeful, self-conscious, playful undertaking)—an undertaking which is by its nature basically expressive; that is, variously searching after and finding the human "in" it. The second basis on which sport and dance are thought fundamentally or qualitatively distinct is similarly reduced to a difference in degree. It is evidently the case that the rules of sport are typically more numerous, elaborate and inflexible than are those of dance. This observation has led to the fashionable notion that dance is basically more creative than sport.[13] Even if this claim goes through, however, it fails to drive a qualitative wedge between sport and dance. The most that can therefore be made of the differences between sport and dance apparently has them distinct as to degree, but nonetheless of the same kind. As such, the two evidently constitute the movement arts, as being those art forms, and only those art forms,[14] which make movement (in the sense earlier ascribed to the "physical" emphasis in sport) their definitive medium of expression.

This leaves physical education which in modern history has undergone the transformation from physical training, in which it was thought an agent of bio-psychological health and fitness; to physical culture, in which it was conceived as an acculturative agent; to physical education itself. Through the first two stages of this development, systems of calisthenic and gymnastic exercise, and the motif of exercise itself, were predominant. Physical education was on the way to becoming itself in these stages, so to speak. With its development to physical education as such, these systems and the basic motif underlying them were left behind, and the possibilities of a genuinely playful treatment of sport and dance moved into the foreground as the dominant, even the constitutive element. Under the terms of this conception, physical education is characterized as sport and dance in pedagogical garb, or sport and dance in the trappings of a formal development toward human fulfillment (a formal development which it is the task of pedagogy to secure). This conception seems superior to the former two by virtue of its drawing the former two into a higher unity, and by virtue of its accounting for our highest experience of physical education in a way that the former two conceptions do not. This conception has not abandoned these other two so much as included them as preliminary notions and showed the way to their distinctly human development. The former two notions are therefore and simply too limited in themselves to satisfy the contemporary view of physical education as an expression of man's highest possibilities. Physical education is thereby conceived as the composite of sport and dance properly so-termed (or authentically undertaken). It is therefore equivalent to the movement arts. The term 'physical education and sport' (which is now widely used to signify the concerns of "physical recreation") is consequently redundant, for it implies a more substantial difference between physical education and sport than can be delivered.

In recent years, such terms as 'anthropokinetics' and 'kinesiology' have been advocated as more suitable to the phenomena taken up by physical education than the term 'physical education' itself. But these effectively refer to the study of man in movement or to the study of a "moving" humanity, a reference previously dismissed as insufficiently discriminating. These terms fail to distinguish endeavors such as sport and dance from others which employ movement only incidentally (e.g., music, drama), in a widely general fashion (e.g., human engineering), or in a mundane way (e.g., house painting, piano moving, truck driving).

With this the circle comes closed, the basic character of sport, dance, exercise, movement, physical education, play, and recreation has been showed, and the key significance of sport has been demonstrated. Even at this, however, only tentative judgments, based significantly on unexamined foundations, have been secured —embryonic provocations for volumes and for another time. If nothing else, the essay has at least demonstrated what is required of such judgments.

Notes

1. The "something else" here refers to "anything" that is the slightest bit different from the "something" it displaces or succeeds, even an "anything" which so closely resembles that "something" so as to be thought synonymous with it. The mere fact that "something" has passed through another moment-expanse is sufficient to call it "something else" in the sense here intended. For this "something else" now has "something" in its experience in a way in which "something" itself does not.

2. This is so even of so-termed "absolute" conditions like temperatureless (absolute zero) and pressureless (absolute vacuum) environments, which are themselves swept up in a universe now widely thought to be moving (on balance, expanding) in "every" moment and throughout "every" expanse.

3. The more primary status of movement, as over and against its conceptual opposite, στασαδ (stasis), is further demonstrated by the terms in which stasis requires movement as a prior notion. The concept of stasis is no more than the result of a vain attempt to say what the contrary of movement is. It is the negative of movement, or the result of trying to say what not-movement is. As such, it depends on movement in a way in which movement itself does not depend on it.

4. This is not, however, to claim that there is nothing but change as such, but that change in the form of displacement and succession is the state in which "everything" finds itself. The formal characteristics of this "everything" nonetheless endure as the substance in which change occurs. Otherwise there would be "nothing" undergoing change. Neither would there be any enduring basis for change itself, let alone any basis for such as moral, aesthetic, and social purpose. Change itself (as well as such purpose for that matter) thereby presupposes that "something" changes.

5. This is not to say that play is, or can be experienced apart from its concrete "attachments," but that insofar as it is experienced, it is experienced as a way of regarding concrete activities, and not as a concrete activity itself. For if this latter were the case (i.e., if it were a concrete activity), we would not think and talk as strictly as we do about playing "things." The linguistic character of play gives at least partial demonstration of this point. Its statuses as a substantive (roughly meaning, light activity), as an intransitive verb (roughly meaning, to move lightly), and as a transitive verb (roughly meaning, to take part in) all imply its descriptive "attachment" to concrete activities per se. It is nearest its strict linguistic and conceptual meaning when used as a participle, or verbal adjective (as in playing "things"), as an adjectival infinitive (as in "something" to be played), or as an adverbial infinitive (as in to play "something" in a certain place, time, way, or to a certain extent).

6. These rules establish the definitive limits of sport, thereby stipulating what is required in order to claim participation in it at all.. As such, they are distinguished from rules of skill which stipulate what must be done in order to participate successfully. Constitutive rules are necessary to sport per se, rules of skill are not.

7. Though these goals may be, and have been

widely put to utilitarian ends, they are not by their nature utilitarian, else they would aim at a much more expedient resolution than they do.

8. The common criterion which distinguishes these categories and makes them mutually exclusive is the number of persons required to claim participation in an activity, and so the number on whom the responsibility for performance directly depends. In individual sports, only one is required; in dual sports, one giving "opposition" to another is required; and in team sports, several giving "opposition" to several others is required. These distinctions are not as empty, inconsequential, and purely quantitative as they first appear. For they establish the qualitative possibilities of personal and interpersonal reference in these activities, and provide the most general, exhaustive, and conclusive means of distinguishing and classifying them. (No such claim of common criterion of distinction, mutual exclusivity, and comprehension is made with respect to the sub-categories of individual, dual, and team sports used here, however. These subcategories ought to be considered instructive, albeit largely unexamined supplements to the larger categories—as useful, if not logically cogent conventions.) Neither are they altogether unproblematic, however. Such as doubles tennis and massed wrestling seem most troublesome. But here one has a massed circumstance which has been upbuilt in the image of, and remains a variation of the dual form of activity. The same form of argument apparently holds in classifying other-than-singles bobsledding, canoeing, figure skating, luge, and rowing as individual sports. In the case of relay events in what are otherwise unequivocally individual sports, one has individual segments of performance which are simply put together. The form of action and interaction remains fundamentally individual.

9. These three forms of sporting activity are considered classical in the sense that they are the most fundamental forms of sporting expression in the three concrete media (aerial, aquatic, and grounded) in which sport has developed. Gymnastics is primarily concerned with the possibilities of sporting movement in the aerial medium, swimming and diving in the aquatic, and track and field athletics in the grounded. This is not to say that gymnastics does not depend on (and operate in) grounded circumstance, that swimming and diving do not depend on (and operate in) aerial and grounded circumstance, or that track and field athletics does not depend on (and operate in) aerial and aquatic circumstance. It is merely to claim that the basic point of whatever use gymnastics might make of grounded conditions (and all the orthodox gymnastics events, balance beam, free exercise, horizontal bar, long horse vault, parallel bars, side horse, and still rings, necessarily make either a direct or indirect such use), it makes for the principal purpose of examining and experiencing aerial possibilities; that whatever use swimming and diving might make of aerial and grounded conditions (and they make

significant use of the former in the recovery phases of the arms in all orthodox strokes except breaststroke and in the breathing phases of all strokes, and of the latter in starting movements of swimming events and in approach and take-off movements of diving events), they make for the principal purpose of examining and experiencing aquatic possibilities; and that whatever use track and field athletics might make of aerial and aquatic conditions (and all orthodox track and field events, running, walking, hurdling, jumping, vaulting, and throwing, make significant use of the former, and steeplechase makes use of the latter), it makes for the principal purpose of examining and experiencing grounded possibilities. Diving is one of two confounding factors here. This is so because its use of aquatic and grounded media is principally for the purpose of examining and experiencing aerial possibilities. It is the aquatic and grounded media which make the aerial possible, not the obverse. As such, diving belongs more so with gymnastics than with swimming. Its traditional alliance is nonetheless retained here. A second confounding factor has to do with classical forms of sporting expression in ice-snow media. Since there are several candidates for this designation (principally, alpine skiing, cross country skiing, figure skating, and speed skating), unlike the case with respect to the other three media, these (with others of their kind) have been put together as comprising the category of individual winter sports.

10. Like such as automobile, motorcycle, and hydroplane racing, shooting too is taken up with a self-propelled mechanical contrivance of sorts. That is to say, the inertia of the projectile in shooting is not rendered solely (not even rendered very much) by the performer or by the performer's manipulation or use of natural (this means mechanical or physical, as distinct from chemical here) forces or energies. The "physical movements" of this sport (and such as automobile, motorcycle, and hydroplane racing) depend heavily (even perhaps primarily) on chemical forces or energies which in significant measure *self*-propel its implements. Its place in this conception of sport is thereby made somewhat dubious. And, of course, its prominent role in biathlon and modern pentathlon also throws them under some suspicion.

11. Nor is it consonant with our experience of either sport or dance to consider sport a dance, drawing attention to the converse possibility.

12. That is, the so-termed "opponent" is typically more conspicuous in sport than in dance. But this is by no means the case in all instances. And even if it were, what results is not a qualitative difference between sport and dance, but a quantitative one.

13. But if this is so on the grounds here adduced, it is so out of a negative concept of creativity as being heightened by a lack of, or a decline in constraint. And while this is likely so in some, even important respects, such a concept has nonetheless to demonstrate its positive side, and to show as well the relation between its negative and posi-

tive sides. Otherwise, the notion of creativity is itself left without differentiations, and is thereby reduced to its own absurdity, or impossibility.

14. Only these highly complex forms of movement expression have interested us sufficiently throughout our historical development to have moved us to making widespread, formal, institutional provision for them. And curiously, the two have undergone a similar formal development (though dance passed through the stages of this development somewhat earlier than sport) in which they have been variously "attached" to "all" of life's integral activities. They have both developed progressively from imitative, sensory, and ordinary forms of expression to representative, imaginative, and extraordinary such forms.

Bibliography

Carlson, Reynold E., Deppe, Theodore R., and MacLean, Janet R. *Recreation in American Life.* Belmont, Calif.: Wadsworth, 1963.

Delattre, Edwin J. "Some Reflections on Success and Failure in Competitive Athletics," *Journal of the Philosophy of Sport.* Vol. 2 (September, 1975), 133–139.

Fraleigh, Warren P. "On Weiss on Records and on the Significance of Athletic Records," *The Philosophy of Sport: A Collection of Original Essays.* Robert G. Osterhoudt (ed.). Springfield, Ill.: Charles C Thomas, 1973.

Huizinga, Johan. *Homo Ludens: A Study of the Play-Element in Culture.* Boston: Beacon Press, 1950.

Kaelin, Eugene F. "The Well-Played Game: Notes Toward an Aesthetics of Sport," *Quest,* No. 10 (May, 1968), 16–28.

Kraus, Richard. *History of the Dance in Art and Education.* Englewood Cliffs, N.J.: Prentice-Hall, 1969.

Kretchmar, R. Scott. "From Test to Contest: An Analysis of Two Kinds of Counterpoint in Sport," *Journal of the Philosophy of Sport,* Vol. 2 (September, 1975), 23–30.

Kupfer, Joseph. "Purpose and Beauty in Sport," *Journal of the Philosophy of Sport,* Vol. 2 (September, 1975), 83–90.

Metheny, Eleanor. *Movement and Meaning.* New York: McGraw-Hill, 1968.

Morgan, William J. "Sport and Temporality: An Ontological Analysis." Unpublished Doctor's dissertation, University of Minnesota, 1975.

Paddick, Robert J. "What Makes Physical Activity Physical?" *Journal of the Philosophy of Sport,* Vol. 2 (September, 1975), 91–101.

Roberts, Terence J. "Sport and the Sense of Beauty," *Journal of the Philosophy of Sport,* Vol. 2 (September, 1975), 91–101.

Sachs, Curt. *World History of the Dance.* Bessie Schonberg (trans.). New York: W. W. Norton, 1937.

Staley, Seward C. *Sports Education: The New Curriculum in Physical Education.* New York: A. S. Barnes, 1939.

Suits, Bernard. "The Elements of Sport," *The Philosophy of Sport: A Collection of Original Essays.* Robert G. Osterhoudt (ed.). Springfield, Ill.: Charles C Thomas, 1973.

Van Dalen, Deobold B. and Bennett, Bruce L. *A World History of Physical Education: Cultural, Philosophical, Comparative.* Second edition. Englewood Cliffs, N.J.: Prentice-Hall, 1971.

White, David A. "Great Moments in Sport:" The One and the Many," *Journal of the Philosophy of Sport,* Vol. 2 (September, 1975), 124–132.

What Is A Game?*

BERNARD SUITS

By means of a critical examination of a number of theses as to the nature of game-playing, the following definition is advanced: To play a game is to engage in activity directed toward bringing about a specific state of affairs, using only means permitted by specific rules, where the means permitted by the rules are more limited in scope than they would be in the absence of the rules, and where the sole reason for accepting such limitation is to make possible such activity.

Prompted by the current interest of social and behavioral scientists in games, and encouraged by the modest belief that it is not demonstrably impossible for philosophers to say something of interest to scientists, I propose to formulate a definition of game-playing.

1. Game-Playing as the Selection of Inefficient Means. Mindful of the ancient canon that the quest for knowledge obliges us to proceed from what is knowable to us to what is knowable in itself, I shall begin with the commonplace that playing games is different from working. Games, therefore, might be expected to be what work, in some salient respect, is not. Let me now baldly characterize work as "technical activity," by which I mean activity in which an agent (as *rational* worker) seeks to employ the most efficient available means for reaching a desired goal. Since games, too, evidently have goals, and since means are evidently employed for their attainment, the possibility suggests itself that games

* From *Philosophy of Science*, 34 (June, 1967), 148-156.

differ from technical activities in that the means employed in games are not the most efficient. Let us say, then, that games are goal-directed activities in which inefficient means are intentionally (or rationally) chosen. For example, in racing games one voluntarily goes all around the track in an effort to arrive at the finish line instead of "sensibly" cutting straight across the infield.

The following considerations, however, seem to cast doubt on this proposal. The goal of a game, we may say, is winning the game. Let us take an example. In poker I am a winner if I have more money when I stop playing than I had when I started. But suppose that one of the other players, in the course of the game, repays me a debt of a hundred dollars, or suppose I hit another player on the head and take all of his money from him. Then, although I have not won a single hand all evening, am I nevertheless a winner? Clearly not, since I didn't increase my money as a consequence of playing poker. In order to be a winner, a sign and product of which is, to be sure, the gaining of money, certain conditions must be met which are not met by the collection of a debt or by felonious assault. These conditions are the rules of poker, which tell us what we can and what we cannot do with the cards and the money. Winning at poker consists in increasing one's money by using only those means permitted by the rules, although mere obedience to the rules does not by itself insure victory. Better and worse means are equally permitted by the rules. Thus in Draw Poker retaining an ace along with a pair and discarding the ace while retaining the pair are both permissible plays, although one is usually a better play than the other. The means for winning at poker, therefore, are limited, but not completely determined by, the rules. Attempting to win at poker may accordingly be described as attempting to gain money by using the most efficient means available, where only those means permitted by the rules are available. But if that is so, then playing poker is a technical activity as originally defined.

Still, this seems a strange conclusion. The belief that working and playing games are quite different things is very widespread, yet we seem obliged to say that playing a game is just another job to be done as competently as possible. Before giving up the thesis that playing a game involves a sacrifice of efficiency, therefore, let us consider one more example. Suppose I make it my purpose to get a small round object into a hole in the ground as efficiently as possible. Placing it in the hole with my hand would be a natural means to adopt. But surely I would not take a stick with a piece of metal on one end of it, walk three or four hundred yards away from the hole, and then attempt to propel the ball into the hole with the stick. That would not be technically intelligent. But such an undertaking is an extremely popular game, and the foregoing way of describing it evidently shows how games differ from technical activities.

But of course it shows nothing of the kind. The end in golf is not correctly described as getting a ball into a hole in the ground, nor even, to be more precise, into several holes in a set order. It is to achieve that end with the smallest possible number of strokes. But strokes are certain types of swings with a golf club. Thus, if my end were simply to get a ball into a number of holes in the ground, I would not be likely to use a golf club in order to achieve it, nor would I stand at a considerable distance from each hole. But if my end were to get a ball into some holes with a golf club while standing at a considerable distance from each hole, why then I would certainly use a golf club and I would certainly take up such positions. Once committed to that end, moreover, I would strive to accomplish it as efficiently as possible. Surely no one would want to maintain that if I conducted myself with utter efficiency in pursuit of this end I would not be playing a game, but that I would be playing a game just to the extent that I permitted my efforts to become sloppy. Nor is it the case

that my use of a golf club is a less efficient way to achieve my end than would be the use of my hand. To refrain from using a golf club as a means of sinking a ball with a golf club is not more efficient because it is not possible. Inefficient selection of means, accordingly, does not seem to be a satisfactory account of game-playing.

2. The Inseparability of Rules and Ends in Games. The objection advanced against the last thesis rests upon, and thus brings to light, consideration of the place of rules in games: they seem to stand in a peculiar relation to ends. The end in poker is not simply to gain money, nor in golf simply to get a ball into a hole, but to do these things in prescribed (or, perhaps more accurately, not to do them in proscribed) ways; that is, to do them only in accordance with rules. Rules in games thus seem to be in some sense inseparable from ends. To break a rule is to render impossible the attainment of an end. Thus, although you may receive the trophy by lying about your golf score, you have certainly not won the game. But in what we have called *technical activity* it is possible to gain an end by breaking a rule; for example, gaining a trophy by lying about your golf score. Whereas it is possible in a technical action to break a rule without destroying the original end of the action, in games the reverse appears to be the case. If the rules are broken the original end becomes impossible of attainment, since one cannot (really) win the game unless he plays it, and one cannot (really) play the game unless he obeys the rules of the game.

This may be illustrated by the following case. Professor Snooze has fallen asleep in the shade provided by some shrubbery in a secluded part of the campus. From a nearby walk I observe this. I also notice that the shrub under which he is reclining is a man-eating plant, and I judge from its behavior that it is about to eat the man Snooze. As I run across to him I see a sign which reads KEEP OFF THE GRASS. Without a qualm I ignore this prohibition and save Snooze's life. Why did I make this (no doubt unconscious) decision? Because the value of saving Snooze's life (or of saving a life) outweighed the value of obeying the prohibition against walking on the grass. Now the choices in a game appear to be radically unlike this choice. In a game I cannot disjoin the end, winning, from the rules in terms of which winning possesses its meaning. I of course can decide to cheat in order to gain the pot, but then I have changed my end from winning a game to gaining money. Thus, in deciding to save Snooze's life my purpose was not "to save Snooze while at the same time obeying the campus rules for pedestrians." My purpose was to save Snooze's life, and there were alternative ways in which this might have been accomplished. I could, for example, have remained on the sidewalk and shouted to Snooze in an effort to awaken him. But precious minutes might have been lost, and in any case Snooze, although he tries to hide it, is nearly stone deaf. There are evidently two distinct ends at issue in the Snooze episode: saving Snooze and obeying a rule, out of respect either for the law or for the lawn. And I can achieve either of these ends without at the same time achieving the other. But in a game the end and the rules do not admit of such disjunction. It is impossible for me to win the game and at the same time to break one of its rules. I do not have open to me the alternatives of winning the game honestly and winning the game by cheating, since in the latter case I would not be playing the game at all and thus could not, *a fortiori*, win it.

Now if the Snooze episode is treated as an action which has one, and only one, end—(Saving Snooze) ampersand (Keeping off the grass)—it can be argued that the action has become, just by virtue of that fact, a game. Since there would be no independent alternatives, there would be no choice to be made; to achieve one part of the end without achieving the other part would be to fail utterly. On such an interpretation of the episode suppose I am congratulated by a grateful faculty for my timely intervention. A perfectly appropriate response would be: "I don't deserve your praise. True, I saved Snooze, but since I walked on the grass it doesn't count," just as though I were to admit to kicking the ball into the cup on the fifth green. Or again, on this interpretation, I would originally have conceived the problem in a quite different way: "Let me if I can save Snooze without walking on the grass." One can then imagine my running as fast as I can (but taking no illegal short-cuts) to the Athletic Building, where I request (and meticulously sign out for) a pole vaulter's pole with which I hope legally to prod Snooze into wakefulness, whereupon I hurry back to Snooze to find him disappearing into the plant. "Well," I remark, not without complacency, "I didn't win, but at least I played the game."

It must be pointed out, however, that this example is seriously misleading. Saving a life and keeping off the grass are, as values, hardly on the same footing. It seems likely that the Snooze episode appears to support the contention at issue (that games differ from technical actions because of the inseparability of rules and ends in the former) only because of the relative triviality of one of the alternatives. This peculiarity of the example can be corrected by supposing that when I decide to obey the rule to keep off the grass, my reason for doing so is that I am a kind of demented Kantian, and thus regard myself to be bound by the most weighty philosophical considerations to honor *all* laws with equal respect. So regarded, my maddeningly proper efforts to save a life would not appear ludicrous but would constitute moral drama of the highest order. But since the reader may not be a demented Kantian, a less fanciful logically identical example may be cited.

Let us suppose the life of Snooze to be threatened not by a man-eating plant but by Professor Threat, who is found approaching the snoozing Snooze with the obvious intention of murdering him. Again I want to save Snooze's life, but I cannot do so (let us say) without killing Threat. However, there is a rule to which I am very strongly committed which forbids me to take another human life. Thus, although (as it happens) I could easily kill Threat from where I stand (with a loaded and cocked pistol I happen to have in my hand), I decide to try to save Snooze by other means, just because of my wish to obey the rule which forbids killing. I therefore run toward Threat with the intention of wresting the weapon from his hand. I am too late and he murders Snooze. This seems to be a clear case of an action having a conjunctive end of the kind under consideration, but one which we are not at all inclined to call a game. My end, that is to say, was not simply to save the life of Snooze, just as in golf it is not simply to get the ball into the hole, but to save his life without breaking a certain rule. I want to put the ball into the hole fairly and I want to save Snooze morally. Moral rules are perhaps generally regarded as figuring in human conduct in just this fashion. Morality says that if something can be done only immorally it ought not to be done at all. *What profiteth it a man, etc.* The inseparability of rules and ends does not, therefore, seem to be a completely distinctive characteristic of games.

3. Game Rules as Not Ultimately Binding. It should be noticed that the foregoing criticism requires only a partial rejection of the proposal at issue. Even though the attack shows that not all things which correspond to the formula are games, it may still be the case that all games correspond to the formula. This suggests that we ought not to reject the proposal, but that we ought first to try to limit its scope by adding to it an adequate differentiating principle. Such a differentia might be provided by noticing a striking difference between the two Snooze episodes. The efforts to save Snooze from the man-eating plant without walking on the grass appeared to be a game because saving the grass strikes us as a trifling consideration when compared with saving a life. But in the second episode, where KEEP OFF THE GRASS is replaced by THOU SHALT NOT KILL, the situation is quite different. The difference may be put in the following way. The rule to keep off the grass is not an ultimate command, but the rule to refrain from killing is. This suggests that, in addition to being the kind of activity in which rules are inseparable from ends, games are also the kind of activity in which commitment to these rules is never ultimate. For the person playing the game there is always the possibility of there being a non-game rule to which the game rule may be subordinated. The second Snooze episode is not a game, therefore, because the rule to which the rescuer adheres, even to the extent of sacrificing Snooze for its sake, is, for him, an ultimate rule. Rules are lines that we draw, but in games the lines are always drawn short of a final end or a paramount command. Let us say, then, that a game is an activity in which observance of rules is part of the end of the activity, and where such rules are non-ultimate; that is, where other rules can always supersede the game rules: that is, where the player can always stop playing the game.

However, consider the following counter-example. Suppose an auto racer. During a race a child crawls out on the track directly in the path of his car. The only way that he can avoid running over the child is to turn off the track and by breaking a rule disqualify himself. He chooses to run over the child, because for him there are no rules of higher priority than the rules of the game. I submit that we ought not, for this reason, to deny that he is playing a game. It no doubt strikes us as inappropriate to say that a person who would do such a thing is (only) playing. But the point is that the driver is not playing in an unqualified sense, he is playing a *game*. And he is evidently playing it more whole-heartedly than the ordinary driver is prepared to play it. From his point of view a racer who turned aside instead of running over the child would have been playing *at* racing; that is, he would not have been a dedicated player. But it would be paradoxical indeed if supreme dedication to an activity somehow vitiated the activity. We do not say that a man isn't really digging a ditch because his whole heart is in it.

However, the rejoinder may be made that, to the contrary, that is just the mark of a game: it, unlike digging ditches, is just the kind of thing which cannot command ultimate loyalty. That, it may be contended, is just the force of the proposal about games under consideration. And in support of this contention it might be pointed out that it is generally acknowledged that games are in some sense essentially non-serious. We must therefore ask in what sense games are, and in what sense they are not, serious. What is believed when it is believed that games are not serious? Not, certainly, that the players of games always take a very light-hearted view of what they are doing. A bridge player who played his cards randomly might justly be accused of failing to take the game seriously; indeed, of failing to play the game at all just because of his failure to take it seriously. It is much more likely that the belief that games are not serious means what the proposal under consideration implies: that there is always something in the life of a player of a game more important than playing the game, or that a game is the kind of thing that a player could always have reason to stop playing. It is this belief which I would like to question.

Let us consider a golfer, George, so devoted to golf that its pursuit has led him to neglect, to the point of destitution, his wife and six children. Furthermore, although George is aware of the consequences of his mania, he does not regard his family's plight as a good reason for changing his conduct. An advocate of the view that games are *not* serious might submit George's case as evidence for that view. Since George evidently regards nothing in his life to be more important than golf, golf has, for George, *ceased to be a game*. And this argument would seem to be supported by the complaint of George's wife that golf is for George no longer a game, but a way of life.

But we need not permit George's wife's observation to go unchallenged. The correctness of saying that golf for George is no longer merely a form of recreation may be granted. But to argue that George's golf playing is for that reason not a game is to assume the very point at issue, which is whether a game can be of supreme importance to anyone. Golf, to be sure, is taking over the whole of George's life. But it is, after all, the game which is taking over his life, and not something else. Indeed, if it were not a game which had led George to neglect his duties, his wife might not be nearly as outraged as she is; if, for example, it had been good works, or the attempt to formulate a definition of game-playing. She would no doubt still deplore such extra-domestic preoccupation, but to be kept in rags because of a game must strike her as an altogether different order of deprivation.

Supreme dedication to a game, as in the cases of the auto racer and George, may be repugnant to nearly everyone's moral sense. That may be granted; indeed, insisted upon, since our loathing is excited by the very fact that it is a game which has usurped the place of ends we regard as so much more worthy of pursuit. Thus, although such behavior may tell us a good deal about such players of games, I submit that it tells us nothing about the games they play. I believe that these observations are sufficient to discredit the thesis that game rules cannot be ultimately binding on game players.[1]

4. Means, Rather than Rules, as Non-Ultimate. I want to agree, however, with the general contention that in games there is something which is significantly non-ultimate, that there is a crucial limitation. But I would like to suggest that it is not the rules which suffer such limitation. Non-ultimacy evidently attaches to games at a quite different point. It is not that the rules which govern a game must be short of ultimate commands, but that the means which the rules permit must be short of ultimate utilities. If a high-jumper, for example, failed to complete his jump because he saw that the bar was located at the edge of a precipice, this would no doubt show that jumping over the bar was not the over-riding interest of his life. But it would not be his refusal to jump to his death which would reveal his conduct to be a game; it would be his refusal to use something like a ladder or a catapult in the attempt. The same is true of the dedicated auto racer. A readiness to lose the race rather than kill a child is not what makes the race a game; it is the refusal to, *inter alia*, cut across the infield in order to get ahead of the other contestants. There is, therefore, a sense in which games may be said to be non-serious. One could intelligibly say of the high jumper who rejects ladders and catapults that he is not serious about getting to

the other side of the barrier. But one would also want to point out that he could be deadly serious about getting to the other side of the barrier *without* such aids; that is, about high-jumping. But whether games as such are less serious than other things would seem to be a question which cannot be answered solely by an investigation of games.

Consider a third variant of Snooze's death. In the face of Threat's threat to murder Snooze, I come to the following decision. I choose to limit myself to non-lethal means in order to save Snooze even though lethal means are available to me and I do not regard myself to be bound by any rule which forbids killing. (In the auto racing example the infield would *not* be filled with land mines.) And I make this decision even though it may turn out that the proscribed means are necessary to save Snooze. I thus make my end not simply saving Snooze's life, but saving Snooze's life without killing Threat, even though there appears to be no reason for restricting myself in this way.

One might then ask how such behavior can be accounted for. And one answer might be that it is unaccountable, that it is simply arbitrary. However, the decision to draw an arbitrary line with respect to permissible means need not itself be an arbitrary decision. The decision to be arbitrary may have a purpose, and the purpose may be to play a game. And it seems to be the case that the lines drawn in games are not actually arbitrary at all. For not only *that* the lines are drawn, but also *where* they are drawn, has important consequences not only for the type, but also for the quality, of the game to be played. It might be said that drawing such lines skillfully (and therefore not arbitrarily) is the very essence of the gamewright's craft. The gamewright must avoid two extremes. If he draws his lines too loosely the game will be dull because winning will be too easy. As looseness is increased to the point of utter laxity the game disappears altogether, since there are then no rules proscribing available means. Thus a homing propellant device could be devised which would insure a golfer a hole in one every time he played. On the other hand, rules are lines that can be drawn too tight, so that the game becomes too difficult. And if a line is drawn very tight indeed the game is squeezed out of existence. Suppose a game in which the goal is to cross a finish line. One of the rules requires the contestants to stay on the track, while another rule requires that the finish line be located at a position such that it is impossible to cross it without leaving the track. The pres-

---

[1] The author has argued for the possibility that life itself is a game in "Is Life a Game We Are Playing?" *Ethics.* Vol. 77, No. 3, April 1967.

ent proposal, therefore, is that games are activities in which rules are inseparable from ends (in the sense agreed to earlier), but with the added qualification that the means permitted by the rules are smaller in scope than they would be in the absence of the rules.

5. Rules are Accepted for Sake of the Activity They Make Possible. Still, even if it is true that the function of rules in games is to restrict the permissible means to an end, it does not seem that this is in itself sufficient to exclude things which are not games. When I failed in my attempt to save Snooze's life because of my unwillingness to commit the immoral act of taking a life, the rule against killing functioned to restrict the means I would employ in my efforts to reach a desired end. What then distinguishes the case of the high jumper and of the auto racer from my efforts to save Snooze morally, or the efforts of a politician to get elected without lying? The answer lies in the reason for obeying rules in the two types of case. In games I obey the rules just because such obedience is a necessary condition for my engaging in the activity such obedience makes possible. But in other activities—e.g., in moral actions—there is always another reason, what might be called an external reason, for conforming to the rule in question; for a moral teleologist, because its violation would vitiate some other end, for a deontologist because the rule is somehow binding in itself. In morals conformity to rules makes the action right, but in games it makes the action.

Further to illustrate this point, two other ways in which rules function may be contrasted with the way in which rules function in games. Rules can be directives to attain a given end (If you want to improve your drive, keep your eye on the ball), or they can be restrictions on the means to be chosen to a given end (Do not lie to the public in order to get them to vote for you). In the latter way morals, for example, often appear as limiting conditions in a technical activity, although a supervening technical activity can also effect the same limitation (If you want to get to the airport in time, drive fast, but if you want to drive safely, don't drive too fast). Consider a ruled sheet of paper. I conform to these rules, when writing, in order to write straight. Now suppose that the rules are not lines on a sheet of paper, but paper walls which form a labyrinth, and while I wish to be out of the labyrinth, I don't wish to damage the walls. The walls are limiting conditions on my coming to be out. Returning to games, consider a third

case. Again I am in the labyrinth, but now my purpose is not to *be* outside (as it might be if Ariadne were waiting for me), but to *get* out of the labyrinth, so to speak, labyrinthically. What is the status of the walls? Clearly they are not means for my coming to be outside the labyrinth because it is not my purpose to (simply) be outside. And if a friend suddenly appeared overhead in a helicopter I would decline the offer of a lift, although I would accept it in the second case. My purpose is to get out of the labyrinth only by accepting the conditions it imposes. Nor is this like the first case. There I was not interested in seeing whether I could write a sentence without breaking a rule (crossing a line), but in using the rules so that I could write straight.

We may therefore say that games consist in acting in accordance with rules which limit the permissible means to a sought end, and where the rules are obeyed just so that such activity can take place.

6. Winning Is Not the End with Respect to which Rules Limit Means. There is, however, a final difficulty. On the one hand to describe rules as operating more or less permissively with respect to means seems to conform to the ways in which we invent or revise games. But on the other hand it does not seem to make sense at all to say that in games there are means for attaining one's end over and above the means permitted by the rules. Consider chess. The end sought by chess players is, it would seem, to win. But winning means putting a chess piece on a square in accordance with the rules of chess. But since to break a rule is to fail to attain that end, what other means are available? It was for just this reason that the first proposal was rejected: using a golf club in order to play golf is not a less efficient, and thus alternative, means for seeking the end in question; it is a (logically) indispensable means.

The objection can be met, I believe, by pointing out that there is an end in chess analytically distinct from winning as an end. Let us begin again, therefore, from a somewhat different point of view and say that the end in chess is, in a very restricted sense, to place one of your pieces on the board in a position such that the opponent's king is, in terms of the rules of chess, immobilized. Now, without going outside the game of chess we may say that the means for bringing about this state of affairs consist in moving the chess pieces. The rules of chess, of course, state how the pieces may be moved; they distinguish between legal and illegal moves. Since the knight, for example, is permitted to move in only a highly restricted manner, it is clear that the permitted means for moving the knight are of less scope than the possible means for moving him. It should not be objected at this point that other means for moving the knight—e.g., along the diagonals—are not really possible on the grounds that such use of the knight would break a rule and thus not be a means to winning. For the present point is not that such use of the knight would be a means to winning, but that it would be a possible (though not permissible) way in which to move the knight so that he would, for example, come to occupy a square such that, according to the rules of chess, the king would be immobilized. A person who made such a move would not, of course, be playing chess. Perhaps he would be cheating at chess. By the same token I would not be playing a game if I abandoned my arbitrary decision not to kill Threat while at the same time attempting to save Snooze. Chess, as well as my third effort to save Snooze's life, are games because of an "arbitrary" restriction of means permitted in pursuit of an end.

The chief point is that the end here in question is not the end of winning the game. There must be an end distinct from winning because it is the restriction of means to this other end which makes winning possible, and also defines, in any given game, what it means to win. In defining a game we shall therefore have to take into account these two ends and, as we shall see in a moment, a third end as well. First there is what might be called the end which consists in a certain state of affairs: a juxtaposition of pieces on a board, saving a friend's life, crossing a finish line. Then, when a restriction of means for attaining this end is made with the introduction of rules, we have

a second end, winning. Finally, with the stipulation of what it means to win, a third end emerges: the activity of trying to win; that is, playing the game. It is noteworthy that in some cases it is possible to pursue one of these ends without pursuing the others and that in some cases it is not. Thus, it is possible to pursue the end of getting as many tricks at bridge as you can without pursuing the end of winning, since you may seek this goal, and also achieve it, by cheating. But it is impossible to seek to win without seeking to take a certain (relative) number of tricks, nor is it possible to seek to play without seeking both of the other ends.

7. The Definition. My conclusion is that to play a game is to engage in activity directed toward bringing about a specific state of affairs, using only means permitted by specific rules, where the means permitted by the rules are more limited in scope than they would be in the absence of the rules, and where the sole reason for accepting such limitation is to make possible such activity.[2,3]

[2] Additional work on the subject of games by the author includes "Games and Paradox" *Philosophy of Science.* Vol. 34, No. 3, September, 1969; "Can You Play a Game Without Knowing It?" *Studies in Philosophy and in the History of Science,* Coronado Press, 1970.

[3] In a paper titled "The Elements of Sport" presented to the Third International Symposium on the Sociology of Sport, the author presented a revised version of the definition advanced in the present article: To play a game is to attempt to achieve a specific state of affairs, using only means permitted by rules, where the rules prohibit use of more efficient in favour of less efficient means, and where such rules are accepted just because they make possible such activity. Or, for short: Playing a game is the voluntary attempt to overcome unnecessary obstacles.

The Nature of Play*

JOHAN HUIZINGA

First and foremost . . . all play is a voluntary activity. Play to order is no longer play: it could at best be but a forcible imitation of it. By this quality of freedom alone, play marks itself off from the course of the natural process. It is something added thereto and spread out over it like a flowering, an ornament, a garment. Obviously, freedom must be understood here in the wider sense that leaves untouched the philosophical problem of determinism. It may be objected that this freedom does not exist for the animal and the child; they *must* play because their instinct drives them to it and because it serves to develop their bodily faculties and their powers of selection. The term "instinct", however, introduces an unknown quantity, and to presuppose the utility of play from the start is to be guilty of a *petitio principii*. Child and animal play because they enjoy playing, and therein precisely lies their freedom.

Be that as it may, for the adult and responsible human being play is a function which he could equally well leave alone. Play is superfluous. The need for it is only urgent to the extent that the enjoyment of it makes it a need. Play can be deferred or suspended at any time. It is never imposed by physical necessity or moral duty. It is never a task. It is done at leisure, during "free time". Only when play is a recognized cultural function—a rite, a

* From *Homo Ludens*. London: Routledge & Kegan Paul, 1950. Copyright 1950 by Roy Publishers. Reprinted by permission of Beacon Press and Routledge & Kegan Paul Ltd.

ceremony—is it bound up with notions of obligation and duty.

Here, then, we have the first main characteristic of play: that it is free, is in fact freedom. A second characteristic is closely connected with this, namely, that play is not "ordinary" or "real" life. It is rather a stepping out of "real" life into a temporary sphere of activity with a disposition all of its own. Every child knows perfectly well that he is "only pretending", or that it was "only for fun". How deep-seated this awareness is in the child's soul is strikingly illustrated by the following story, told to me by the father of the boy in question. He found his four-year-old son sitting at the front of a row of chairs, playing "trains". As he hugged him the boy said: "Don't kiss the engine, Daddy, or the carriages won't think it's real". This "only pretending" quality of play betrays a consciousness of the inferiority of play compared with "seriousness", a feeling that seems to be something as primary as play itself. Nevertheless, as we have already pointed out, the consciousness of play being "only a pretend" does not by any means prevent it from proceeding with the utmost seriousness, with an absorption, a devotion that passes into rapture and, temporarily at least, completely abolishes that troublesome "only" feeling. Any game can at any time wholly run away with the players. The contrast between play and seriousness is always fluid. The inferiority of play is continually being offset by the corresponding superiority of its seriousness. Play turns to seriousness and seriousness to play.

Play may rise to heights of beauty and sublimity that leave seriousness far beneath. Tricky questions such as these will come up for discussion when we start examining the relationship between play and ritual.

As regards its formal characteristics, all students lay stress on the *disinterestedness* of play. Not being "ordinary" life it stands outside the immediate satisfaction of wants and appetites, indeed it interrupts the appetitive process. It interpolates itself as a temporary activity satisfying in itself and ending there. Such at least is the way in which play presents itself to us in the first instance: as an intermezzo, an *interlude* in our daily lives. As a regularly recurring relaxation, however, it becomes the accompaniment, the complement, in fact an integral part of life in general. It adorns life, amplifies it and is to that extent a necessity both for the individual—as a life function—and for society by reason of the meaning it contains, its significance, its expressive value, its spiritual and social associations, in short, as a culture function. The expression of it satisfies all kinds of communal ideals. It thus has its place in a sphere superior to the strictly biological processes of nutrition, reproduction and self-preservation. This assertion is apparently contradicted by the fact that play, or rather sexual display, is predominant in animal life precisely at the mating-season. But would it be too absurd to assign a place *outside* the purely physiological, to the singing, cooing and strutting of birds just as we do to human play? In all its higher forms the latter at any rate always belongs to the sphere of festival and ritual—the sacred sphere.

Now, does the fact that play is a necessity, that it subserves culture, or indeed that it actually becomes culture, detract from its disinterested character? No, for the purposes it serves are external to immediate material interests or the individual satisfaction of biological needs. As a sacred activity play naturally contributes to the well-being of the group, but in quite another way and by other means than the acquisition of the necessities of life.

Play is distinct from "ordinary" life both as to locality and duration. This is the third main characteristic of play: its secludedness, its limitedness. It is "played out" within certain limits of time and place. It contains its own course and meaning.

Play begins, and then at a certain moment it is "over". It plays itself to an end. While it is in progress all is movement, change, alternation, succession, association, separation. But immediately connected with its limitation as to time there is a further curious feature of play: it at once assumes fixed form as a cultural phenomenon. Once played, it endures as a new-found creation of the mind, a treasure to be retained by the memory. It is transmitted, it becomes tradition. It can be repeated at any time, whether it be "child's play" or a game of chess, or at fixed intervals like a mystery. In this faculty of repetition lies one of the most essential qualities of play. It holds good not only of play as a whole but also of its inner structure. In nearly all the higher forms of play the elements of repetition and alternation (as in the *refrain*), are like the warp and woof of a fabric.

More striking even than the limitation as to time is the limitation as to space. All play moves and has its being within a play-ground marked off beforehand either materially or ideally, deliberately or as a matter of course. Just as there is no formal difference between play and ritual, so the "consecrated spot" cannot be formally distinguished from the play-ground. The arena, the card-table, the magic circle, the temple, the stage, the screen, the tennis court, the court of justice, etc., are all in form and function play-grounds, i.e. forbidden spots, isolated, hedged round, hallowed, within which special rules obtain. All are temporary worlds within the ordinary world, dedicated to the performance of an act apart.

Inside the play-ground an absolute and peculiar order reigns. Here we come across another, very positive feature of play: it creates order, *is* order. Into an imperfect world and into the confusion of life it brings a temporary, a limited perfection. Play demands order absolute and supreme. The least deviation from it "spoils the game", robs it of its character and makes it worthless. The profound affinity between play and order is perhaps the reason why play, as we noted in passing, seems to lie to such a large extent in the field of aesthetics. Play has a tendency to be beautiful. It may be that this aesthetic factor is identical with the impulse to create orderly form, which animates play in all its aspects. The words we use to denote the elements of play belong for the most part to aesthetics, terms with which we try to describe the effects of beauty: tension, poise, balance, contrast, variation, solution, resolution, etc. Play casts a spell over us; it is "enchanting", "captivating". It is invested with the noblest qualities we are capable of perceiving in things: rhythm and harmony.

The element of tension in play to which we have just referred plays a particularly important part. Tension means uncertainty, chanciness; a striving to decide the issue and so end it. The player wants something to "go", to "come off"; he wants to "succeed" by his own exertions. Baby reaching for a toy, pussy patting a bobbin, a little girl playing ball—all want to achieve something difficult, to succeed, to end a tension. Play is "tense", as we say. It is this element of tension and solution that governs all solitary games of skill and application such as puzzles, jig-saws, mosaic-making, patience, target-shooting, and the more play bears the character of competition the more fervent it will be. In gambling and athletics it is at its height. Though play as such is outside the range of good and bad, the element of tension imparts to it a certain ethical value in so far as it means a testing of the player's prowess: his courage, tenacity, resources and, last but not least, his spiritual powers—his "fairness"; because, despite his ardent desire to win, he must still stick to the rules of the game.

These rules in their turn are a very important factor in the play-concept. All play has its rules. They determine what "holds" in the temporary world circumscribed by play. The rules of a game are absolutely binding and allow no doubt. Paul Valéry once in passing gave expression to a very cogent thought when he said: "No scepticism is possible where the rules of a game are concerned, for the principle underlying them is an unshakable truth. . . ." Indeed, as soon as the rules are transgressed the whole play-world collapses. The game is over. The umpire's whistle breaks the spell and sets "real" life going again.

The player who trespasses against the rules or ignores them is a "spoil-sport". The spoil-sport is not the same as the false player, the cheat; for the latter pretends to be playing the game and, on the face of it, still acknowledges the magic circle. It is curious to note how much more lenient society is to the cheat than to the spoil-sport. This is because the spoil-sport shatters the play-world itself. By withdrawing from the game he reveals the relativity and fragility of the play-world in which he had temporarily shut himself with others. He robs play of its *illusion*—a pregnant word which means literally "in-play" (from *inlusio, illudere* or *inludere*). Therefore he must be cast out, for he threatens the existence of the play-community. The figure of the spoil-sport is most apparent in boys' games. The little community does not enquire whether the spoil-sport is guilty of defection because he dares not enter into the game or because he is not allowed to. Rather, it does not recognize "not being allowed" and

calls it "not daring". For it, the problem of obedience and conscience is no more than fear of punishment. The spoil-sport breaks the magic world, therefore he is a coward and must be ejected. In the world of high seriousness, too, the cheat and the hypocrite have always had an easier time of it than the spoil-sports, here called apostates, heretics, innovators, prophets, conscientious objectors, etc. It sometimes happens, however, that the spoil-sports in their turn make a new community with rules of its own. The outlaw, the revolutionary, the cabbalist or member of a secret society, indeed heretics of all kinds are of a highly associative if not sociable disposition, and a certain element of play is prominent in all their doings.

A play-community generally tends to become permanent even after the game is over. Of course, not every game of marbles or every bridge-party leads to the founding of a club. But the feeling of being "apart together" in an exceptional situation, of sharing something important, of mutually withdrawing from the rest of the world and rejecting the usual norms, retains its magic beyond the duration of the individual game. The club pertains to play as the hat to the head. It would be rash to explain all the associations which the anthropologist calls "phratria"—e.g. clans, brotherhoods, etc.—simply as play-communities; nevertheless it has been shown again and again how difficult it is to draw the line between, on the one hand, permanent social groupings—particularly in archaic cultures with their extremely important, solemn, indeed sacred customs—and the sphere of play on the other.

The exceptional and special position of play is most tellingly illustrated by the fact that it loves to surround itself with an air of secrecy. Even in early childhood the charm of play is enhanced by making a "secret" out of it. This is for *us*, not for the "others". What the "others" do "outside" is no concern of ours at the moment. Inside the circle of the game the laws and customs of ordinary life no longer count. We are different and do things differently. This temporary abolition of the ordinary world is fully acknowledged in child-life, but it is no less evident in the great ceremonial games of savage societies. During the great feast of initiation when the youths are accepted into the male community, it is not the neophytes only that are exempt from the ordinary laws and regulations: there is a truce to all feuds in the tribe. All retaliatory acts and vendettas are suspended. This temporary suspension of normal social life on account of the sacred play-season has numerous traces in the more advanced civilizations as well. Everything that pertains to saturnalia and carnival customs belongs to it. Even with us a bygone age of robuster private habits than ours, more marked class-privileges and a more complaisant police recognized the orgies of young men of rank under the name of a "rag". The saturnalian licence of young men still survives, in fact, in the ragging at English universities, which the *Oxford English Dictionary* defines as "an extensive display of noisy and disorderly conduct carried out in defiance of authority and discipline".

The "differentness" and secrecy of play are most vividly expressed in "dressing up". Here the "extra-ordinary" nature of play reaches perfection. The disguised or masked individual "plays" another part, another being. He *is* another being. The terrors of childhood, open-hearted gaiety, mystic fantasy and sacred awe are all inextricably entangled in this strange business of masks and disguises.

Summing up the formal characteristics of play we might call it a free activity standing quite consciously outside "ordinary" life as being "not serious", but at the same time absorbing the player intensely and utterly. It is an activity connected with no material interest, and no profit can be gained by it. It proceeds within its own proper boundaries of time and space according to fixed rules and in an orderly manner. It promotes the formation of social groupings which tend to surround themselves with secrecy and to stress their difference from the common world by disguise or other means.

Sport and Play:
Suspension of the Ordinary*

KENNETH L. SCHMITZ

Sport and play are familiar, but their meaning is not obvious. Play is perhaps as old as man himself, and some will say older. Sport has undergone a remarkable development in some civilizations. It is pursued today by millions in the highly technological societies. Sport is sometimes firmly distinguished from play, and it certainly contains other factors. Nevertheless, the following reflection will suggest that sport is primarily an extension of play, and that it rests upon and derives its central values from play. On this basis it will be maintained that a generous acceptance of the play element in sport is essential for the full realization of this latter form of human behaviour.

The variety of play poses a grave difficulty in understanding it. Its very unity is problematic. Is there a single phenomenon of play which has sufficient unity to be called a special form of human behaviour? The present reflection moves within the context of certain uses not exclusive to English in which the word "play" occurs. Children play in the yard, waves play on the beach, lovers engage in erotic play, an actor plays a part, a musician plays an instrument, a footballer plays a game, a bettor plays the horses, and the gods play with men. The meanings are various; some are peripheral, extended or metaphorical uses. I think, however, that a central core of meaning remains which points towards an indeterminate yet coherent form of human behaviour. This complex structure I call the phenomenon of play.

Wittgenstein poses the difficulty when he lists a wide range of uses of the word "game." He thinks that the variety shows that there is no essence common to all games but only a family resemblance which permits a chain of different uses. I sympathize with much of what Wittgenstein says about the search for a common essence at all costs. Nevertheless, I think that he assumes too strong a doctrine of essence and too exacting a conception of language before he goes on to his refutation. He seems to tie the doctrine of essence to the doctrine of substance. Now this is an understandable conjunction in the light of much of traditional philosophy, but I do not think it is a necessary or a wise one. It might be said that I set out here to clarify the "essence" of play, but I certainly do not think that I will have established a "substance" of play. I have mentioned a "central core" and a "structure," but it may be more helpful to bear in mind more fluid and dynamic metaphors than the traditional figure of a static structure, idea or form. Gabriel Marcel often speaks of a phenomenon as present in varying degrees along a continuum. Or we might even picture an element as more or less present and more or less pure in a series of chemical solutions.[1] But these are only metaphors.

* Presented at the annual meeting of the American Association for the Advancement of Science, Dallas, Texas, December, 1968.

[1] For example, G. Marcel, *The Mystery of Being* (Gifford Lectures, 1949-50), Regnery, Chicago, 2 vols., n.d.

Nor should we be surprised if the same word is extended to activities which do not share an important central meaning. Ordinary usage is the usage of ordinary men, and not that of scientists or philosophers. Family resemblances suffice. It is enough in ordinary speech that one important similarity hold between a clear instance of play, such as children's frolic, and an extended usage, such as piano playing. Thus we speak of ball-players and easily transfer the vocabulary of play and sport to events such as war-games where the factor of contest so heavily weighs. Although the usage is clear enough, further thought may uncover reasons for the frequent association of contest with play but not its necessity for all forms of play. Then, too, the contest in war-games may prove alien in meaning and psychological tone to the contest which occurs in sporting games.

When reflective analysis seeks to isolate the phenomenon of play it must recognize still other hazards. The difficulty of bringing play to reflective clarity is a difficulty which all immediate and obvious phenomena share. Just as in emotion, for example, so too in play, we live under the spell of peculiar immediacy. We throw ourselves into the spirit of the frolic or game, and when reflection itself becomes an ingredient in playfulness it takes on the character of immediacy, serving the values and objectives of the game. Moreover, play compounds the difficulty by revealing itself in a way that is secretive and shy. It can dodge the determined attentions of reflection by encouraging an amused contempt for it, or by permitting itself to be banished to the years of growing-up. An adult and work-oriented thought finds it easy to neglect or to misrepresent it, as though it were not worthy of "serious" attention. It resists analysis and preserves its essential meaning by turning our accounts of it away from itself to some alien value. Of course, we must recognize the biological and psychological value of play, in relaxation and escape, in rest and exercise, in education and character-formation. But unless play is nothing but these functions, we cannot understand them fully without understanding *it*. The present intent, then, is to clarify the spirit of play, to determine its appropriate forms, and to characterize the element of play in sport.

There is a thicket of other difficulties, too. Play hides obscurely within a host of very complex phenomena and behaviours and is subtle enough to be easily confused with other forms. For a full analysis, it would be necessary to say what play is not. It seems easiest to see that play is not work, and yet it may call sometimes for very great effort. War may highlight the difference, for like work, war is serious, but like play it is non-productive. The words "conquest" and "victory" belong to the vocabulary of war. The first is said easily enough of work, and the second of play. Some forms of play also resemble war in having the element of contest in them; but the essence of war is deadly contest, it is heavy with death. The grave risk of life is not excluded from play, but if life is risked for some alien value, no matter how high, or if death is certain, the spirit of play is extinguished. There is a certain lightness about play which it shares with other forms of leisure. To be sure, play is not the same as good humour, for although it may be fun, it is not necessarily funny. G. K. Chesterton caught the mood when he remarked that certain affairs were too important to be taken seriously. Play consists in what we may call "non-serious" importance. Still, it cannot be equated simply with pleasure or amusement. Indeed, a full analysis of play would have to make room within it for ingredients of pain and discomfort. It would have to be asked, too, whether a high degree of cruelty, as in the ancient bear-baiting or the gladiatorial games, crushes, perverts or merely tempers the spirit of play.

Such an extended analysis of play is not appropriate here, and I turn instead to sketch out, briefly and tentatively, the positive character of this elusive blithe spirit.

The Varieties of Play. Play can be considered under four general varieties: frolic, make-believe, sporting skills and games. The least formal play is simple spontaneous frolic, and this is associated especially with the very young. It is that aspect of play which is found also in young animals, and its occasional appearance in adult humans seems to manifest the feature of neoteny so pronounced in man. Such play among kittens and puppies, or something very like play, may well be a kind of training along with a desire to satisfy curiosity and to express plain high spirits. It is usually intense and brief and tends to dissipate itself with the outburst of energy that makes it possible. It is an immediate and unreflecting expression of a kind of animal joy, a kicking off of the normal patterns of behaviour, purposeless and without constraint. "Horsing around" illustrates the manner in which the play-world can erupt for a brief moment. A practical joke can trigger a spontaneous display. Someone from the group splashes cold water upon the others lying at leisure in sun and sand, and an impromptu "battle" begins, with little or no declared object and with fluid changing of sides. It is a quicksilver form of play, dashing off now in one direction, now in another, fragmenting and rejoining forces in new combinations for new momentary objectives.

A second more or less informal variety of play is that of make-believe or "just pretending." This, too, is commonest with children but not exclusive to them. There is, of course, daydreaming, a sort of playing with images, roles and situations, though this tends to diminish with adult life or is translated into artistic creativity. Among adults the carnival such as the Mardi Gras, the parade such as the Santa or homecoming parade, and costume parties are examples of this variety of play, intermixed with elements of frolic. It is interesting that some form of the mask or costume is used as a means by which the adult can enter the play-world. In its secular shape as in its religious origin, the mask is a device for suspending the everyday world. The child, on the other hand, needs no such device and with nothing at all can create for himself the world which his playful imagination gives to him. There are usually no well-defined and explicit rules for pretending games, though the roles assumed determine a rough and approximate fittingness. One child is quick to tell another that she is out of character, and the adult who goes to a ball dressed as Bugs Bunny will find his part already somewhat defined for him. Such playfulness, however, is quite different from a theatrical role in which the part is already drawn *a priori* and the actor is expected to interpret and manifest it by using the words and situations provided beforehand by the playwright. What is uppermost in the play of the theatre is representation, whereas in play itself a rough approximation serves merely to suggest and maintain the illusion proper to it. On stage the play is for the sake of presentation, whereas in make-believe the representation is for the sake of play. More generally, it may be said that art and aesthetic experience centre upon the embodiment and expression of meaning, whereas play is for the sake of a certain form of action. In the ballet, for example, action is subordinated to gesture, but in genuine play, mimicry and expression are either incidental or for the sake of the action.

The more formal varieties of play take two styles: skills and games. The first style includes surfboarding, sailing, horse-riding, mountain-climbing, hiking and similar play activities. It calls for knowledge, skill and a certain endurance; so, at least in an elementary way, does the bouncing of a ball, jumping with a pogo stick, yawing a Yo-Yo and skipping rope. The final style of play is completely formal, such as the games of baseball, card-playing and the like. Both styles of play are contests. The former require the mastery of a skill in conformance with natural forces, such as the behaviour of wind and water or the motion of ball and rope. They may even have rudimentary rules. In the truly formal games, however, rules predominate, and although they are determined by agreement, they are held as absolutely binding. Even in solitaire one cannot actually *win* the game if he cheats. Cheating in play is the counterpart of sin in the moral order. It seeks the good of victory without conforming to the spirit of the game and the rules under which alone it is possible to possess it. In the flowery language of a bygone era: the crown of victory sits hollow upon the head of a cheat, who has excluded himself from the values of the game-world and can only enjoy the incidental fruits that sometimes attend a victory. This is quite apart from any moral do's or don'ts, and is written into the very texture of the game-world. In any case, the rules of play differ from those of morality. We can take up the game or leave it, but the rules of morality oblige without any conditionality. Moral rules apply within a context of human action and values that is not that of play and that may touch directly upon the issues of life and death.

In each of these four varieties of play different features predominate: in the frolic the aspect of spontaneous celebration, in imaginative pretense the aspect of creativity, in skill and game the aspect of contest. These aspects are met with in non-play situations too: celebration in worship, creativity in art and contest in work and war. It remains, therefore, to mark out their peculiar quality in the play-world and to indicate its ontological character.

Play as Suspension of the Ordinary World.[2] The spirit of play may be carried over into many activities and even subordinated to other purposes, but it is manifested and realized most perfectly in the four varieties distinguished above. The essence of play comes into existence through the decision to play. Such a constitutive decision cannot be compelled and

[2] See Eugen Fink, *Spiel als Weltsymbol*, Kohl-hammer, Stuttgart, 1960.

is essentially free. Through it arises the suspension of the ordinary concerns of the everyday world. Such a decision does not simply initiate the playing but rather constitutes it. That is, it does not stand before the playing as winding a mechanical toy stands before its unwinding performance, but rather it underlies and grounds the entire duration of play. This duration may be interrupted or ended at any time, and in this sense the play-world is fragile, ceasing to be either because of the intrusion of the natural world of ordinary concerns, the loss of interest on the part of the players, or the completion of the play-objective. Devices are sometimes used for entrance into and maintenance of the play-spirit, but they are subordinate to the essential demands of play. In a prevalent adult form of contemporary play, nightclubbing, which intends to resemble the frolic, alcohol is almost methodically used to make the transition from the ordinary world somewhat easier. The constant threat of the price tag at the end of the evening naturally makes the suspension of ordinary concerns rather more difficult. It goes without saying that too much alcohol brings about the demise of play, as do drugs, for play seems to demand a deliberate maintenance of itself in keeping with the voluntary character of its founding decision. Play may be a kind of madness, but it is self-engendered and self-maintained.

Inasmuch as the play-decision suspends ordinary concerns, it breaks open a new totality. The world of play with its own non-natural objectives and formalities may be said to transcend the natural world and the world of everyday concern. Of course, it must reckon with natural laws and cannot suspend their real effective impact. Players tire and drop out of the game or are injured; or there just isn't time for a last set of tennis or bridge; or the little girls playing house are called in for supper. Moreover, some forms of play, such as surfboarding or mountain-climbing, deliberately set for their objectives the conquest of natural forces. What is common to these and all forms of play is that natural processes do not determine the significance of the play. The player does not follow natural forces as such. Whereas the worker often follows them in order to redirect them as in cultivation, the player may resist them, ignore them as far as possible or create a new order of significance whose elements are non-natural, as in word-games. The surfer follows them in order to wrest from them a carefree moment of exhilarating joy; the archer takes them into

account in order to hit a target of his own proposing; and the chess-player moves within a set of spatial possibilities that are ideal in themselves and only indicated by the board and chessmen.

Religion, art and play are rightly spoken of as ways of transcending the strictly natural world. Religion, however, does not suspend the world of nature. Quite the contrary, in its historical forms, it turns back from a sacred and alien distance towards nature in order to reawaken and restore it to its original freshness and creativity. Art and aesthetic experience transcend the natural world in the embodiment and expression of concrete, symbolic meaning. Art suspends the natural and puts it out of play when it gives ultimate value to transnatural objectives. Kant, of course, speaks of a certain detachment or disinterestedness. The sign of the transcendence of play over the natural world is manifest by a certain excess which characterizes its spirit. There is in it an uncalled-for exhilaration, a hilarity in the contest and in the mood of celebration. Like art and religion, play is not far from the feast, for art celebrates beauty and religion celebrates glory, but play celebrates the emergence of a finite world that lies outside and beyond the world of nature while at the same time resting upon it.

The Play-world as a Distinctive Order. The space and time of play are not contiguous with natural space and time. The little child creates an area in the room in which battles are fought, seas sailed, continents discovered, in which animals roam and crops grow. Adults create the playing field which is a space directed according to the objectives and rules of the game. A ball driven to the right of a line is "foul," another landing beyond a certain point is "out of play." In chess the knight alone can jump and the bishop can only move diagonally. Play-space is not at all relative in most games and to the extent to which arbitrary rules are invented to that extent the space becomes more determinate and more absolute. Players hold willingly to the rules or those who do not have officials to encourage them in the most formal sports. This maintenance of the absolutely binding force of the rules is a free acceptance flowing out of and essentially one with the play-decision, and with the suspension of the natural ordinary world and the substitution of a new order. The laws of natural forces are put to use in an extraordinary way within an extraordinary world inspired by a motive that has suspended the ordinary interests of everyday life.

2

The structured order of play-space is especially evident in those games in which a single or double point in the play-space is the key to the contest, the privileged space of the goals, target or finishing-line. So, too, play-time is not contiguous with ordinary time, though it must frequently bow to it. In ice hockey sixty minutes of play-time are not sixty minutes of clock-time, and in baseball play-time is simply nine innings or more. Of course, natural space and time are the alien boundaries that ring about and mark the finitude of human play, but the play has its own internal boundaries set by the objectives and rules of the game. When a ball is out of bounds in many games the game-time stops also. Men set the objectives and rules of play and yet there is a certain sense in which the play-objective, freely chosen, sets its own basic rules. Play seems to begin by abandoning forms of everyday behaviour, but it maintains that abandonment in a positive and determinate way by creating a new space and time with new forms and rules of behaviour that are not determined by or functional within the everyday world but which nevertheless have a positive meaning of their own. Within its boundaries and objectives the play-world exhibits a totality of meaning and value that is strikingly complete and perfect. Play reveals itself as transnatural, fragile, limited perfection.

The suspension of the natural world and its subordination to the game or its sublimation into the play context can be described as the suppression of the real, where "reality" is restricted to the natural and ordinary world. Play then builds an illusion. Huizinga notes that the Latin word for play (*ludus*) is closely related to the word for illusion (*inlusio*).[2] The "inactuality" of play is most evident in the imaginative play of make-believe. This suspension of the "real" world by means of a play-decision releases a world of "unreality" which needs no justification from outside itself. It is a self-sealed world, delivering its own values in and for itself, the freedom and joy of play. As a piece of fine art needs no other defence than itself, and as the feast need exist for no other reason than its own values, so too play, though its claims must be balanced within the whole man against those of "reality," receives justification only through and in itself. As colour cannot validate its existence and meaning except to one who sees, so play cannot vindicate itself except to one who plays. To

[2] *Homo Ludens: a study of the play element in culture,* (1944), Beacon, Boston, 1955, p. 36. See also Fink, *op. cit.,* pp. 66 ff.

[3] Huizinga, *op. cit.,* p. 4.

anyone else it appears superfluous. The stern Calvin Coolidge, it is said, once snorted that going fishing was childish, which only proved to fishermen that he was absurd. Play has its own built-in finality. It is in this sense objectless; it has no other object than itself.

Nevertheless, an adequate philosophy can free the mind from an exclusive preoccupation with the natural world and open it out onto all the modes of being. Each is seen to have its value. Like religion and art, play embodies a significance that is not fully grasped in clear concepts. As an analysis does not replace a poem or a painting, so a description of its rules is no substitute for play. But an analysis may open the mind to the genuine reality of play. The proper vehicle of meaning in play is action and in this it is much closer to ritual and myth than to scientific concepts. Play is meaning embodied in action; it is "significant form"[3] precisely as human behaviour. The world which opens out through the play-decision is a world of possibilities closed off from the natural and ordinary world. Measured against the ordinary world the world of possibility opened up by play seems inactual and illusory; but measured in terms of being itself, it is a radical way of being human, a distinctive mode of being. It is a way of taking up the world of being, a manner of being present in the world in the mode of creative possibility whose existential presence is a careless joyful freedom.

I suggest, then, that there is a phenomenon of play which is an indeterminate yet coherent mode of human behaviour. It comes to be through a decision which does not simply initiate or occasion play, but which founds and underlies it. It is a decision which is freely taken and maintained, either spontaneously or deliberately. It is a decision which seeks to secure certain values for human consciousness and human existence, a certain meaning and a certain freedom. It may be called an activity of maintaining an illusion, if we speak in terms which still give primacy to the natural world. But it may also be called an activity of suspension, whereby the natural forces while not abrogated are dethroned from their primacy. More positively, it may be called an activity of constitution, which breaks open distinctive possibilities of meaning, freedom and value. It has no other essential objective than those implicit in the founding decision. It has its own time and space, boundaries and objectives, rewards and penalties. It is a distinctive way, voluntary and finite, of man's being-in-the-world. Playing in the world, man recovers himself as a free and transcendent being.

The Play-element in Sport. Two factors

are especially prominent in sport: the first is the emphasis on good performance, and the second is the element of contest. If sport consisted simply of performance and contest, however, scholarship examinations would be reported in the sporting pages. Examinations are liable to be deadly serious and to be related directly to educational objectives which are part of the natural and social world.

Sport may be carried on at various levels of competence and preparedness, from the unplanned street game to the carefully planned amateur or professional sporting event. In the former, natural ability and past experience determine the proficiency of the maneuvers. Planned events are usually preceded by exercises for general conditioning and precise training. These preparations are directed towards the performance of activities within a non-natural space and time and in accord with more or less formally specified rules. The excellence of the performance is judged within a matrix of values that flow from the decision to play this or that kind of game.

The performance, moreover, is for the sake of the contest, either against natural forces, such as in the high jump, or against other players, as in track meets. In some sports, there is only one contestant, as in hunting; but in most, as in team games, a contestant pits himself also against other players. The performance is tested by the contest of player against player, and the verdict is sealed by the victory.

It may seem that the play element is not essential to sport. Thus, for example, the sport of hunting lies very close to the natural needs of man. Moreover, it has little of formal rules. The various game laws are not to be confused with sporting rules, for they are meant to conserve the natural supply of game as a condition for further hunting. They are laws, not rules. Of course, if two huntsmen vie with each other for the largest or the quickest bag, we say that they have made a game out of it. Here again, they have imposed upon the natural value, namely, the food procured, a game-value, the prize of victory. Such a contest, however, is to be distinguished from the contest of bucks seeking a mate or tycoons seeking a fortune. It is imaginable that the latter might be taken up in a *spirit* of play, but it is not properly playful in its *form*. We see here a distinction between the forms of play and the spirit which inhabits them. This spirit can sometimes animate certain other forms of behaviour. Thus a man may bet in order to win and pay off the mortgage, or he may bet in order to risk something valuable to him. Only the latter is animated by a spirit of play. Even it is no longer play if it is compulsive, for it may then be the sublimation of the wish to totter between life and death.

In addition to good performance and contest, then, spontaneous creative freedom is inherent in play. This suggests that sport can be carried out without the spirit of play. Nevertheless, in the life of individuals and in the history of the race, sport emerges from play as from an original and founding existential posture. Sport is free, self-conscious, tested play which moves in a transnatural dimension of human life, built upon a certain basis of leisure. Sport is in its origin and intention a movement into transcendence which carries over from the founding decision to play and which builds upon that decision an intensified thrust towards the values of self-consciousness tested through performance, competition and victory. There is certainly a return to seriousness in the discipline of formal sport. There is training, performance and competition. But the objectives of sport and its founding decision lie within play and cause sport to share in certain of its features—the sense of immediacy, exhilaration, rule-directed behaviour, and the indeterminacy of a specified outcome.

Sport can be demanding, but its essence is as delicate as any perfume and can be as readily dissipated. There are three abuses which can kill the spirit of play within sport and reduce sport to something less than its fullest human possibilities.

The first abuse is the exaggeration of the importance of victory. I do not refer to the will to win, which must be strong in any highly competitive sport. Still, such a will must be situated within a more generous context—the desire to perform as well as it is humanly possible. Many factors not under the control of players or judges may determine the ultimate victor. Such an awareness does not tarnish the prize, but situates it properly within a limited and qualified texture. Victory in sports is not absolute, and it should not be allowed to behave like the absolute. The policy of winning at all costs is the surest way of snuffing out the spirit of play in sport. The fallout of such a policy is the dreary succession of firings in college and professional sport. Such an emphasis on victory detaches the last moment from the whole game and fixes the outcome apart from its proper context. It reduces the appreciation of the performance, threatens the proper disposition towards the rules and turns the contest into a naked power struggle. The upshot is a brutalization of the sport. And so, the sport which issued from the play-decision, promising freedom and exhilaration, ends dismally in lessening the humanity of players and spectators.

The second abuse stems from the rationalization of techniques within a sport when the rationalization is promoted by an exaggerated sense of the value of efficiency. Good performance is important and the best performance is a desirable ideal. A coach has always to deal with a definite group of individual players. He must assess their potential for the game, combining firmness with good judgment and enthusiasm with restraint. Hard coaching is to be expected, but under pressure of competition it is tempting to let moderation give way to an uninterrupted drive for limitless proficiency. An abstract tyranny of the possible may drive players beyond what they should be asked to give, compelling them to spend what they neither have nor can afford. Driven beyond their natural capacities, they lose the spirit of play, and the values which are supposed to be the initial and perhaps even the paramount reason for taking up the sport. There is a subtle and difficult difference between such tyrannic proficiency and the will to excel which every competitor must have and which leads him to pit his body and personality with and against others. There is a difference between a tyrant and a coach who rightly demands the best his players can put forth. There is a difference, too, between a rationalization which sacrifices everything to technical competence and a reasonable improvement of techniques of training and performance which lift a sport to new accomplishments. Such a merely technical drive is more than likely in our age which tends to over-rationalize all life in the name of technical perfection. The deepest problems in our technological society centre about salvaging, promoting and developing truly human possibilities. Sport stands in a very sensitive position. It can be part of the drive to dehumanization, or in a very direct and privileged way, to the recapture of human values and human dignity. An ultimate and limitless demand for proficiency forced upon players and sport at the cost of all other values including those of play will diminish all who participate—players, staff and spectators.

The first and second abuses are internal threats which arise from detaching victory or performance from the context of play. The third abuse arrives from outside what is essential to sport. It arises with the presence of spectators and threatens to alienate the sport from its play-objectives and values. Such an alienation becomes even more likely when the commercial possibilities of a sport are exploited. The genuine essence of play cannot be present when it is play only for the spectators, as in the gladiatorial contests of the Roman circus in which contestants were often compelled against their wishes to face wild beasts or even one another. One of the requirements is that the participants also take up the activity in a spirit of play. In commercial sport, the spectators usually attend the game in a spirit of play, though some attend simply with friends or to be seen. The players, on the other hand, are under contract, though it is under contract precisely "to play." It seems an oversimplification, however, to discount professional sport as play merely because the players are paid. We do not call a work of fine art non-art simply because it is commissioned. Moreover, the distinction between amateur and professional is a social one, distinguishing those who pursue a vocation from those who pursue an avocation. Olympic sport claims to reflect the time when some games were part of the culture of a "gentleman." Amateurs today are of three kinds: the occasional players who are not very serious in their pursuit of the sport; those who, like many bowlers or curlers, are serious devotees of the sport but not under contract to play it; and those would-be pros who are not yet skilled enough to play the sport under contract. On the side of the professional player what threatens the purity of the spirit of play is the compulsion implied in the contractual obligation to render services at given times, to practise in order to maintain and improve skills, and to participate in games as required. But these demands are intrinsic to many games. The threat lies even more in the nature of the binding force. In professional sport it does not lie in interest in the game itself but rather is reinforced and ultimately enforced by values not intrinsic to the game. Perhaps the clearest distinction is between the wage the pro earns and the win or loss of the game. Win or lose, for a time at least he is paid a wage for services delivered; but he gets the victory only when "the gods of the game" smile upon him. Play ceases when the primary reasons for undertaking it are alien to the values of the play-world itself. Values intrinsic to the play-world include not letting down one's own teammates in team games, not begging off the contest because of personal discomfort, taking pleasure in performing activities within the rules of the game, prizing the victory and its symbols. Values that lie outside the play-world include agreement to deliver services for wages earned, abiding by a contract because of fear of being sued, playing out games in order not to be barred from further league participation, finishing out a sports career in order to achieve social and economic standing upon ceasing to play. These motives are not unworthy; they are simply not motives of play. A player may respect the values of play without directly experiencing them, as when he finishes out his sports' career as ably as possible in order to fulfill the possibilities of the game and thereby allow other participants and spectators to share in the values of the game. Heroism in sport often arises through the determination of a player to maintain the importance of the play-world even in the face of disturbances from the "real" world, such as painful injuries, private worries, physical exhaustion, or even fading interest, although the fan tends to look upon the latter as a betrayal. On the side of the spectator in professional and even in other organized sport, what threatens the purity of the spirit of play is the reduction of the players to hirelings, and the game to something which is expected to deliver to the spectator a period of pleasure for money paid. The commercialization of sport can, of course, be a way of seeing that the quality and abundance of playing is increased; but it can and often does simply pervert sport into just another profitable pleasure industry. Many things give pleasure. Some of them can be bought. The play-world is not one of them. Over-commercialization of sport disillusions the spectator and risks defeating the objectives of commercialization.

The play-world in general offers itself to anyone who wishes to enter it, either as participant or as spectator. But to receive the gift of play he must take up the values of the game as important in and for themselves. He may get angry with "his" team when it plays badly and boast of it when it plays well; but he will not view the players simply as objects employed to give him a pleasurable spectacle. This is a purely objectivist viewpoint and a form of reductionism. It is easy for a spectator to drift into this attitude, because his relation to the game is only partial. He bears no responsibility, and he lives the risks and thrills, defeats and victories in a moving but not a completely involved way. The player is committed with his body and plunges in as one participant; the spectator participates as the whole team, but indirectly. Nevertheless, play calls for and can achieve a vantage point which undercuts the distinction of the purely subjective and the purely objective, in which I am here and they are there. The fan enjoys a special complicity with his team and easily transfers the symbolic value of the victory to himself and his group. He feels himself in some sense one with the participants of the game. What unites them is the particular form of the play-world, and the importance of its objectives and values.

In sum, then, sport can nourish the spirit of objectivity, for it contains a native generosity with which it seeks excellence of form and action in obedience to conventional rules and submits freely to the award of victory or defeat according to those rules. In so doing, sport manifests a distinctive mode of human life, combining creative freedom with disciplined order for the sake of skilled competition and earned victory. In the engagement the player must encounter his opponent not as an enemy in war but as one whose excellence challenges him and makes possible his own best performance. Players and spectators discover in a new dimension the significance of competitors, team and fans. The sharp difference of subject and object is bridged by the common context and objectives. A fan may surprise himself applauding an exceptionally fine play against his own team, or at least unhappily admiring it. At a race-meet fans from several schools spontaneously urge on the front runner who seems able to beat the existing record, even though he will beat their own runners. It is a victory of man against time and space and himself. Of course, the spectator can be treated as one who needs bread and circuses, but wiser sports managers will try to transform an appetite for constantly renewed sensations into an experience of community. The radical breaking-down of more traditional ties has seen the rise of massive spectator sports. Is it not possible that the attraction of sport for non-players lies in the invitation to experience freedom, meaning and excellence in the context of a free community of individuals bound together by a common appreciation for the values of the game? In that experience of free community men discover new possibilities of human excellence and reach out to recover a fuller meaning of themselves.

The Classification of Games*

ROGER CAILLOIS

The multitude and infinite variety of games at first causes one to despair of discovering a principle of classification capable of subsuming them under a small number of well-defined categories. Games also possess so many different characteristics that many approaches are possible. Current usage sufficiently demonstrates the degree of hesitance and uncertainty: indeed, several classifications are employed concurrently. To oppose card games to games of skill, or to oppose parlor games to those played in a stadium is meaningless. In effect, the implement used in the game is chosen as a classificatory instrument in the one case; in the other, the qualifications required; in a third the number of players and the atmosphere of the game, and lastly the place in which the contest is waged. An additional over-all complication is that the same game can be played alone or with others. A particular game may require several skills simultaneously, or none.

Very different games can be played in the same place. Merry-go-rounds and the diabolo are both open-air amusements. But the child who passively enjoys the pleasure of riding by means of the movement of the carousel is not in the same state of mind as the one who tries as best he can to correctly whirl his diabolo. On the other hand, many games are played without implements or accessories. Also, the same implement can fulfill different functions, depending on the game played. Marbles are generally the equipment for a game of skill, but one of the players can try to guess whether the marbles held in his opponent's hand are an odd or even number. They thus become part of a game of chance.

This last expression must be clarified. For one thing, it alludes to the fundamental characteristic of a very special kind of game. Whether it be a bet, lottery, roulette, or baccara, it is clear that the player's attitude is the same. He does nothing, he merely awaits the outcome. The boxer, the runner, and the player of chess or hopscotch, on the contrary, work as hard as they can to win. It matters little that some games are athletic and others intellectual. The player's attitude is the same: he tries to vanquish a rival operating under the same conditions as himself. It would thus appear justified to contrast games of chance with competitive games. Above all, it becomes tempting to investigate the possibility of discovering other attitudes, no less fundamental, so that the categories for a systematic classification of games can eventually be provided.

After examining different possibilities, I am proposing a division into four main rubrics, depending upon whether, in the games under consideration, the role of competition, chance, simulation, or vertigo is dominant. I call these *agôn, alea, mimicry,* and *ilinx,* respectively. All four indeed belong to the domain of play. One *plays* football, billiards, or chess (*agôn*); rou-

* Reprinted with permission of The Macmillan Company from *Man, Play, and Games* by Roger Caillois, translated by Meyer Barash. Copyright © 1961 by The Free Press of Glencoe, Inc.; and with permission of © Editions Gallimard.

lette or a lottery (*alea*); pirate, Nero, or Hamlet (*mimicry*); or one produces in oneself, by a rapid whirling or falling movement, a state of dizziness and disorder (*ilinx*). Even these designations do not cover the entire universe of play. It is divided into quadrants, each governed by an original principle. Each section contains games of the same kind. But inside each section, the different games are arranged in a rank order of progression. They can also be placed on a continuum between two opposite poles. At one extreme an almost indivisible principle, common to diversion, turbulence, free improvisation, and carefree gaiety is dominant. It manifests a kind of uncontrolled fantasy that can be designated by the term *paidia*. At the opposite extreme, this frolicsome and impulsive exuberance is almost entirely absorbed or disciplined by a complementary, and in some respects inverse, tendency to its anarchic and capricious nature: there is a growing tendency to bind it with arbitrary, imperative, and purposely tedious conventions, to oppose it still more by ceaselessly practicing the most embarrassing chicanery upon it, in order to make it more uncertain of attaining its desired effect. This latter principle is completely impractical, even though it requires an ever greater amount of effort, patience, skill, or ingenuity. I call this second component *ludus*.

I do not intend, in resorting to these strange concepts, to set up some kind of pedantic, totally meaningless mythology. However, obligated as I am to classify diverse games under the same general category, it seemed to me that the most economical means of doing so was to borrow, from one language or another, the most meaningful and comprehensive term possible, so that each category examined should avoid the possibility of lacking the particular quality on the basis of which the unifying concept was chosen. Also, to the degree that I will try to establish the classification to which I am committed, each concept chosen will not relate too directly to concrete experience, which in turn is to be divided according to an as yet untested principle.

In the same spirit, I am compelled to subsume the games most varied in appearance under the same rubric, in order to better demonstrate their fundamental kinship. I have mixed physical and mental games, those dependent upon force with those requiring skill or reasoning. Within each class, I have not distinguished between children's and adults' games, and wherever possible I have sought instances of homologous behavior in the animal world. The point in doing this was to stress

the very principle of the proposed classification. It would be less burdensome if it were perceived that the divisions set up correspond to essential and irreducible impulses.

Fundamental Categories

Agôn. A whole group of games would seem to be competitive, that is to say, like a combat in which equality of chances is artificially created, in order that the adversaries should confront each other under ideal conditions, susceptible of giving precise and incontestable value to the winner's triumph. It is therefore always a question of a rivalry which hinges on a single quality (speed, endurance, strength, memory, skill, ingenuity, etc.), exercised, within defined limits and without outside assistance, in such a way that the winner appears to be better than the loser in a certain category of exploits. Such is the case with sports contests and the reason for their very many subdivisions. Two individuals or two teams are in opposition (polo, tennis, football, boxing, fencing, etc.), or there may be a varying number of contestants (courses of every kind, shooting matches, golf, athletics, etc.). In the same class belong the games in which, at the outset, the adversaries divide the elements into equal parts and value. The games of checkers, chess, and billiards are perfect examples. The search for equality is so obviously essential to the rivalry that it is reestablished by a handicap for players of different classes; that is, within the equality of chances originally established, a secondary inequality, proportionate to the relative powers of the participants, is dealt with. It is significant that such a usage exists in the *agôn* of a physical character (sports) just as in the more cerebral type (chess games for example, in which the weaker player is given the advantage of a pawn, knight, castle, etc.).

As carefully as one tries to bring it about, absolute equality does not seem to be realizable. Sometimes, as in checkers or chess, the fact of moving first is an advantage, for this priority permits the favored player to occupy key positions or to impose a special strategy. Conversely, in bidding games, such as bridge, the last bidder profits from the clues afforded by the bids of his opponents. Again, at croquet, to be last multiplies the player's resources. In sports contests, the exposure, the fact of having the sun in front or in back; the wind which aids or hinders one or the other side; the fact, in disputing for positions on a circular track, of finding oneself in the inside or outside lane constitutes a crucial test, a trump or disadvantage whose influence may be considerable. These inevitable imbalances are negated or modified by drawing lots at the beginning, then by strict alternation of favored positions.

The point of the game is for each player to have his superiority in a given area recognized. That is why the practice of *agôn* presupposes sustained attention, appropriate training, assiduous application, and the desire to win. It implies discipline and perseverance. It leaves the champion to his own devices, to evoke the best possible game of which he is capable, and it obliges him to play the game within the fixed limits, and according to the rules applied equally to all, so that in return the victor's superiority will be beyond dispute.

In addition to games, the spirit of *agôn* is found in other cultural phenomena conforming to the game code: in the duel, in the tournament, and in certain constant and noteworthy aspects of so-called courtly war.

In principle, it would seem that *agôn* is unknown among animals, which have no conception of limits or rules, only seeking a brutal victory in merciless combat. It is clear that horse races and cock fights are an exception, for these are conflicts in which men make animals compete in terms of norms that the former alone have set up. Yet, in considering certain facts, it seems that animals already have the competitive urge during encounters where limits are at least implicitly accepted and spontaneously respected, even if rules are lacking. This is notably the case in kittens, puppies, and bear cubs, which take pleasure in knocking each other down yet not hurting each other.

Still more convincing are the habits of bovines, which, standing face to face with heads lowered, try to force each other back. Horses engage in the same kind of friendly dueling: to test their strength, they rear up on their hind legs and press down upon each other with all their vigor and weight, in order to throw their adversaries off balance. In addition, observers have noted numerous games of pursuit that result from a challenge or invitation. The animal that is overtaken has nothing to fear from the victor. The most impressive example is without doubt that of the little ferocious "fighting" willow wrens. "A moist elevation covered with short grass and about two meters in diameter is chosen for the arena," says Karl Groos.[1] The males gather

[1] Karl Groos. *The Play of Animals*. English translation. New York: D. Appleton & Co., 1898, p. 151.

there daily. The first to arrive waits for an adversary, and then the fight begins. The contenders tremble and bow their heads several times. Their feathers bristle. They hurl themselves at each other, beaks advanced, and striking at one another. *Never is there any pursuit or conflict outside the space delimited for the journey.* That is why it seems legitimate for me to use the term *agôn* for these cases, for the goal of the encounters is not for the antagonist to cause serious injury to his rival, but rather to demonstrate his own superiority. Man merely adds refinement and precision by devising rules.

In children, as soon as the personality begins to assert itself, and before the emergence of regulated competition, unusual challenges are frequent, in which the adversaries try to prove their greater endurance. They are observed competing to see which can stare at the sun, endure tickling, stop breathing, not wink his eye, etc., the longest. Sometimes the stakes are more serious, where it is a question of enduring hunger or else pain in the form of whipping, pinching, stinging, or burning. Then these ascetic games, as they have been called, involve severe ordeals. They anticipate the cruelty and hazing which adolescents must undergo during their initiation. This is a departure from *agôn*, which soon finds its perfect form, be it in legitimately competitive games and sports, or in those involving feats of prowess (hunting, mountain climbing, crossword puzzles, chess problems, etc.) in which champions, without directly confronting each other, are involved in ceaseless and diffuse competition.

Alea. This is the Latin name for the game of dice. I have borrowed it to designate, in contrast to *agôn*, all games that are based on a decision independent of the player, an outcome over which he has no control, and in which winning is the result of fate rather than triumphing over an adversary. More properly, destiny is the sole artisan of victory, and where there is rivalry, what is meant is that the winner has been more favored by fortune than the loser. Perfect examples of this type are provided by the games of dice, roulette, heads or tails, baccara, lotteries, etc. Here, not only does one refrain from trying to eliminate the injustice of chance, but rather it is the very capriciousness of chance that constitutes the unique appeal of the game.

Alea signifies and reveals the favor of destiny. The player is entirely passive; he does not deploy his resources, skill, muscles, or intelligence. All he need do is await, in hope and trembling, the cast of the die. He risks his stake. Fair play, also sought but now taking place under ideal conditions, lies in being compensated exactly in proportion to the risk involved. Every device intended to equalize the competitors' chances is here employed to scrupulously equate risk and profit.

In contrast to *agôn*, *alea* negates work, patience, experience, and qualifications. Professionalization, application, and training are eliminated. In one instant, winnings may be wiped out. *Alea* is total disgrace or absolute favor. It grants the lucky player infinitely more than he could procure by a lifetime of labor, discipline, and fatigue. It seems an insolent and sovereign insult to merit. It supposes on the player's part an attitude exactly opposite to that reflected in *agôn*. In the latter, his only reliance is upon himself; in the former, he counts on everything, even the vaguest sign, the slightest outside occurrence, which he immediately takes to be an omen or token—in short, he depends on everything except himself.

Agôn is a vindication of personal responsibility; *alea* is a negation of the will, a surrender to destiny. Some games, such as dominoes, backgammon, and most card games, combine the two. Chance determines the distribution of the hands dealt to each player, and the players then play the hands that blind luck has assigned to them as best they can. In a game like bridge, it is knowledge and reasoning that constitute the player's defense, permitting him to play a better game with the cards that he has been given. In games such as poker, it is the qualities of psychological acumen and character that count.

The role of money is also generally more impressive than the role of chance, and therefore is the recourse of the weaker player. The reason for this is clear: *Alea* does not have the function of causing the more intelligent to win money, but tends rather to abolish natural or acquired individual differences, so that all can be placed on an absolutely equal footing to await the blind verdict of chance.

Since the result of *agôn* is necessarily uncertain and paradoxically must approximate the effect of pure chance, assuming that the chances of the competitors are as equal as possible, it follows that every encounter with competitive characteristics and ideal rules can become the object of betting, or *alea*, e.g. horse or greyhound races, football, basketball, and cock fights. It even happens that table stakes vary unceasingly during the game, according to the vicissitudes of *agôn*.[2]

Games of chance would seem to be peculiarly human. Animals play games involving competition, stimulation, and excess. K. Groos, especially, offers striking examples of these. In sum, animals, which are very much involved in the immediate and enslaved by their impulses, cannot conceive of an abstract and inanimate power, to whose verdict they would passively submit in advance of the game. To await the decision of destiny passively and deliberately, to risk upon it wealth proportionate to the risk of losing, is an attitude that requires the possibility of foresight, vision, and speculation, for which objective and calculating reflection is needed. Perhaps it is in the degree to which a child approximates an animal that games of chance are not as important to children as to adults. For the child, play is active. In addition, the child is immune to the main attraction of games of chance, deprived as he is of economic independence, since he has no money of his own. Games of chance have no power to thrill him. To be sure, marbles are money to him. However, he counts on his skill rather than on chance to win them.

Agôn and *alea* imply opposite and somewhat complementary attitudes, but they both obey the same law—the creation for the players of conditions of pure equality denied them in real life. For nothing in life is clear, since everything is confused from the very beginning, luck and merit too. Play, whether *agôn* or *alea*, is thus an attempt to substitute perfect situations for the normal confusion of contemporary life. In games, the role of merit or chance is clear and indisputable. It is also implied that all must play with exactly the same possibility of proving their superiority or, on another scale, exactly the same chances of winning. In one way or another, one escapes the real world and creates another. One can also escape himself and become another. This is *mimicry*.

Mimicry. All play presupposes the temporary acceptance, if not of an illusion (indeed

[2] For example, in the Balearic Islands for jai alai, and cockfights in the Antilles. It is obvious that it is not necessary to take into account the cash prizes that may motivate jockeys, owners, runners, boxers, football players, or other athletes. These prizes, however substantial, are not relevant to *alea*. They are a reward for a well-fought victory. This recompense for merit has nothing to do with luck or the result of chance, which remain the uncertain monopoly of gamblers; in fact it is the direct opposite.

this last word means nothing less than beginning a game: *in-lusio*), then at least of a closed, conventional, and, in certain respects, imaginary universe. Play can consist not only of deploying actions or submitting to one's fate in an imaginary milieu, but of becoming an illusory character oneself, and of so behaving. One is thus confronted with a diverse series of manifestations, the common element of which is that the subject makes believe or makes others believe that he is someone other than himself. He forgets, disguises, or temporarily sheds his personality in order to feign another. I prefer to designate these phenomena by the term *mimicry*, the English word for mimetism, notably of insects, so that the fundamental, elementary, and quasi-organic nature of the impulse that stimulates it can be stressed.

The insect world, compared to the human world, seems like the most divergent of solutions provided by nature. This world is in contrast in all respects to that of man, but it is no less elaborate, complex, and surprising. Also, it seems legitimate to me at this point to take account of mimetic phenomena of which insects provide most perplexing examples. In fact, corresponding to the free, versatile, arbitrary, imperfect, and extremely diversified behavior of man, there is in animals, especially in insects, the organic, fixed, and absolute adaptation which characterizes the species and is infinitely and exactly reproduced from generation to generation in billions of individuals: e.g. the caste system of ants and termites as against class conflict, and the designs on butterflies' wings as compared to the history of painting. Reluctant as one may be to accept this hypothesis, the temerity of which I recognize, the inexplicable mimetism of insects immediately affords an extraordinary parallel to man's penchant for disguising himself, wearing a mask, or *playing a part*—except that in the insect's case the mask or guise becomes part of the body instead of a contrived accessory. But it serves the same purposes in both cases, viz. to change the wearer's appearance and to inspire fear in others.

Among vertebrates, the tendency to imitate first appears as an entirely physical, quasi-irresistible contagion, analogous to the contagion of yawning, running, limping, smiling, or almost any movement. Hudson seems to have proved that a young animal "follows any object that is going away, and flees any approaching object." Just as a lamb is startled and runs if its mother turns around and moves toward the lamb without warning, the lamb

trails the man, dog, or horse that it sees moving away. Contagion and imitation are not the same as simulation, but they make possible and give rise to the idea or the taste for mimicry. In birds, this tendency leads to nuptial parades, ceremonies, and exhibitions of vanity in which males or females, as the case may be, indulge with rare application and evident pleasure. As for the oxyrhinous crabs, which plant upon their carapaces any alga or polyp that they can catch, their aptitude for disguise leaves no room for doubt, whatever explanation for the phenomenon may be advanced.

Mimicry and travesty are therefore complementary acts in this kind of play. For children, the aim is to imitate adults. This explains the success of the toy weapons and miniatures which copy the tools, engines, arms, and machines used by adults. The little girl plays her mother's role as cook, laundress, and ironer. The boy makes believe he is a soldier, musketeer, policeman, pirate, cowboy, Martian,[3] etc. An airplane is made by waving his arms and making the noise of a motor. However, acts of mimicry tend to cross the border between childhood and adulthood. They cover to the same degree any distraction, mask, or travesty, in which one participates, and which stresses the very fact that the play is masked or otherwise disguised, and such consequences as ensue. Lastly it is clear that theatrical presentations and dramatic interpretations rightly belong in this category.

The pleasure lies in being or passing for another. But in games the basic intention is not that of deceiving the spectators. The child who is playing train may well refuse to kiss his father while saying to him that one does not embrace locomotives, but he is not trying to persuade his father that he is a real locomotive. At a carnival, the masquerader does not try to make one believe that he is really a marquis, toreador, or Indian, but rather tries to inspire fear and take advantage of the surrounding license, a result of the fact that the mask disguises the conventional self and liberates the true personality. The actor does not try to make believe that he is "really" King Lear or Charles V. It is only the spy and the fugitive who disguise themselves to really deceive because they are not playing.

Activity, imagination, interpretation, and

[3] As has been aptly remarked, girls' playthings are designed to imitate practical, realistic, and domestic activities, while those of boys suggest distant, romantic, inaccessible, or even obviously unreal actions.

mimicry have hardly any relationship to *alea*, which requires immobility and the thrill of expectation from the player, but *agôn* is not excluded. I am not thinking of the masqueraders' competition, in which the relationship is obvious. A much more subtle complicity is revealed. For nonparticipants, every *agôn* is a spectacle. Only it is a spectacle which, to be valid, excludes simulation. Great sports events are nevertheless special occasions for *mimicry*, but it must be recalled that the simulation is now transferred from the participants to the audience. It is not the athletes who mimic, but the spectators. Identification with the champion in itself constitutes *mimicry* related to that of the reader with the hero of the novel and that of the moviegoer with the film star. To be convinced of this, it is merely necessary to consider the perfectly symmetrical functions of the champion and the stage or screen star. Champions, winners at *agôn*, are the stars of sports contests. Conversely, stars are winners in a more diffuse competition in which the stakes are popular favor. Both receive a large fan-mail, give interviews to an avid press, and sign autographs.

In fact, bicycle races, boxing or wrestling matches, football, tennis, or polo games are intrinsic spectacles, with costumes, solemn overture, appropriate liturgy, and regulated procedures. In a word, these are dramas whose vicissitudes keep the public breathless, and lead to denouements which exalt some and depress others. The nature of these spectacles remains that of an *agôn*, but their outward aspect is that of an exhibition. The audience are not content to encourage the efforts of the athletes or horses of their choice merely by voice and gesture. A physical contagion leads them to assume the position of the men or animals in order to help them, just as the bowler is known to unconsciously incline his body in the direction that he would like the bowling ball to take at the end of its course. Under these conditions, paralleling the spectacle, a competitive *mimicry* is born in the public, which doubles the true *agôn* of the field or track.

With one exception, *mimicry* exhibits all the characteristics of play: liberty, convention, suspension of reality, and delimitation of space and time. However, the continuous submission to imperative and precise rules cannot be observed—rules for the dissimulation of reality and the substitution of a second reality. *Mimicry* is incessant invention. The rule of the game is unique: it consists in the actor's fascinating the spectator, while avoiding an error that might lead the spectator to break the spell. The spectator must lend himself to the illusion without first challenging the décor, mask, or artifice which for a given time he is asked to believe in as more real than reality itself.

Ilinx. The last kind of game includes those which are based on the pursuit of vertigo and which consist of an attempt to momentarily destroy the stability of perception and inflict a kind of voluptuous panic upon an otherwise lucid mind. In all cases, it is a question of surrendering to a kind of spasm, seizure, or shock which destroys reality with sovereign brusqueness.

The disturbance that provokes vertigo is commonly sought for its own sake. I need only cite as examples the actions of whirling dervishes and the Mexican *voladores*. I choose these purposely, for the former, in technique employed, can be related to certain children's games, while the latter rather recall the elaborate maneuvers of high-wire acrobatics. They thus touch the two poles of games of vertigo. Dervishes seek ecstasy by whirling about with movements accelerating as the drumbeats become ever more precipitate. Panic and hypnosis are attained by the paroxysm of frenetic, contagious, and shared rotation.[4] In Mexico, the *voladores*—Huastec or Totonac—climb to the top of a mast sixty-five to one hundred feet high. They are disguised as eagles with false wings hanging from their wrists. The end of a rope is attached to their waists. The rope then passes between their toes in such a way that they can manage their entire descent with head down and arms outstretched. Before reaching the ground, they make many complete turns, thirty according to Torquemada, describing an ever-widening spiral in their downward flight. The ceremony, comprising several flights and beginning at noon, is readily interpreted as a dance of the setting sun, associated with birds, the deified dead. The frequency of accidents has led the Mexican authorities to ban this dangerous exercise.[5]

It is scarcely necessary to invoke these rare and fascinating examples. Every child very well knows that by whirling rapidly he reaches a

[4] D. Depont and X. Coppolani. *Les Confréries religieuses musulmanes* (Algiers, 1887), pp. 156-159, 329-339.

[5] Description and photographs in Helga Larsen. "Notes on the Volador and Its Associated Ceremonies and Superstitions," *Ethnos*, 2, No. 4 (July, 1937), 179-192, and in Guy Stresser-Péan. "Les origines du volador et du comelagatoazte," *Actes du XXVIII Congres International des Américanistes*, Paris, 1947, 327-334. . . .

centrifugal state of flight from which he regains bodily stability and clarity of perception only with difficulty. The child engages in this activity playfully and finds pleasure thereby. An example is the game of teetotum[6] in which the player pivots on one foot as quickly as he is able. Analogously, in the Haitian game of *maïs d'or* two children hold hands, face to face, their arms extended. With their bodies stiffened and bent backward, and with their feet joined, they turn until they are breathless, so that they will have the pleasure of staggering about after they stop. Comparable sensations are provided by screaming as loud as one can, racing downhill, and tobogganing; in horsemanship, provided that one turns quickly; and in swinging.

Various physical activities also provoke these sensations, such as the tightrope, falling or being projected into space, rapid rotation, sliding, speeding, and acceleration of vertilinear movement, separately or in combination with gyrating movement. In parallel fashion, there is a vertigo of a moral order, a transport that suddenly seizes the individual. This vertigo is readily linked to the desire for disorder and destruction, a drive which is normally repressed. It is reflected in crude and brutal forms of personality expression. In children, it is especially observed in the games of hot cockles, "winner-take-all," and leapfrog in which they rush and spin pell-mell. In adults, nothing is more revealing of vertigo than the strange excitement that is felt in cutting down the tall prairie flowers with a switch, or in creating an avalanche of the snow on a rooftop, or, better, the intoxication that is experienced in military barracks—for example, in noisily banging garbage cans.

To cover the many varieties of such transport, for a disorder that may take organic or psychological form, I propose using the term *ilinx*, the Greek term for whirlpool, from which is also derived the Greek word for vertigo (*ilingos*).

This pleasure is not unique to man. To begin with, it is appropriate to recall the gyrations of certain mammals, sheep in particular. Even if these are pathological manifestations, they are too significant to be passed over in silence. In addition, examples in which the play element is certain are not lacking. In order to catch their tails dogs will spin around until they fall down. At other times they are seized by a fever for running until they are exhausted. Antelopes, gazelles, and wild horses

are often panic-stricken when there is no real danger in the slightest degree to account for it; the impression is of an overbearing contagion to which they surrender in instant compliance.[7]

Water rats divert themselves by spinning as if they were being drawn by an eddy in a stream. The case of the chamois is even more remarkable. According to Karl Groos, they ascend the glaciers, and with a leap, each in turn slides down a steep slope, while the other chamois watch.

The gibbon chooses a flexible branch and weighs it down until it unbends, thus projecting him into the air. He lands catch as catch can, and he endlessly repeats this useless exercise, inexplicable except in terms of its seductive quality. Birds especially love games of vertigo. They let themselves fall like stones from a great height, then open their wings when they are only a few feet from the ground, thus giving the impression that they are going to be crushed. In the mating season they utilize this heroic flight in order to attract the female. The American nighthawk, described by Audubon, is a virtuoso at these impressive acrobatics.[8]

Following the teetotum, *maïs d'or*, sliding, horsemanship, and swinging of their childhood, men surrender to the intoxication of many kinds of dance, from the common but insidious giddiness of the waltz to the many mad, tremendous, and convulsive movements of other dances. They derive the same kind of pleasure from the intoxication stimulated by high speed on skis, motorcycles, or in driving sports cars. In order to give this kind of sensation the intensity and brutality capable of shocking adults, powerful machines have had to be invented. Thus it is not surprising that the Industrial Revolution had to take place before vertigo could really become a kind of game. It is now provided for the avid masses by thousands of stimulating contraptions installed at fairs and amusement parks.

These machines would obviously surpass their goals if it were only a question of assaulting the organs of the inner ear, upon which the sense of equilibrium is dependent. But it is the whole body which must submit to such treatment as anyone would fear undergoing, were it not that everybody else was seen struggling to do the same. In fact, it is worth watching people leaving these vertigo-inducing machines. The contraptions turn people pale and

---

[6] [*Toton* in the French text. M.B.]

[7] Groos, *op. cit.*, p. 208.

[8] *Ibid.*, p. 259.

dizzy to the point of nausea. They shriek with fright, gasp for breath, and have the terrifying impression of visceral fear and shrinking as if to escape a horrible attack. Moreover the majority of them, before even recovering, are already hastening to the ticket booth in order to buy the right to again experience the same pleasurable torture.

It is necessary to use the word "pleasure," because one hesitates to call such a transport a mere distraction, corresponding as it does more to a spasm than to an entertainment. In addition, it is important to note that the violence of the shock felt is such that the concessionaires try, in extreme cases, to lure the naive by offering free rides. They deceitfully announce that "this time only" the ride is free, when this is the usual practice. To compensate, the spectators are made to pay for the privilege of calmly observing from a high balcony the terrors of the cooperating or surprised victims, exposed to fearful forces or strange caprices.

It would be rash to draw very precise conclusions on the subject of this curious and cruel assignment of roles. This last is not characteristic of a kind of game, such as is found in boxing, wrestling, and in gladiatorial combat. Essential is the pursuit of this special disorder or sudden panic, which defines the term vertigo, and in the true characteristics of the games associated with it: viz. the freedom to accept or refuse the experience, strict and fixed limits, and separation from the rest of reality. What the experience adds to the spectacle does not diminish but reinforces its character as play.

The Nature of Sport: A Definitional Effort*

JOHN W. LOY, JR.

Sport is a highly ambiguous term having different meanings for various people. Its ambiguity is attested to by the range of topics treated in the sport sections of daily newspapers. Here one can find accounts of various sport competitions, advertisements for the latest sport fashions, advice on how to improve one's skills in certain games, and essays on the state of given organized sports, including such matters as recruitment, financial success, and scandal. The broad yet loose encompass of sport reflected in the mass media suggests that sport can and perhaps should be dealt with on different planes of discourse if a better understanding of its nature is to be acquired. As a step in this direction we shall discuss sport as a game occurrence, as an institutional game, as a social institution, and as a social situation or social system.

I. SPORT AS A GAME OCCURRENCE

Perhaps most often when we think of the meaning of sport, we think of sports. In our perspective sports are considered as a specialized type of game. That is, a sport as one of the many "sports" is viewed as an actual game occurrence or event. Thus in succeeding paragraphs we shall briefly outline what we consider to be the basic characteristics of games in general. In describing these characteristics we shall continually make reference to sports in particular as a special type of game. A game we define as any form of playful competition

* From *Quest*, X (May, 1968), 1-15.

whose outcome is determined by physical skill, strategy, or chance employed singly or in combination.[1]

IA. "Playful." By "playful competition" we mean that any given contest has one or more elements of play. We purposely have not considered game as a subclass of play,[2] for if we had done so, sport would logically become a subset of play and thus preclude the subsumption of professional forms of sport under our definition of the term. However, we wish to recognize that one or more aspects of play constitute basic components of games and that even the most highly organized forms of sport are not completely devoid of play characteristics.

The Dutch historian Johan Huizinga has made probably the most thorough effort to delineate the fundamental qualities of play. He defines play as follows:

Summing up the formal characteristics of play we might call it a free activity standing quite consciously outside "ordinary" life as being "not serious," but at the same time absorbing the player intensely and utterly. It is an activity connected with no material interest, and no profit can be gained by it. It proceeds within its own proper boundaries of time and space according to fixed rules and in an orderly manner. It promotes the formation of social groupings which tend to surround themselves with secrecy and to stress their differences from the common world by disguise or other means (Huizinga, 1955, p. 13).

Caillois has subjected Huizinga's definition to critical analysis (Caillois, 1961, pp. 3-10) and has redefined play as an activity which is free, separate, uncertain, unproductive, and governed by rules and make-believe (*Ibid.*, pp. 9-10). We shall briefly discuss these qualities ascribed to play by Huizinga and Caillois and suggest how they relate to games in general and to sports in particular.

IA1. "Free." By free is meant that play is a voluntary activity. That is, no one is ever strictly forced to play, playing is done in one's free time, and playing can be initiated and terminated at will. This characteristic of play is no doubt common to many games, including some forms of amateur sport. It is not, however, a distinguishing feature of all games, especially those classified as professional sport.

IA2. "Separate." By separate Huizinga and Caillois mean that play is spatially and temporally limited. This feature of play is certainly relevant to sports. For many, if not most, forms of sport are conducted in spatially circumscribed environments, examples being the bullring, football stadium, golf course, race track, and swimming pool. And with few exceptions every form of sport has rules which precisely determine the duration of a given contest.

IA3. "Uncertain." The course or end result of play cannot be determined beforehand. Similarly, a chief characteristic of all games is that they are marked by an uncertain outcome. Perhaps it is this factor more than any other which lends excitement and tension to any contest. Strikingly uneven competition is routine for the contestants and boring for the spectators; hence efforts to insure a semblance of equality between opposing sides are a notable feature of sport. These efforts typically focus on the matters of size, skill, and experience. Examples of attempts to establish equality based on size are the formation of athletic leagues and conferences composed of social organizations of similar size and the designation of weight classes for boxers and wrestlers. Illustrations of efforts to insure equality among contestants on the basis of skill and experience are the establishment of handicaps for bowlers and golfers, the designation of various levels of competition within a given organization as evidenced by freshman, junior varsity, and varsity teams in scholastic athletics, and the drafting of players from established teams when adding a new team to a league as done in professional football and basketball.

IA4. "Unproductive." Playing does not in itself result in the creation of new material goods. It is true that in certain games such as poker there may occur an exchange of money or property among players. And it is a truism that in professional sports victory may result in substantial increases of wealth for given individuals. But the case can be made, nevertheless, that a game *per se* is non-utilitarian.[3] For what is produced during any sport competition is a game, and the production of the game is generally carried out in a prescribed setting and conducted according to specific rules.

IA5. "Governed by rules." All types of games have agreed-upon rules, be they formal or informal. It is suggested that sports can be distinguished from games in general by the fact that they usually have a greater variety of norms and a larger absolute number of formal norms (i.e., written prescribed and proscribed norms).[4] Similarly, there is a larger number of sanctions and more stringent ones in sports than in games. For example, a basketball player must leave the game after he has committed a fixed number of fouls; a hockey player must spend a certain amount of time in the penalty box after committing a foul; and a football player may be asked to leave the game if he shows unsportsmanlike conduct.

With respect to the normative order of games and sports, one explicit feature is that they usually have definite criteria for determining the winner. Although it is true that some end in a tie, most contests do not permit such an ambivalent termination by providing a means of breaking a deadlock and ascertaining the "final" victor. The various means of determining the winner in sportive endeavors are too numerous to enumerate. But it is relevant to observe that in many sport competitions where "stakes are high," a series of contests is held between opponents in an effort to rule out the element of chance and decide the winner on the basis of merit. A team may be called "lucky" if it beats an opponent once by a narrow margin; but if it does so repeatedly, then the appellations of "better" or "superior" are generally applied.

IA6. "Make-believe." By the term make-believe Huizinga and Caillois wish to signify that play stands outside "ordinary" or "real" life and is distinguished by an "only pretending quality." While some would deny this characteristic of play as being applicable to sport, it is interesting to note that Veblen at the turn of the century stated:

> Sports share this characteristic of make-believe with the games and exploits to which children, especially boys, are habitually inclined. Make-believe does not enter in the same proportion into all sports, but it is present in a very appreciable degree in all (Veblen. 1934, p. 256).

Huizinga observes that the "'only pretending' quality of play betrays a consciousness of the inferiority of play compared with 'seriousness'" (Huizinga, 1955, p. 8). We note here that occasionally one reads of a retiring professional athlete who remarks that he is "giving up the game to take a real job"[5] and that several writers have commented on the essential shallowness of sport.[6] Roger Kahn, for example, has written that:

The most fascinating and least reported aspect of American sports is the silent and enduring search for a rationale. Stacked against the atomic bomb or even against a patrol in Algeria, the most exciting rally in history may not seem very important, and for the serious and semi-serious people who make their living through sports, triviality is a nagging, damnable thing. Their drive for self-justification has contributed much to the development of sports (Kahn, 1957, p. 10).

On the other hand, Huizinga is careful to point out that "the consciousness of play being 'only pretend' does not by any means prevent it from proceeding with the utmost seriousness" (Huizinga, 1955, p. 8). As examples, need we mention the seriousness with which duffers treat their game of golf, the seriousness which fans accord discussions of their home team, or the seriousness that national governments give to Olympic Games and university alumni to collegiate football?[7,8]

Accepting the fact that the make-believe quality of play has some relevance for sport, it nevertheless remains difficult to empirically ground the "not-ordinary-or-real-life" characteristic of play. However, the "outside-of-real-life" dimension of a game is perhaps best seen in its "as-if" quality, its artificial obstacles, and its potential resources for actualization or production.

IA6(a). In a game the contestants act as if all were equal, and numerous aspects of "external reality" such as race, education, occupation, and financial status are excluded as relevant attributes for the duration of a given contest.[9]

IA6(b). The obstacles individuals encounter in their workaday lives are not usually predetermined by them and are "real" in the sense that they must be adequately coped with if certain inherent and socially conditioned needs are to be met; on the other hand, in games obstacles are artificially created to be overcome. Although these predetermined obstacles set up to be conquered can sometimes attain "life-and-death" significance, as in a difficult Alpine climb, they are not usually essentially related to an individual's daily toil for existence.[10]

IA6(c). Similarly, it is observed that in many "real" life situations the structures and processes needed to cope with a given obstacle are often not at hand; however, in a play or game situation all the structures and processes necessary to deal with any deliberately created obstacle and to realize any possible alternative in course of action are potentially available.[11]

In sum, then, games are playful in that they typically have one or more elements of play: freedom, separateness, uncertainty, unproductiveness, order, and make-believe. In addition to having elements of play, games have components of competition.

IB. "Competition." Competition is defined as a struggle for supremacy between two or more opposing sides. We interpret the phrase "between two or more opposing sides" rather broadly to encompass the competitive relationships between man and other objects of nature, both animate and inanimate. Thus competitive relationships include:

1. competition between one individual and another, e.g., a boxing match or a 100-yard dash;
2. competition between one team and another, e.g., a hockey game or a yacht race;
3. competition between an individual or a team and an animate object of nature, e.g., a bullfight or a deer-hunting party;
4. competition between an individual or a team and an inanimate object of nature, e.g., a canoeist running a set of rapids or a mountain climbing expedition; and finally,
5. competition between an individual or team and an "ideal" standard, e.g., an individual attempting to establish a world land-speed record on the Bonneville salt flats or a basketball team trying to set an all-time scoring record. Competition against an "ideal" standard might also be conceptualized as man against time or space, or as man against himself.[12]

The preceding classification has been set forth to illustrate what we understand by the phrase "two or more opposing sides" and is not intended to be a classification of competition *per se*. While the scheme may have some relevance for such a purpose, its value is limited by the fact that its categories are neither mutually exclusive nor inclusive. For instance, an athlete competing in a cross-country race may be competitively involved in all of the following ways: as an individual against another individual; as a team member against members of an opposing team; and as an individual or team member against an "ideal" standard (e.g., an attempt to set an individual and/or team record for the course).[13]

IC. "Physical skill, strategy, and chance." Roberts and Sutton-Smith suggest that the various games of the world can be classified

. . . on the basis of outcome attributes: (1) games of *physical skill*, in which the outcome is determined by the players' motor activities; (2) games of *strategy*, in which the outcome is determined by rational choices among possible courses of action; and (3) games of *chance*, in which the outcome is determined by guesses or by some uncontrolled artifact such as a die or wheel (Roberts and Sutton-Smith, 1962, p. 166).

Examples of relatively pure forms of competitive activities in each of these categories are weight-lifting contests, chess matches, and crap games, respectively. Many, if not most, games are, however, of a mixed nature. Card and board games, for instance, generally illustrate a combination of strategy and chance. Although chance is also associated with sport, its role in determining the outcome of a contest is generally held to a minimum in order that the winning side can attribute its victory to merit rather than to a fluke of nature. Rather interestingly it appears that a major role of chance in sport is to insure equality. For example, the official's flip of a coin before the start of a football game randomly determines what team will receive the kickoff and from what respective side of the field; and similarly the drawing of numbers by competitors in track and swimming is an attempt to assure them equal opportunity of getting assigned a given lane.

ID. "Physical prowess." Having discussed the characteristics which sports share in common with games in general, let us turn to an account of the major attribute which distinguishes sports in particular from games in general. We observe that sports can be distinguished from games by the fact that they demand the demonstration of physical prowess. By the phrase "the demonstration of physical prowess" we mean the employment of developed physical skills and abilities within the context of gross physical activity to conquer an opposing object of nature. Although many games require a minimum of physical skill, they do not usually demand the degree of physical skill required by sports. The idea of "developed physical skills" implies much practice and learning and suggests the attainment

of a high level of proficiency in one or more general physical abilities relevant to sport competition, e.g., strength, speed, endurance, or accuracy.

Although the concept of physical prowess permits sports to be generally differentiated from games, numerous borderline areas exist. For example, can a dart game among friends, a horseshoe pitching contest between husband and wife, or a fishing contest between father and son be considered sport? One way to arrive at an answer to these questions is to define a sport as any highly organized game requiring physical prowess. Thus a dart game with friends, a horseshoe pitching contest between spouses, or a fishing contest between a father and son would not be considered sport; but formally sponsored dart, horseshoe, or fishing tournaments would be legitimately labelled sport. An alternative approach to answering the aforementioned questions, however, is to define a sport as an institutionalized game demanding the demonstration of physical prowess. If one accepts the latter approach, then he will arrive at a different set of answers to the above questions. For this approach views a game as a unique event and sport as an institutional pattern. As Weiss has rather nicely put it:

A game is an occurence; a sport is a pattern. The one is in the present, the other primarily past, but instantiated in the present. A sport defines the conditions to which the participants must submit if there is to be a game; a game gives rootage to a set of rules and thereby enables a sport to be exhibited (1967, p. 82).

II. SPORT AS AN INSTITUTIONALIZED GAME

To treat sport as an institutionalized game is to consider sport as an abstract entity. For example, the organization of a football team as described in a rule book can be discussed without reference to the members of any particular team; and the relationships among team members can be characterized without reference to unique personalities or to particular times and places. In treating sport as an institutionalized game we conceive of it as distinctive, enduring patterns of culture and social structure combined into a single complex, the elements of which include values, norms, sanctions, knowledge, and social positions (i.e., roles and statuses).[14] A firm grasp of the meaning of "institutionalization" is necessary for understanding the idea of sport as an institutional pattern, or blueprint if you will, guiding the organization and conduct of given games and sportive endeavors.

The formulation of a set of rules for a game or even their enactment on a particular occasion does not constitute a sport as we have conceptualized it here. The institutionalization of a game implies that it has a tradition of past exemplifications and definite guidelines for future realizations. Moreover, in a concrete game situation the form of a particular sport need not reflect all the characteristics represented in its institutional pattern. The more organized a sport contest in a concrete setting, however, the more likely it will illustrate the institutionalized nature of a given sport. A professional baseball game, for example, is a better illustration of the institutionalized nature of baseball than is a sandlot baseball game; but both games are based on the same institutional pattern and thus may both be considered forms of sport. In brief, a sport may be treated analytically in terms of its degree of institutionalization and dealt with empirically in terms of its degree of organization. The latter is an empirical instance of the former.

In order to illustrate the institutionalized nature of sport more adequately, we contrast the organizational, technological, symbolic, and educational spheres of sports with those of games. In doing so we consider both games and sports in their most formalized and organized state. We are aware that there are institutionalized games other than sports which possess characteristics similar to the ones we ascribe to sports, as for example chess and bridge; but we contend that such games are in the minority and in any case are excluded as sports because they do not demand the demonstration of physical prowess.

IIA. "Organizational sphere." For present purposes we rather arbitrarily discuss the organizational aspects of sports in terms of teams, sponsorship, and government.

IIA1. "Teams." Competing sides for most games are usually selected rather spontaneously and typically disband following a given contest. In sports, however, competing groups are generally selected with care and, once membership is established, maintain a stable social organization. Although individual persons may withdraw from such organizations after they are developed, their social positions are taken up by others, and the group endures.[15]

Another differentiating feature is that as a rule sports show a greater degree of role differentiation than games do. Although games often involve several contestants (e.g., poker), the contestants often perform identical activities and thus may be considered to have the same roles and statuses. By contrast, in sports involving a similar number of participants (e.g., basketball), each individual or combination of just a few individuals performs specialized activities within the group and may be said to possess a distinct role. Moreover, to the extent that such specialized and differentiated activities can be ranked in terms of some criteria, they also possess different statuses.

IIA2. "Sponsorship." In addition to there being permanent social groups established for purposes of sport competition, there is usually found in the sport realm social groups which act as sponsoring bodies for sport teams. These sponsoring bodies may be characterized as being direct or indirect. Direct sponsoring groups include municipalities which sponsor Little League baseball teams, universities which support collegiate teams, and business corporations which sponsor AAU teams. Indirect sponsoring groups include sporting goods manufacturers, booster clubs, and sport magazines.

IIA3. "Government." While all types of games have at least a modicum of norms and sanctions associated with them, the various forms of sport are set apart from many games by the fact that they have more—and more formal and more institutionalized—sets of these cultural elements. In games rules are often passed down by oral tradition or spontaneously established for a given contest and forgotten afterwards; or, even where codified, they are often simple and few. In sports rules are usually many, and they are formally codified and typically enforced by a regulatory body. There are international organizations governing most sports, and in America there are relatively large social organizations governing both amateur and professional sports. For example, amateur sports in America are controlled by such groups as the NCAA, AAU, and NAIA; and the major professional sports have national commissioners with enforcing officials to police competition.

IIB. "Technological sphere." In a sport, technology denotes the material equipment, physical skills, and body of knowledge which are necessary for the conduct of competition and potentially available for technical improvements in competition. While all types of games require a minimum of knowledge and often a minimum of physical skill and material equipment, the various sports are set apart from many games by the fact that they typically require greater knowledge and involve higher levels of physical skill and necessitate more material equipment. The technological aspects of a sport may be dichotomized into those which are intrinsic and those which are extrinsic. Intrinsic technological aspects of a sport consist of the physical skills, knowledge, and equipment which are required for the conduct of a given contest *per se*. For example, the intrinsic technology of football includes: (a) the equipment necessary for the game—field, ball, uniform, etc.; (b) the repertoire of physical skills necessary for the game—running, passing, kicking, blocking, tackling, etc.; and (c) the knowledge necessary for the game—rules, strategy, etc. Examples of extrinsic technological elements associated with football include: (a) physical equipment such as stadium, press facilities, dressing rooms, etc.; (b) physical skills such as possessed by coaches, cheer leaders, and ground crews; and (c) knowledge such as possessed by coaches, team physicians, and spectators.

IIC. "Symbolic sphere." The symbolic dimension of a sport includes elements of secrecy, display, and ritual. Huizinga contends that play "promotes the formation of social groupings which tend to surround themselves with secrecy and to stress their difference from the common world by disguise or other means" (1955, p. 13). Caillois criticizes his contention and states to the contrary that "play tends to remove the very nature of the mysterious." He further observes that "when the secret, the mask or the costume fulfills a sacramental function one can be sure that not play, but an institution is involved" (1961, p. 4).

Somewhat ambivalently we agree with both writers. On the one hand, to the extent that Huizinga means by "secrecy" the act of making distinctions between "play life" and "ordinary life," we accept his proposition that groups engaged in playful competition surround themselves with secrecy. On the other hand, to the extent that he means by "secrecy" something hidden from others, we accept Caillois's edict that an institution and not play is involved.

IIC1. The latter type of secrecy might well be called "sanctioned secrecy" in sports, for there is associated with many forms of sport competition rather clear norms regarding approved clandestine behavior. For example, football teams are permitted to set up enclosed practice fields, send out scouts to spy on opposing teams, and exchange a limited number of game films revealing the strategies of future opponents. Other kinds of clandestine action such as slush funds established for coaches and gambling on games by players are not always looked upon with such favor.[16]

IIC2. A thorough reading of Huizinga leads one to conclude that what he means by secrecy is best discussed in terms of display and ritual. He points out, for example, that "the 'differentness' and secrecy of play are most vividly expressed in 'dressing up'" and states that the higher forms of play are "a contest *for* something or a representation *of* something"—adding that "representation means display" (1955, p. 13). The "dressing-up" element of play noted by Huizinga is certainly characteristic of most sports. Perhaps it is carried to its greatest height in bullfighting, but it is not absent in some of the less overt forms of sport. Veblen writes:

> It is noticeable, for instance, that even very mild-mannered and matter-of-fact men who go out shooting are apt to carry an excess of arms and accoutrements in order to impress upon their own imagination the seriousness of their undertaking. These huntsmen are also prone to a histrionic, prancing gait and to an elaborate exaggeration of the motions, whether of stealth or of onslaught, involved in their deeds of exploit (1934, p. 256).

A more recent account of "dressing-up" and display in sports has been given by Stone (1955), who treats display as spectacle and as a counterforce to play. Stone asserts that the tension between the forces of play and display constitute an essential component of sport. The following quotation gives the essence of his account:

> Play and dis-play are precariously balanced in sport, and, once that balance is upset, the whole character of sport in society may be affected. Furthermore, the spectacular element of sport, may, as in the case of American professional wrestling, destroy the game. The rules cease to apply, and the "cheat" and the "spoilsport" replace the players.
>
> The point may be made in another way. The spectacle is predictable and certain; the game, unpredictable and uncertain. Thus spectacular display may be reckoned from the outset of the performance. It is announced by the appearance of the performers—their physiques, costumes, and gestures. On the other hand, the spectacular play is solely a function of the uncertainty of the game (p. 98).

In a somewhat different manner another sociologist, Erving Goffman, has analyzed the factors of the uncertainty of a game and display. Concerning the basis of "fun in games" he states that "mere uncertainty of outcome is not enough to engross the players" (1961, p. 68) and suggests that a successful game must combine "sanctioned display" with problematic outcome. By display Goffman means that "games give the players an opportunity to exhibit attributes valued in the wider social world, such as dexterity, strength, knowledge, intelligence, courage, and self-control" (*Ibid.*). Thus for Goffman display represents spectacular play involving externally relevant attributes, while for Stone display signifies spectacular exhibition involving externally non-relevant attributes with respect to the game situation.

IIC3. Another concept related to display and spectacle and relevant to sports is that of ritual. According to Leach, "ritual denotes those aspects of prescribed formal behavior which have no direct technological consequences" (1964, p. 607). Ritual may be distinguished from spectacle by the fact that it generally has a greater element of drama and is less ostentatious and more serious. "Ritual actions are 'symbolic' in that they assert something about the state of affairs, but they are not necessarily purposive: i.e., the performer of ritual does not necessarily seek to alter the state of affairs" (*Ibid.*). Empirically ritual can be distinguished from spectacle by the fact that those engaged in ritual express an attitude of solemnity toward it, an attitude which they do not direct toward spectacle.

Examples of rituals in sport are the shaking of hands between team captains before a game, the shaking of hands between coaches after a game, the singing of the national anthem before a game, and the singing of the school song at the conclusion of a game.[17]

IID. "Educational sphere." The educational sphere focuses on those activities related to the transmission of skills and knowledge to those who lack them. Many if not most people learn to play the majority of socially preferred games in an informal manner. That is, they acquire the required skills and knowledge associated with a given game through the casual instruction of friends or associates. On the other hand, in sports, skills and knowledge are often obtained by means of formal instruction. In short, the educational sphere of sports is institutionalized, whereas in most games it is not. One reason for this situation is the fact that sports require highly developed physical skills as games often do not; to achieve proficiency requires long hours of practice and qualified instruction, i.e., systematized training. Finally, it should be pointed out that associated with the instructional personnel of sport programs are a number of auxiliary personnel

such as managers, physicians, and trainers—a situation not commonly found in games.

III. SPORT AS A SOCIAL INSTITUTION

Extending our notion of sport as an institutional pattern still further, we note that in its broadest sense, the term sport supposes a social institution. Schneider writes that the term institution

. . . denotes an aspect of social life in which distinctive value-orientations and interests, centering upon large and important social concern . . . generate or are accompanied by distinctive modes of social interaction. Its use emphasizes "important" social phenomena; relationships of "strategic structural significance" (1964, p. 338).

We argue that the magnitude of sport in the Western world justifies its consideration as a social institution. As Boyle succinctly states:

Sport permeates any number of levels of contemporary society, and it touches upon and deeply influences such disparate elements as status, race relations, business life, automotive design, clothing styles, the concept of the hero, language, and ethical values. For better or worse it gives form and substance to much in American life (1963, pp. 3-4).

When speaking of sport as a social institution, we refer to the sport order. The sport order is composed of all organizations in society which organize, facilitate, and regulate human action in sport situations. Hence, such organizations as sporting goods manufacturers, sport clubs, athletic teams, national governing bodies for amateur and professional sports, publishers of sport magazines, etc., are part of the sport order. For analytical purposes four levels of social organization within the sport order may be distinguished: namely, the primary, technical, managerial, and corporate levels.[18] Organizations at the primary level permit face-to-face relationships among all members and are characterized by the fact that administrative leadership is not formally delegated to one or more persons or positions. An example of a social organization associated with sport at the primary level is an informally organized team in a sandlot baseball game.

Organizations at the technical level are too large to permit simultaneous face-to-face relationships among their members but small enough so that every member knows of every other member. Moreover, unlike organizations at the primary level, organizations at the technical level officially designate administrative leadership positions and allocate individuals to them. Most scholastic and collegiate athletic teams, for example, would be classified as technical organizations with coaches and athletic directors functioning as administrative leaders.

At the managerial level organizations are too large for every member to know every other member but small enough so that all members know one or more of the administrative leaders of the organization. Some of the large professional ball clubs represent social organizations related to sport at the managerial level.

Organizations at the corporate level are characterized by bureaucracy: they have centralized authority, a hierarchy of personnel, and protocol and procedural emphases; and they stress the rationalization of operations and impersonal relationships. A number of the major governing bodies of amateur and professional sport at the national and international levels illustrate sport organizations of the corporate type.

In summary, the sport order is composed of the congeries of primary, technical, managerial, and corporate social organizations which arrange, facilitate, and regulate human action in sport situations. The value of the concept lies in its use in macro-analyses of the social significance of sport. We can make reference to the sport order in a historical and/or comparative perspective. For example, we can speak of the sport order of nineteenth-century America or contrast the sport order of Russia with that of England.

IV. SPORT AS A SOCIAL SITUATION

As was just noted, the sport order is composed of all social organizations which organize, facilitate, and regulate human action in sport situations. Human "action consists of the structures and processes by which human beings form meaningful intentions and, more or less successfully, implement them in concrete situations" (Parsons, 1966, p. 5). A sport situation consists of any social context wherein individuals are involved with sport. And the term situation denotes "the total set of objects, whether persons, collectivities, culture objects, or himself to which an actor responds" (Friedsam, 1964, p. 667). The set of objects related to a specific sport situation may be quite diverse, ranging from the elements of the social and physical environments of a football game to those associated with two sportniks[19] in a neighborhood bar arguing the pros and cons of the manager of their local baseball team.

Although there are many kinds of sport situations, most if not all may be conceptualized as social systems. A social system may be simply defined as "a set of persons with an identifying characteristic plus a set of relationships established among these persons by interaction" (Caplow, 1964, p. 1). Thus the situation represented by two teams contesting within the confines of a football field, the situation presented by father and son fishing from a boat, and the situation created by a golf pro giving a lesson to a novice each constitutes a social system.

Social systems of prime concern to the sport sociologist are those which directly or indirectly relate to a game occurrence. That is to say, a sport sociologist is often concerned with why man gets involved in sport and what effect his involvement has on other aspects of his social environment. Involvement in a social system related to a game occurrence can be analyzed in terms of degree and kind of involvement.

Degree of involvement can be assessed in terms of frequency, duration, and intensity of involvement. The combination of frequency and duration of involvement may be taken as an index of an individual's "investment" in a sport situation, while intensity of involvement may be considered an index of an individual's "personal commitment" to a given sport situation.[20]

Kind of involvement can be assessed in terms of an individual's relationship to the "means of production" of a game. Those having direct or indirect access to the means of production are considered "actually involved" and are categorized as "producers." Those lacking access to the means of production are considered "vicariously involved" and are categorized as "consumers." We have tentatively identified three categories of producers and three classes of consumers.

Producers may be characterized as being primary, secondary, or tertiary with respect to the production of a game. (1) "Primary producers" are the contestants who play the primary roles in the production of a game, not unlike the roles of actors in the production of a play. (2) "Secondary producers" consist of those individuals, who while not actually competing in a sport contest, perform tasks which have direct technological consequences for the outcome of a game. Secondary producers include club owners, coaches, officials, trainers, and the like. It may be possible to categorize secondary producers as entrepreneurs, managers, and technicians. (3) "Tertiary producers" consist of those who are actively involved in a sport situation but whose activities have no direct technological consequences for the outcome of a game. Examples of tertiary producers are cheerleaders, band members and concession workers. Tertiary producers may be classified as service personnel.

Consumers, like producers, are designated as being primary, secondary, or tertiary. (1) "Primary consumers" are those individuals who become vicariously involved in a sport through "live" attendance at a sport competition. Primary consumers may be thought of as "active spectators." (2) "Secondary consumers" consist of those who vicariously involve themselves in a sport as spectators via some form of the mass media, such as radio or television. Secondary consumers may be thought of as "passive spectators." (3) "Tertiary consumers" are those who become vicariously involved with sport other than as spectators. Thus an individual who engages in conversation related to sport or a person who reads the sport section of the newspaper would be classified as a tertiary consumer.

In concluding our discussion of the nature of sport we note that a special type of consumer is the *fan.* A fan is defined as an individual who has both a high personal investment in and a high personal commitment to a given sport.

NOTES

1. This definition is based largely on the work of Caillois (1961) and Roberts and others (1959). Other definitions and classifications of games having social import are given in Berne (1964) and Piaget (1951).
2. As have done Huizinga (1955), Stone (1955), and Caillois (1961).
3. Cf. Goffman's discussion of "rules of irrelevance" as applied to games and social encounters in general (1961, pp. 19-26).
4. E.g., compare the rules given for games in any edition of Hoyle's *Book of Games* with the NCAA rule book for various collegiate sports.
5. There is, of course, the amateur who gives up the "game" to become a professional.
6. For an early discussion of the problem of legitimation in sport, see Veblen, 1934, pp. 268-270.
7. An excellent philosophical account of play and seriousness is given by Kurt Riezler (1941, pp. 505-517).
8. A sociological treatment of how an individual engaged in an activity can become "caught up" in it is given by Goffman in his analysis of the concept of "spontaneous involvement" (1961, pp. 37-45).

9. For a discussion of how certain aspects of "reality" are excluded from a game situation, see Goffman's treatment of "rules of irrelevance." Contrariwise see his treatment of "rules of transformation" for a discussion of how certain aspects of "reality" are permitted to enter a game situation (1961, pp. 29-34).
10. Professional sports provide an exception, of course, especially such a sport as professional bullfighting.
11. Our use of the term "structures and processes" at this point is similar to Goffman's concept of "realized resources" (1961, pp. 16-19).
12. Other possible categories of competition are, of course, animals against animals as seen in horse racing or animals against an artificial animal as seen in dog racing. As noted by Weiss: "When animals or machines race, the speed offers indirect testimony to men's excellence as trainers, coaches, riders, drivers and the like—and thus primarily to an excellence in human leadership, judgment, strategy, and tactics" (1967, p. 22).
13. The interested reader can find examples of sport classifications in Hesseltine (1964), McIntosh (1963), and Sapora and Mitchell (1961).
14. This definition is patterned after one given by Smelser (1963, p. 28).
15. Huizinga states that the existence of permanent teams is, in fact, the starting-point of modern sport (1955, p. 196).
16. Our discussion of "sanctioned secrecy" closely parallels Johnson's discussion of "official secrecy" in bureaucracies (1960, pp. 295-296).
17. For an early sociological treatment of sport, spectacle, exhibition, and drama, see Sumner (1960, pp. 467-501). We note in passing that some writers consider the totality of sport as a ritual; see especially Fromm (1955, p. 132) and Beisser (1967, pp. 148-151 and pp. 214-225).
18. Our discussion of these four levels is similar to Caplow's treatment of small, medium, large, and giant organizations (Caplow, 1964, pp. 26-27).
19. The term sportnik refers to an avid fan or sport addict.
20. Cf. McCall and Simmons (1966, pp. 171-172).

REFERENCES

Berne, Eric. *Games People Play,* New York: Grove Press, 1964.
Beisser, Arnold R. *The Madness in Sports.* New York: Appleton-Century-Crofts, 1967.
Boyle, Robert H. *Sport—Mirror of American Life.* Boston: Little, Brown, 1963.
Caillois, Roger. *Man Play and Games,* tr. Meyer Barash. New York: Free Press, 1964.
Caplow, Theodore. *Principles of Organization.* New York: Harcourt, Brace and World, 1964.

Fromm, Erich. *The Sane Society*. New York: Fawcett, 1955.

Goffmann, Erving. *Encounters*. Indianapolis: Bobbs-Merrills, 1961.

Hesseltine, William B. "Sports," *Collier's Encyclopedia*, 1964.

Huizinga, Johan. *Homo Ludens—A Study of the Play-Element in Culture*. Boston: Beacon Press, 1955.

Johnson, Harry M. *Sociology: A Systematic Introduction*. New York: Harcourt, Brace, 1960.

Kahn, Roger. "Money, Muscles—and Myths," *Nation*, CLXXXV (July 6, 1957), 9-11.

Leach, E. R. "Ritual," in *A Dictionary of the Social Sciences*, ed. Julius Gould and William L. Kolb. New York: Free Press, 1964.

Lüschen, Gunther. "The Interdependence of Sport and Culture." Paper presented at the National Convention of the American Association for Health, Physical Education and Recreation, Las Vegas, 1967.

McCall, George J., and J. L. Simmons. *Identities and Interactions*. New York: Free Press, 1966.

McIntosh, Peter C. *Sport in Society*. London: C. A. Watts, 1963.

Piaget, Jean. *Play, Dreams and Imitation in Childhood*, tr. C. Gattegno and F. M. Hodgson. New York: W. W. Norton, 1951.

Riezler, Kurt. "Play and Seriousness," *The Journal of Philosophy*, XXXVIII (1941), 505-517.

Roberts, John M., and others. "Games in Culture," *American Anthropologist*, LXI (1959), 597-605.

————, and Brian Sutton-Smith. "Child Training and Game Involvement," *Ethnology*, 1 (1962), 166-185.

Sapora, Allen V., and Elmer D. Mitchell. *The Theory of Play and Recreation*. New York: Ronald Press, 1961.

Schneider, Louis. "Institution," in *A Dictionary of the Social Sciences*, ed. Julius Gould and William L. Kolb. New York: Free Press, 1964.

Smelser, Neil J. *The Sociology of Economic Life*. Englewood Cliffs, N. J.: Prentice-Hall, 1963.

Stone, Gregory P. "American Sports: Play and Display," *Chicago Review*, IX (Fall 1955), 83-100.

Sumner, William Graham. *Folkways*. New York: Mentor, 1960.

Torkildsen, George E. "Sport and Culture." M.S. thesis, University of Wisconsin, 1957.

Veblen, Thorsten. *The Theory of the Leisure Class*. New York: Modern Library, 1934.

Weiss, Paul. "Sport: A Philosophic Study." Unpublished manuscript, 1967.

Toward a Non-Definition of Sport*

FRANK McBRIDE

What I propose to do here is assemble some reminders for a particular purpose.[1] The reminders concern the nature and limitations of definition in general and definition of 'sport' in particular. The purpose is to discourage attempts at defining the concept of sport. I shall discuss the following claims:

A. Neither the intension nor the extension of the concept sport is concise.
B. Attempts to limit concisely the intension of the concept sport will either fail or end up as stipulative.
C. The concept sport is ordinarily employed in a wide variety of ways, i.e. has a wide variety of usages, or meanings.
D. Philosophers of sport ought not waste their time attempting to define 'sport.'

You will note that the first three of these claims are descriptive while the fourth is normative. I take the descriptive claim statements to be true, although I don't expect to establish this in each case in an incontrovertible manner. And further, if claim statements A, B, and C, taken together, are true, I take this to be strong support for the normative claim, claim D.

One final note before considering the claims. Most of what I have to say here concerns lexical or conventional definition, i.e. reports of how words are and have been employed. This can be contrasted with the stipulative or contrived definition. I have no quarrel with those who *openly* define in the latter manner, for

*From *The Journal of the Philosophy of Sport*, II (Sept., 1975), 4–11.

example, the scientist in a description of research or the logician in the interpretation of a system of propositional calculus. By all means let 'logical connection' mean what the behaviorist wants it to mean and let 'x' stand for anything at all or nothing. What I do quarrel with is for the stipulative definition to be masqueraded as conventional. It may satisfy someone's compulsion for precision or order but is at best misleading and at worst deceitful.

Claim A: Neither the Intension nor the Extension of the Concept Sport is Concise

Let me stipulate what I mean by "intension" and "extension." The *intension* of a word consists of the property or properties a thing must possess to belong to the class of things designated by that word (more simply, the criteria for inclusion in the set). The *extension* of a word consists of the class of things to which that word refers (more simply, the members of the set). (7:pp. 90–91) The intension of 'triangle' for example, consists of the properties of a) having three sides, and b) having three interior angles equal to 180 degrees. The extension of 'triangle' consists of the class of all geometric figures possessing these properties. I do not wish to defend the integrity of this distinction. I merely find it useful.

In the above cited example we also find a classic example of a concept whose boundaries are concisely drawn and whose membership is clearly limited. There are, for example (if we are willing to remain for a few more minutes in a pre-Einsteinian world), no borderline cases. Every conceivable geometric figure either is or is not a triangle, and we have accepted ways of determining which individuals are members of the set and which are not. That is to say, both the intension and the extension of the concept triangle are concise.

A concept may be thought of as vague when either the intension or the extension cannot be concisely limited. The four possibilities for a concept being vague and/or concise are as follows:

1. The extension is concisely limited but the intension is vague, e.g. 'human.' (7:p. 94)
2. The intension is clearly limited but the extension is vague, e.g. 'identical.' (Examples are hard to come by here. Certain ethical expressions might qualify, e.g. 'justice.')
3. Both the extension and intension are concisely limited, e.g. 'triangle.'
4. Neither the extension nor the intension are concisely limited, e.g. 'games.'[2]

The claim with respect to 'sport' is thus the stronger possibility, that both the intension and the extension of the concept are vague. For the moment I shall content myself with presenting examples of two ways in which this vagueness occurs. Later on consideration of claim B will center around the difficulties of specifying the intension of 'sport.' The factual data mentioned in the consideration of claim C will direct further attention to the extensional vagueness difficulties.

Fishing, fencing, skiing, wrestling, track and field, swimming, auto racing, scuba diving, rock climbing, and thoroughbred racing are sports. They are not games. Badminton, football, curling, baseball, golf, tennis, field hockey, bowling, and basketball are sports and they are, also, games. An anthropologist or an ordinary language analyst would not find this to be particularly interesting, let alone perplexing. This just happens to be the way it is, and that is that. For the neo-Aristotelian, the essentialist, however, a problem is set. The question that must be answered is of course *why*? Why are some sports games and some sports not games? The question would eventuate in a search for the common and peculiar features that define the concept sport, or games, or both. But this leads us into consideration of claim B. What I want to do here, painful as it may be is *stop*, to resist the compulsion to pursue the *why* question; to recognize that the why question is vain. As we have seen, the instances of the extension of 'sport' are varied in

at least two fundamental ways, some are games and some are not games.

The second example speaks more to the intensional vagueness claim. Most of us are familiar with the expression, "I do not consider that a sport." I would, for example, be ready at any moment to say this, and with sincerity, regarding dog fighting, cock fighting, bull fighting, and a number of forms of hunting and fishing. There are times when I would want to say it with respect to boxing, football, and field hockey. Once again the why question would seem legitimate *and in this case it is*. Someone who takes one of these to be the sport of sports might, for example, legitimately request a reason *and get one in response*. My response, or anyone's would most likely be something like: "The elements of cruelty or sadism go beyond the limits of sport." More precisely what is being said is that the elements of cruelty or sadism go beyond the limits of sport *as I or someone else conceives of them*. The point I wish to make is this: in at least a limited number of cases *the boundaries of sport are both logical and psychological*. What is sport for one may not be for another. What is sport for some may not be for others. I would contend that this discrepancy extends into the culture itself, into the language, into the employment of the expression "sport." We might be able to achieve unanimity with respect to certain clearcut examples of what is and what is not sport. I would doubt, however, that the borderline between would be empty.

Claim B: Attempts to Limit Concisely the Intension of the Concept Sport Will Either Fail or End Up as Stipulative

The kind of failure I have in mind here is being too narrow or too broad. A definition is too narrow if it excludes instances that would ordinarily (conventionally) be included. A definition is too broad if it includes instances that would ordinarily (conventionally) not be included. To illustrate I take the example of 'games.' If we restrict the definition to 'activities played with a ball' we have excluded badminton, curling, and ice hockey, to mention only a few activities that are ordinarily included. If, on the other hand, our definition includes only 'having rules and player(s)' we have included the stock market, the symphony orchestra, the local thespian group, and perhaps other instances that would not ordinarily be included. It should be pointed out that a definition may, at one and the same time, be both too narrow and too broad. For example, the first definition of games, above, allows for the inclusion of any random ball playing by dog, man, or cat. I do not think that all of this would ordinarily be admitted.

The strategy employed here will be as follows: 1) suggest a defining property or properties of sport, 2) test for narrowness (abbreviated as tn), 3) test for broadness (abbreviated as tb). A single counter-example will be sufficient to invalidate a definition. The exercise will not be (could not be) exhaustive.

Definition #1: having rules.

tn: I am not certain that the practical mandates, the sort of rules of thumb, associated with fishing, skiing, and rock climbing would count as rules; at least not in the same sense as the rules for ball sports, for example.

tb: The tn difficulty may be ignored. Quite obviously as a single defining feature "having rules" is too broad. After all, hospitals, armies, jails, and schools also have rules, and we wouldn't want to include these, or the activities ordinarily associated with them, as sports. For the sake of argument let us admit "having rules" as a common property of sports. We found that as a single defining feature the definition was too broad. Let us attempt now to find another property that, when combined with this first property, will provide a statement of the intension of 'sport' that will stand the test of counter-example. Let us try the following:

Definition #2: voluntary and having rules.

tn: No exclusion, although it would still probably be thought of as sport if Jack Nicklaus were ordered by the PGA to play in the Sioux City Open.

tb: The tn difficulty may be ignored. A number of valid counter-examples can be conjured up, e.g. an all volunteer army. The definition is too broad.

For the sake of further argument let us admit "voluntary and having rules" as properties common to all sports. These properties may be common but, as we found above, they are not peculiar to sport, i.e. the definition was too broad. Let us add a third feature to our definition:

Definition #3:   voluntary, having rules, and involving a test of how bodily excellent a person can be.[3]

tn: Certain forms of fishing and hunting could hardly be said to test how bodily excellent a person can be. Nor do the owners or players at the race track test themselves in this way. The definition is too narrow.

tb: The volunteer army activity might well provide such a test. The circus acrobat or the stunt man must also be included. The definition is also too broad.

Having eliminated the most recent additional property as neither common nor peculiar, we are now back to definition #2 which, as you will recall, requires a bit of shoring up. But I am weary of the whole dreary business. What I want to say is something like this: *The whole undertaking is in principle wrong-headed!* You cannot take a concept that is as a matter of fact (a matter of language, a matter of culture) vague and make it precise by presenting an essentialist definition of the concept. As Wittgenstein put it: "We do not know the boundaries because none have been drawn." (10:69)

Finally, there is a difference between locating boundaries and drawing boundaries. The former is a descriptive task, the latter normative. What I am trying to show is that what boundary there is between what is and what is not sport is blurred. Attempts to indicate it concisely fall under the category of *drawing boundaries* not locating them. I would call such a definition stipulative.

Claim C: The Concept Sport is Ordinarily Employed in a Wide Variety of Ways, i.e., Has a Wide Variety of Usages, or Meanings

None of us need much reminding on this point. This job has been done before, by many. (4:pp. vii–58) For openers, I would suggest a peek at *The Oxford English Dictionary.* (6:pp. 655–659) This report of usage of the expression "sport" and derivative concepts takes us back almost six centuries. It requires almost five full pages, fine print, three columns to the page. All in all there are one-hundred-twenty-seven different usages reported: noun—26, verb—31, and 70 derivative usages (each of which incorporates the expression "sport").[4] Some of these ways of using the concept have faded into antiquity, perhaps from a lack of use, but a great many continue in one way or another in present usage. To illustrate, I have selected eight different noun usages dating from 1617 to 1892 and have contrasted them with what might be considered contemporary employments. The method of analysis of what I have taken to be contemporary usages is, I think, quite similar to that employed by the lexicographers in putting together the *OED*. Essentially (if I dare use that expression), it involves two steps: 1) finding (or in my case conjuring up) a statement wherein the ex-

And of course we have said nothing about land, league, or subject. The point of this kind of analysis is 1) to explicate the meaning of an expression in a given context, and 2) to show that an expression has different meanings in different contexts. In the examples below I have inserted the substitutions for 'sport' inside the parentheses following the statements.

Employment Cited in OED:	Contemporary Employment:
1. (1a, 1821) "great sport to them was jumping in a sack." (fun, entertainment)	It was great sport to watch the kittens play. (fun, entertainment)
2. (1b, 1617) "Italians love a fearful wench, that oftens flies from Venus sport." (amorous, dalliance, or intercourse)	She sure messed up his fancy sporting coat. (courting, amorous pursuits) (from the folk song "Monongahela Sal")
3. (1c, 1787) "The higher an angler goes up the Thames . . . the more sport, and the greater variety of fish he will meet with." (fishing activity)	Old Blue is an excellent sport dog. (hunting)
4. (4, 1671) "On this they voted it a libel, and to be burned by the hangman. Which was done but the sport was, the hangman burned the Lord's order with it." (jest, joke)	It was just in sport. (jest, play)
5. (5a, 1780) "The high sport was to burn the jails." (pastime, diversion)	Tennis, the sport of kings. (pastime, diversion)
6. (5b, 1871) "In such a state of things hunting might be a sport, as war might be a sport." (game)	The sport of billiards . . . (game)
7. (7a, 1697) "But oh! Commit not thy prophetic mind to flitting leaves, the sport of ev'ry wind." (play thing)	The wind sported with her gown. (played)
8. (8a, 1892) " 'Unhappy, Mr. Collings, the victim of a thousand sports,' I murmured, americanizing my language for the nonce." (gamblers)	Give me a sporting chance. (fair, as in gaming)

pression of interest appears, and 2) substituting another expression (or other expressions) that will not change the meaning of the statement in any important way.[5] The only qualification for participation in this game is to be a speaker of English. Let us take a dry run with the concept of "dry" (as it happens to be handy):

a. Anyone for a dry martini?
b. My throat is so dry, I can hardly swallow.
c. Smith has a rather dry sense of humor.

Acceptable substitutions might be as follows:

a. tart, non-sweet
b. parched, devoid of moisture
c. unemotional, impersonal

I do not hold any particular brief for the substitutions put forward here (although I and the lexicographers that compiled the *OED* agree on several of them). What is important is that speakers of English *in general* agree. The matter could be decided in minutes within any qualified group.

Claim D: Philosophers of Sport Ought Not Waste their Time Attempting to Define 'Sport'

Claims A and B speak mainly to the question of vagueness, claim C to that of ambiguity. Taken together the claim is that the concept of sport is both vague and ambiguous, and to a considerable extent. While the argument for this claim, claim D, rests primarily on the vagueness problem, the ambiguity factor enters the picture in a significant way. It would in principle be possible to specify the intension and extension of each different employment of a highly ambiguous concept *provided each of those employments were concise.* I have tried to point out that this proviso is not applicable to 'sport.' But even if it were applicable, imagine the immensity of the task of attempting to limit the one-hundred-twenty-seven different employments of the concept. Imagine having to try out as many counter-examples as you could conjure up for each of those employments. And then of course the question arises as to whether we could consider the result a *definition.* Certainly not in the usual sense.

I am reminded of the scene in Lewis Carroll's *Sylvie and Bruno Concluded* where Meine Herr tells of having constructed a map with a scale of 1:1, i.e. one mile to one mile. (2:pp. 616–617) Would we want to call such a monstrosity *a map?* We might carry the analogy a step further: In Carroll's tale the 'map' was never spread out. The farmers objected that it would shut out the sunlight. I wonder if our multi-volumed "definition" of 'sport' would ever be used *as a definition?* But we may forget all of this nonsense. The concept of sport is, along with being highly ambiguous, also extremely vague. *It cannot be defined,* at least not in the way we have been speaking of definition. I should point out that this is an analytic claim. I *am not* saying that it, 'sport,' cannot be defined because it is too arduous a task, i.e. like the claim in the statement: "Dhaulagiri cannot be climbed." What I am saying is that it is logically impossible to define the concept. The problem is one of logic not of logistics. Definition is fine for the precise concept, but it will not fit the facts of the life of the imprecise concept.

Epilogue

Perhaps we should rejoice that 'sport' is not a precise concept. If it were, we would probably not be considering matters such as this and it is highly unlikely that there would exist a society such as ours. As Michael Scriven puts it: ". . . when a precise definition *is* possible, one may be sure the term defined is either a new technical term or one not of great importance for scientific or philosophical issues . . ." (8:p. 8) Justus Hartnack, in speaking of Witt-

genstein's attack on essentialism, puts it even stronger when he says, "It is arguable that *no* concept of philosophical interest can be defined." (5:p. 71)

But then, that too may be a waste of time. I am reminded of a poem by Stephen Crane:

I Saw a Man

I saw a man pursuing the horizon
Round and round they sped.
I was disturbed at this;
I accosted the man.
"It is futile," I said,
"You can never . . ."
"You lie," he cried.
And ran on. (3:p. 892)

NOTES

[1] This, according to Wittgenstein, is what the work of the philosopher consists in. (10:127)
[2] This was Wittgenstein's example; the concept at the focal point of his criticism of essentialism. (10:68–71)
[3] I have borrowed this feature from Weiss. (9:p. 143)
[4] It may be of interest to the reader to note that 'play' and its derivative forms outranks 'sport' in different employments 176 to 127.
[5] Alston (1:pp. 10–11) and Strawson, among others, have found this method of analysis useful.

Bibliography

1. Alston, William P. *Philosophy of Language.* Englewood Cliffs, N.J.: Prentice-Hall, Inc., 1964.
2. Carroll, Lewis (pseud.). "Sylvie and Bruno Concluded," *The Complete Works of Lewis Carroll. Alexander* Woolcott (ed.). New York: Random House, no date.
3. Ciardi, John (ed.). *An Introduction to Literature.* Boston: Houghton Mifflin, Inc., 1959.
4. Gerber, Ellen W. (ed.). *Sport and the Body: A Philosophical Symposium.* Philadelphia: Lea and Febiger, 1972.
5. Hartnack, Justus. *Wittgenstein and Modern Philosophy.* Maurice Cranston (trans.). Garden City, N.Y.: Doubleday and Co., Inc., 1965.
6. *The Oxford English Dictionary,* Vol. 10. London: Clarendon Press, 1970.
7. Salmon, Wesley C. *Logic.* Englewood Cliffs, N.J.: Prentice-Hall, Inc., 1963.
8. Scriven, Michael. *Primary Philosophy.* New York: McGraw-Hill Book Co., 1966.
9. Weiss, Paul. *Sport: A Philosophic Inquiry.* Carbondale: Southern Illinois University Press, 1969.
10. Wittgenstein, Ludwig. *Philosophical Investigations.* 3rd Ed., Translated by G. E. M. Anscombe. New York: The Macmillan Co., 1958.

Some Aristotelian Notes on the Attempt to Define Sport*

WILLIAM J. MORGAN

The purpose of this paper is to disarm the non-essentialist argument—a term which has been appropriated to designate the arguments advanced respectively by Kleinman (13: pp. 29–34), Fogelin (8: pp. 58–61), and McBride (16: pp. 4–11)—that "sport" cannot be defined because of the multiple meanings it carries as a concept. The present attempt to discredit the non-essentialist argument follows two convergent lines of argument both of which draw their argumentative force from Aristotle's theory of "focal meaning" enunciated in the middle books of the *Metaphysics*. First of all, it will be argued that the non-essentialist's claim that sport is an ambiguous concept rests on an oversimplistic theory of predication that undermines their argument: a theory founded on the simple dichotomy of synonymy (univocal predication) and homonymy (equivocal predication) which, in itself, is incapable of handling a multi-edged concept such as sport. On this first arm of our argument then, it will be maintained that what the non-essentialist argument actually succeeds in demonstrating in this case is not what it ostensibly set out to demonstrate, namely, the inherent ambiguity of the concept sport, but rather the inappropriateness of the conceptual apparatus it tacitly employed to treat this concept. Secondly, by introducing a *tertium quid*, Aristotle's theory of "focal meaning," the further attempt will be

*From *The Journal of the Philosophy of Sport*, IV (Fall, 1977), 15–35.

made to show how this revised theory of predication—which provides a significant alternative to the narrow synonymy-homonymy schema—allows us to treat sport in a non-ambiguous way by tracing the systematic interconnections of its various meanings. The conclusion thus aimed at is that the endeavor to define sport is not the empty enterprise the non-essentialists would have us believe that it is but, on the contrary, manifests itself as a viable philosophic venture, and, moreover, one that persists in consonance with the fundamental charge of philosophic inquiry.

I

The seeds of the non-essentialist position (a position which we have ascribed to the respective works of Kleinman, Fogelin, and McBride) were sown in an early essay by Graves wherein he observed that: "There are few words in the English language which have such a multiplicity of divergent meanings as the word sport." (9: p. 877) The crux of the non-essentialist's case that sport is an inherently ambiguous concept, and resultantly an indefinable concept, thus rests principally on the point that sport is predicated of a diverse series of activities which house an equally diverse series of meanings. In this vein, Kleinman maintains that the "open" way in which sport is used and practiced precludes any attempt to close the conceptual limits of this word by establishing, through definition, its necessary and sufficient properties. Fogelin, in turn, cites the great diversity in which the word sport is used in daily parlance, taking special note of the fact that sport lacks any clearly distinguishable conceptual boundaries. And although McBride sharpens the charge that sport is an ambiguous word by tracing the source of this ambiguity to its "intensional" (the criteria in virtue of which a particular member is granted admission to a discrete class of things) and "extensional" (the actual members which comprise a set) vagueness, both of these claims draw their impetus from the commonly indiscriminate manner in which sport is used in ordinary language, a usage that takes on a variety of contextual meanings.

It should be made clear at the outset that what the non-essentialists are not arguing against is the overt "stipulation" of the meaning of a term which occurs, for example, in science when the scientist, for the purpose of communicative precision, specifies the exact meanings of the terms he employs in his investigation. Rather, the force of their argument is directed against those who covertly stipulate the meaning of a term and then proceed to parade this stipulative definition as a conventional one (a conventional definition, of course, being one that conforms to the canons of ordinary usage). And what the seek to show specifically with respect to the word sport is that any attempt to conceptually specify the limits of this concept cannot succeed because it is an imprecise concept, i.e., one whose conceptual edges are blurred. Consequently, any endeavor to house all activities that carry the name sport under one neat category, the genus sport, yields at best a "confused and obscure genus," one that invariably is either too broad (such that activities not commonly thought of as sportive enterprises are granted admission into the realm of sport) or too narrow (such that activities commonly regarded as sportive ones are denied admission into the realm of sport).

On this account then, the persistent attempt to locate the precise boundaries of sport, to ferret out its essential core of meaning, is castigated as a capitulation to wishful thinking, more specifically, a capitulation to an unwarranted 'craving' for generality and precision. Such efforts, it is argued, spring from what Kant has designated as the "natural tendency of human beings to abuse their conceptual apparatus in an attempt to make it yield substantive truth." (8: p. 61) In more technical terms, this natural disposition to misuse our conceptual apparatus, that disposition which

allegedly underlies the attempt to render precise an imprecise concept such as sport, leads to what Fogelin calls the error of *a priori empiricism*: deciding something *must* be the case in lieu of any supporting empirical inquiry. The most common manifestation of this error occurs when a favored sporting activity is signalled out for attention and made the touchstone for deciding whether or not an activity is a sport. The problem with this procedure, so the non-essentialists argue, is that it involves an arbitrary choice (its arbitrary character, of course, stems from the idiosyncratic foundation of this decision) and one, therefore, which invariably conflicts with what other people regard as standard cases thereby touching off a dispute about the fundamental nature of sport. The error evident here is that disputes of this sort are based on confusing our individual decision to view sport in this manner with the essential nature of sport itself.

Marshalling all of these arguments together, the non-essentialists conclude that sport is an indefinable concept, one that resists a concise definition because of its endemic ambiguity. Hence, the effort to define sport is considered to be a futile endeavor. That is to say, it is not the case that this definitional task is simply too difficult to accomplish, but that 'it necessarily cannot be accomplished. Accordingly, Kleinman and McBride take this claim to be an analytic truth, one that is necessarily, as opposed to contingently, true, and one, therefore, that cannot be dislodged by empirical inquiry. From this conclusion issues the normative caveat that sport philosophers ought not waste their time on such vapid definitional enterprises—indeed the entire enterprise is rejected wholesale as a pseudo-problem generated by an uncritical craving for precision—but should instead address their attention to more pressing philosophic matters.

One further move, however, must be made to fully certify the non-essentialists' case against the definability of sport. This additional move is prompted by the following question: does not the mere fact that we call all these activities by the common name sport entitle us to the conclusion that there must be some common thread of meaning that runs through all of them? Pressed by this disclaimer, the non-essentialists resort to the last arm of their argument, Wittgenstein's notion of "family resemblances."[1] Following Wittgenstein's injunction to 'look' and 'see' and not merely to presume that there must be some essential element shared by all activities that bear the name sport, the non-essentialists argue that what we in fact find when we scan these multifarious activities is an overlapping of characteristics that form a complex network of similarities. We find, then, no common essence but a "family of resemblances" in which the degree of similarity is closest when we consider adjacent members of the family and furthest apart when we consider distant members of the family. This way of accounting for the manifold predication of sport thus obviates the need to resort to a common essence thereby securing the non-essentialist's conclusion that sport cannot be defined because it lacks an essential core of meaning. And, moreover, it also shows that calling all these activities by the name sport is not a practice without any apparent rhyme or reason; for it is because we can detect these similarities that we call all those activities that have them as their characteristics by the same name.

II

The attempt to overturn the non-essentialist's argument that sport is an indefinable concept must first await a full-blown examination of the conceptual model that undergirds this attempt: namely, Aristotle's theory of "focal meaning." In order to present a fully satisfactory account of Aristotle's theory of "focal meaning," however, it will be necessary to show how this theory critically emerges from his early philosophic work in which we find him operating with a rather primitive version of the synonymy-homonymy schema.

Appropriating the legacy bequeathed to him by Socrates' and Plato's celebrated search for essences (the former in terms of definition, the latter in terms of a theory of Forms), Aristotle embarked on a similar path of thought. His search for essences, however, was tempered from the outset by a critical spirit which reared its head at the very beginning of his sojourn: namely, his criticism of Plato's theory of Forms. Although Aristotle mounted a vast array of arguments against Plato's theory of Forms, most of which were rehearsed in the form of *aporiae* in the opening books of the *Metaphysics*, the principal argument he employed, and the one that served as the point of departure for his own investigations, was the "third man" argument (an argument so named because members of the Academy seized on the Form "man" as their stock example in criticizing Plato's theory). Plato himself raised a version of this argument in *Parmenides* (23: 131e–132b), but it was Aristotle

who explicitly sketched out this argument in an early essay entitled "On Ideas." One possible formalization of this argument goes something like this:

1. a, b, c, are particulars which comprise the set F (set I).
2. all members of set I are called F in virtue of F-ness. (This has subsequently been called the one over many assumption, henceforth referred to as the O.M. assumption.)
3. F-ness is not itself a member of set I. (This has subsequently been called the non-identity assumption, henceforth referred to as the N.I. assumption.)
4. F-ness is itself F. (This has subsequently been called the self-predication assumption, henceforth referred to as the S.P. assumption.)
5. F-ness and members of set I form a second set of F's (set 2).
6. all members of set II are F in virtue of one and the same Form, F-ness2 (O.M. thesis).
7. F-ness2 is not a member of set II (N.I. thesis).
8. F-ness2 is itself F (S.P. thesis).
9. F-ness2 ‡ F-ness.

The inference Aristotle draws from this argument is precisely this: regardless of the Form one substitutes here the result will always be the same, the generation of a vicious regress.[2] Now the damage wrought by this argument cannot be underestimated; for if the argument goes through unscathed it vitiates Plato's search for essences, his attempt to isolate the 'one over the many.' Fully cognizant of this devastating consequence, Aristotle realized that one of the premises of Plato's account must be dropped. And since it was his intent not to abandon the search for essences initiated by his philosophic predecessors, for he was as well convinced of the philosophic propriety of this venture, the 'one over many' assumption is retained by Aristotle.[3] Hence, Aristotle's reassumption of an essentialist posture was critically coupled with the realization that either the S.P. assumption or the N.I. assumption must be abandoned lest his own pursuit of essences suffer the same fate as Plato's. The first step Aristotle took toward the resolution of this problem occurred in the *Categories* where he focused his attention on the development of a new theory of predication, a focus based on the premise that Plato's endeavor to locate essences could be certified as a legitimate philosophic exercise only by critically revising the logic of predication that served as the foundation for this endeavor.

Guided by the errors he noted in the logic of predication underlying Plato's theory of Forms—more specifically, those errors associated with the self-predication and non-identity assumptions of his theory—Aristotle devoted his early logical treatise, the *Categories,* to a detailed examination of the general subject of predication.[4] Our specific interest in this work, however, stems from his discovery of the fundamental difference in the logic of the following two statements: (1.) 'Socrates is a man,' (2.) 'Socrates is pale.'[5] In the first instance, we have a case of what is called strong or synonymous predication. The marks of strong predication are that both the name and the definition (*logos*) can be predicated of the subject. (3: 1ª6) What is said of the subject here then, that he is a man, is essentially true of the subject; such that, in the absence of this characteristic the subject would cease to be what it is, i.e. what it is in its very essence. In the latter statement, on the other hand, 'Socrates is pale,' we have an exemplar case of weak predication, or what Aristotle formally calls homonymous predication. In this instance, only the name and not the definition can be predicated of the subject. (3: 1ª1) The point Aristotle makes here is that to say 'Socrates is pale' is not to predicate anything essential of Socrates, but merely to state something that incidentally happens to be true of Socrates. Thus, if Socrates lost this attribute, by blushing for example, the absence of this feature would in no significant way affect what Socrates essentially 'is.'

As can readily be gleaned from our above discussion, in the case of strong (synonymous) predication Aristotle does allow for a version of the self-predication assumption in that man is man in the sense in which we say 'Socrates is a man.' But, on pain of regress, he doesn't allow a full strain non-identity assumption to hold here; for man is not something different than what Socrates 'is.' The predicate man, then, names not some disparate ideal thing, Plato's error, but a sort, or class of things. Consequently, as the designator of a class of things, its very existence is contingent upon the existence of the individual members it names. In weak (homonymous) predication, on the other hand, Aristotle denies the self-predication assumption; pale is not pale in the same sense in which we say 'Socrates is pale.' This initial denial, in turn, leads him to accept the non-identity thesis here; for 'paleness' is not the same sort of thing that Socrates 'is.'

Thus, working from this rather austere synonymy-homonymy model of predication, Aristotle was able to ferret out cases of strong predication from cases of weak predication. On this scheme then, either something is predicated univocally of its subject (in which case both the name and the definition can be said of the subject) or equivocally of its subject (in which case only the name and not the definition can be said of the subject). In this way, he was able to recast the dilemma in Plato's theory of Forms raised by his faulty logic of predication: either the Form and its nominates carry their name in a univocal fashion and thus are identical with one another, or the use of the same word to name the Form and its nominates is a mere equivocation. It now remains to be seen what important implications he adduces from this early account of predication.

Perhaps the most important implication to be noted here, from our expository standpoint at any rate, is how this theory of predication influences Aristotle's treatment of the subject 'being.' The extent and precise nature of this influence can readily be discerned in Aristotle's charge that his predecessors' search for the common element(s) of all existing things is in principle futile and wrong-headed; for the main argument he supplies for this claim is that 'being' is homonymous, has a great variety of contextual meanings. (4: 992ᵇ 18–24) Thus, Aristotle's denial of any universal science of being qua being is directly linked to his employment of the synonymy-homonymy model of predication here, a model which when invoked with respect to 'being' begets the conclusion that 'being' is an ambiguous concept. Although this charge regarding the vain character of the attempt to locate the common element(s) of 'being' includes virtually all of Aristotle's philosophic predecessors, the principal target he has in mind here is Plato's master-science of 'being,' a science Plato called "dialectic" which he appears to have sketched out in the middle books of the *Republic.* And the main charge Aristotle brings against this so-termed super-science, recasting the previous point, is that it overlooked the fact that the word 'being' is ambiguous.[6] Put in more direct terms, Aristotle viewed Plato's master-science of 'being' as a pseudo scientific enterprise precisely because it was insensitive to the ambiguous status of this concept, the fact that the term 'being' educes many diverse shades of meaning which cannot be concisely delimited for the purposes of scientific investigation.

Thus, on the grounds that 'being' is an ambiguous concept, a classification prompted by his underlying synonymy-homonymy conceptual matrix, Aristotle categorically rejects the possibility of any general science of 'being.' 'Being,' therefore, cannot be conceived as a genus of some sort because it is an equivocal concept. Indeed, working on the premise that 'being' is homonymous, Aristotle goes into yet more detail why the genus model won't work here:

> it is not possible that . . . being should be a single genus of things; for the differentia of any genus must . . . have being . . . but it is not possible for the genus taken apart from its species (any more than for the species of the genus) to be predicated of its proper differentia; so that if . . . being is a genus, no differentia will . . . have being. (4: 998^b 20–28)

The more technical point Aristotle makes here is that the universality commonly attributed 'being' cannot be that of a genus; for 'being' can be predicated of everything whereas a genus cannot be predicated of its differentiae.[7] The absurd consequence that accrues from the designation of 'being' as a genus is that the 'being' of its differentiae must be paradoxically denied. This consequence cannot be averted by simply violating the order of relation which obtains between a genus and its differentiae and allowing the genus to be predicated of its proper differentiae; for if this were so, the differentia would contain the genus thus confounding the disparate meanings intended by the respective use of these terms— that is, the differentia by definition cannot be said to contain a genus.

Following on the heels of Aristotle's polemic against any general science of 'being' (a polemic he waged throughout the early logical treatises, the *Posterior Analytics,* and the opening books of the *Metaphysics*), his subsequent declaration in book four of the *Metaphysics* that there is indeed a universal science of 'being' that treats of 'being qua being' (a general science which is to be distinguished from the special sciences that partition off a certain segment of 'being' for investigation) comes as no small surprise. This sudden reversal stems from his newly formed contention that 'being' has been prematurely assigned an ambiguous rating, a contention based on the realization that the synonymy-homonymy account of predication he has been operating with thus far is

not sophisticated enough to handle a polychrestic term like 'being.' The substantive arsenal behind this new claim for a general science of 'being,' however, rests on his discovery of a *tertium quid,* a model of predication called "focal meaning" which can accommodate itself to words or, more correctly, the things designated by such words, that fall outside the narrow province of the synonymy-homonymy schema. By introducing this new theory, then, Aristotle is able to meet his own objections concerning the ambiguity of 'being' thereby setting the stage for the construction of a general science of 'being.'

Aristotle's discovery of "focal meaning" was accomplished not by relinquishing his previous critical stance that words like 'being' take on a variety of meanings and definitions according to the context in which they are used, sustaining his earlier veto of the genus model as a viable paradigm of predication for such terms, but by pointing out that these diverse contextual meanings are, in fact, logically affiliated with one another. He does this by showing that the different senses the word 'being' assumes can all be explained as variations of one primary sense of the word. This primary sense of the word is so-called because it turns up as a constituent element in all the definitions we affix to the manifold senses of 'being.' Aristotle's point here can best be illustrated by considering one of the favorite examples he uses to explain this theory, the concept of 'medicine.'

The concept medicine, argues Aristotle, can be used and, consequently, understood in a number of different ways. It can be used, for example, to refer to the science of medicine, or to a medical person, or to a medical instrument. And although it is certainly true that the word medicine, as it is used above, answers to different definitions according to the specific context in which it is used, it seems fair to say as well that it is not merely being used equivocally either. For all these respective uses of the concept refer back to one common core of meaning which is to be regarded as the primary meaning of the term, in this case the meaning indicated by the science of medicine itself. That is to say, we call an individual a medical person only because he/she is a practitioner of the science of medicine. Similarly, an instrument is designated as a medical instrument only in virtue of the fact that it is used by a medical person to further implement the science of medicine. In each case then, we are entitled to predicate the concept of medicine of some person or thing be-

3

cause it refers back to, and variously qualifies, the primary meaning denoted by the science of medicine.

Applying this model directly to 'being,' Aristotle similarly argues that the divergent senses of 'being' all refer back to one central point of reference, that point of reference in virtue of which the multifarious meanings of 'being' can be systematically ordered. In this case, the central point of reference turns out to be substance; for in order to explain such things as qualities, affections, privations, etc., one must first account for that which has these various determinations as its attributes: namely, substance. As he thus argues:

> . . . there are many senses in which a thing is said to be, but all refer to one starting point; some things are said to be because they are substances, others because they are affections of substance, others because they are a process towards substance, or destructions or privations or qualities of substance. (4: 1103ª 25–1003ᵇ 20)

Consequently, all items in categories other than substance are said 'to be' only insofar as they can be certified as bonafide attributes of substance. By means of this "reductive operation," then, Aristotle was able to successfully parry his previous charge regarding the ambiguity of 'being' thereby laying the foundation for a general science of 'being.' And this general science of 'being' was to include not only a study of substance but as well a study of how the subsidiary senses of 'being' relate to 'being' in its foremost sense (substance). Thus, on this revised account, we have a science not only when we have an exact definition that can be predicated of all the members of a particular class without qualification (synonymous predication), but also in the case in which things, and their respective meanings, are systematically related to one central point of reference (focal meaning). As Aristotle remarks: "For not only in the case of things which have one common notion [synonymy] does the investigation belong to one science, but also in the case of things which are related to one common nature [focal meaning]; for even these in a sense have one common notion." (4: 1003ᵇ 13–15)

III

Following the main drift of Aristotle's argument sketched out above, and in accord with one arm of the non-essentialist's argument, it is argued that the concept sport does not qualify as a candidate for synonymous predication. The reason for this is, of course, that sport is a polychrestic term, a word that harbors many nuances of meaning, and as such, a word that cannot be made to fit a synonymous model of predication without inducing some distortion in the process. Consequently, any attempt to render sport as a genus of some sort (the latter, of course, being a paradigmatic case of synonymy) must be abandoned owing to the fact that it cannot account for the multiple meanings predicated of sport. The generic unity needed to provide a suitable definition of sport, then, as the non-essentialists correctly argue, cannot be supplied by simply lumping all these divergent meanings under the genus sport; for at best such an effort yields a "confounded genus," one that does not resolve the issue at hand (the definability or indefinability of sport), but in some sense exacerbates this problem in virtue of it being an equivocal as opposed to a univocal genus, and thus, strictly speaking, not a genus at all.

However, if we more closely follow Aristotle's lead on this point, an even more devastating case than that made by the non-essentialists can be brought against the genus model with respect to sport. That is, reconsidering Aristotle's argument that 'being' cannot be a genus because 'being' can be predicated of everything whereas a genus cannot be predicated of its differentiae, a similar case can be made (in a modified sense, of course, given that the extension of sport, though of sufficient magnitude to warrant the use of Aristotle's argument here, does not parallel that of 'being') that the extensional limits of sport preclude treating it as a genus because doing so entails that it cannot be predicated of its proper differentiae. Succinctly put, the point to be made here is that if sport is passed off as a type of genus it cannot be applied to its differentiae—whether the differentiae we draw up here concerns the number of people engaged in a particular sport (in which case we generate the following sub-classes: individual sports, dual sports, team sports), or the use of a pivotal implement such as a ball (in which case we simply partition sport off into two classes: ball games and non-ball games), or the natural element(s) in which a sporting venture is conducted (in which case we divide sports into such classes as water sports, snow sports, ice sports, aerial sports, field sports, etc.)—without ensnaring the classification scheme in insuperable problems. For when the attempt is made to apply the genus sport to one of its differentiae, say ball-games, the unhappy result that ensues is that the differentia concerning ball-games can now be said to contain the genus sport thereby short-circuiting the entire classification effort. Secondly, a point which is merely a corollary of the first, in predicating sport of any one of its differentiae one must correlatively deny all other possible species of sport that fall outside the boundaries of the chosen species (the chosen species being, of course, the one marked off by the differentia selected for consideration) entrance into the genus; for if we, for example, once again attach the predicate sport to the differentia concerning ball-games (remembering that such a move submerges the genus into the differentia), all other species of sport that have a different differentia (namely, in this case all sporting activities that do not use a ball in the conduct of their activity) are denied admittance into the genus. And since it seems plausible to maintain that the extension of sport clearly exceeds the conceptual compass marked off by any one differentia, the undeniable conclusion that forces itself upon us is that sport cannot be treated as a genus.

It is readily apparent from our above remarks that we stand in fundamental agreement with the non-essentialists on the point that sport cannot be treated as a synonymous concept. But it is here that our ways must part. For unlike the non-essentialists we are not yet ready to consign sport to the ever expanding bin of ambiguous concepts. On the contrary, the assessment of sport as an ambiguous term is, on our view, a premature move that is based on a fundamental over-simplification: namely, an over-simplistic theory of predication which recognizes only cases of synonymy and homonymy. Thus, following Aristotle's discovery of a *tertium quid*, we will attempt to show that sport involves neither a strict case of synonymy nor a simple case of homonymy, but rather a case of "focal meaning."

Inasmuch as it is our intent here only to suggest the feasibility of defining sport under the conceptual model of "focal meaning" proposed by Aristotle, and not to undertake an independent and exhaustive analysis of the common root-experience of sport (a task which clearly takes us outside the thematic confines drawn for the present essay), the attempt to demonstrate that sport exemplifies a case of focal meaning will be made by borrowing from the results of Joseph Esposito's investigation that the central experience of sport is the experience of "possibility." (7: pp. 137–146) On Esposito's analysis, then, the core experience of sport lies in the rather unique encounter with possibility it offers the self; for if we survey the different sport forms before us what we find peculiar to each is the presence of an artificially contrived challenge which the self attempts to overcome. And it is precisely this challenge, this contrived attempt to overcome unnecessary obstacles, that provides the self with an opportunity to exercise human possibilities not available in everyday life situations.[8] As Esposito remarks: "To the player, the game, if properly constructed, presents . . . an opportunity to experience possibility . . . the sportive player enjoys a situation where all the fascination of encountering the possible exists." (7: pp. 141–44)

Using the idiom of "possibility" as our focal point, the following hierarchical scheme suggests itself. First of all, that which counts in the purest sense as a sportive activity are those instances of sport which allow for an unmediated (in the sense of being unconstrained by external impinging factors whether the source of that external constraint be another opponent, one's teammate, an animate non-human, or an inanimate mechanical device) pursuit of one's possibilities.[9] On this account, then, only individual sporting activities (swimming, diving, skiing, track and field, cross-country, gymnastics, archery, bowling, golf, weightlifting, figure skating, single's sculling, cycling), in which the resolve to seek out and actualize one's possibilities is directly contingent on the response of the individual athlete, qualify in the strictest sense as sportive endeavors. Next in line are the dual sports (including the combative dual sports such as boxing, fencing, and wrestling, and the court dual sports such as tennis, badminton, etc.) in which one's encounter with its possibilities is by and large dependent upon the performance of one's opponent. After these, we have team sports (football, basketball, baseball, soccer, lacrosse, ice hockey, field hockey, rugby, water polo, rowing, and yachting) in which one's projection of its possibilities is tempered not only by the response of one's opponents but as well by the performance of one's fellow teammates. And finally, we have those sports which rely rather heavily on the performance of either an animate non-human (equestrian events, polo) or an inanimate mechanical device (auto racing, airplane racing, etc.) for the conduct of their activity, thereby diminishing still further the role played by the individual athlete in this evocation of possibility.

The central reference point of this hierarchical scheme is, of course, the element of possibility and the extent to which one's projection of its possibilities is mediated by external impinging factors. And the point to be made here, using Aristotle's model of "focal meaning" as our conceptual frame of reference, is this: despite the fact that as one moves either up or down the hierarchy the contextual setting and, resultantly, the precise manner in which one encounters its possibilities (whether independently, in which case we have virtually a complete expression of one's possibilities for Being, or contingently, in which case we have a considerably diminished expression of one's possibilities for Being) varies, each instance of sport is so named because it contains a moment of possibility that is experienced by the player, an experience which lies at the heart of these diverse sporting ventures and serves to define them. This central moment of possibility, moreover, is not simply a common element that merely happens to be shared by all these activities—in the same sense, for instance, in which these sporting forms share human movement as the medium of their respective activities, a medium peculiar not only to sport but to all human movement phenomena, e.g., dance, exercise, etc.—but an essential element that distinguishes sport from other enterprises human beings commonly engage in. To reiterate our previous point, then, although each of the above mentioned sport forms answers to different definitions given their variant contextual structures, it is because this element of possibility turns up as an integral component of these definitions that we can predicate the word sport of them without equivocation, that is, without ensnaring our account in a case of mere ambiguity.

It should be further noted in this regard that the classification scheme of "focal meaning" provides us with a ready way of handling the metaphorical predication of sport. Metaphorical usage, it will be remembered, involves the contrived reassignment of the literal meaning of a term for the express purpose of evoking new shades of meaning. Put more succinctly, metaphor is a form of usage whereby the literal meaning of a term is purposely extended and stretched beyond its literal bounds. So rendered, it is apparent that the type of predication operative here is of an incidental sort. That is, reimporting the concept sport as our frame of reference, the meanings predicated of sport in this fashion are intended to exceed the literal province of meanings peculiar to this concept, that province of meanings which is regarded as the essential meaning of the term. Viewed from this standpoint, some of the modern contextual paraphrases McBride proposes

for sport, such as the phrase "Give me a sporting chance," can be accounted for (as all such metaphorical uses can be) as metaphorical extensions of this concept which incidentally qualify the primal (essential) meaning of sport, a meaning we have suggested, following Esposito's lead, resides in the esoteric sense of possibility aroused in sport.

The crucial point to be observed here, however, is that the metaphorical extension of a term is always a matter of qualifying a well established meaning, one regarded as the literal (essential) meaning of a term. Hence, metaphorical usage presupposes that the concept it modifies must possess an underlying unity of meaning. In the absence of such an underlying unity, metaphorical extension is simply out of the question, i.e., doomed to failure since there is no common thread of meaning to be qualified. As Midgley adroitly points out:

> Metaphor . . . is an epidiascope projecting enlarged images of a word's meaning; turn the word around and you get different pictures, but where we don't grasp the underlying unity we get no metaphor at all. (18: p. 249)

Consequently, those who unabashedly seize on the fact that the word sport is commonly used in a metaphorical manner in the hopes of demonstrating the equivocal status of this concept, taking special note of the proliferation of meanings generated by this type of predication, disarm their own argument; for in showing up the metaphorical fertility of this word they unwittingly grant the very presupposition of metaphorical usage that undermines their own argument: namely, the necessity of the concept having a clearly discernible underlying unity of meaning.

IV

The intent of the above discussion has been to suggest that sport is an expression that has "focal meaning," i.e., one primary meaning—in our example, the notion of possibility—which serves as the normative guide for systematically ordering all its other meanings. So treated, it was argued, contra the non-essentialists, that sport is not an ambiguous word that carries a vast array of unrelated meanings, but rather that all its meanings are logically affiliated with one another and can be variously explained as derivative uses of a primary use. In thus showing that sport should not be partitioned off as a simple case of ambiguity, we have swept away in the process the main objection marshalled by the non-essentialists against defining sport. As such, the prospect of presenting a suitable definition of sport, along the lines sketched above, once again posits itself as a viable alternative provided, of course, we do not fall into the trap of attempting to spin out such definitional efforts under the aegis of a synonymy-homonymy conceptual model, a model ill-suited for the task.

Before closing our discussion on this point, however, one further objection yet remains to be mounted by those of a non-essentialist persuasion. This is the objection Fogelin and McBride would likely raise, that we have subtly passed through a stipulative definition of sport for a conventional one. And the evidence they would most likely cite here is the activities that would be excluded from the conceptual ken of sport if an exemplar such as "possibility" was used (e.g., dog racing and cock fighting would be excluded owing to an absence of human possibility), activities, many of which, according to the canons of conventional language, are readily granted admission into the sportive realm. On the face of this evidence, the charge likely to be lodged is that we have arbitrarily redefined sport thereby circumventing, not resolving, the problems raised by the non-essentialists with respect to the attempt to define sport. The definability of sport would thus, on this rejoinder at any rate, still appear to be a problematic issue. In the effort to parry this "stipulative" charge, three further points of argument will need to be considered.

The first thing to be noted, recasting our main argument, is that the thrust of the non-essentialist's "stipulative" rejoinder draws its vitality and argumentative force from the synonymy-homonymy conceptual model that undergirds it. That is to say, it is only on the basis of this predication model that the "stipulative" charge gets off the ground in the first place. For on finding sport to be a word that belies a synonymous rendering, the only recourse left on this predication scheme is that sport is an equivocal concept and, therefore, a concept that cannot be defined in other than a "stipulative" manner. Accordingly, any definition proffered of sport is immediately written off as a "stipulative" one given the either/or alternatives prescribed by the synonymy-homonymy paradigm. The problem evident here, however, is that the charge rests on a logical error. To be more precise, it rests on an unduly narrow predication account, one that in recognizing only strict cases of synonymy and simple cases of homonymy closes itself off to cases that properly fall outside the am-

bit of its conceptual framework. It is thus argued that under the influence of this austere synonymy-homonymy bifurcation the non-essentialist's analysis is led awry by prompting it to yield, at best, premature claims and, at worst, patently false ones: in this case, the alleged indefinability of sport.

The second objection to be raised against the "stipulative" rejoinder is that it is based on yet another logical error—one which as we shall shortly see is not entirely unrelated to the first, namely, the *petitio principi* fallacy. The objection here, then, is simply that the non-essentialist argument begs the question in its endeavor to certify the conclusion that sport can be defined only in a stipulative manner. This error raises its head most decisively in McBride's paper, specifically in the section where he considers the problems that beset the attempt to concisely specify the "intension" of sport. On this account, each respective effort to locate the "intensional" boundaries of sport, in all three such efforts are made, falls short either because it fails the test for broadness, or the test for narrowness, or both of the aforementioned tests. The problem with McBride's analysis, however, is that his uncritical acceptance of the conventional way in which sport is used commits him at the outset to accept such a wide assortment of activities as legitimate sporting activities (thereby widening the "extensional" limits of sport to an unmanageable degree) that any attempt to precisely specify the "intension" of this concept cannot succeed. To be sure, this is exactly the claim McBride works so hard to achieve, but the point is that nowhere does this claim follow as a conclusion from an argument, rather it is merely assumed, and as such, never explicitly argued for but apparently offered up as a tenet of our faith in the truth value of ordinary language.

The third and last line of argument to be levelled against the non-essentialist's "stipulative" retort is that it is a one-sided account, and as such, a dispenser of half-truths. The source of its one-sidedness in this regard can be traced to the non-essentialist's unqualified acceptance of conventional discourse as the normative guide for our talk and, consequently, our thought, about sport. Although this uncritical reliance on conventional language had something to do with the second objection we raised against the "stipulative" rejoinder, it will here be independently signalled out as a further substantial point of argument that underlies the "stipulative" rebuttal advanced by the non-essentialists. Hence, if we are to fully escape the wrath of the "stipulative" charge, we must directly contend with the ordinary language premise packed into their "stipulative" rejoinder.

To begin with, in conceding a half-truth status to the non-essentialist argument in this context, we are admitting that their argument is not completely without substance. That is to say, a certain measure of truth is to be granted their argument in this vein. And this measure of truth concerns the salutary influence the non-essentialist position exerts on those among us who qualify as "definition mongers," i.e., those who simply insist on essences and precise definitions while ignoring altogether any problems of ambiguity. This unalloyed quest for absolute certitude must, of course, be critically tempered, and it seems plausible to suggest that a sympathetic reading of the non-essentialist argument does much to curb this surfeited appetite. But, it seems equally incontrovertible that the 'craving for ambiguity and fragmentation,' the active searching out of ambiguity and the official sanctioning of such ambiguity (making one who engages in such a search a puzzle-monger of sorts), must also be critically tempered lest our concepts self-destruct before our very eyes no longer having any semblance of a unified meaning. To lead one's investigation in either direction, certitude or ambiguity, is to destroy that parity which on the one hand guards against unduly speculative ventures and on the other hyper-critical accounts. And in orienting their argument in the latter direction, as evidenced by their full blown adoption of ordinary language as the standard for our talk about sport (a form of language literally fraught with ambiguity), we are charging the non-essentialists with violating this parity assumption. Further critical elaboration is in order here.

To briefly reiterate our previous point, it is our express position that the non-essentialist's "stipulative" argument is suspect in that it can be viewed as surrendering to a certain 'craving for ambiguity' in virtue of its acceptance of conventional (ordinary) language as the prototype for determining whether or not something qualifies as a sporting activity. The charge being pressed here, then, is that the non-essentialist account suffers from an imbalance, a one-sided emphasis on ordinary language which contaminates their analysis from the outset. For just as the non-essentialists advise us, correctly it is suspicioned, to heed Kant's caveat that man has a natural penchant for abusing his conceptual apparatus in the endeavor "to make it yield substantive truth," we are equally well advised, according to the view presently being put forth, to heed Heidegger's caveat that man exhibits as well a natural penchant for engaging in what he calls "idle talk"—that form of talk indigenous to our everyday conventional discourse. "Idle talk," following in the main Heidegger's analysis, is a rather loose and uncritical type of conversing —one concerned neither with completeness nor correctness of expression—which understands and interprets everything from the taken-for-granted stance everyday man assumes in his daily dealings in the world. As such, the act of disclosure (communication) evinced in this taken-for-granted posture towards the world perverts itself into an act of covering up in virtue of its failure to penetrate the familiarity by which we understand the world in our daily round of activities, a familiarity which prevents us from entering into a more fundamental relationship with that which is talked about.[10] Now, to choose to ignore this common penchant to discourse via "idle talk," is to be insensitive about language in a quite different sense than that noted by the non-essentialists: namely, to overlook the rather obvious limitations and inconsistencies of conventional language. Thus, on our account, to let stand as legitimate uses of the word sport whatever man's everyday palaver so indicates, is nothing short of a philosophic embarrassment; for the implied assumption packed into this view is that philosophic analysis has no insight to offer on its own concerning such matters. What is more, the non-essentialist's complete reliance on ordinary language (excluding Kleinman, of course) presages the literal negation of philosophy, at least in its traditional and contemporary continental forms, whereby philosophy is reduced to the mundane task of merely reporting on ordinary usage without pretense of usurping its normative authority.[11]

In rejecting the ordinary language premise of the non-essentialist's stipulative rejoinder on the grounds that it is a residuum of a one-sided account, one whose consequences we find untenable, we are clearly not advocating the counter-position that ordinary language about sport is to be completely discounted—a move which would make us fully vulnerable to the "stipulative" charge—but only that its limitations be recognized thereby de-absolutizing it as the standard for our understanding of the world in general and sport in particular. What in effect is being called for here, then, a call which delivers us from the wrath of the "stipulative" epitaph, is not the arbitrary stipulation of the meaning of the term sport, but rather a full-scaled determination of the meaning of this word. Such a full blown determination of meaning is not simply a matter of arbitrarily picking an exemplar case of sport as the standard for determining whether or not something qualifies as a sporting activity (after a Platonic fashion), nor is it a matter of simply consulting our ordinary talk about our sporting experiences (after a Wittgensteinian fashion); rather, it entails a rigorous and exhaustive examination of this phenomenon, one that is open to and critical of all the facets of our experience of the sportive realm including those disclosed to us in ordinary language.

V

In accord with the line of argument sketched out in our introductory remarks, it was argued that the non-essentialist's claim that sport is an indefinable concept is suspect in that it rests on an unduly narrow synonymy-homonymy predication model, a conceptual model that cannot accommodate itself to polychrestic words of the kind exemplified by sport. On the basis of this initial line of argument, then, it was concluded that the non-essentialist account missed its intended mark; for it demonstrated not that sport is an indefinable concept but only that the conceptual paradigm of synonymy and homonymy is ill-suited for the task. The more substantive point to be posited from this line of inquiry, however, incorporating our second line of argument (Aristotle's theory of "focal meaning"), is precisely this: that sport can indeed be defined provided the conceptual model we employ for such a definitional quest includes Aristotle's doctrine of "focal meaning," or something like it, as its *tertium quid*.

Notes

1. Although Fogelin is the only author herein considered that actually invokes Wittgenstein's notion of "family resemblances" to explain his continued use of the generic name sport in his analysis, it is clear that both McBride and Kleinman (though the latter would perhaps insist on a phenomenological as opposed to a linguistic route to such a notion) would also need to resort to such a device in light of their decision to retain the common name sport in their respective inquiries. For in lieu of such a conceptual device, and further recognizing that both adhere to the view that sport lacks any central core of meaning, an explanation is still left wanting as to why both continue to employ the generic name sport, a practice which suggests, implicitly at any rate, that the concept sport does in fact possess the central core of mean-

ing they deny it has. At very least, the plural form (sports) is called for here in order to reflect the divergent pluralism of meanings both Kleinman and McBride find with respect to sport.

2. In all fairness to Plato's account, however, Allen has recently argued that an auxiliary premise is needed to get the regress of the ground, a premise that certifies Plato's so-termed self-predication assumption (F-ness is itself F) as an assumption that genuinely entails self-predication. As he notes: "Plato . . . accepts the following thesis; some (perhaps all) entities which may be designated by a phrase of the form 'the F itself', . . . may be called F. So the Beautiful Itself will be beautiful, . . . But this thesis does not, by itself, imply self-predication; for that, an auxiliary premise is required. . . . This premise is that a predicate of the type '. . . is F' may be applied univocally to F particulars and to the F itself, so that when . . . we say that a given act is just, and that Justice is just, we are asserting that both have identically the same character." (2: pp. 168–69) Allen later goes on to argue that this additional premise, one crucial to the generation of the regress, cannot in fact be tacked on to Plato's theory on the grounds that in Plato's account the predicate is applied equivocally, as opposed to univocally, thereby averting any problems of self-predication.

3. The non-essentialists resolve this problem, of course, by eliminating the O.M. assumption altogether. For those who chose not to follow this latter route, however, it bears mentioning that both the N.I. and S.P. assumptions are needed to generate the regress and, therefore, that dropping one of these premises is all that is required to prevent the regress.

4. The word "category" is itself derived from the Greek *Katêgoria* which means 'to say something about something,' 'to predicate something of a subject.' As such, the *Categories* is, in effect, a study of what it is to predicate something of a subject. In saying this, however, we should also make it clear from the outset that Aristotle's interest in the *Categories* is not with words *per se*, but rather with the things such words refer to.

5. Henceforth, the exposition of Aristotle's theory of "focal meaning" must claim a rather obsequious reliance on G.E.L. Owen's following three essays: "Logic and Metaphysics in Some Earlier Works of Aristotle," (21: pp. 163–190) "Aristotle on the Snares of Ontology," (20: pp. 69–95) "The Platonism of Aristotle." (22: pp. 147–174)

6. The shift made here from saying 'being' is homonymous to saying that 'being' is an homonymous word must not, of course, blind us to the previously mentioned point that Aristotle's focus is on nonlinguistic items (the things designated by words) and not linguis-

tic items *per se* (words in lieu of their reference to things). The shift, however, is a quite natural one taking the reasonable view that language is the medium in which homonymy is expressed.

7. In Aristotle's schema, differentiae are subsidiary marking devices that divide off one class of things from another. They are subsidiary in the sense that the primary mechanism by which one class of things is partitioned off from another is accomplished by citing their secondary substances, for Aristotle, their respective genera and species.

8. A few additional remarks need to be made here. First of all, the reader should be reminded that our use of Esposito's notion of "possibility" as the suggested focal point was intended only to be an illustrative example, and as such, was incorporated merely to illustrate how we might handle the concept sport under the tutelage of Aristotle's theory of "focal meaning." Consequently, one may quarrel altogether with our use of this example, or perhaps find particular fault with it, but if one is going to disarm our argument the substantial point that needs to be addressed is precisely this: whether or not the conceptual model this example of "possibility" was meant to illustrate ("focal meaning") offers us a way out of the definitional dilemma posed by the non-essentialists; a dilemma which, as we have observed, draws its argumentative firepower from the synonymy-homonymy bifurcation that underlies it. Our remaining remarks will concern the example itself. Firstly, because Esposito indiscriminately shifts his attention from games to sport it will be necessary to contextualize his thesis somewhat in order to more specifically accommodate the sportive realm. And this contextualization consists simply in this: that in sport this element of possibility is experienced within a structured competitive setting and is accompanied by the display of psychomotor skill involving a rather significant (as opposed to incidental) employment of the body. Secondly, although Esposito fails to specify as concisely as we would like the precise sense of possibility he contends is evoked by sport, his preliminary remarks concerning this matter make at least this much clear: the type of possibility excited by sport is of a peculiarly human sort. As such, and in the interests of avoiding mis-interpretation on this point (insofar as this is possible in lieu of a more in-depth examination), this distinctively human sense of possibility aroused in sport must be distinguished from the following two types of possibility: logical and empirical possibility. Logical possibility, that which is contradictory or not, covers such a vast expanse of possible action, argues Stack. that it disqualifies itself as a viable normative guide for the projection of human possibilities. (26: p. 17) That is to say, as Aristotle for one noted, one does not concern oneself in one's

human conduct with that which is logically possible as such, but only with that which one has the potentiality to actualize. Similarly, this sportive sense of possibility must also be distinguished from empirical possibility, that modality of possibility which concerns itself with what 'may or may not happen' with respect to physical phenomena based on the knowledge of known empirical laws governing such phenomena. Insofar as we speak of man as a physical being having specific physical capacities, this notion of possibility extends, as it does for all biological phenomena, to the human domain. But the connection observed here is at best a tangential one in that it takes into account only man's physical possibilities ignoring by fiat what for the present may be called man's spiritual capacities. On this view, man's realization of his inherent potentialities is considered exclusively from a biological perspective, and thus, can be indiscriminately likened, e.g., to the maturation of a flower or a tree. Hence, since both of these modalities of possibility refer only incidentally to the human realm (neither calling attention primarily nor uniquely to this realm), they are to be distinguished from human possibility and, by implication, sportive possibility.

9. No claim for originality can be made here for all that we are doing at this point is merely duplicating, *mutatis mutandis,* Robert Osterhoudt's fine classification of sport developed in his incisive essay, "An Hegelian Interpretation of Art, Sport, and Athletics." (19: pp. 346–47) The only observable difference in our account is that the above classification is based on the category of possibility as opposed to the Hegelian categories of the spiritual and the sensuous employed by Osterhoudt, categories which the present author as yet is not prepared to embrace.

10. "Idle talk" gives rise, then, to an implicit operationalization of language whereby linguistic items, and their nominates, are identified with a particular function(s) in a given sociocultural system. In this way, the meanings of concepts are ensconced within an established universe of discourse, one that parallels the established reality, and thereby understood exclusively in terms of their (established) functional use. The nature of this functional use, and the reality it is based on, lie, of course, outside the conceptual horizon of ordinary language. What is thus achieved by the functionalization of concepts vis à vis ordinary discourse is nothing less than the blunting of the content of our conceptual vocabulary; for as Marcuse has noted: "Prior to its operational usage, the concept *denies* the identification of the thing with its function; it distinguishes that which the thing *is* from the contingent functions of the thing in the established reality." (14: p. 95)

11. To be sure, ordinary language philosophers of the likes of Wittgenstein were not only aware

of this consequence (the negation of philosophy in its traditional form), but actively worked to ratify it, fully convinced that traditional philosophy, in its insatiable quest for absolute certitude, represented a mis-guided form of philosophic thinking. On this account, then, traditional philosophy is castigated as a form of thinking gone awry, as a type of philosophic thinking that generates pseudo-philosophic problems which divert our attention from more pressing philosophic issues. As Marsh has recently pointed out, however, even Wittgenstein himself wavers on the point whether or not philosophy is entitled to expurgate ordinary usage. As he remarks: "Wittgenstein seems inconsistent on the point whether philosophy has the right to critically improve on ordinary language. At times he says that an attempt to make the boundaries sharper and more exact by universal essences is a violation of ordinary, actual usage and, therefore, is more or less arbitrary and incorrect. . . . At other times he talks about the 'grammar' of certain expressions like 'knowing' in a different way in which he suggests that the philosopher does indeed have the right to improve on ordinary language. . . . It is, for instance, never correct to use 'knowing' for expressions like 'knowing one's pain' because such expressions are redundant, an error in such cases is impossible. It is always correct, on the other hand, to use 'knowing' in cases where error is conceivable." (15: p. 251)

Bibliography

1. Abbagnano, Nicola. *Critical Existentialism.* Translated by Nino Langiulli. Garden City, New York: Doubleday Co., 1969.
2. Allen, R. E. "Participation and Predication in Plato's Middle Dialogues." *Plato, Metaphysics and Epistemology: A Collection of Critical Essays.* Edited by Gregory Vlastos. Garden City, New York: Doubleday Co., 1971.
3. Aristotle. *Categories and De Interpretatione.* Translated by J. L. Ackrill. Oxford: Oxford University Press, 1963.
4. Aristotle. *Metaphysics. The Basic Works of Aristotle.* Edited by Richard McKeon. New York: Random House, 1941.
5. Burke, Richard. "Work and Play." *Ethics,* 82 (Oct., 1971), 33–47.
6. Elliot, R. K. "Aesthetics and Sport." *Readings in the Aesthetics of Sport.* Edited by H. T. A. Whiting and D. W. Masterson. London: Lepus Books, 1974.
7. Esposito, Joseph L. "Play and Possibility." *Philosophy Today,* 18 (Summer, 1974), 137–46.
8. Fogelin, R. J. "Sport: The Diversity of the Concept." *Sport and the Body: A Philosophical Symposium.* Edited by Ellen Gerber. Philadelphia: Lea and Febiger, 1972.
9. Graves, H. "A Philosophy of Sport." *Contemporary Review,* 78 (Dec., 1900), 877–93.
10. Heidegger, Martin. *Being and Time.* Translated by John MacQuarrie and Edward Robinson. New York: Harper and Row, 1962.
11. Huizinga, Johan. *Homo Ludens: A Study of the Play Element in Culture.* Boston: Beacon Press, 1970.
12. Keating James. "Sportsmanship as a Moral Category." *Ethics,* 75 (Oct., 1964), 25–35.
13. Kleinman, Seymour. "Toward a Non-Theory of Sport." *Quest,* (May, 1968), 29–34.
14. Marcuse, Herbert. *One-Dimensional Man.* Boston: Beacon Press, 1966.
15. Marsh, James. "The Triumph of Ambiguity: Merleau-Ponty and Wittgenstein." *Philosophy Today,* 19 (Fall, 1975), 243–55.
16. McBride, Frank. "Toward a Non-Definition of Sport." *Journal of the Philosophy of Sport,* 2 (Sept., 1975), 4–11.
17. Metheny, Eleanor. *Connotations of Movement in Sport and Dance.* Dubuque, Iowa: William C. Brown Co., 1965.
18. Midgley, Mary. "The Game Game." *Philosophy: The Journal of the Royal Institute of Philosophy,* 49 (July, 1974), 231–53.
19. Osterhoudt, Robert. "An Hegelian Interpretation of Art, Sport and Athletics." *The Philosophy of Sport: A Collection of Original Essays.* Edited by Robert G. Osterhoudt. Springfield, Illinois: Charles C Thomas, 1973.
20. Owen, G. E. L. "Aristotle On the Snares of Ontology." *New Essays on Plato and Aristotle.* Edited by Renford Bambrough. New York: Humanities Press, 1966.
21. Owen, G. E. L. "Logic and Metaphysics in Some Earlier Works of Aristotle." *Aristotle and Plato in the Mid-Fourth Century.* Edited by I. During and G. E. L. Owen. Goteborg: Almquist and Wiksell, 1957.
22. Owen, G. E. L. "The Platonism of Aristotle." *Proceedings of the British Academy,* 51 (1965), 147–74.
23. Plato. *Parmenides. The Collected Dialogues of Plato.* Edited by Edith Hamilton and Huntington Cairns. New Jersey: Princeton University Press, 1969.
24. Plato, *Phaedo. The Collected Dialogues of Plato.* Edited by Edith Hamilton and Huntington Cairns. New Jersey: Princeton University Press, 1969.
25. Robinson, Richard. "Socratic Definition." *The Philosophy of Socrates: A Collection of Critical Essays.* Edited by Gregory Vlastos. Garden City, New York: Doubleday Co., 1971.
26. Stack, George J. "Subjective Possibility." *Personalist,* (Winter 1972), 14–24.
27. Strang, Colin. "Plato and the Third Man." *Plato, Metaphysics and Epistemology: A Collection of Critical Essays.* Garden City, New York: Doubleday Co., 1971.
28. Vlastos, Gregory. "The Third Man Argument in the *Parmenides.*" *Philosophical Review,* 63 (1954), 289–301.
29. Wittgenstein, Ludwig. *Philosophical Investigations.* Translated by G. E. M. Anscombe. Oxford: Oxford University Press, 1953.

BIBLIOGRAPHY ON THE NATURE OF SPORT

Avedon, Elliot M. and Sutton-Smith, Brian. *The Study of Games.* New York: John Wiley & Sons, 1971.

Blumenfield, Walter. "Observations Concerning the Phenomenon and Origin of Play." *Philosophy and Phenomenological Research,* I (June, 1941), 470–478.

Bowen, Wilbur P. and Mitchell, Elmer D. "The Philosophy of Play" in The *Theory of Organized Play.* New York: A. S. Barnes, 1927.

Brooks, J. D., and Whiting, H. T. A. *Human Movement: A Field of Study.* Lafayette, Ind.: Bart Publishers, 1973.

Browne, Evelyn. "An Ethological Theory of Play." *Journal of Health, Physical Education, and Recreation,* 39 (September, 1968), 36–39.

Caillois, Roger. "Unity of Play; Diversity of Games." *Diogenes,* 19 (Fall, 1957), 92–121.

Caillois, Roger. "Play and the Sacred" in *Man and the Sacred.* Translated by Meyer Barash. Illinois: Free Press of Glencoe, 1959.

Caillois, Roger. *Man, Play, and Games.* Translated by Meyer Barash. New York: Free Press of Glencoe, 1961.

Carlisle, R. "The Concept of Physical Education." *Proceedings of the Annual Conference of the Philosophy of Education Society of Great Britain.*

Champlin, Nathaniel. "Are Sports Methodic?" *The Journal of the Philosophy of Sport,* IV (Fall, 1977), 104–116.

Chase, Stuart. "Play." *Whither Mankind.* Edited by Charles A. Beard. New York: Longmans, Green and Company, 1928.

Cox, Harvey. "Faith as Play" in *The Feast of Fools: A Theological Essay on Festivity and Fantasy.* Cambridge: Harvard University Press, 1969.

Dearden, R. F. "The Concept of Play." *The Concept of Education.* Edited by R. S. Peters. London: Routledge & Kegan Paul, 1967.

Ehrmann, Jacques. "Homo Ludens Revisited." *Game, Play, Literature.* Edited by Jacques Ehrmann. Boston: Beacon Press, 1971.

Fogelin, Robert J. "Sport: The Diversity of the Concept." Unpublished paper presented at the annual meeting of the American Association for the Advancement of Science, Dallas, Texas, December, 1968.

Fox, Larry. "A Linguistic Analysis of the Concept 'Health' In Sport." *Journal of the Philosophy of Sport,* II (September, 1975), 31–35.

Giddens, A. "Notes on the Concept of Play and Leisure." *Sociological Review,* 12 (March, 1964), 73–89.

Graves, H. "A Philosophy of Sport." *Contemporary Review,* LXXVII, (December, 1900), 877–893.

Grazia, Sebastion de. *Of Time, Work, and Leisure.* New York: Twentieth Century Fund, 1962.

Groos, Karl. *The Play of Man.* New York: D. Appleton, 1901.

Gulick, Luther Halsey. "Psychological, Pedagogical, and Religious Aspects of Group Games." *Pedagogical Seminary* (now *Journal of Genetic Psychology*), 6 (1899), 135–151.

Gulick, Luther Halsey. *A Philosophy of Play.* New York: Charles Scribner's Sons, 1920.

Huizinga, Johan. *Homo Ludens.* London: Routledge & Kegan Paul, 1950.

Jeu, Bernard. "*What is Sport?*" Diogenes, 80 (1972), 150–163.

Jolivet, Regis. "Work, Play, Contemplation." Translated by Sister M. Delphone. *Philosophy Today,* V (Summer, 1961), 114–120.

Kaplan, Max. "Games and Sport as Leisure" in *Leisure in America: A Social Inquiry.* New York: John Wiley & Sons, 1960.

Keating, James W. "Sportsmanship as a Moral Category." *Ethics,* LXXV (October, 1964), 25–35.

Keating, James W. "The Urgent Need for Definitions and Distinctions." *Physical Educator,* 28 (March, 1971), 41–42.

Kleinman, Seymour. "*Toward a Non-Theory of Sport.*" Quest, X (May, 1968), 29–34.

Krug, Orvis. "The Philosophical Relationship Between Physical Education and Athletics." Unpublished Ed. D. dissertation, New York University, 1–58.

Loy, John Jr. "The Nature of Sport: A Definitional Effort." *Quest,* X (May, 1968), 1–15.

Manser, Anthony. "Games and Family Resemblances." *Philosophy,* XVII (July, 1967), 210–255.

McBride, Frank. "Toward a Non-Definition of Sport." *Journal of the Philosophy of Sport,* II (Sept., 1975), 4–11.

Melvin, Bruce L. "Play, Recreation, and Leisure Time." *Proceedings of the Sixty-Third Annual Meeting of the College Physical Education Association.* Washington, DC, 1960.

Metheny, Eleanor. "This 'Thing' Called Sport." *Journal of Health, Physical Education, and Recreation,* 40 (March, 1969), 59–60.

Miller, David L. *Gods and Games: Toward a Theology of Play.* New York: World Publishing Company, 1970.

Morgan, William J. "Some Aristotelian Notes on the Attempt to Define Sport." *Journal of the Philosophy of Sport,* IV (Sept., 1977), 15–35.

Neale, Robert E. *In Praise of Play.* New York: Harper & Row, 1969.

Osterhoudt, Robert. *An Introduction to the Philosophy of Physical Education and Sport.* Champaign, Illinois: Stipes Publishing Company, 1977.

Osterhoudt, Robert G., Ed. *The Philosophy of Sport.* Springfield, Illinois: Charles C Thomas, 1973.

Paddick, Robert J. "What Makes Physical Activity Physical?" *Journal of the Philosophy of Sport,* II (Sept., 1975), 12–22.

Paddick, Robert Joseph. "The Nature of a Field of Knowledge in Physical Education." Unpublished Master's thesis, University of Alberta, 1967.

Patrick, G. T. W. "The Play of a Nation." *Scientific Monthly*, 13 (October, 1921), 350–362.

Petrie, Brian Malcom. "Physical Activity, Games, and Sport: A System of Classification and an Investigation of Social Influences Among Students of Michigan State University." Unpublished Ph.D. dissertation, Michigan State University, 1970.

Potter, Stephen. "The Game Itself" in *The Theory and Practice of Gamesmanship*. New York: Bantam Books, 1965. (First published New York: Holt, Rinehart and Winston, 1948).

Renshaw, Peter. "The Nature of Human Movement Studies and Its Relationship with Physical Education." *Quest*, XX (June, 1973), 79–86.

Roberts, John M., Arth, Malcom J. and Bush, Robert R. "Games in Culture." *American Anthropologist*, 61 (August, 1959), 597–605.

Rossi, Ernest Lawrence. "Game and Growth: Two Dimensions of our Psychotherapeutic Zeitgeist." *Journal of Humanistic Psychology*, 7 (Fall, 1967), 139–154.

Roszak, Theodore. "Forbidden Games." Wayne State University Graduate *Comment*, X (1967), 25–34. (Reprinted in *Sport in the Socio-Cultural Process*. Edited by M. Marie Hárt. Dubuque, Iowa: WM. C. Brown, 1972).

Sapora, Allen V. and Mitchell, Elmer D. "Definitions and Characteristics of Play and Recreation" in *The Theory of Play and Recreation*. Third Edition. New York: Ronald Press, 1948.

Schmitz, Kenneth L. "Sport and Play: Suspension of the Ordinary." Unpublished paper presented at the annual meeting of the American Association for the Advancement of Science, Dallas, Texas, December 28, 1968.

Slusher, Howard S. *Man, Sport and Existence*. Philadelphia: Lea & Febiger, 1967.

Steinbeck, John. "Then My Arm Glassed Up." *Sports Illustrated*, 23 (December 20, 1965), 94–102.

Stone, Gregory P. "Some Meanings of American Sport." College Physical Education Association. *Proceedings of the 60th Annual Meeting*. Columbus, Ohio, 1957. (Reprinted in *Sport and American Society*. Edited by George H. Sage. Massachusetts: Addison-Wesley, 1970).

Stone, Gregory P. "Some Meanings of American Sport: An Extended View." *Aspects of Contemporary Sport Sociology*. Proceedings of C.I.C. Symposium on the Sociology of Sport. Edited by Gerald S. Kenuon. Illinois: The Athletic Institute, 1969.

Suits, Bernard. "The Elements of Sport." *The Philosophy of Sport: A Collection of Original Essays*. Edited by Robert G. Osterhoudt. Illinois: Charles C Thomas, 1973.

Suits, Bernard. "What is a Game." *Philosophy of Science*, 34 (June, 1967), 148–156.

Suits, Bernard. "Words on Play." *Journal of the Philosophy of Sport*, IV (Sept., 1977), 117–131.

Sutton-Smith, Brian. "A Formal Analysis of Game Meaning." *Western Folklore*, XVIII (January, 1959), 13–24.

Thomas, Duane. "Sport: The Conceptual Enigma." *Journal of the Philosophy of Sport*, III (Sept., 1976), 35–41.

VanderZwagg, Harold J. "Sport: Existential or Essential?" *Quest*, IXX (May, 1969), 47–56.

VanderZwagg, Harold J. "Sports Concepts." *Journal of Health, Physical Education, and Recreation*, 41(March, 1970), 35–36.

VanderZwagg, Harold J. *Toward a Philosophy of Sport*. Reading, Mass.: Addison-Wesley, 1972.

Vernes, Jean-Rene. "The Element of Time in Competitive Games." Translated by Victor A. Velen. *Diogenes*, 50 (September, 1965), 25–42.

Weiss, Paul. "Records and the Man." *Philosophic Exchange*, 1 (Summer, 1972), 89–97.

SECTION II

Sport and Metaphysical Speculations

One of the major issues addressed by philosophy concerns the question "what is the fundamental nature or constitution of reality?" The field of inquiry formally committed to the study of this question is known as metaphysics. Simply defined then, metaphysics is the study of reality. But it hardly needs to be said that other forms of inquiry, most notably the natural and social sciences, deal with the reality-question as well. Hence, the principal difference between metaphysical and scientific inquiry lies not so much in the question itself but rather in the breadth in which the question is considered. That is, although it is certainly true that science deals with reality, it always does so in quite discrete ways: partitioning off various strata of reality for critical study (e.g., the biological sciences of physics and chemistry examine respectively the structural and functional properties of reality). Metaphysics, on the other hand, does not fragment the reality-question, and thus the analysis corresponding to it, into such discrete segments, but rather retains the comprehensive flavor of the question by considering it in its most general form. Metaphysics is best defined, then, by the synoptic intent it brings to this question, an intent that presupposes the highest order of generality.

The question regarding the general nature of reality can itself be asked in three more definite ways. First, one can ask what is reality with regard to nature or the world. This branch of metaphysics carries the formal name of cosmology. Secondly, one can ask what is reality with regard to a divine entity or condition. This form of metaphysical inquiry is

formally known as theology. And third, one can inquire into the nature of reality from the standpoint of human existence. This latter type of study is called ontology. However, because cosmological investigations have been, for the most part, preempted by the far-reaching advances of modern science, and because theology has insulated itself as a separate area of inquiry in the contemporary epoch, the field of ontology has assumed the forefront of metaphysical inquiry. Not surprisingly, the preeminence of this latter type of metaphysical study has duly recorded itself in the literature concerning metaphysics and sport, and accordingly, in the readings selected for this edition (all of which consider the being-status of sport from the standpoint of human existence).

Clearly one of the classical pieces of work in this area is Eugen Fink's "The Ontology of Play." The basic thesis Fink advances in this essay is that play is a fundamental, irreducible, mode of human existence, one that, although far removed from the plane of reflective thought, presupposes a certain self-conscious awareness of our being-human. The selection from Sartre entitled "Play and Sport," extracted from Part IV of his *magum opus Being and Nothingness*, presents one of the most provocative accounts of play in the literature. Sartre's discussion of play is preceded by a lengthy analysis which argues that virtually all of our human strivings (work, science, art) can be reduced to the general category of desire known as "having": that category which establishes the self's (*pour soi*) basic relation to objects or things (*en soi*) as one in which the former seeks to possess, appropriate, dominate, own, or use the latter. Yet, according to Sartre, there remains one human enterprise which apparently cannot be subsumed under this possessive relationship. And that enterprise is play whose goal is not to possess the object(s) of its concern but to provide expressive outlet for the realization of the player's unique subjectivity. But on closer inspection, argues Sartre, even play discloses itself to be at bottom "possessive" towards the world of objects and things. Netzky's essay, "Playful Freedom: Sartre's Ontology Reappraised," presents a critical rejoinder to Sartre's imputation of an appropriative element to play, and in so doing, opens up the possibility of a genuine, supramundane form of existence: namely, playful existence.

In "Athletics and Angst: Reflections on the Philosophical Relevance of Play," Hyland develops an ontology of play based on Martin Heidegger's major work *Being and Time*. Hyland's basic thesis is that in the exigencies of the sportive contest many issues of life itself are brought into sharp relief. One of the more important, but less obvious, of such issues is that sport offers an opportunity to experience oneself as a complete (whole) human being in a world that furnishes, for the most part, only fragmented experiences of one's self. In "Play and Possibility," Joseph Esposito argues that the core experience of play, when considered most fundamentally from the player's perspective, is the experience of "possibility." According to this view then, play activities are contrived human settings which are structured in such a way that the player is confronted with a variety of possibilities in the form of obstacles or challenges to be overcome. The purpose of the game is precisely to confront the player with such possibilities.

Morgan's "An Analysis of the Futural Modality of Sport" exacts an account of sport in terms of the future dimension of human time. In this regard, he argues that sport is rooted in a distinctive (non-everyday) projection of the future. Morgan concludes that the special status of sport's futural orientation allows the self to experience its temporality in a fulfilled manner as opposed to the empty and inconsequential way in which such temporality is experienced in training, and by extension, everyday life. Algozin's essay, "Man and Sport," argues the view that our fascination with sport can ultimately be traced to our human yearning for what he calls "unalienated action." Because most of our everyday activities are of the alienated variety, according to Algozin, people thirst for activities such as sport; for

insofar as the sportive situation clearly marks off success (victory) from failure (defeat) and makes provision for the fulfillment of these tangible goals, it qualifies as a form of unalienated activity.

Jaspers' "Limits of the Life-Order: Sport" and Harper's "Man Alone" both discuss sport from the perspective of humanity's so-termed contemporary predicament wherein the self finds itself at the mercy of the masses, bereft of any semblance of individuality and identified exclusively with the daily function it performs in and for mass-life. On Jaspers' account, there is a certain tension manifest in the individual's life between the desire to safeguard existence, which leads one in the direction of mass-life, and the desire to express existence, which leads one in the direction of selfhood. Interestingly enough, Jaspers treats sport in terms of both elements of this dyadic impulse structure. On the one hand, sport is described as giving vent to the self-preservative impulse, and on the other, as making provision for the expression of one's individuality. Harper, however, stakes a greater claim for sport arguing, in effect, that sport can and does allow the self to break the fetters of its public existence and fully realize itself as a unique, singular being. For Harper the potential for this experience of the self in sport is linked to the state of solitude engendered in the latter whereby the self is pressed to accept personal responsibility for its acts, and in so doing, to come to grips with the self revealed therein.

The last two essays of this section, Gerber's "Identity, Relation and Sport" and Hyland's "Competition and Friendship," focus their central attention on the development of individuality through a meaningful encounter with the significant "others" of the sport situation. In the first of these pieces, Gerber develops an account of sport as a dialogical relation between players, a relation, moreover, that exhibits all the essential features of Buber's authentic I–Thou relationship. In the second, Hyland examines the relation between competitive play and friendship, a relation not altogether unproblematic given that competition in play often leads to alienation as opposed to friendship. He concludes in this regard, based on a conception of human nature as both monadic and relational, that not only are competition and friendship compatible in the play sphere, but that competitive encounters steeped in friendship represent the highest forms of competitive play.

The readings included herein thus explore the nature of sport in terms of various elements of the human condition. The principal question at issue is simply this: what is the reality—status of sport? The question itself can be variously framed: What is the fundamental nature of sport? What form of being is peculiar to sport? What are the essential features of sport? How can sport be likened to or distinguished from other kindred human movement phenomena (play, exercise, game, dance)? What relation obtains between sport and other human strivings (on the intramundane level of everyday existence and the supramundane level of science, art, religion and philosophy)? The whole array of issues considered in metaphysical inquiry also present themselves for critical inspection when focused more specifically on sport. Thus, such themes as the mind—body relation, finitude, infinitude, time, space and freedom become viable topics of inquiry for those interested in the metaphysics of sport.

Basically, there are three ways or approaches one can take in attempting to answer such questions. (These approaches are by no means exclusive to metaphysics but characterize the whole field of philosophic inquiry and thus extend to the other major areas of philosophy: knowledge and value.) First of all, one may develop the implications of major philosophic schools of thought (naturalism, realism, idealism, pragmatism, existentialism, . . .) for issues central to sport. Second, one may develop the implications of the philosophic systems advanced by major philosophers (e.g., Plato, Aristotle, Kant) for issues of specific interest to sport. And last, one may simply launch into a direct philosophic examination of one or more of the issues cited above. Because of the philosophic acumen and originality presupposed by the latter approach, it is clearly the most difficult of the three.

Those interested in a further study of sport from the metaphysical perspective will find ample reading material in this area. A brief sketch of some of the major work dealing with this topic includes the following. Hyland (1977) interprets play as a natural (in the Aristotelian sense) human stance rooted in "responsive openness." Morgan's essay (1976) attempts to develop some directives for constructing an ontology of sport. Novak's recent book (1976) argues that sport qualifies as a form of natural religion. Lawton (1976) ties Novak's work on sport to his other writings all of which point, according to the author, to a developing theology of culture. Garrett (1976) investigates the particular sport of baseball in terms of the categories of articulation and perspective.

Roochnik's essay (1975), in a similar vein to Hyland's work, suggests that play is best regarded as a stance people assume toward various activities and, in turn, that sport is one particularly meaningful place in which human beings can play. Herman (1975) rejects a mechanistic interpretation (one developed by Descartes and refined by Skinner in his conception of operant behaviorism) of life in general and sport in particular. Fraleigh (1975) takes a look at some of the different senses of purpose commonly attributed to sporting activity. Meier (1975) considers the potential for authentic existence in sport. Morgan (1975) examines sport from the perspective of human time. Hinman (1974) develops a comprehensive interpretation of Nietzsche's musings on man and the world from the standpoint of play. Gebauer (1973) forges a characterization of sport as a reconstructed world with its own peculiar meaning context. Krell (1972) provides an indepth examination of Fink's analysis of play focusing on his conception of human play and world play. Weiss (1969) considers the metaphysical status of sport in the closing chapter of his book. Metheny (1968) analyzes the basic character of the kindred phenomena of movement, sport, exercise and dance.

Harper (1971) and Thompson (1967) approach this subject from the methodological perspective of phenomenology. Both have written dissertations which are extensive analyses of aspects of the human condition in a specific sport situation. The search for being through the medium of sport is the focus of Slusher's major work (1967). Slusher takes up this topic again in a later essay (1972) arguing that sport should be conducted in such a manner that it allows the athlete to fully realize his individual potential.

The most comprehensive work on sport and relation is Kretchmar's dissertation (1971) in which he develops an account of the "other" in sport. In more recent work (1975, 1973), Kretchmar refines his early work on relation in sport looking more specifically at the competitive strife and the types of personal and interpersonal relations generated therein. Meier (1976) analyzes two forms of interpersonal communication, exemplified by the expressions "kinship of the rope" and "loving struggle," integral to the sport of mountain climbing. Kleinman (1975) also considers the relation that obtains between the self and the "other" within the competitive framework of sport.

Fraleigh (1973) investigates the different forms of freedom available to the participant in sport. Coutts (1968) and Slusher (1967) critically examine this issue as well.

Although metaphysical analysis has all too often been dismissed as a lofty exercise of abstract cognition that has little, if any, import for the so-termed "real" world, of interest only to those of a similar abstract cast of mind, a more serious perusal of this matter reveals the reverse of this assertion to be true. That is, when the issue is pressed more fully it is apparent that the various ways in which we envisage the nature of sport, our ideas about what sort of "thing" it is, reflect themselves in the actual way we regard sport. By and large then, the worth of our lived involvement in sport, of our practice and conduct of it, is contingent on the worth of the ideas that undergird this involvement. Unfortunately, more often than not our notion of what sport "is" has been determined by popular acclaim, a state of affairs that no doubt has much to do

with its present corrupt state. This latter point notwithstanding, it is precisely in terms of the apparent close relation between our thoughts about the nature of something and our regard for that thing(s) that the relevance of metaphysics reveals itself; for in assuming a metaphysical posture towards (say) sport no abstract flight away from the "real" world context of this phenomenon is intended, but rather a more critical and abiding basis for this sphere of action. What generally gets confused for abstract indifference with respect to metaphysics in this regard is the metaphysician's refusal to leave matters concerning this lived context of experience to the caprice and artifice of popular opinion. In this sense, metaphysics represents one of the most fundamental ways in which the world in general and sport in particular can be addressed, and paradoxically, efforts to have it banished as unduly abstract at bottom show themselves to be flights, of the most pernicious sort, away from "reality."

The Ontology of Play*

EUGEN FINK

In an age characterized by the noise of the machine, the role of play, in the structure of human life becomes more and more apparent. Not only the expert analysts of civilization, educators and specialists in anthropology as well are agreed on this point. Modern man himself has become aware of the importance of play. Contemporary literature and the passionate interest in games and sports are evidence enough. For modern man play is a vital-impulse with its own value and sphere of activity, participated in for its own sake. It is a kind of reward for the unpleasantness that goes with material progress in modern technocracy. It is also seen as a means of rejuvenating one's inner vitality, a return to the morning freshness of life at its origin, to the source of one's creative powers. In human history there have certainly been times a good deal more gay, more relaxed, more given to play than our own; when there was more play, when men had more leisure and were more familiar with the Muses. However no other age has had so many possibilities and occasions for play. Never has there been such a systematic exploitation of life on a grand scale. Playfields and stadiums are in the original plans of cities. Games in vogue in different countries are brought to international com-

* From *Philosophy Today*, 4 (Summer, 1960), 95-110. English translation by Sister M. Delphine from *Oase des Glucks Gedanken zu einer Onto-logie des Spiels*. Freiburg in Br.: Alber-Verlag, 1957.

petitions. Playing materials are mass-produced. But it is still in question whether our age has reached a deep understanding of the nature of play. Can we evaluate the many meanings of the term or thoroughly penetrate the aspect of being in the phenomenon-play? Do we know what constitutes play and specifies it from the philosophic point of view?

We want to consider that strange and very particular mode of being that characterizes the play of man, to conceptualize the elements that make up its being and give rough draft of the speculative concept of play. To some this subject may seem dry and abstract. We would surely prefer something of the very atmosphere of play with a lightness of touch in treating the subject, stressing its creative fullness, its over-flowing richness and its inexhaustible attraction. A brilliant essay could be written, a game with the reader discovering the hidden sense of words and ideas through the surprise effect of a play on words; something pertaining to a literary *genre* rather than a treatise on play. In using a serious approach there is the feeling of betraying the very nature of play. Philosophy, as with Plato, has made contributions poetic-wise in the domain of speculative thought. A consideration of play in the same vein might achieve the same end, since the subject itself is provocative of a sublime play of the spirit. But such a treatment demands something of the Attic wit. Our consideration, therefore, will be simple, with no pretence to poetry. It will be in three parts: a preliminary characterization of the phenomenon-play; the analysis of its structure; the relation of play and being.

I

Play is a vital fact which each of us knows subjectively. Everyone has taken part in play and can speak of it from experience. It is hardly necessary to make it the subject of scientific research to discover it and to disengage it from other phenomena. Play is universally known. Each of us understands it in its many forms. Our experience is all the evidence we need. Each of us has been a player. Moreover, familiarity with play is more than individual. It is a public act in which all can participate. Play is an accepted and ever recurring fact of the social world. We live through abandon[ing] ourselves to it, we recognize it as an ever possible act. Through play we find ourselves no longer imprisoned and isolated on our own individuality. In play we are assured of a social contact of particular intensity. All play, even that which seems to turn in upon oneself, such as that of the solitary child, has a social dimension. The fact that we actually live ourselves into the act of play, approaching it as something interior to ourselves, makes man as the subject of the attribute-play. However does man alone play? Can we say that animals play, the vitality of each living creature expressing itself exteriorly in a sort of joy of living? Biology, it is true, presents us with some interesting cases of animal behavior which occasionally resemble the play of human beings. It would be a mistake, however, to consider these on the same plane in terms of constituent elements, as if surface resemblance presupposes identity in mode of being. We can certainly formulate a biological concept of behavior in play which would link man and animal from the point of view of animality. But this would say nothing about the mode of being behind the exterior manifestations which resemble each other. We cannot proceed with the discussion from this point of view until the question of the ontological mode of being of man and animal is clarified. In our opinion human play possesses a meaning and exclusiveness of its own. Only a halting metaphor can be used to apply it to the case of either animals or the ancient gods. In the final analysis, what is important is the way in which the term "play" is applied, the fullness of meaning attributed to it, its delimitation in terms of reference, the conceptual penetration we give it.

We propose the question of human play,

beginning with the fact such as moments of play, we are freed by it, we understand it in our daily experience. Play does not enter into our lives as simply as vegetative processes. It is always a process that has a meaning, a lived experience. All our life consists in enjoying this act (which does not require reflexive consciousness). Generally, if we give ourselves over to play, we are far from reflection. And yet, all play presupposes the awareness of our own activity. There is a current and rather pedestrian view of play, a sort of vulgar interpretation: that play is nothing more than a phenomenon on the margin of human life, a peripheral fact, an occasional sort of thing. The more important moments of our existence lie elsewhere. We consistently hear it opposed to the serious occupations of life that are filled with a sense of responsibility; it is referred to as "recreation," "relaxation," and "diversion." It is claimed that life finds its fulfillment in the difficult pursuit of knowledge, in moral excellence or a professional attitude of mind, in prestige, in dignity and honor, in power, prosperity and similar goals. Play, on the other hand, seems to be like an occasional break, a pause that highlights the more genuine and serious aspects of life, like a dream opposed to being awake. From time to time, it is argued, man should slip from under the yoke of slavery, free himself from the shame of always starting over, lift the weight of the daily grind, quit watching the clock—for a more leisurely pace, perhaps even squandering time. In the economy of life "tension" alternates with "relaxation," business with leisure. We prescribe for ourselves "weeks of hard work" and "holidays for merry-making." Thus play seems to have a legitimate but quite restricted place in the vital rhythm man has set himself. Play is an *ergänzung*, a supplementary thing, a recreative pause, a surcease from burdens, a ray of light over the darker and severe landscape of life. By force of habit we limit play by contrasting it to the seriousness of life, to an attitude of moral commitment, to work—to all the prosaic things of reality. We identify it with frolic, with flight toward the regions of imagination, away from the hard realities of life to dreams and utopia. It exists just to keep man from succumbing to the modern world of work, from forgetting how to laugh amid moral rigorism, from becoming the prisoner to duty. Analysts of civilization recommend play to ward off disasters. It takes on a therapeutic value against the ills of the soul. But the question is, how does such advice understand the very nature of play? As a peripheral phenomenon in contrast to the serious? Can we never look at it except in terms of work, of a drive against odds? Is there not within us a little of that divine detachment of spirit, of the joyous buoyancy of play that joins us to the "birds of the air" and the "lilies of the field?" Is play only for preventing psychic disorders that trouble men in the modern world? As long as we accept such implications, "play and work," "play and the realities of life," play cannot be thought of in its proper sense and in its true ontological dimensions. It remains in the shadow of phenomena seemingly opposed to it, which obscure and deform it. It is considered as the non-serious, the non-obligatory, the non-authentic, as mere idleness. It is precisely by the very way in which its salutary effects are praised that we prove our estimation of it as a marginal phenomena, a peripheral counterbalance or as a sort of ingredient adding flavor to the insipidity of our existence.

It is even doubtful that such a view gives an adequate understanding of play as phenomenon. It is true that the behavior of adults shows less and less of the grace natural to play. Too often their games are nothing more than an organized escape from boredom. An adult seldom plays naturally. But for a child, play is the undisturbed center of existence. It is the very stuff of child-life. As age forces him to leave this center, the rude storms of life get the upper hand. Duty, care and work use up the vital energies of the adolescent. As the serious side of life asserts itself, the importance of play diminishes. We usually consider how we can educate the child to pass smoothly from a being who plays into one that works. We present work to the child under the aspect of play, as a methodical and disciplinary game where the burden becomes unnoticeably heavier little by little. The point is to keep a maximum of spontaneity, imagination and initiative as in play, to create a kind of joy in work. This well-known pedagogical experience is based on the general conviction that while play is inherent in man, especially during childhood, it occupies a less conspicuous place with the advancement of age. The play of the child shows more freely certain traits characteristic of human play. It is more ingenuous, less equivocal and dissimulating than the play of adults. The child knows little about the seduction of masquerading. It plays in all innocence. But how much hidden play is disguised in the serious affairs of the adult world, in honors, social conventions; how much hidden drama in the meeting of lovers. Everything considered, per-

haps we would not want to say that ideal play is that of the child. The adult can also play, but in a different way that is more furtive, more masked. If we take our notion of play from the world of the child alone, we misunderstand its nature, fall into equivocation. In fact, the domain of play extends from the little girl's playing with a doll to the tragedy. Play is not only a peripheral manifestation of human life, it is not a contingent phenomenon that emerges upon occasion. In essence, it comes under the ontological dispositions of human existence. It is a fundamentally existential phenomenon. It is not derived from any other manifestation of life. To oppose play to any other phenomenon is to risk misunderstanding it. On the other hand, we must recognize that the fundamental phenomena which are decisive in human existence are all interlaced and intertwined. They never appear isolated or juxtaposed against one another. They interpenetrate, interinfluence. Each has a hold over the whole of man. To throw light upon the reciprocal influence of the moments of existence, the tensions and harmonies, is the task of an anthropology not limited to the description of biological, psychic and intellectual facts, but which penetrates by intuition the paradoxes of lived existence.

Man, at every stage of existence, is marked by the all-pervasive proximity of death, inescapable. And in so far as he has a body and sensitive life, he is affected by his relations to the earth which both resists him and yields its riches. The same is true of domination and love, all his dealings with his fellowmen. In his essence man is mortal; by nature he works, he struggles, and by the same count, he plays. Death, work, domination, love and play, these are the elements of the patterns which we find in human existence, so enigmatic and ambiguous. And if Schiller says, ". . . A man is whole only when he plays," it is also true to say that he is whole only when he works, struggles, opposes death and loves. We cannot draw up principles for an interpretation of human existence without referring to these fundamental phenomena. It will be sufficient to say in passing, though, that all of them are manifested in changing, enigmatically and ambiguous ways. The principal reason is that man is exposed and abandoned and at the same time watched over and protected. He is not completely carried along by instinct like the animal, nor is he as free as the immaterial angel. His is a freedom in the midst of a nature which binds him to an obscure tendency which permeates his being. And he simply integrates it into his knowledge of his own existence. On the other hand, free acts completely control his life. Because of this mingling of self-expression and repression, his existence is a continual tension within the self. We live within ourselves constantly preoccupied with ourselves. Only the vital being, of whom it can be said that "into his being he goes with his own being," can die, work, struggle, love and play. Only such a being is in touch with surrounding reality and the total environment—the world. To be related to self, to understand being and to reveal oneself to the world, this triple moment is known perhaps less easily in play than in the other fundamental phenomena of human existence.

But that is why play exists. It is act in its spontaneity, acting in its very activity, the living impulse. Play is life that moves within its own orbit. However, the moving forces of play do not coincide with the other forces of human life. For in all action other than play— whether it be the simple "praxis" which has its end in itself or the production of the artist (*poiesis*) where the end is the work—there is essentially implied a tendency toward the end of man, toward beatitude, toward *Eudaimonía*. We are busy finding the virtuous path to the fullness of life. For us life is a "task." Consequently, at no moment can we be said to have a place of rest. We are aware of the fact that we are "travelers." The violence of our vital project constantly lifts us out of the established moment to carry us toward a life of virtue and happiness. Thus we are compelled to attain *Eudaimonía,* though we are not in agreement as to what it is. We are not only moved by aspirations that uplift us, we are not at rest until we can give the one and only "interpretation" of this happiness. It is one of the paradoxes of human existence that in the incessant pursuit of *Eudaimonía* we never attain it; we cannot be happy in the sense of perfect achievement in this life. While we breathe, our life is caught in a vertiginous cascade. We are carried forward by the desire to perfect and complete our fragmentary being. We live in terms of the future. We experience the present moment as a preparation, as a stage, as a passing phase. This strange "futurism" of man's life is bound up with his fundamental character. We are not a simple fact like plants and animals. We force ourselves to find a "meaning" in our existence. We must understand the reason for our life on earth. It is a demon-like urge which drives man to search for an interpretation of his earthly journey, a passion of the soul. Something with-

in makes man search for the source of his grandeur as well as his misery. No other creature is troubled in his very being by the question of the mysterious meaning of his existence. The animal cannot and God has no need to ask the question. All human response to the question of the meaning of life means that man has an end which will finally be attained. With most men the position is not explicit, but their conduct is directed by the basic idea which they form of the "supreme good." The different ends which permeate our daily life are ordered in terms of a principle which harmonized their oppositions and indicates the final end. Particular ends are linked to what the community considers the absolute end of man.

Within this architectonic ordering of ends all human work is carried on. The serious side of life is developed, authentic attitudes are produced and confirmed. But the tragic element in man's situation is that he cannot guarantee in any absolute sense his final end by his own efforts. When the major question of his existence is brought up, he gropes in the night unless a superhuman power comes to his aid. That is why the confusion of Babel reigns among men as soon as we ask what can be the true end, the destination, the true happiness of human nature. This is also why unrest, anxiety and uncertainties are characteristic of human life.

But play fits into this situation in a way quite different from any other human activity. It stands out in remarkable relief to all that characterizes life teleologically. It cannot be expressed in terms of the architectonic complex of ends. It does not fall under the final end as do other actions. Its activity is not disturbed by the fundamental uncertainties which we take into account in interpreting happiness. If we compare play to the rest of life with its impetuous dynamism, its provoking orientation toward the future, play appears as a serene "presence" with a meaning sufficient to itself. It is like an oasis of happiness found in the desert of our questing, which in itself recalls the punishment of Tantalus. Play enraptures us. During play we are momentarily freed from the daily grind and, as it were, magically transported to another planet where life seems more light, more carefree, more happy. We often hear that play is a gratuitous activity, without finality. This is not exactly the case. Considered as a whole, play is determined by an internal end and we will discover in its different stages the particular ends which form a whole. However, the immanent end of play is not directed as that of the other activities of man toward the supreme end. The activity of play has only internal finalities which do not transcend it. This brings to mind that particular form of play that is seen in terms of its physical attraction: military formation. For the sake of our well being, play is here found in an adulterated form, an activity in view of an end other than its own. Play is here in terms of ends extraneous to its nature and it is not easy to see just how much value comes from it as play. It is precisely because play in an unadulterated form is self-sufficient that it possesses a complete and firmly established meaning which makes it possible for man to find in it an asylum in time where time itself is no longer that torrent which carries us forward. It is rather a respite with a spark of eternity in it. It is apparently the child, therefore, who plays best. Again it is the child who knows that relation to time most intimately of which the poet Rilke speaks:

O childhood hours, behind whose make-believe
Was hid more than the past and before us lay
No future to contend. Though we dreamed, 'tis true
Of growing up and were perhaps in haste to be well grown,
More was it for the love of being those
Who had no other merit than being grown.
While yet not hid from life, we tasted joy
Which gives repose and were suspended thence
In an interval between the universe and play, a place,
From all eternity, chosen for the pure event.
                    (Rilke, *Duineser Elegien—*
                              Vierte Elegie)

For the adult, play is a strange oasis, a place of rest filled with dreaming along the relentless, pressing course of life. Play gives us a "presence." But it does not reach into the silent depths of the soul where we listen to the eternal breathing of the universe and contemplate pure images in the stream of passing things. Play is activity, creative force, and still it is near what is unchangeable and eternal. Play breaks the continuity of life's course, its coherence which determines the final end. It cuts across the groove in which life ordinarily runs. It sees things "at a distance." However, in seeming to subtract from the unified current of life, it sets up a relation in a meaningful manner: the representation which it gives of it. When, as is the custom, we do not restrict play by relating it to work, to reality, to the serious, to the authentic, we commit the fault of not placing it with the other phenomena of

existence. For play is itself a fundamental phenomenon of existence, just as original and basic in itself as death, work and domination. Only it is not linked to the other fundamental phenomena in a common pursuit of the ultimate end. It confronts them, as has been pointed out, to use them representationally. We play with the serious, the authentic, the real. We play with work and struggle, love and death. We even play with play.

II

Let us look at the matter a little more closely. In making the initial step in understanding this valuable concept of play, we must examine the articulations and the structure of the whole of play just as it is.

We can indicate at first sight, as an essential element of play, that it is a passion of the soul. We can say that all man is and does is colored by either one or the other states of the soul—joy, sadness or the gray tone of indifference. Play, at least in its source, has the coloring of joy. Joy reigns in it as undisputed master at each moment, carrying it forward and giving it wings. As soon as the joy is gone, the action disappears. This does not mean that throughout the duration of play we must be gay and in good humor. The joy arising from play is a singular pleasure, difficult to put your finger on. It does not resemble the pleasures of the senses in the relaxation of the body or the physical intoxication with speed. On the other hand, neither is it a purely spiritual delight, sheer intellectual joy. It is a joy rooted in a most special creative activity, open to many interpretations. It can include a profound sadness, a tragic suffering. It can embrace the most striking contraries. The pleasure which accompanies tragic action from one end to the other draws its power of ecstasy and emotion, mixed with terror and rapture, from the reign of the dreadful. The representation of horror is the source of the pleasure. Play transfigures even the mask of the Gorgon.

What is that strange pleasure which drastically mixes contraries, overlapping one with the other, leaving joy in the first place? However moved to tears we may be, we smile at the comedy and tragedy which are our life and which the play represents to us. Does the pleasure of play include the suffering and grief thus presented to us in this evocation because the action refers to past afflictions and time has softened them? Or is it that the turning back of the wheel of time alleviates the living bitterness, the sorrows formerly so real? By no means. In play we do not experience "real pain"—and, yet, the emotion of play gives rise to a strange type of pain which, actually but not really, moves us, seizes us, touches us, shakes us. The sorrow is only played, but even modified by play it is still a power that moves us. It has this capacity only because the delights of play include it. This delight is indispensable to the activity of play. We cannot compare it to other known forms of functional pleasure. It is true that we always feel a sense of well-being unrelated to any object whenever we do not submit our life passively but offer our being with spontaneous initiative, direct it in assuming responsibilities and mold it in creative processes. The creative quality of existence is in itself a "surge forward." But the fulfillment of play is accompanied by a pleasure which we cannot compare with the joys experienced in any other action or psychic urge. The pleasure in play is grounded not only in the element of creative spontaneity— it is also the ecstasy which accompanies our entry into any "universe," into the objective world. It is not only the pleasure experienced in playing, but a joyous attitude with regard to play as well.

A second step in studying the structure of play is to point out the meaning play establishes. Each type of play, as far as we can see, establishes a certain meaning. But purely physical movement, exercising arms and legs by repeating certain rhythms is not play in the strict sense of the word. It is simply confusing to call play such behavior as that of relaxing indulged in by young animals and children. These movements bring no meaning whatsoever to their author. We can speak of play only when the meaning of a specific end creatively accompanies such movements. Furthermore, in a particular game, we must distinguish between the intrinsic meaning of play —the meaningful bond between things, actions and played relations—and the external meaning, the meaning of play for those who initiate it and take part in it, as well as the meaning it is supposed to have for the spectators. It is evident that there are games which include spectators as spectators (such as games at the circus), and games which exclude them.

We might mention a third element in play: the community element. Play is a fundamental possibility of social life. To play is to play together, to play with others; it is a deep manifestation of human community. Play is not, as far as its structure is concerned, an individual and isolated action; it is open to our neighbor as partner. There is no point in underlining

the fact that we often find solitary players playing alone at personal games, because the very meaning in play includes the possibility of other players. The solitary player is often playing with imaginary partners. The community of play does not necessarily require real persons present. It is enough for a real player to have a real game and not merely an imagined one.

Another essential element is that of the rule in play. Play is established by a commitment and bound to it; it is limited by whatever concerns the arbitrary modification of any action. It is not entirely free. There is no play without a commitment agreed upon and accepted. However, the rule of play is not a law; the commitment is not irrevocable. Even in the course of play, we can change the rule with the permission of partners. However, then the modified rule holds and fixes the course of what can be done by either. We all know the difference between traditional games where we adopt rules already formulated and the improvised games that are just made up. The community of play has to come to an agreement about the rules of the latter. We might expect these improvised games to be the most popular, since they leave the field open to imagination and permit the development and free reign of pure possibilities. But this is not necessarily the case. The act of being bound to a pre-established rule is often a positive experience with its own delights. This may seem strange, but it is explained by the fact that traditional games are often bound up with collective imagination, with self-commitments rooted in the deep primordial patterns of common experience. A number of children's games, which may seem naive, are in fact rudiments of certain magical practices of antiquity.

Each type of play demands equipment. Each of us knows about playthings, but it is still hard to define them. We do not have to enumerate all possible types, but we must know their nature or at least recognize that here is a problem. Playthings do not make up a definite world of their own, as is the case with things that are made. According to nature (in the larger sense of that which exists in itself), these are not artificial objects if man has not made them. It is only by his own work that man produces artificial things. He is the artisan (technités) of a human environment. He cultivates the earth, tames the animals, makes tools. A tool is an artificial thing that human work has formed. We can distinguish artificial things from natural things, but they are one and the same in being on the plane of the same universal reality which includes them all.

Though a plaything can be an artificial object, it is not necessarily so. Just a piece of wood, a fallen branch, can function as a doll. The hammer, which, by its very form, is the will of man imposed on an assemblage of wood and iron, belongs just as the wood, the iron, and the man himself, to one and the same order of reality. It is not so with playthings. Seen from the exterior, that is from the point of view of those who do not play, it is evidently a fragmentary object of the real world. It is simply something that holds a child's attention. The doll is a product of the toy industry, it is a mannequin made up of material and a piece of wire or of plastic. We can buy it at a certain price; it is merchandise. But seen with the eyes of a little girl who plays, the doll is a child and the small girl is its mother. Perhaps it is not as though the child thought the doll were actually a living child, for she is not under a false impression nor apt to confuse the nature of things. She possesses, on the contrary, a simultaneous knowledge of the doll as such and its meaning in play. The child who plays lives in two worlds. What makes a thing a toy—gives the essence of toy— is something rather magical. It endows an everyday thing with a kind of mysterious being. It is then infinitely more than a simple means of amusement, more than a thing which one must put together and keep in hand. Human play has need of playthings. Above all, in his specifically human actions, man is not free to bypass things. He needs them. He cannot ignore the hammer in his work, the sword for conquest, the couch for love, the lyre if he be a poet, an altar for religion— and playthings for play.

Each plaything symbolizes the totality of real things. To play is to take an explanatory attitude toward being at all times. Reality is concentrated in the plaything in the form of a single thing. All play is an attempt to have the plaything yield to the vital energy of man so that he might test symbolically the totality of the resistance of being. But human play not only comes under the magical intimacy with playthings. We must look a little closer at the notion of the player, for we are in the presence of a very particular type of "schizophrenia," of the duality of man; which of course is not pathological. The player who engages in play performs a precise action in terms of the real world, quite recognizable. However, as to the meaning and intrinsic context of play he assumes a role. It then becomes necessary to distinguish between the real man who "plays" and the man charged with a role within the context of play. There is a real basis for saying that the player loses himself in his role. He lives his role with a very particular intensity and, for that reason, not in the manner of an hallucination where we cannot distinguish "reality" from "illusion." The player can renounce his role. Even at times he is necessarily engrossed, the consciousness of his double existence does not abandon him. He lives in two worlds, but not through distraction or want of concentration. The duality belongs to the very nature of play.

The structural elements we have thus listed are all present in the fundamental concept, "the world of play" (*Spiel welt*). All play is a magical creation in the world of play. It is here that the player assumes a role, that the community of play alternately distributes the roles, that the rules of play are imposed and that the plaything takes on meaning. The world of play is an imaginary sphere. It is a difficult problem, therefore, to clarify its essential structure. We play in the world which we call real, but in so doing, we create for ourselves another world, a mysterious one. This is not just nothing and still it is not something real either. In the world of play we act according to our role; but in this world imaginary persons live, as the "child" which takes on body and life, but which is nothing more than a doll or even a piece of wood in reality. In projecting a world of play, the player disguises himself as a creature of that "world," losing himself in the project, becoming that person whose role he has assumed and moving, for the present, in the midst of things and among partners who belong to such a world of play. Confusion might arise here for in imagination we think of things of the world of play in themselves as "realities" and even the distinction between reality and illusion can frequently be re-adjusted.

But it does not follow that the real things in our daily world are veiled or even masked by the superimposition of the world of play to the point that we no longer recognize them. This is not at all the case. The world of play does not interpose a wall between us and being that surrounds us. Strictly speaking, the world of play has neither place nor duration but operates in interior space and time proper to it. However when we play we use real time and have real space besides. But we do not pass by continuous transition from the space of the world of play to that we ordinarily occupy. The same holds for time. The strange interlacing of spheres of the world of reality and that of play cannot be explained by any other example known of spatial-temporal proximity. The world of play is not suspended in a domain of pure imagination. It always possesses a real theatre. However, it is never a real thing among other real things. But real objects are indispensable to it as props. This is to say that the imaginary character of the world of play cannot be reduced to purely subjective illusion, nor defined as fancy not affecting us except interiorly and unable to make its appearance in the world of real things.

We come now to the fundamental characteristics of play. Human play is a creation through the medium of pleasure of a world of imaginary activity. It is the singular joy of "appearances" (*Freud am Schein*). Play is always characterized by an element of representation. This element determines its meaning. It then effects a transfiguration; life becomes peaceful. We are freed little by little, and we eventually discover that we have been redeemed from the weight of real life. Play lifts us from a situation of fact, from an imprisonment depressing by nature, and by means of fantasy helps us enjoy passing through a multitude of "possibilities," without imposing on us the necessity of making a choice. In playing man lives out two extremes of existence. One puts man at the peak, gives him an almost unlimited power of creation, establishes a freedom that is impossible in reality. The player feels himself master of his own creations, play becomes a possibility scarcely limited by human freedom. At the highest point in play freedom prevails. But we also find in play the contrary of freedom (a facet of being taken perhaps from the real world) which can bring about a sort of alienation from enchantment, even to the point of coming under the demonical power of the mask. Play can conceal the Appolonian clarity of free ipseitas as well as the Dionysian inebriation which accompanies a certain abandonment of human personality.

Man's relationship to the enigmatic "appearances" of the world of play, to the sphere of the imaginary, is ambiguous. Play is a phenomenon for which we cannot easily find adequate categories. It is perhaps a dialectic much concerned with not reducing paradoxes to a dead level, which would let us for that very reason experience the tantalizing ambiguity of dialectic. The great philosophers have insisted on the eminent meaning of play. If common sense does not recognize this it is because play means nothing more to it than a lack of seri-

ousness and authenticity, because it sees in play only pointless activity. Hegel, however, said that in its indifference and extreme lack of seriousness, play is the unique and most sublime expression of true seriousness. And Nietzsche in *Ecce homo*: "I do not know of any other method than play for facing the most important tasks."

Can play be explained if it is not seen purely and simply as an anthropological phenomenon? Could it be that our consideration has gone beyond man? Does this mean that we must study the behavior of play as it involves other creatures also? The problem is really that of knowing whether or not we can understand play in its ontological structure without limiting it by paying attention to the sphere of the imagination. Whether play is something man alone can do is a question which remains open and depends on whether man the player is still bound to the human world or if he has entered a superhuman world.

From the beginning, play is a symbolic act of representation, in which human life interprets itself. The most ancient games are magical rites, the principal liturgical cultures of primitive man, expressing his being-in-the-world in which he represents his destiny, commemorates the events of birth and death, weddings, war, the chase and work. The manner of symbolic representation in magical games draws its elements from the simple world around men just as he draws upon the nebula world of the imagination. In primitive times, play was not practiced so much as an act in its pleasure-giving aspect as is the case for those isolated individuals or groups, who periodically detach themselves from the social group to inhabit their own little isle of passing happiness. Originally, play was the strongest unifying force. It found a community quite different, it is true, from that of the living and the dead, the governing and governed, and even from that based on the family. The community of play of primitive man included all the forms and structures of common life that we have enumerated and it is called forth a reliving of all the elements of life. This reached its high point with the community keeping festival. The ancient feast was more than a popular form of rejoicing. It was reality itself —hoisted to the world of magic—the reality of human life in all its relations. It was a liturgical spectacle where man experienced the proximity of the gods, heroes, the dead, and where he found himself in the presence of all the beneficent and dreadful powers of the universe. Primitive play had deep contacts with religion. The community *en fête* included the spectators, the mysteries and epics; here the exploits and sufferings of the gods and man were passed in review. What was represented was nothing less than the whole universe.

III

In attempting to reduce the structure of play to a certain number of fundamental concepts, such as the climate of play, community of play, rule of play, plaything, and the world of play, we often used the word "imaginary." An equivalent of this word would be "appearing-to-be." However, in this term *is* concentrated a remarkable intellectual aporia, a dead end. We understand the term "appearing-to-be" in its strictest sense when it operates in concrete determined situations. But it is still a difficult and complicated matter to say precisely what we mean by it. The most important philosophic questions and considerations are involved in the most everyday things and words. The concept "appearing-to-be" is altogether as obscure and indefinable as that of "being." And the two concepts are related to each other in an intricate, perplexing and even inextricable manner; they interpenetrate and intermingle in their application. In thinking all this out we get further and further into the labyrinth of being.

With the question of the "appearing-to-be," in so far as it is related to the domain of human play, we ask a truly philosophic problem. Play is a "creative producing." Its effect, that is in the world of play, is exercised in the sphere of the "appearing-to-be," a field in which we can hardly expect consistency. The "appearing-to-be" of the world of play cannot be dismissed simply by calling it nothingness. We actually move within it when we play. We live in it at times, certainly, a life that is as free and fanciful as that of a dream, but sometimes we give ourselves over to it with genuine zeal. At times such an "appearing-to-be" has a presence and suggestive force more powerful and impressive than the everyday affairs which are quite banal in their very seriousness. What then is the imaginary? Where should we locate this strange "appearing-to-be," what is its condition? On the determination of that place and condition depends, in great part, the understanding of the ontological nature of play.

We are in a habit of speaking of "appearings-to-be" in various acceptations of the term. For example we think of the exterior appearance of things, of their superficial aspect, of their frontal aspect, and the like. That which "appears-to-be" pertains to what is represented as the shell pertains to the nut and as the substance to its manifestation. More often we speak of an "appearing-to-be" as in the case of a subjective fallacious interpretation, of an erroneous opinion, of a confused representation. In this case, we who interpret reality poorly have within us a semblance of that which resides in the subject. But there is also a subjective "appearing-to-be" with a legitimate place within us. It is a product of the imagination and does not relate to the categories of truth and error as does the representation and objects represented. With these abstract distinctions we can formulate our question. Which "appearing-to-be" is in the world of play? The outer appearance of things? A fallacious representative? A phantasm produced within us? We cannot deny that in play as a whole imagination manifests itself and unfolds in a particular manner. However, is the world of play nothing more than a product of the imagination? We might find an easy way out by saying that the imaginary universe that is the world of play exists uniquely in the human imagination and cite accordingly the case of hallucination and individual imaginary occurrences which have been united into collective hallucination or "intersubjective fantasy." To play, however, is always to use playthings. Anyone who considers the nature of a plaything will attest that play does not come into our life only in a purely interior manner, for it cannot escape being related to the objective exterior world. The world of play consists in both subjective elements of the imagination and objective ones or real ones. The imagination is known as the psychic power. We recognize the dream as such, as well as interior percepts and various imaginary contents. But what is the significance of the objective or real "appearing-to-be"? It exists in the reality of curious things which, without doubt, are in themselves something of reality and yet contain an element of un-reality. This may seem both singular and astounding. However, this is commonly known, though we ordinarily do not speak of it in terms so involved and abstract. All that is needed is simply images presented objectively, as a poplar on the shore of a lake projecting its reflection over the mirroring surface of the water. The reflections themselves make up part of the whole of the optic phenomenon, which consists of real things and the light which envelops them. Things exposed to light project their shadows. The trees on the bank are reflected in the lake, a smooth and highly polished metal surface reflects the objects around it. What is reflected? As an image it is real; it is a real reproduction of a real tree, its source. But it is "in" (or "as") image that the tree is represented. It appears to be on the surface of the water, but in such a way that it springs from the medium of the reflection and is not there in reality. An "appearing-to-be" of that nature is a kind of being apart. As a constituent element of its reality it possesses a specifically unreal element. It resides on the surface of another being which is simply real. The reflection of the poplar does not hide the surface of the water which it covers and which serves it as a mirror. The reflections of the poplar are there as reflection, a real thing known in itself and an unreal poplar in the sphere of reflection. This may seem sophistic; however, this fact is in everyone's experience and easily distinguished, for it is of daily occurrence. The doctrine of being of Plato, which has profoundly influenced western philosophy, takes as a model at decisive moments in his elucidation, the notion of image in terms of shadow and reflection and thus interprets the structure of the universe.

There is more than a simple parallel between the real "appearing-to-be" (reflection and the like), and the work of play. The real "appearing-to-be" is by priority counted as a structural element in the world of play. To play is real behavior, which includes what we call a "reflection," the attitudes which the world of play portions out according to the roles one takes in it. When all is taken together, the possibility that a man might construct a real "appearing-to-be" proper to a world of play depends, in a great measure, on the fact that such already exists in nature. Man not only knows how to make artificial objects generally, but he knows how to produce things which properly belong to an "appearing-to-be-that-is." He projects imaginary worlds of play. The little girl raises the body of material composition, doll, to the sphere of her "living child" by an act of the imagination, and with it herself to the role of "mother." Real things are always involved in the world of play; but they take on the character of a real "appearing-to-be"; sometimes even they are related to a subjective "appearing-to-be" which comes from the human spirit. Play is a creation with limited possibilities in the magical world of appearances.

The problem of explaining how the real and unreal interlace in human play requires untiring effort. The ontological determination of play leads us into the chief questions of philos-ophy, to being and nothingness, to the "appearing-to-be" and becoming. We see that the expression, "the unreality of play," is both hasty and superficial, unless understood in terms of the enigmatic world of the imaginary. But we ask, what human and what cosmic meaning does the imaginary have? Is it a limited sphere in the midst of real things? Is the strange country of the unreal that exalted place where we call upon the presence of the "essences" of all things? In the magical reflection which operates in the world of play, it is not important which isolated object (for instance the plaything) becomes *symbol*. It represents another thing. Human play (even if we no longer recognize it as such after a while) is the symbolic action which puts us in the presence of the meaning of the world and of life.

The ontological problems which play poses for us do not exhaust the questions which have been brought up concerning the mode of being of the world of play and the symbolic value of playthings or of the action of play. In the history of thought, there have been those who have not only tried to conceive of the being of play, but also have dared an unheard of inversion of the process, concluding that the meaning of being springs from play. This is what I would call the speculative concept of play. In short, speculation is the characterization of the nature of being which takes for its point of departure the metaphorical consideration of a being. It is a conceptual formula of the essence of the world developed from a model within that world. The philosophers have used and perhaps abused models of this kind: Thales, of water; Plato, of light; Hegel, of the spirit; and the like. But the clarifying force of these models do not depend on the arbitrary choice of each of these thinkers. It is important, above all, to know whether or not the whole of being can be found in reflection in a single isolated being. In the measure in which the cosmos reproduces itself metaphorically in something which makes up part of the world in terms of structure and imprint, a key-phenomenon of philosophy can be discovered from which a speculative formula of the world can be developed.

As far as that goes, the phenomenon of play is a manifestation distinguished by the fundamental character of symbolic representation. Could it be then that play is a spectacle which might represent the whole as in parable, producing a clarifying and speculative metaphor of the world? One philosopher has had the courage or rather the temerity to think so. At the dawn of European thought, Heraclitus had formulated the sentence: "The course of the world is a child who plays at moving his pawns —a kingship of childhood." (Frg. 52, Diels.) And about twenty-five centuries later in the history of thought, we find in Nietzsche: "Becoming and disappearing, constructing and destroying, without moral imputation, with an eternally childlike innocence, behold what is reserved in the world for the souls that play, those of the artist and the child." "The world is Zeus' play . . ." (*Die Philosophie im tragischen Zeitalter der Griechen.*)

The depth of such a concept has its danger and its power of seduction, for it impels one to an esthetic interpretation of the world. But the strange formula of the world through which the totality of being is viewed as a game could be made to bear out the fact that play is not an anodyne, a peripheral or even puerile phenomenon, that we mortals are oriented to play in a mysteriously fundamental sense, precisely because we can produce magically things that testify to our creative power and our glory. If the essence of the world were thought of as play, it would follow that man is the only being within the immensity of the universe who can understand the infinity of the whole and respond accordingly. This is nothing more than recovering for himself the sense of the infinite, that eludes him, that he might be able to reach to the source of his being.

The opening up of human existence to the abyss of being by means of play, to being as a whole, which is also a form of play, is a theme that has inspired the poet Rilke:

So long as you merely catch, what you yourself
Toss up—'tis only skill of a minor range.
Only when you suddenly catch the ball
Thrown by your eternal Companion of play
Against your center, in a perfect gesture,
In one of the arcs, traced against the great bridge
    of God
Does knowing how to seize it really count—
Not for yourself, but for the world. And if, per-
    chance,
You had the force and courage to return it—
Why then, 'tis no miracle;
But if lacking the strength and courage, you still
Have thrown it, as the Year throws the birds,
The southward seeking birds to the Young
    Warmth
Of the land beyond the seas—then first
In such a feat do you really play the game.
Do not bother to throw again.
Be not disturbed. Out of your hands it springs
Like a Meteor and settles in its proper sphere.
(Translation of Fritz Klatt in *Rainer Maria Rilke*,
p. 79.)

When philosophers and poets stress the power and meaning of play as a profound human reality, perhaps we should remember the words that warn us that we will not enter into the kingdom of heaven unless we become like little children.

*Play and Sport**

JEAN-PAUL SARTRE

There remains one type of activity which we willingly admit is entirely gratuitous; the activity of *play* and the "drives" which relate back to it. Can we discover an appropriative drive in sport? To be sure, it must be noted first that play as contrasted with the spirit of seriousness appears to be the least possessive attitude; it strips the real of its reality. The serious attitude involves starting from the world and attributing more reality to the world than to oneself; at the very least the serious man confers reality on himself to the degree to which he belongs to the world. It is not by chance that materialism is serious; it is not by chance that it is found at all times and places as the favorite doctrine of the revolutionary. This is because revolutionaries are serious. They come to know themselves first in terms of the world which oppresses them, and they wish to change this world. In this one respect they are in agreement with their ancient adversaries, the possessors, who also come to know themselves and appreciate themselves in terms of their position in the world. Thus all serious thought is thickened by the world; it coagulates; it is a dismissal of human reality in favor of the world. The serious man is "of the world" and has no resource in himself. He does not even imagine any longer the possibility of *getting out of* the

world, for he has given to himself the type of existence of the rock, the consistency, the inertia, the opacity of being-in-the-midst-of-the-world. It is obvious that the serious man at bottom is hiding from himself the consciousness of his freedom; he is in *bad faith* and his bad faith aims at presenting himself to his own eyes as a consequence; everything is a consequence for him, and there is never any beginning. That is why he is so concerned with the consequences of his acts. Marx proposed the original dogma of the serious when he asserted the priority of object over subject. Man is serious when he takes himself for an object.

Play, like Kierkegaard's irony, releases subjectivity. What is play indeed if not an activity of which man is the first origin, for which man himself sets the rules, and which has no consequences except according to the rules posited? As soon as a man apprehends himself as free and wishes to use his freedom, a freedom, by the way, which could just as well be his anguish, then his activity is play. The first principle of play is man himself; through it he escapes his natural nature; he himself sets the value and rules for his acts and consents to play only according to the rules which he himself has established and defined. As a result, there is in a sense "little reality" in the world. It might appear then that when a man is playing, bent on discovering himself as free in his very action, he certainly could not be concerned with *possessing* a being in the world. His goal, which he aims at through sports or pantomime or games, is to attain himself as a certain being, precisely the being which is in question in his being.

The point of these remarks, however, is not to show us that in play the desire to *do* is irreducible. On the contrary we must conclude that the desire to do is here reduced to a certain desire to be. The act is not its own goal for itself; neither does its explicit end represent its goal and its profound meaning; but the function of the act is to make manifest and to present to *itself* the absolute freedom which is the very being of the person. This particular type of project, which has freedom for its foundation and its goal, deserves a special study. It is radically different from all others in that it aims at a radically different type of being. It would be necessary to explain in full detail its relations with the project of being-God, which has appeared to us as the deep-seated structure of human reality. But such a study can not be made here; it belongs rather to an *Ethics* and it supposes that there has been a preliminary definition of nature and the role of purifying reflection (our descriptions have hitherto aimed only at *accessory* reflection); it supposes in addition taking a position which can be *moral* only in the face of values which haunt the For-itself. Nevertheless the fact remains that the desire to play is fundamentally the desire to be.

Thus the three categories "to be," "to do," and "to have" are reduced here as everywhere to two; "to do" is purely transitional. Ultimately a desire can be only the desire *to be* or the desire *to have*. On the other hand, it is seldom that play is pure of all appropriative tendency. I am passing over the desire of achieving a good performance or of beating a record which can act as a stimulant for the sportsman; I am not even speaking of the desire "to have" a handsome body and harmonious muscles, which springs from the desire of appropriating objectively to myself my own being-for-others. These desires do not always enter in and besides they are not fundamental. But there is always in sport an appropriative component. In reality sport is a free transformation of the worldly environment into the supporting element of the action. This fact makes it creative like art. The environment may be a field of snow, an Alpine slope. To see it is already to possess it. In itself it is already apprehended by sight as a symbol of being.[1] It represents pure exteriority, radical spatiality; its undifferentiation, its monotony, and its whiteness manifest the absolute nudity of substance; it is

[1] See section III.

the in-itself which is only in-itself, the being of the phenomenon, which being is manifested suddenly outside all phenomena. At the same time its *solid* immobility expresses the permanence and the objective resistance of the In-itself, its opacity and its impenetrability. Yet this first intuitive enjoyment can not suffice me. That pure in-itself, comparable to the absolute, intelligible plenum of Cartesian extension, fascinates me as the pure appearance of the not-me; What I wish precisely is that this in-itself might be a sort of emanation of myself while still remaining in itself. This is the meaning even of the snowmen and snowballs which children make; the goal is to "do something out of snow"; that is, to impose on it a form which adheres so deeply to the matter that the matter appears to exist for the sake of the form. But if I approach, if I want to establish an appropriative contact with the field of snow, everything is changed. Its scale of being is modified; it exists bit by bit instead of existing in vast spaces; stains, brush, and crevices come to individualize each square inch. At the same time its solidity melts into water. I sink into the snow up to my knees; if I pick some up with my hands, it turns to liquid in my fingers; it runs off; there is nothing left of it. The in-itself is transformed into nothingness. My dream of appropriating the snow vanishes at the same moment. Moreover *I do not know what to do* with this snow which I have just come to see close at hand. I can not get hold of the field; I can not even reconstitute it as that substantial total which offered itself to my eyes and which has abruptly, doubly collapsed.

To ski means not only to enable me to make rapid movements and to acquire a technical skill, nor is it merely to *play* by increasing according to my whim the speed or difficulties of the course; it is also to enable me to *possess* this field of snow. At present *I am doing something to it*. That means that by my very activity as a skier, I am changing the matter and meaning of the snow. From the fact that now in my course it appears to me as a slope to go down, it finds again a continuity and a unity which it had lost. It is at the moment connective tissue. It is included between two limiting terms; it unites the point of departure with the point of arrival. Since in the descent I do not consider it in itself, bit by bit, but am always fixing on a point to be reached beyond the position which I now occupy, it does not collapse into an infinity of individual details but is *traversed toward* the point which I assign myself. This traversal is not only an activity of movement; it is also and especially a synthetic activity of organization and connection; I spread the skiing field before me in the same way that the geometrician, according to Kant, can apprehend a straight line only by drawing one. Furthermore this organization is marginal and not focal; it is not for itself and in itself that the field of snow is unified; the goal, posited and clearly perceived, the object of my attention is the spot at the edge of the field where I shall arrive. The snowy space is massed underneath implicitly; its cohesion is that of the blank space understood in the interior of a circumference, for example, when I look at the black line of the circle without paying explicit attention to its surface. And precisely because I maintain it marginal, implicit, and understood, it adapts itself to me, I have it well in hand; I pass beyond it toward its end just as a man hanging a tapestry passes beyond the hammer which he uses, toward its end, which is to nail an arras on the wall.

No appropriation can be more complete than this instrumental appropriation; the synthetic activity of appropriation is here a technical activity of utilization. The upsurge of the snow is the matter of my act in the same way that the upswing of the hammer is the pure fulfillment of the hammering. At the same time I have chosen a certain point of view in order to apprehend this snowy slope: this point of view is a determined *speed*, which emanates from me, which I can increase or diminish as I like; through it the field traversed is constituted as a definite object, entirely distinct from what is would be at another speed. The speed organizes the ensembles at will; a specific object does or does not form a part of a particular group according to whether I have or have not taken a particular speed. (Think, for example, of Provence seen "on foot," "by car," "by train," "by bicycle." It offers as many different aspects according to whether or not Béziers is one hour, a morning's trip, or two days distant from Narbonne: that is, according to whether Narbonne is isolated and posited for itself with its environs or whether it constitutes a coherent group with Béziers and Sète, for example. In this last case Narbonne's *relation to the sea* is directly accessible to intuition; in the other it is denied; it can form the object only of a pure concept.) It is I myself then who give form to the field of snow by the free speed which I give myself. But at the same time I am acting upon *my matter*. The speed is not limited to imposing a form on a matter given from the outside; it *creates* its matter. The snow, which sank under my weight when

I walked, which melted into water when I tried to pick it up, solidifies suddenly under the action of my speed; it supports me. It is not that I have lost sight of its lightness, its non-substantiality, its perpetual evanescence. Quite the contrary. It is precisely that lightness, that evanescence, that secret liquidity which hold me up; that is, which condense and melt in order to support me. This is because I hold a special relation of appropriation with the snow: *sliding*. This relation we will study later in detail. But at the moment we can grasp its essential meaning. We think of sliding as remaining on the surface. This is inexact; to be sure, I only skim the surface, and this skimming in itself is worth a whole study. Nevertheless I realize a synthesis which has depth. I realize that the bed of snow organizes itself in its lowest depths in order to hold me up; the sliding is action *at a distance*; it assures my mastery over the material without my needing to plunge into that material and engulf myself in it in order to overcome it. To slide is the opposite of taking root. The root is already half assimilated into the earth which nourishes it; it is a living concretion of the earth; it can utilize the earth only by making itself earth; that is, by submitting itself, in a sense, to the matter which it wishes to utilize. Sliding, on the contrary, realizes a material unity in depth without penetrating farther than the surface; it is like the dreaded master who does not need to insist nor to raise his voice in order to be obeyed. An admirable picture of power. From this comes that famous advice: "Slide, mortals, don't bear down!" This does not mean "Stay on the surface, don't go deeply into things," but on the contrary, "Realize syntheses in depth without compromising yourself."

Sliding is appropriation precisely because the synthesis of support realized by the speed is valid only for the slider and during the actual time when he is sliding. The solidity of the snow is effective only for me, is sensible only to me; it is a secret which the snow releases to me alone and which is already no longer true *behind my back*. Sliding realizes a strictly individual relation with matter, an historical relation; the matter reassembles itself and solidifies in order to hold me up, and it falls back exhausted and scattered behind me. Thus by my passage I have realized that which is unique *for me*. The ideal for sliding then is a sliding which does not leave any trace. It is sliding on water with a rowboat or motor boat or especially with water skis which, though recently invented, represent from this point of view the ideal limit of aquatic sports. Sliding on snow is already less perfect; there is a trace behind me by which I am compromised, however light it may be. Sliding on ice, which scratches the ice and finds a matter already organized, is very inferior, and if people continue to do it despite all this, it is for other reasons. Hence that slight disappointment which always seizes us when we see behind us the imprints which our skis have left on the snow. How much better it would be if the snow re-formed itself as we passed over it! Besides when we let ourselves slide down the slope, we are accustomed to the illusion of not making any mark; we ask the snow to behave like that water which secretly it is. Thus the sliding appears as identical with a continuous creation. The speed is comparable to consciousness and here symbolizes consciousness.[2] While it exists, it effects in the material the birth of a deep quality which lives only so long as the speed exists, a sort of reassembling which conquers its indifferent exteriority and which falls back like a blade of grass behind the moving slider. The informing unification and synthetic condensation of the field of snow, which masses itself into an instrumental organization, which is *utilized,* like the hammer or the anvil, and which docilely adapts itself to an action which understands it and fulfills it; a continued and creative action on the very matter of the snow; the solidification of the *snowy mass* by the sliding; the similarity of the snow to the water which gives support, docile and without memory, or to the naked body of the woman, which the caress leaves intact and troubled in its inmost depths—such is the action of the skier on the real. But at the same time the snow remains impenetrable and out of reach; in one sense the action of the skier only develops its *potentialities. The skier makes it produce* what it can produce; the homogeneous, solid matter releases for him a solidity and homogeneity only through the act of the sportsman, but this solidity and this homogeneity dwell as properties enclosed in the matter. This synthesis of self and not-self which the sportsman's action here realizes is expressed, as in the case of speculative knowledge and the work of art, by the affirmation of the right of the skier over the snow. It is *my* field of snow; I have traversed it a hundred times, a hundred times I have through my speed effected the

birth of this force of condensation and support; it is *mine.*

To this aspect of appropriation through sport, there must be added another—a difficulty overcome. It is more generally understood, and we shall scarcely insist on it here. Before descending this snowy slope, I must climb up it. And this ascent has offered to me another aspect of the snow—resistance. I have realized this resistance through my fatigue, and I have been able to measure at each instant the progress of my victory. Here the snow is identical with *the Other,* and the common expressions "to overcome," "to conquer," "to master," etc. indicate sufficiently that it is a matter of establishing between me and the snow the relation of master to slave. This aspect of appropriation which we find in the ascent, exists also in swimming, in an obstacle course, etc. The peak on which a flag is planted is a peak which has been *appropriated.* Thus a principal aspect of sport—and in particular of open air sports—is the conquest of these enormous masses of water, of earth, and of air, which seem *a priori* indomitable and unutilizable; and in each case it is a question of possessing not the element for itself, but the type of existence in-itself which is expressed by means of this element; it is the homogeneity of substance which we wish to possess in the form of snow; it is the impenetrability of the in-itself and its nontemporal permanence which we wish to appropriate in the form of the earth or of the rock, etc. Art, science, play are activities of appropriation, either wholly or in part, and what they want to appropriate beyond the concrete object of their quest is being itself, the absolute being of the in-itself.

Thus ontology teaches us that desire is originally a desire *of being* and that it is characterized as the free lack of being. But it teaches us also that desire is a relation with a concrete existent in the midst of the world and that this existent is conceived as a type of in-itself; it teaches us that the relation of the for-itself to this desired in-itself is appropriation. We are, then, in the presence of a double determination of desire: on the one hand, desire is determined as a desire to be a certain being, which is the *in-itself-for-itself* and whose existence is ideal; on the other hand, desire is determined in the vast majority of cases as a relation with a contingent and concrete in-itself which it has the project of appropriating.[3]

[2] We have seen in Part Three the relation of motion to the for-itself.

[3] Except where there is simply a *desire to be*—the desire to be happy, to be strong, etc.

Playful Freedom:*
Sartre's Ontology Re-appraised

RALPH NETZKY

I

Sartre's ontology has been interpreted in a variety of ways, but all of these seem to share one common characteristic—an emphasis upon "seriousness." In the following essay I will speculatively suggest that this, much discussed but frequently mis-interpreted, system of being really culminates in a theory of play.

The key to the significance of play in Sartre's ontology lies in a generally neglected passage of *Being and Nothingness*.[1] This passage occurs within the section on "Existential Psychoanalysis." Sartre is here in the process of developing his claim that all human desire is reducible ultimately to the desire to be—specifically the desire for the unity of being-for-itself (human consciousness) with being-in-itself (all other forms of being). This represents, of course, man's unrealizable project of being god. Illustrating this claim, Sartre has previously argued that the desire for knowledge is ultimately reducible to the desire to have, or possession. And he will soon insist that this desire to have is itself fundamentally expressive of the desire to be. It is in this connection that he examines the nature of play. Is it too merely an expression of this same desire, in particular the desire to have and thus of the all encompassing desire to be? Or is play a unique category of human experience, one

*From *Philosophy Today*, Carthagena Station, Celina, Ohio, 45822, XVIII (Summer, 1974), 125–136.

that can not be neatly fitted into this scheme? Sartre writes,

"Play, indeed, like Kierkegaardian irony, releases subjectivity. What is play, actually, if not an activity of which man is the ground and source in which man poses the rules to himself, and which can only have consequences according to the rules posed? As soon as man realizes that he is free and wishes to use this freedom, which is moreover able to be his anguish, his activity is play; he is, indeed, the first principle of play, in it he escapes to his own domain, he poses to himself the value and the rules of his acts, and he only allows himself to be satisfied according to the rules that he himself has posed and defined. For this reason there is a 'diminishing of the reality,' of the world."[2]

Before exploring Sartre's subsequent discussion of play, it seems necessary to unpack some of the concepts initially outlined in this very suggestive passage. I will begin with a more general discussion, relating these ideas, when appropriate, to treatments of play by other writers; the paper will then return more specifically to Sartre's text in order to fill in the details. How is play, following the clues provided by Sartre above, to be understood philosophically? What is its meaning for human experience?

According to Sartre play is fundamentally linked to human freedom. It springs from and reflects human subjectivity. This means that play can not be understood apart from choice, since choice expresses this freedom. Illustrating the founding of play in freedom, then, is the fact that I can only *choose* to play. Conceivably I can be *compelled* to labor, or to sing, or to eat, or to fornicate, and to die—but not to play. "Play to order is no longer play; it could at best be but a forcible imitation of it," writes Johannes Huizinga, in one of the few systematic treatments of the subject of play.[3] And I can stop playing whenever I choose. Play is, thus, essentially characterized by free choice, more so it seems than any other form of human experience.

Sartre also indicates that in play man *uses* freedom. How more specifically is this the case? The way this seems to occur is that in play we posit, even if only temporarily, our surpassing of the material necessities that normally limit human existence, or as Sartre describes it, our "situation." Play re-apprehends such necessities of our "situation" as labor, death, etc. in the realm of freedom. This is what Sartre calls the "diminishing of the reality of the world" that occurs in play. In contrast to these necessary demands which normally haunt our existence, play is purely gratuitous. It is beyond cause or reason. In other words, play posits our transcendence over these necessities, these brute facts of our situation; in this way, play affirms, or even exhibits, human freedom. "In play there is something 'at play' which transcends the immediate needs of life."[4] This is one of the most important distinguishing characteristics of play.

I have, along with Sartre, emphasized that freedom is the source and meaning of play. Play should, nevertheless, be clearly distinguished from pure caprice. Not surprisingly this difference lies in the presence of rules in play, but the function of these rules is not quite as simple as we might first assume. Play consists in a surpassing of the necessities of our situation; but the effects of the latter are not entirely absent here; the rules in play may be viewed as symbolically representing these necessities. In play, however, these demands of my situation are reapprehended by freedom: they are, in a sense, present, but we are aware that they are ultimately "harmless." The reason is, as Sartre observes, that in play I am the source and ground of the rules, rules as representing the necessities of my situation. It is only my *choice* that gives them their efficacy. The rules limit the scope of my action, but it is an ultimately self-imposed limitation. In most areas of existence these demands of our situation are like rocks and shoals against which we often flounder; moving within the limitations imposed by rules in play, we have

at least a non-thematic awareness that we are "safe." The rules are our creations. In other words, in most cases necessity is the ground of freedom; in play freedom is the ground of necessity. Heidegger characterizes *Dasein* (or human consciousness) as "*thrown* being-unto-death" (it. mine): in play, I am the thrower.

How more specifically do rules represent my situation within play? Are we able to make this relationship more concrete? Human existence demands that I *must* labor, I must die, I must respond to certain conditions imposed upon me by society. Likewise, when playing football, for example, I (or we) must gain ten yards in four downs, I must not cross the line of scrimmage before the ball is centered; and there are a host of other restrictions within which I move when playing this game. Play is, in this manner, a drama, a microcosm, demands similar to those of daily non-playful existence are, in play, re-created in miniature. But the difference is that here, in play, not only must I respond to these rules—I have also created them; I have endowed them with their power by *choosing* to play football. And I also have the power to make them "disappear" instantly, since at any time I am able to choose to stop playing. In other areas of existence these demands are inexorably thrust down before me. I cannot escape. There is no choice. In play all is founded in choice. This contrast reveals why the element of mockery, of taunting, is so essential to play. Since the necessities characterizing my everyday situation, as represented by the rules, are here harmless, I am, in play, teasing them mocking them; I am taunting them with my freedom. It is this element which lifts an activity from the "serious" world into the realm of play. More literally, this fundamental feature of play might be termed the *non-necessity of the necessary.*

Providing a further example of the essential function of rules in play are the varying contexts in which the activity of hunting occurs. Primitive man hunted for the sake of survival. He was not hunting for sport or play. Therefore he probably had no qualms about killing any game that he happened to encounter, including young or crippled animals. Hunting for what is known as sport, or play, in modern times is, on the other hand, hedged in by a wide variety of rules.[5] For example, as a sportsman, the hunter would not bag very young or lame animals—and unless he were a complete boor, he would not desire to sneak into the zoo at night to make his kills. Hunting can be, then, either necessary and serious—or playful; and it is primarily the presence of freely chosen, self posited, rules that distinguishes it as the latter. Most other forms of play would appear to be similarly defined.

I have been speaking as if play must contain rules. Certain discussions appear, nevertheless, to suggest the possibility of play without rules; at least they distinguish between rule-governed and ruleless play. Following Jean Piaget, John D. Caputo writes,

"To play, in many languages, means to swing, to wave, to flutter. The paradigm instance of such play, then, is that of the child. . . We ought to distinguish this sense of play from another but distinct idea: play as a game with rules. The game with rules, according to Jean Piaget, is a more rational behavior persisting throughout adulthood. In this play the rules are freely accepted, but must be adhered to rigorously. To break the rules (cheating) in a game with rules is to destroy the essential playfulness of the game."[6]

While we would certainly agree with this affirmation of the importance of rules, as defining the game, the distinction here between rule-governed and ruleless play seems in one sense too narrow, and in another too wide. First it is interesting to note that there is only one root word for both "play" and "game" in Piaget's own French language. Play seems, in this respect, to be identified with playing a game; and a game must contain rules. More specifically the structure of certain forms of children's play may not be as complex as that of chess, for example, but this does not mean that they are without rules. A very simple child's activity is kite-flying. (Adults have also been known to indulge in this practice, either on their own or taking over from an inept child.) Yet kite-flying, as rudimentary as it is, involves at least two very definite rules: a) the kite must remain above the ground; b) it must stay attached to the string. An even simpler instance of the type of play to which Piaget appears to refer is the act of jumping over a brook. However, this too involves one obvious rule: that of not landing in the brook. The extent of rules in play may, then, actually be more far reaching than the above discussion acknowledges.

The combined scope of the two categories of play (child's and adult type play) as delineated by Piaget, may also be too wide. Does this description leave room for what we often think of as pure caprice? The more elementary pole of movements mentioned here seem to approach very closely to what social scientists term mere "behavior," in contrast to "meaningful behavior" or "action."[7] And it is evident that if play is to be understood as a distinct, recognizable, form of human experience, it must certainly be meaningful. Those forms of children's activities cited above that do not contain at least very simple rules may, then, possibly fall outside of the province of meaningful, and thus playful, behavior. This is why I would concur with what Sartre implies by including the posting of rules in his definition of play; that, even if they should be very primitive in nature, play does inherently involve rules.[8]

Following from the preceding discussion may be questions concerning the exact range of play. Specifically, which forms of experience would be labelled play, and which would not? First we should note that play, in the current meaning of the term, is not necessarily limited to specific recreational activities; we might also be able to playfully adopt certain social roles, and even to assume a playful attitude toward life itself. The question of the relationship between play, sport, and games might also be raised here. To what degree are these terms synonymous, to what extent do they refer to different forms of activity? There seems, however, to be little need to examine this issue in great detail for our present purposes. Very briefly, it is hard to see how an activity could be properly called a "game" or "sport" unless it is first play; and we are concerned primarily with the latter. Play seems to be the broadest term of the three, and we are using "sport" and "game" in the sense of particular forms of play.[9]

Wherever its exact boundary may lie, it is clear that play must be understood as an autonomous category of human experience. Play can not be used merely as a means to some other allegedly higher goal—if it is to remain play. As affirming freedom, in the manner in which we have suggested, play must be its own end. This fact is illustrated by the situation of the professional athlete. Suppose it is argued that, because an athlete earns his livelihood at a particular sport, playing this sport is here subsumed under the category of work. He is playing *for the sake of* making money. I would, however, dispute the possibility of such an interpretation; rather, to the extent that he participates in the sport primarily for financial gain, our aspiring Joe Namath, or Bobby Riggs, is no longer playing. The play element vanishes. He is, purely and simply, working. In this respect play and work are dialectical opposites: a given activity may be experienced as play, at one time, at another time as work, but this activity can not be experienced as both play and work simultaneously. Again, following Sartre, play has been described as the transcendence of the realm of necessity of which work, or labor, is an integral part. In the very stimulating article referred to previously, Richard Burke defines the ideal social order as one in which work and play are integrated, in which work is seasoned with play, and play with work.[10] But, while these may be closely alternated with each other, this should not blur the fact that the two are essentially separate categories of experience. We work because it is necessary; play is by definition unnecessary.

The autonomy of play can be illustrated in other areas of experience as well. For example motives that are primarily religious would also seem to obliterate the play element in a given activity. Dancing and singing would, in most cases, be considered forms of play; but when, as in certain religions, they are used as ritual with the "higher" aim of appeasing the deity (or deities), song and dance would lose, on our interpretation, their character of play. Capturing this idea somewhat poetically, Edward Mooney writes, "While we are engaged in sports, ceremony, or dance (as forms of play) the rewards appear to be intrinsic, coming from the pursuit itself . . . flowering in the life we bring to it, and nourished by the life we in turn receive."[11] When they are used merely as means within the larger process of religious worship, the final rewards of singing and dancing are not intrinsic, they become extrinsic to the activity itself; as subordinated to a more "ultimate" end, singing and dancing are here no longer independent categories of experience. This is why they are not, in this context, playful. Or singing and dancing here aim at "increasing" rather than "diminishing" as in play, the reality, the necessity (recalling Sartre's earlier description) of the world.

Elaborating upon Sartre's initial sketch, I have characterized play as primarily an affirmation of human choice and freedom, one that transcends and mocks the demands that normally comprise our situation: and finally I have suggested that these demands are re-apprehended in play through the rules, rules as the non-necessity of the necessary. Where does this interpretation fit within the larger framework of Sartre's thought? What significance does Sartre himself attach to his initial, and very provocative, comments concerning the nature of play? I will now examine these issues, before briefly hinting at the wider philosophical implications of such an interpretation.

II

Our account indicates that play is an exultation of human freedom: specifically, in Sartre's terminology, play would be a thrust on the part of consciousness, as being-for-itself, as freedom, away from the demands of our situation and from the solidity and opacity of things, or being-in-itself. And we have seen how Sartre's initial remarks concerning play provide the basis for this interpretation. The direction of Sartre's analysis is, however, suddenly shifted. Play too is swept into the ontological juggernaut. It is reduced to a mere mode within the all-encompassing desire to be, or the project of being god: this means that play is understood merely as another expression of the desire of consciousness as translucent being-for-itself to *unite* with the solidity and opacity of being-in-itself. Sartre tries to accomplish this by claiming that play primarily manifests the desire to appropriate, which in turn reduces ultimately to an expression of this desire-to-be.

"The fact remains, nevertheless, that the desire to play is fundamentally desire of being . . . in the sporting act itself there is an appropriative component . . . The surroundings may be a field of snow, an Alpine slope. To see it is already to possess it. In itself it is already seized by sight as a symbol of being . . . The meaning of skiing isn't only to make rapid movements and to acquire technical skill, neither is it any longer to play by increasing my speed according to my whim, or by making the course more difficult; it is rather to allow me to possess this field of snow."[12]

Emphasizing appropriation, in this manner, is what allows Sartre to conclude that play is "fundamentally desire of being." And it is this emphasis upon what is supposed to be the basic appropriative element in play that we will question. Is this consistent with Sartre's opening remarks concerning the meaning of play? I strongly doubt whether this is the case.

Certain of Sartre's own comments seem to specifically challenge his subsequent treatment of play. He remarks, "Indeed it is necessary to notice first that play, in opposing itself to the spirit of seriousness, seems to be the least possessive attitude of all; it strips the real of its reality."[13] How is play quickly reduced, then, to an expression of this same desire to possess? Part of the confusion here seems to be generated by the particular examples of play activities that Sartre chooses for analysis; he selects skiing and mountain climbing. Are these not, however, particularly slanted toward the appropriative factor? In skiing and mountain climbing the self bluntly pits itself against the natural environment, and obviously we do often speak in this connection of "conquest," or "possession," of this environment. But are these really representative forms of play? It would seem far more difficult to claim that appropriation is the predominant desire if we examine such play activities as competing in a race, kite flying, or performing in a symphony concert.[14] If the desire to possess is present in such activities, it would seem to be very much in the background. It would appear rather far-fetched to claim that in kite-flying I desire to *possess* the air, or that in competing in a race my primary aim is possession of the ground. Each activity instead posits necessities, in the form of rules (in music this would correspond to the relations of harmony etc.), and each allows a surpassing of this necessity, because of achievement within the domain of these rules. Thus while the desire to possess might be present to a limited extent in these forms of play (other than skiing and mountain climbing), there is little reason to believe that possession is the dominant theme of such activities. Yet Sartre never really considers this question, appearing to assume all along that an analysis of skiing and mountain climbing is equally applicable to all of the many forms of play.

And is the desire to possess really fundamental even within, for example, skiing? Attempting to defend the view that skiing should be understood primarily in terms of the desire to appropriate, Sartre presents a detailed and characteristically penetrating phenomenological analysis of this sport. I have suggested that, even if this analysis should be fully valid, it does not necessarily hold true for other forms of play. And while Sartre's investigation of the act of skiing is too lengthy to trace in detail here, it is questionable whether the specific conclusion that he draws from this analysis is itself valid. Again, briefly, Sartre insists that when gliding over the snow, in the act of skiing, I desire to assimilate this snow; I desire to make it mine, while still retaining its permanence and solidity as being-in-itself. I wish ". . . this in-itself to be related to me in the form of an emanation of myself."[15] Could this conclusion not be reversed, however, with equal plausibility? This occurs when (while still viewing it from the same methodological perspective) we briefly analyze the act of skiing in terms of our preceding description of the nature of play. On such an interpretation the aim of travelling over the snow would be *separation* instead of assimilation, *escape* rather than possession. In other words the significance of this gliding is that the snow could, at any moment, engulf me—but I am always eluding its grasp; I am just out of reach—it closes in behind me, but my motion carries me beyond its permanence and opacity. Instead of wishing to *assume* the being of this in-itself, I am, thus, teasing, taunting, this being; I am asserting my freedom, my transcendence over it. Is this not an equally plausible interpretation of the meaning of skiing as a form of play?

If the above sounds at times like a lurid tale from Kafka, that may just be one of the features inherent in phenomenological analysis. And it is not necessarily intended as a final judgment upon the meaning of skiing or similar sports. This brief description has merely been advanced as a possible alternative to Sartre's account, and it seems at least ostensibly plausible. But the important point here is that if skiing is not directly representative of all forms of play, and if Sartre's conclusion concerning the meaning of skiing is itself questionable (in the way I have suggested), then the grip of the project of being would be broken. It would no longer be all-encompassing. Sartre has maintained that all human activity is explicable in terms of this project of being. On our interpretation, play would be at least one category of human experience that could not be explained in these terms. Consciousness as freedom and subjectivity would not in play seek to unite its being with the being of the in-itself. More aptly consciousness would affirm the extent to which it escapes this very being, positing its separation, its freedom from it. If Sartre describes the project of being god (the desire of consciousness as being-for-itself to found itself in the in-itself) as the desire to be, according to our approach play manifests the opposite of such a project—play expresses the desire not to be. Play affirms and celebrates the extent to which, as for-itself, consciousness is *not* the opacity and solidity of the in-itself. This is evidenced by the way in which play is light, giddy, anxious. It is a celebration of freedom—an affirmation of the non-necessity of the necessary (as discussed previously). To the extent that play has ontological significance, then, this would appear to lie in its expression of the desire *not* to be.

The above is necessarily conjectural, but it is the logical outcome of the view that I have been developing throughout this paper. And, again, what is perhaps the strongest support for this interpretation is provided by Sartre himself. It is he who, at the beginning of his discussion of this topic, hints at the ontological uniqueness of play (as outlined immediately above) without, unfortunately, ever following up this suggestion. This occurs specifically when Sartre indicates that an understanding of the significance of play presages his *Ethics*, an ethics of freedom. He writes,

"This particular type of project (play) which has freedom as its goal and foundation warrants a special study. It is indeed radically different from all others in that it aims at a radically different type of being. It is, certainly, necessary to explain in full detail its connection with the project of being god which has appeared to us as the profound structure of human reality. But this study can not be conducted here; it refers us indeed to an *Ethics*, and it supposes that we have given a preliminary definition of the nature and role of purifying reflection (up to this point our description has only been concerned with accomplice reflection). It would also require us to take a position which would have to be understood as *moral*, in regard to the values that haunt the For-itself."[16]

Sartre suggests, then, that this *Ethics* might interpret consciousness in a manner that is radically different from the project of being god—the project that especially dominates the latter part of *Being and Nothingness*. Although our description of play, as expressing the desire *not* to be, is never specifically articulated by Sartre, it appears to be in accord with the outline of this *Ethics*.

In sum, I have suggested that play is an autonomous, but rule-governed, affirmation of human freedom, mocking the necessities that inevitably characterize our existence: as expressing the desire not to be, play posits the non-necessity of the necessary. I make no claims to completeness in this respect, to revealing all of the implications of play for Sartre, or for existentialism in general. There is still much work to be done. This account has succeeded, however, to the extent that it has established the general importance of play in Sartre's ontology, to the degree that it has

removed some of the obscurity previously surrounding this suggestive theme.

REFERENCES

1. Jean-Paul Sartre, *L'Etre et le néant; Essai d'ontologie phénoménologique* (Paris, Gallimard, 1943). Subsequently this book will be referred to as L. E. The English translation of this work by Hazel Barnes, *Being and Nothingness; An Essay on Phenomenological Ontology* (New York, Washington Square Press, 1966) will be referred to as *B.N.*
2. *L.E.* p. 669, *B.N.*, p. 711.
3. Johannes Huizinga, *Homo Ludens: A Study of the Play Element in Culture* (New York, Harper and Row, 1970), p. 6.
4. *Ibid.*, p. 1.
5. This is not intended to morally sanction hunting for what is called "sport;" it is merely used as a, hopefully, illuminating example.
6. John D. Caputo, "Being, Ground and Play in Heidegger's Philosophy," *Man and World*, Vol. III, no. 1, p. 37.
7. See, for example, May Brodbeck (ed.), *Readings in the Philosophy of the Social Sciences* (New York, The Macmillan Company, 1968) especially Chapter I.
8. *L.E.* p. 669, *B.N.* p. 711.
9. This is examined in more detail in Richard Burke's "Work and Play," *Ethics*, vol. 82, pp. 33-47.
10. *Ibid.*, p. 47.
11. Edward F. Mooney, "Nietzsche and the Dance," *Philosophy Today*, Vol. XIV, no. 1¼, p. 39.
12. *L.E.* pp. 670-671, *B.N.* pp. 710-711.
13. *L.E.* p. 669, *B.N.* pp. 710-711.
14. I would, in accord with the writers referred to above, include music and possibly art too, within our description of play; but we can not explore this point here.
15. *L.E.* p. 671, *B.N.* p. 713.
16. *L.E.* p. 670, *B.N.* p. 712. Sartre also indicates the direction such an *Ethics* would take at the very end of *Being and Nothingness*, *L.E.* p. 722, *B.N.* p. 768. The problems Sartre would face in creating such a work are discussed in Thomas C. Anderson's "Is a Sartrean *Ethics* Possible?", *Philosophy Today* Vol. 14, Summer 1970, pp. 116-140.

Athletics and Angst:
Reflections on the Philosophical Relevance of Play

DREW A. HYLAND

But yield who will to their separation,
My object in living is to unite
My avocation and my vocation
As my two eyes make one in sight.
Only where love and need are one
And the work is play for mortal stakes,
Is the deed ever really done
For Heaven and the future's sakes.
        ROBERT FROST: "Two Tramps in Mud Time"

An acquaintance of mine once said to me, in a state of considerable inebriation, "The trouble with women is they've never been out on the football field, back on their own two yard line, where they had to hold the line or lose the game." There is probably a kernel of truth in this, not about women but about being on one's own two-yard line. For my own experience with athletics has suggested to me that many athletic contexts function in part as writ-large images of life itself.[1] That is, many of the recurring themes and issues of life are magnified and made explicit in the exigencies of a contest. This occurs on several levels. On a fairly obvious level, one finds the element of competition, so integral an aspect of human being, brought forth as the urgent issue that it truly is. Similarly with such themes as working with others, being a good winner and loser, staying in good physical health, all the reasons usually and rightfully offered by proponents of athletics every day. But on a somewhat less obvious level, this same phenomenon occurs, this same magnification and making explicit of

the issues of life itself. To suggest just one example: I believe we could say that athletics offers something which, on the aesthetic level, all great art offers, and which may be one of the ultimate sources of appeal to human being of both art and athletics: a suggestion of a completed theme in a life characterized by the most radical and decisive partiality. It should be obvious how art accomplishes this. I am concerned here with athletics. It could be said that our day-to-day lives are shot through with incompleteness—jobs left undone, aspirations unfulfilled, human frustrations everywhere. In the midst of this partiality, athletics, by the very fact that the game has a time limit, impose a momentary if arbitrary possibility of completeness, a theme of life begun and brought to fulfillment. This completeness, even if arbitrary, may bring to focus that which is obscured by the seeming interminableness of our day-to-day lives. Part of my intention in this paper, then, is to offer some suggestions as to the relevance of athletic games to an understanding of man.

In this regard, it is worth noting that the various "movements" in contemporary philosophy have been notably silent on this theme, possibly because of their confidence that anything like athletics could in principle have nothing to do with the "serious" pursuit of philosophy, possibly also because their conception of philosophy makes them incapable of dealing with such a concrete aspect of human experience. In the case of at least one such "movement," however, "existential phenomenology" so-called, such silence is, unnecessary. For I believe that existential phenomenology, specifically of the sort which Heidegger employs in *Being and Time*, can reveal much about the meaning of athletics for human being. For that reason, I propose to adopt a basically Heideggerian framework in my analysis of athletics.

At the same time, I believe we shall discover in the Heideggerian mode, that the Heideggerian-phenomenological method itself both reveals and conceals, that while the method is certainly capable of revealing much, it also necessarily conceals certain aspects of experience. However, since I myself am not an existential phenomenologist (nor, to be sure, a positivist) I shall not hesitate to make a value judgment on this revealing-concealing of phenomenology. Instead of suggesting that it is a necessary consequence of the revealing-concealing happening of Being in the 20th century, I shall suggest that it constitutes an inadequacy in the Heideggerian-phenomenological method. I hope that my effort will be both play-ful and ser-ious.

One of the most common dissatisfactions with *Being and Time* (indeed with many works in existential phenomenology) is that notwithstanding its claim to analyze concrete human experience, it is an immensely abstract work. In an effort to overcome this objection, I propose to begin by taking as my material for analysis the most concrete possible experience, the last few minutes of a particular basketball game in which I played. An analysis of the structure of that experience will, I hope, be fruitful; but first, it will be necessary to describe in some detail that experience.

Basketball has long had a deep effect on my life, from my first game in junior high school, when I was sick with nervousness the whole day of the game, through high school, when on those occasions when we lost or I had not played well, I refused to attend school the following day, to my years on the basketball team at Princeton University, where the increase in my own maturity and the people with whom I played gave the game an even deeper, yet less obsessive meaning than it had had before. The particular experience I wish to relate involves the last basketball game I played for Princeton, in fact the last four minutes of that game. We had won the Ivy League all three years, but this was the best team on which I had ever played. After winning the League Championship, we had been

invited to play in the N.C.A.A. Championship tournament, and had surprised everyone except ourselves by winning the first game. We were now in the Eastern quarter-finals, against St. Joseph's College, a team which was ranked among the top ten teams in the country and which was heavily favoured to beat us. The game was played in the Coliseum in Charlotte, North Carolina, a large fieldhouse with 13,500 seats, all filled, of whom most of the occupants were cheering for us, probably because we were such underdogs. The game had gone much as expected. St. Joseph's, bigger and stronger, had gradually pulled away from us until, with about five minutes left in the game, they had about a fifteen point lead. I had been in and out of the game several times, alternating with my brother, Art, who, although only a sophomore, was already bigger and a much better player than me. With about five minutes left, Artie committed a foul, and the coach sent me in to take his place. I reported to the scorer and knelt along the sideline, awaiting a pause in the game so that I could go in. As I waited, the pressure relaxed a bit, and my thoughts wandered, not definitely, but vaguely, over my whole experience of basketball that year, and all years.

It had been an eventful and meaningful year. As a team, we had developed a closeness both on and off the court which is rare, and which probably added to our success. We were all clubmates in the same eating club. Three of the members of the team were also my roommates, a fourth, my brother. We had, through temperament and interest, I suppose, developed a friendship, a rapport, such as I had never known before, nor have I experienced since.

Early in the season, our coach, "Cappy" Cappon, whom we all respected in deep measure, suffered a severe heart attack, and we had won the league championship largely by remembering all that he had previously taught us. Coupled with that loss, Don Swan, the captain of the team and one of my roommates, had been nearly killed in the first tournament game two nights before when he had taken a spill and landed on his head. He was in a hospital in New York City.

I reflected, vaguely as I say, on these people, and on this game, as I awaited a pause. These reflections, and especially this game, were given a deeper sense of urgency and meaning by the realization that the four remaining minutes were probably to be the last four minutes I was to play with this team, these people. Yes, I would continue to live with them, probably know some of them all my life, even play basketball with them in pickup games; but not like this; not with the peculiar unity and closeness that had gone with playing on an organized team, where more, it seemed, was at stake. If I had had time to continue reflecting, I might have become sad; but the whistle blew, and I entered the game.

Even as Heidegger speaks of becoming "lost" in the world of the everyday[2]—and one must hope, despite his protestations, that he speaks here pejoratively—so one can speak of becoming "lost" in a game—but here most emphatically *not* pejoratively. In the game about which I am speaking I became "lost" in the game in the sense that my involvement was total. One thinks here of Spinoza's discussions of the unity of one's own power of activity with the power of activity of nature. All the activity of my mind, indistinguishable now from the activity of my body, became involved in, yet determinative of, the rhythm and flow of the game. I became part of it in a way that is not expressed by saying that *I* was a participant *in* the game. Such language draws too arbitrary a dichotomy between my own activity and the game. Perhaps foremost among the characteristics of these moments of total involvement is the extraordinary experience of time. The "hour" is irrelevant; so too is the arbitrary fact that a game happens to last forty minutes. Rather, time has its meaning almost exclusively in terms of past, present, and future. But what was "past" was only what I had done in the game so far, and it was all encompassed into what I did right now, and what I did now was wholly directed towards what was to happen in the next play. The past, present, future were all drawn into my activity, into the action of the game. I remember that we began to catch up, that we stole the ball again and again, scoring each time, so that the pandemonium of the spectators made more forceful still the excitement of knowing that we were catching up. I stole the ball twice, scored both times, told myself to push harder in effort. We kept coming on, driven by the intensity of the game itself, intensified still further by the indefinite but pervasive roar of the crowd. As St. Joseph's was coming down the court I ran to deflect a pass, turned to throw the ball to a teammate alone for an easy shot, when the referee's whistle blew. When I had hit the ball in the air and run to retrieve it, he called me for an "air dribble." St. Joseph's was awarded the ball. I looked at the scoreboard for the first time since I had entered the game. There were

twelve seconds left. We were losing by one point, one point which, if the referee had not blown his whistle, would have been our margin of victory instead of defeat.

It was not really sadness that pervaded the locker room as we sat there, mostly glancing at each other and back to the floor. Nor was it depression, bitterness, anger. There was something simple, a sense of oneness between us all, which both had to terminate, yet would always be; a silent calmness that bespoke a deep realization; something had come to an end.

II

Let me begin my Heideggerian analysis of this experience with two of the most obviously relevant issues, space and time. To take space first; it is immediately clear, and commensurate with the phenomenological view, that what is not of primary relevance here is my so-called "objective" location in the world, that I happened to be in Charlotte, North Carolina (instead of, say, Durham), that the game was played in *this* gym (rather than some other) even that the size of the floor on which the game was played was some one hundred feet by fifty. Rather, the space that was relevant *was* relevant in terms of the game itself. In the game, I "experienced" space in terms of how tired I got running from one end to the other, whether a teammate was close enough to me to throw an accurate pass, whether I was close enough to the basket to take a good shot, and most significantly, in terms of the boundary lines, outside of which the game no longer continued. To be sure, at any given moment of the game I happened to be so many feet or inches from the basket, the boundaries, my teammates. But that was not the criterion in terms of which I decided to shoot or not, in terms of which the game took on its meaning. Far more relevant was whether I was across the half-court line, whether my teammate had a better opportunity for a shot. One can even go into some of the details of Heidegger's discussion of spatiality and note such factors as the "de-severing" character of my participation in the game and the "directionality" involved. What better examples could be given of the de-severing character of Dasein's spatiality than that of a basketball player dribbling up a court, looking to see what teammates are open for a shot, or whether an opening is developing for him to take a shot himself? Similarly, the directionality involved in the space of the game was understood in terms of which basket I was defending, which attacking, on which side of the court most of my teammates happened to be, whether the basket was to my right or left. It never occurs to any basketball player to determine that the "objective" direction of the basket he is defending is south-southwest. The space involved in this or any basketball game, then, reaffirms Heidegger's conviction that to the space which is experienced by Dasein in his being, "present-at-hand" "objective" space is often largely irrelevant. The space, the "Da" in which I found meaning was determined by the exigencies of the game itself.

Closely related to the spatiality of the game is what Heidegger would call the ready-to-hand character of the equipment used. An "objective" observer might note that the circumference of all regulation basketballs is 22 inches, that every basket is 10 feet high, that every regulation basketball floor is made of wood. But because of the nature of the game every basketball player is sensitive to a whole range of factors which an objective observer might consider insignificant and perhaps even unnoticeable. The relative resilience of the floor, the "feel" of the backboard, the lighting in the gym, the slipperiness of the ball take on great importance only because of the nature of the game. One's "circumspective concern" in the game determines the "meaning" of the equipment we employ, and indeed of our environment. Basketball, or any game, exemplifies this clearly.

It is equally clear that the phenomenological account of time is relevant to my basketball experience. As I indicated earlier, anything like "objective" time cannot possibly account for my experience of time in the game. The game must have taken about two hours to play. Of what relevance is that? In that game, the past, present, and future were not disjuncted and understood as something separate from *me*. Rather, past, present, and future were understood as gathered together in a unity which was the unity of the game, and of my activity in the game. The "past" of the game was brought into the present as what I was doing *now*. My particular activity now *was* only as the action of the game *was*, and the action of the game always culminated in the present. Likewise, the future was gathered into the present in that all my activity was directed fully to the future, but to the *future* of the *game*, and of my continued activity in that game. Any athlete knows what I mean here. As I played, I played always *toward*

what was to be next, not any definite shot or act, but toward any possibility that the game—and I—would realize. But all this direction, *to* what was to be, out of what had been, was gathered into my playing as I was playing *now*. Thus, I did not, so to speak, pause and calculate my next move, I *played*, and my play was the game and what was to be the game. At the same time, in broader terms, I had a "history," a past which included my long interest in basketball, which had contributed to my being in that situation, in that game. Still, and in keeping with Heidegger's analysis, it was the future toward which my being in the game was primarily oriented. This phenomenon corresponds clearly to that future orientation of Dasein which Heidegger calls "Being-ahead-of-itself."

Heidegger's notion of "Being-ahead-of-itself" clarifies another aspect of my experience, which he would refer to as possibility. He characterizes human being as ahead-of-itself in terms of its possibilities for being, possibilities which are *definite* possibilities for being what we are. This very sense of Being-ahead-of-itself in terms of possibility pervaded my basketball experience. All my playing was ahead-of-itself because it was directed towards the possibilities of my activity, which would in turn be the possibilities of the game. These possibilities were definite, definite because I was playing *basketball*, in this place, with *this* team. They were not definite in the sense of a calculated "next I will take a jump shot," which would have been, in terms of the basketball game, an inauthentic experience. Yet the experience that I described was not *just* in terms of the four minutes of the game, but included my reflections before I entered, and afterwards, in the locker room. On this level too, possibility was essential to my experience. For as I knelt along the sideline, although my reflections were of what had been (e.g., my coach's heart attack, my teammates), these reflections were occasioned by and directed to the future. They served to intensify my awareness of what was about to happen, intensify my awareness of the possibilities, definite possibilities for being, which lay immediately before me. At the same time they centered on one possibility which was in a way the most definite of all, that it might be the last time I played on this team, with these people. My reflections centered on the impending finality of the game I was about to play, and this sense of finality gave my playing a sense of urgency and importance which it had rarely had before. On a slightly different level, within the game itself, all my activity was directed and determined by one ultimate possibility, that the game would end. This, clearly, is the ultimate possibility of any game, but it is only in moments of genuine involvement that one becomes aware of its importance.

Both these levels of possibility have close affinities with what Heidegger calls the ultimate possibility of authentic being, Being-towards-death. It was Heidegger's remarks on Being-toward-death that clarified for me the overpowering sense of urgency that I found in that basketball game. For authentic Dasein, Being-toward-death is the ultimate possibility, the possibility that *that* Dasein might not be. This possibility is certain, yet indefinite as to the "when" it might become actual. Likewise in my experience, the possibility of *not* playing on that team, *not* playing that game, was certain, yet indefinite, in the same way. Similarly, the fact that the game had an imminent end gave it the meaning it had. A game without an end would be no game. The same may be true with life. And this brings us to the closely related issue of finitude.

One of the most important aspects of Being-toward-death as Heidegger elucidates it is its revelation of Dasein's radical finitude. Heidegger's remarkable suggestion is that our lives take on the meaning they do precisely *because* we are finite, not in spite of that fact. This finitude has two basic modes, first, that Dasein dies, second, that Dasein is always situated, always in a "place," and so never in all places. Again, the basketball game reflects and magnifies both forms. The finitude of the situation is manifested, for example, in the boundaries of the court. When I or the ball move outside the boundaries, the game stops. The court is the basketball player's "world." Its meaning *is* within the bounds. Similarly my own limitations had a special meaning in that situation. At 5′9″, I necessarily was a backcourt man rather than a center or forward. My possibilities in the game were therefore oriented *toward,* say, playmaking, and so *not* toward, say, rebounding. The finitude of death is reflected in the fact that the game has an end, and that the end is that *toward* which, in a sense, the game is always oriented. It is nowadays fashionable to congratulate such men as Sartre and Camus for their sunburst that because we die, life is absurd. The basketball game suggests precisely the reverse. The end makes the game rational. Death enables life to take on meaning. It offers us a stake.[3]

It should now be obvious that the kind of involvement that I had in that game was a mode of what Heidegger calls Being-in-the-world.[4] I suggested in my description of the game that the relation between my own being and that of the game was much too close to say simply that *I* played *in* the game. Such a distinction suggests too radical a separation between *my* being as one *playing* the game and the game itself. *My* being *was* in terms of my being part of the game, and the game took on *its* being in part, through my participation. To suggest that that game, or any game, was nothing more than the activity of each of the players would be inadequate; equally so to suggest that the game would have had the same meaning, or any meaning, *without* those particular players in that particular situation. Heidegger takes pains to show that the existentiale of Being-in-the-world undercuts the traditional subject-object dichotomy, that such a dichotomy can only inadequately characterize Dasein's relation to world. He is surely right.

There remains to discuss the importance in that game of the other players involved, both my own teammates and those against whom I was competing. The relevant Heideggerian existentiale here is of course "Being-with" as "solicitude" (Fürsorge). I indicated in my descriptive section that the friendships that had developed on our team contributed to the deep meaning that the game had for me. If we had not been so close, the game undoubtedly would not have had the same meaning, much less if I had been playing with strangers in a pickup-game. Similarly, my orientation toward the St. Joseph players was a mode of solicitude. I did not, could not, comport myself toward them as I did toward, say, the ball and the basket. They were other human beings, some of whom, in fact, I had come to know personally in other encounters. Yet here we were playing against them, in competition with them. It would be easy but entirely wrong to identify this encounter in competition as alienation. For even in this "important" game, as in all genuine play, the competition is never alienation. If it were, cheating, trying to hurt the opposing players, in short doing *anything* to overcome the opposition, understood, supposedly, as a threat to my freedom, would be the rule. Instead, even though both teams wanted to win, rules were still obeyed; the competition was in a context of sportsmanship. It is not too much to say that the sportsmanlike competition in athletics offers to man an image of an encounter with others, even in the context of opposition, which avoids the alienation on which Heidegger and the other existentialists dwell so endlessly, and about which I shall presently have more to say.[5]

III

By now I hope these two broad theses have been established: that reflection on play *is* relevant to a philosopher's effort to "know thyself" and that the Heideggerian phenomenological framework is indeed insightful in such a reflection. In establishing these theses, it might also have come to pass that play itself was established as a worthwhile enterprise, even if only to offer material for phenomenological investigations. But to paraphrase Heidegger, "revealing and concealing are the same," and so it is necessary to observe that the Heideggerian phenomenological method does not seem to adequately "save the phenomena." Let us begin with a more thorough discussion of "Being-with."

It is important to note that Heidegger includes his discussion of Being-with and solicitude in his analysis of Dasein's "everydayness,"[6] and that when he turns to a consideration of "authenticity" all Dasein's relations to other Dasein become utterly irrelevant as, with anticipatory resoluteness, he faces up alone to his ultimate possibility.[7] The strong implication is that all of one's dealings with others, either positive or negative, are part of the mode of "Fallenness," when one is lost in the world of "The They." When one is "Angst-voll" and authentic, one is *alone*. This attitude, even more forcefully maintained by Sartre, contributes to the excessive emphasis in existentialism on individuality, and the accompanying conviction that the most fundamental stance that man takes toward "the other" is one of *alienation*. But my basketball experience suggests quite the contrary.[8] It is fair to say that that experience, indeed my whole experience with basketball, has been deeply meaningful, meaningful in good measure because it led me to precisely that experience—a recognition of one's kind of being—which the existentialists call authentic. Yet that meaning occurred in such a way that possibly the most decisive "existentiale" was Being-with. The meaning of that game arose in terms of positive modes of Being-with, both the close kinship with my teammates and the sportsmanlike competition with the opposition. This is confirmed by a consideration of the ways in which these positive modes can on occasion break down in athletic competition. Fights occasionally break out; but when such explicit modes of alienation arise, the game is ruined, it is not a game

at all. Similarly, we have all known and been frustrated by teammates who would seem to play with anticipatory resoluteness; for them their teammates pale into irrelevance; not how the team fares but how *they* do is what counts. They play alone, no matter how many men are on the team. But interestingly, we would likely label this mode of participation inauthentic. The Heideggerian account reverses itself. The basketball game situation suggests that meaning of the sort that leads to authentic awareness of one's human being can occur in a context of encounter, an encounter which can even be a kind of opposition.[9] Perhaps the most obvious of all instances of this is love. But what we call love is one manifestation of what Plato called Eros. It has been noted,[10] and it is true enough, that Eros is Plato's word for Care (Sorge). But in substituting the "value-less" phenomenologically descriptive term Care for Plato's Eros, Heidegger apparently neglected to remember that the intentional character of human being means that man's most primordial mode of being is encounter, and that that encounter can be, and often is, with other men.

But possibly the most conspicuous absence from my Heideggerian analysis has been the all-important mood of Angst. There was no sense of being in a nothing in which I no longer had anything to hold onto for support. To be sure, my orientation was toward the possibility of the end of the game and of an experience—I have already related this to Being-toward-death—but I was hardly "Angst-voll." There was no calling into question of my whole being, no placing it in a void where it would be forced to take on itself or else fall back into the tranquillity of "The They." An essential characteristic of Angst as Heidegger describes it is uncanniness (Unheimlichkeit), a feeling of "no longer being at home." Yet in that experience playing basketball—and to judge from my own experience, in all play situations—I *was* at home in a way that I rarely feel at other times. Playing first reveals to man the true meaning of home.

And yet, if "authenticity" as the term is used by the existentialists signifies something like self-knowledge, a coming to explicit awareness of one's own being and one's place in the "world," then my experience with basketball, my experience with play generally, has been "authentic." I hope I have documented this. If so, then it looks as if "Angst" is not the only stance out of which authenticity can emerge. Two questions then arise; what is there about the play experience which can occasion self-knowledge, and why might Heidegger have overlooked it? I have already adumbrated my answer to the first question. Certainly *one* of the primary qualities of my experience which contributed to its having meaning was what Heidegger calls Being-with, or what I have called encounter. That game—all games—offered a variety of encounters which were revelatory of the kind of encounter possible in life, and so revelatory of one of the primary modes of human being. While many aspects of that experience closely fit Heidegger's framework, it now appears that Angst was replaced by encounter. And this is possible, again, because both Angst and encounter are manifestations, one "positive," one "deficient," of what Plato called Eros.

If so, why does Heidegger overlook this possibility? I believe we can now suggest the following. Interpreters of Heidegger, both pro and con, invariably follow the master in making the mood of Angst the core of any discussion about "authenticity." But it now seems that Angst is derivative of a far more basic position of Heidegger's. I refer to the fact that, by placing his prior discussion of Being-with in his analysis of "Everydayness" and so in *contrast* to authenticity, Heidegger has closed off in advance the possibility of encounter as a path to authenticity. I have already related this to an excessive concern with individuality on the part of Heidegger and the existentialists generally. Once encounter has been closed off as an occasion for authenticity, Heidegger is thrown back on the individual as the sole source of insight into himself. And what is that mood in which we are literally most individual? It is *loneliness,* which comes close to being a synonym for Angst. Thus, the crucial reason for the centrality of Angst in Heidegger's analysis—and at the same time, as the play experience reveals, his decisive mistake—is the prior rejection of encounter as one other possible occasion for that self-knowledge in which we truly become "our own selves" (eigentlich).[11]

IV

Heidegger rightly characterizes genuine self-awareness, as man's mode of transcendence. And it is transcendence, precisely the finite transcendence of self-awareness, that breaking free from the unreflective wallowing in our everyday lives, that man seeks and sometimes precariously achieves. No doubt Angst can occasion that transcendence. But I believe I have documented another occasion for a similar transcendence in my analysis of one experience in a basketball game. In play, we break out of the rut of our ordinary lives. Play thus adumbrates a deeper way of breaking out of the everyday, of achieving transcendence through encounter. Perhaps this is what Plato had in mind when he has the Athenian Stranger say in the *Laws* (803eff)

I say that it is necessary to be serious with the serious, but not with the not serious. God is worthy of all seriousness, but man is constructed as a plaything of the gods, and this is the best part of him. All of us then, men and women alike, must live accordingly and spend our lives making our play as beautiful as possible . . . We should pass our lives playing certain games—sacrifice, song, and dance—so that we will be able to propitiate the gods . . .

In play man comes close to the gods. No wonder, then, that Socrates characterizes all writing about the highest things, poetry and even philosophy as the playfulness of the most intelligent men (*Phaedrus*, 276dff, 277eff). The Platonic reaction to Heidegger and the other Angst-voll existentialists might well be: "These men are playing; but not playfully."

FOOTNOTES

1. But like all images, both similar and different, and so doubly instructive.
2. Heidegger, Martin, *Sein und Zeit,* Tubingen: Max Nemeyer Verlag, 1963, e.g. pp. 126, 127.
3. Death, obviously enough, does not guarantee meaning. My point is that only within a context of finitude is it *possible* for meaning to emerge.
4. I believe one could go further, and characterize my being in that game as "ahead-of-itself-Being-already-in (the world) as Being-alongside (entities encountered within-the-world)" or Care (*Sein und Zeit,* e.g. p. 192—Marquarrie and Robinson translation, p. 237).
5. It is tempting to close by noting an analogue to Heidegger's distinction between authenticity and inauthenticity, namely, that many, indeed most of my basketball experiences were not as meaningful as this one, although others were. But I suspect the primary difference, in such a non-intellectual activity as basketball was one of intensity of immersion. To be sure, "authentic" experiences, for Heidegger, are probably more intense than the "tranquilizing" placidness of the everyday. But to characterize intensity as the *essential* difference between authenticity and inauthenticity would be to commit the same mistake as those who claim that because, under conscious-expanding drugs, colors, sounds, and feelings are more intense, they are therefore more authentic. That view is vulgar, even if not always hedonism.

6. Heidegger, *Sein und Zeit,* p. 113 ff.
7. *Ibid.,* p. 235 ff, p. 305 ff, et al.
8. Others have generalized this, I believe rightly, to all play. Cf. Wm. Sadler, "Play: A Basic Human Structure Involving Love and Freedom," in *Review of Existential Psychology and Psychiatry,* Volume VI, No. 3, Fall, 1966, p. 242. One might argue that the play situation is irrelevant because not as real, not as important as our "working" lives, when we are *serious* (and grim). I hope my discussion has already refuted this. But in any case, such a concession to the Protestant Ethic hardly becomes the Neo-Paganism of our post-Christian "happening."
9. Gabriel Marcel has brought home forcefully a similar point against Sartre, but in a different way. Cf. "Existence and Human Freedom" in *The Philosophy of Existentialism,* New York: Citadel Press, pp. 46-90.
10. Rosen Stanley, "Heidegger's Interpretation of Plato" in *The Journal of Existentialism,* Volume VII, No. 28, Summer, 1967, p. 279.
11. In this regard, it is instructive to consider Socrates, whose explicit and constant endeavor was to know himself, but who nevertheless spent his life talking to—and loving—other people. From the absence of Angst from my basketball experience, the absence of such concomitant themes as "guilt" and "anticipatory resoluteness" becomes understandable.

Play and Possibility*

JOSEPH L. ESPOSITO

General accounts of game-playing have been advanced from various perspectives within the social sciences. From the sociological and psychological point of view, social play is regarded, in fact, as serious business—a primitive rehearsal for socialized activity (Huizinga), modeling behavior in children, sacred activity gone secular, etc. Caillois, for example, claims that "games and toys are historically the residues of culture."[1] Games re-enact cosmic and social dramas whose meanings have long been forgotten; the wish for heavenly conquest becomes the greasy pole; football, the titanic struggle between opposing forces over possession of the solar globe; kite-flying, the soul's quest to escape the body; hopscotch, the labyrinth; chess, the drama of medieval life; and monopoly, I would imagine, practice in how to get on in civil society.

The social function of games has also been the subject of considerable study. Correlations between culture and social structures have been sharpened by comparative studies of the degree of cheating allowed by cultures in their games. It has been claimed, for example, that it is characteristically Anglo-Saxon to have a game (golf) in which the possibilities of cheating are unlimited but in which the game immediately loses its point once the rules are violated. Social opportunity has been tied to the idea of being a "good sport"; sportsmanship and the premium it places on self-discipline is supposed to result from an upper-

class which need no longer hope to achieve economic success. In these circumstances, playing with dignity becomes nearly everything; winning, not very much.

Social attitudes toward games of chance are supposed to reflect deep-seated commitments on the part of a society to a certain theory of history and the way rewards are distributed. In opposing lotteries, a society is supposed to be saying that it is not wise to look for success apart from intended and disciplined effort.

Such sociological accounts of games are, for the most part, informative and, sometimes, even enlightening. That there is some legitimacy to the approach can be seen simply by noting the connection between certain kinds of games and the audience they attract. In this limited sense, Caillois is correct in noting that "games discipline instincts and institutionalize them."[2]

There is also a large body of philosophically uninteresting material on games—primarily games involving athletic competition—which emphasizes the benefits of being educated physically. Fitness, readiness, good citizenship, the proper attitude—these are the rewards of sport, looked at from the psycho-developmental point of view.

In my view, however, in neither the sociological nor psychological approaches to game-playing is there anything like a treatment which explains what it is specifically in a game-playing situation which makes that form of human activity so prevalent. One reason for this, I think, is that not enough attention has been given to the players' point of view. In

*From *Philosophy Today*, Carthagena Station, Celina, Ohio 45822. XVIII, (Summer, 1974), 137–146.

short, what has not been asked is what is in the game-situation which makes players want to engage themselves within it. All of the classification of the forms of play (for example, games of competition, chance, mimicry, vertigo) only tangentially touch upon what I shall characterize below as the common-root experience of all game-playing, an experience which any reflective participant recognizes as the essential point of game-playing, and which even the more unreflective participants can be made to see if probed in the proper manner.

Work is often contrasted to play, the implication being that play is an escape from the rigors of highly structured activity directed toward a practical goal. Work involves the routine; play is the special event. Work is serious; play is engaged in for fun. This is the view we would expect to be plausible to someone who is a part of an industrial culture. For the economic demands of that culture are such that a person can only play games after his work for the day or week has been completed. It could then easily become apparent in such a context that the essential point of game-playing must be relaxation, entertainment, or excitement. I suspect that there are people who take up one form of game-playing or another just for these reasons. Their behavior may be explained as one more of the indications of social imitation in mass society or as the result of successful recruitment by "leisure industry." However, they are not likely to take on interest in game-playing for any reason that would sustain such activity for very long. What would be lacking again is that root-experience I shall now attempt to characterize. In what follows I set out an element which appears to me characteristic of nearly all game-playing and then suggest in what way game-playing can be seen as a fundamentally integral human activity—one which may tie together and explain the plausibility of the other approaches.

Children have been noted to make up games out of the context of the moment. Rules are established, the "game" is played, and soon a verdict of success or failure is brought in. Then the "game" is finished, in many cases never repeated again. A child might decide that he "loses" if he steps on any of the cracks in the sidewalk pavement. A challenge is set up. And even if the stakes are pronounced as high ("Step on a crack—Break your mother's back!") no other sanction than the failure of staying off the crack itself is necessary for the playing of the game. In what could be called the "primal condition" of game-playing the child plays

against himself. He sets up his own rules, assesses his performance against the rule-structured situation, and passes a verdict on himself. Beyond this the game can take on a social context. The children can compete against each other; they can make the game an occasion for hurling insults, strengthening allegiances, and so forth.

Analogously, game-playing in college and professional sports can take on a social meaning that may be charged with all sorts of emotional tensions, tensions which are, from the standpoint of the primal condition of play, really beside the point. Fan allegiance surely makes possible the use of athletics as a factor in achieving self-identity and self-awareness. For example, the growth of new major cities produced a corresponding growth in professional teams as a way these cities attempted to achieve in a short time an almost Hegelian-self-consciousness. But again, in none of this can we find the reasons games are played, even by professional athletes. True, a game would nowise be an object of such widespread interest unless it presented a challenge with which the fan wanted to associate himself. But his doing so may have nothing whatsoever to do with his appreciation, which may, in fact, be lacking, of what it is like to play the game itself. He may simply want a bit of the glory his own allegiance helps produce to rub off on himself. Those attracted to games because they present situations embodying the primal condition would play them even without an audience. The social effects of games are themselves socially determinate and, so, do not shed light, in my view, on the nature of game-playing. With respect to this social context of games, Caillois' remark that "games generally attain their goal only when they stimulate an echo of complicity," surely misrepresents the more important reasons games are played.[3] Games are created, not because of something that happens in the audience, but because of something the players themselves experience. Without such an experience, games would lose their point. Caillois' remark, indicative of most accounts of game-playing, fails to distinguish between the differing standpoints of player and audience.

The player of games, if reflective about what he is doing, realizes that even beyond the success of winning the game, there is the interest he takes in the very act of playing itself. It is this interest that is difficult to understand from the view of the spectator who sees the activity of play only as a means to realizing the object of the game. To the player, the game, if properly constructed, presents not so much a challenge—in the usual sense of the word—as an opportunity to experience possibility. Games, in other words, are contrived situations, the purpose of which is to heighten and bring into focus the interplay between possibility and actuality. Each form of play, if my view is correct, should contain within it a moment when possibility can be acutely felt by the player.

Plessner has argued that "play is always playing with something that also plays with the player . . ."[4] This point is correct, at least, in characterizing games played with elastic objects. In this case, it is the player's interaction with an object difficult to control that establishes the moment of possibility: in golf and tennis it is the moment of impact of ball and club or racquet; in basketball it is the moment of impact of ball and rim; in football, the handoff, kick or pass; and in soccer, the kick. The unpredictable bounce of the ball then creates almost immediate new situations for interaction and so also new possibilities.

Plessner's remark also can be made to apply to games played with nature. Rock-climbing is sport and not simply healthy exercise because it contains a moment of possibility—the foothold or grasp on the rock which might give way without notice. In sport-fishing it is the strike of the fish at the lure or bait. (Sporting fish, such as trout or bluefish, are those which attack suddenly and often unpredictably.) When nature has occasion to play with us, as also in sailing, surfing, hunting, gliding, etc., then these activities go beyond mere leisure activity and become occasions of sportive play.

My characterization of play as an encounter with possibility, unlike Plessner's, also has application to games of imitation. The moment to be sought by the child or actor playing someone else is that moment when he really feels he has become that person. Actors certainly speak of this struggle to make the role come alive, and children sometimes seem to behave as if they are momentarily convinced they are someone else. It is the difficulty of affecting such a transition and the clear possibility of failure which make games of imitation such a challenge to the imitator himself.

To anyone who observes game-playing activity from a non-participant point of view, the player's experience of possibility goes unnoticed. To such a person the interest players take in games is often fanatical or silly. Why, he asks, should someone walk around hitting a ball, spend hours shooting baskets with a basketball, entice fish with objects at the end

of a line, or climb a mountain "because it is there?" The player himself, so long as he remains addicted to the experience of possibility contained in the situations of the game he plays, is left unmoved by such a criticism. The actual physical activity of the game—running, walking, moving pieces on a board, etc.—is of secondary importance to the player. He thinks nothing of sitting in a chair for hours or running furiously; his goal is the confrontation with possibility created out of the rules and structures of the game and his performance within that structure.

Existentialist philosophers have argued that what is most characteristic of human existence is what I have called "the experience of possibility." In such an experience they see the source of our understanding of temporality, value, guilt, love and death. "Higher than actuality stands *possibility*," notes Heidegger in *Being and Time*.[5] In less cryptic terms this means that a large part of the meaning of human experience is derived from the structuring that experience is given in time. Ortega y Gasset characterized this capacity to see experience as an unfolding of interlocking events as man's essentially historical nature; for Heidegger, it results from man's being as *Dasein*.

Heidegger distinguishes the sense of "possibility" I am referring to here from "modal possibility." The latter is either what is logically possible or what is "merely" possible ("the contingency of something present-at-hand").[6] In either of these latter cases we judge something to be possible from an abstract standpoint. The former kind of possibility, however, is something more important to us: "Possibility, as an *existentiale*, does not signify a free-floating potentiality-for-Being in the sense of the 'liberty of indifference' (*libertas indifferentiae*). In every case *Dasein*, as essentially having a state-of-mind, has already got itself into definite possibilities. As the potentiality-for-Being which [it] *is*, it had let such possibilities pass by; it is constantly waiving the possibilities of its Being, or else it seizes upon them and makes mistakes. But this means that *Dasein* is Being-possible which has been delivered over to itself—*thrown possibility* through and through."[7]

What Heidegger seems to be saying is that not all of our possibilities are regarded with equal seriousness. Some possibilities we could entertain as courses of actions are "merely" possible; we have no actual concern to tie them into the fabric of our experience. Still others present occasions for momentous decisions—they become specifically *our* possibilities and so become the object of serious concern. Perhaps nothing is so important an object of seriousness than a lost possibility. No reality may be felt as intensely as the unreality of what was not but should have been. *Existentiale* possibilities, in short, must be ones in which we have a stake through concern; in other words, ones in which failure (making mistakes) is an issue for us.

In *Being and Time* Heidegger argues that the experience of possibility is something *Dasein* seeks to avoid. Such avoidance becomes another occasion in the life of *Dasein* when the ontic and ontological become reversed. *Dasein* simply denies that its possibilities are real possibilities for itself. In Heidegger's words, "This levelling off of *Dasein's* possibilities to what is proximally at its everyday disposal also results in a dimming down of the possible as such. The average everydayness of concern becomes blind to its possibilities, and tranquillizes itself with that which is merely 'actual.' "[8] This desire to become undiscriminating about possibilities to philosophers like Kierkegaard, Sartre and Berdyaev, among others, is supposed to result from the burden of our freedom to choose the possible. The stakes in life itself are too high for us, they argue. Bad faith, inauthentic existence, the false stance of objectivity, and "slavery" (Berdyaev) are the responses we make to this situation. The institutionalization of human experience in the form of culture and civilization is supposed to mitigate our feeling of uneasiness in the face of possibility. The basis for this burden of confronting possibilities in life is precisely supposed to be in the condition that nothing is literally repeated in life. Having a conception of life, as we do, we see those possibilities which are an issue for us as demanding a timely response. This means that regret and guilt become part of the stakes of choosing in life, notably the result of mistakes.

Life itself could probably be played as a game were it not for the fact that most of us feel that death is an untimely imposition on life and not its natural culmination. The possibility of having no further possibilities, to use Heidegger's expression, reads back into the decision we make in the process of living a meaning etched in anxiety and dread. Everydayness helps to sanitize the implications of death by announcing national and other social purposes which have a seeming durability personal life does not have. What is missing in life as a whole, however, is any clear, unambiguous sense of what the rules of conduct are or how success is to be gauged. Then also in life

there is not a final summing up and resolution of the effort by the players themselves, something I think essential to game-playing.

To those who believe in a life beyond life, it is possible to regard life as a single rule-governed episode, say, for example, the journey of a soul toward its salvation. Huizinga has noted this connection between the forms of play and the sacred forms of ritual and myth.[9] So also has Santayana.[10] In the game of salvation there can be winners and losers. And the importance theologians give to the fine points in a doctrinal controversy suggests that they hold the tenets of creeds with the same regard as rules of any games must be held by those who play the game.

Kierkegaard argued that it was in the ethical and religious attitudes that the experience of the possible was most threatening to us. Aesthetic and intellectual attitudes were adopted, in his view, precisely in order to avoid the former attitudes: "Ethically regarded, reality is higher than possibility. The ethical proposes to do away with the disinterestedness of the possible by making existence the infinite interest."[11] Morality requires that certain possibilities have a demand on us to be actualized. These are the possibilities which, Kierkegaard is saying, have a greater status than the merely possible or, at least, ought to have if we are to be moral beings. They are possibilities which are supposed to engender dread in us.

In religion the dread of freedom is characterized by Kierkegaard as the experience of the demoniacal. And overcoming the demoniacal through resolute faith is the affirmation of freedom. One of the ways the demoniacal appears—a way appropriate to the present discussion—is in the sudden: "In case the demoniacal were something somatic," Kierkegaard writes, "there never would be the sudden. When a fever, insanity, etc., come back again, one discovers at last a law, and this law in some degree annuls the sudden. But the sudden recognizes no law. It does not properly belong among natural phenomena but is . . . the expression of unfreedom."[12] It is not an accident, Kierkegaard observes, that Mephistopheles appears suddenly in dramatization of *Faust*. His actions must not be continuous and, therefore, understandable.

In the religious attitude, Kierkegaard suggests, we have an example of the desire to overcome the fear of the possible by affirming the victory achieved by the "knight of faith" over the demoniacal. Precisely the opposite account of religion has been given by Feuerbach: religion closes off freedom and the possibility through its reification of value into a heteronomous structure which then is grasped, even if with passionate conviction, only by means of an act of accepting faith. It becomes a game where more effort is given to interpreting the rules than in playing the game, with the effect that daily ritual diminishes and intellectualized creeds take precedence. Of course, Kierkegaard also attacked intellectualized religion, but to Feuerbach and, more recently, to Santayana, his emphases on internal resolve would give little opportunity for one to experience the encounter with the possible in a playful manner.[13] To Feuerbach and Santayana the use of symbol and ritual afforded the opportunity to act out "salvation," i.e., experience religious value, in concrete, sensuous terms. Kierkegaard noted that mime was sometimes capable of capturing the sudden.[14] He should have realized that it could be possible to overcome the sudden in the same fashion—through mimic forms of religious ritual, what are usually called religious "celebrations" today.

Sportive playing is not burdened with difficulties of the religious or ethical attitude. Religion attempts to schematize all of life and so takes on too much. Aside from monastics most of us do not play the game of salvation throughout the daily course of our lives. The secular game, on the other hand, is of more modest design. It takes place within spatial and temporal confines more fit for human comprehension. Even beyond this, however, its most ingenious feature is that it produces a genuine experience of the possible where there is really, from life's standpoint, nothing at stake. Here the player can have his cake and eat it too. Unlike the religious drama, which is a matter of life or death where ultimate consequences weigh so heavily on the players, the sportive player enjoys a situation where all the fascination of encountering the possible exists, but where he can also assure himself that it is only a game. William James' observation that in certain cases faith in a fact can create that fact has application here. The player gives his total commitment to the game-situation created out of the rules, and in so doing he makes the possibilities of action within the game possibilities that are an issue for him.

Kierkegaard and other existentialists have enjoined us to face the possibilities in our daily lives courageously, even while telling us how burdensome that could be. "If I were to wish for anything," Kierkegaard wrote, "I should not wish for wealth and power, but for the passionate sense of the potential, for the eye which, ever young and ardent, sees the possible. Pleasure disappoints, possibility never. And what wine is so foaming, what so fragrant, what so intoxicating, as possibility!"[15] The possibilities in game-playing are such for the player that they do not disappoint him, at least, so long as the player makes the commitment to the game situation. Game-playing, then, might be seen as the opportunity to experience genuine, yet benign, possibilities outside the context of daily life. This notion can help tie together several of the more prevalent accounts of game-playing. For some players, interacting with the possibilities of sportive play can serve as a rehearsal for dealing with life's possibilities. For them it is true that sport builds character. For others, the orderliness and lack of ambiguity in game-playing makes this form of play an escape from practical living—hence, the view of sportive play as leisure activity.[16] In either case the game remains the circumstance in which the outcome of actions lies within the game itself. How the player integrates his activity as a player with the other forms of activity in which he is engaged will depend largely on the character of the player himself. However, such social consequences of game-playing, as noted earlier, which comprise a great deal of the study of play, really do not explain the essential purposes of play in the manner I have here attempted.

Eugen Fink and Howard Slusher have both advanced theories of play somewhat similar to the one I have given. Both contend, in the words of Fink, that play is "an essential element of man's ontological make up."[17] In general, however, they devote most of their effort to a description of *consequences* of the experience of the possible without emphasizing the centrality of the experience itself. Fink, for example, emphasizes the spontaneity of play and the experience of "human timelessness in time . . . a glimpse of eternity."[18] Pure spontaneity, as Dewey often noted, does not have in it the makings of a constructive experience. The goal of the player is not spontaneity itself, but rather the reward of alert action—that is, encountering and quickly controlling possible events. It is the player's timely reaction to desired or undesired possibilities that makes spontaneity an asset in play. He seeks the goal of spontaneous action—viz., a satisfying measure of himself against possible contingencies. The timelessness of play should actually be characterized as the timeliness of action in the play situation. Rather than a sense of timelessness, the player experiences the effects of time's passage in games where events usually occur suddenly, or can (as in chess).

Slusher's account of sportive play largely hinges on his view that in sport, particularly competitive sport, the player gets the opportunity to be purely a self engaged in the act of becoming—self-transcendence, to use Sartre's term. "To open oneself up, and, in the process, transcend the self is one potential contribution of sport," Slusher notes.[19] The body as object is transcended toward the body as pure activity; awareness of the other as co-player becomes transcended toward the awareness of coexistence of all players into a team, what Heidegger and Sartre characterize as the experience of "being-with."[20]

Sport, in my view, does make such forms of transcendence possible; *how* it does this has been the subject of my concern. It is precisely one's opening oneself to *possibilities* that produces the feeling of achievement or failure so essential to the awareness of having become something one was not at an earlier point. There is no opportunity for such mental, physical or social transcendence in games which are either too easy or too difficult, in games, in other words, in which the player overwhelms the possibilities of the game or the possibilities of the game overwhelm the player.

REFERENCES

1. Roger Caillois, *Man, Play, and Games*, trans. Meyer Barash, Free Press, (New York, 1961), p. 58.
2. *Ibid.*, p. 55.
3. *Ibid.*, p. 39.
4. Helmuth Plessner, *Laughing and Crying*, trans. J. S. Churchill and M. Grene, Northwestern Univ. Press, (Evanston, 1970), p. 77.
5. Martin Heidegger, *Being and Time*, trans. John Macquarrie and Edward Robinson, Harper and Row (New York, 1962), p. 63 (H38).
6. *Ibid.*, p. 183 (H143).
7. *Ibid*, p. 183 (H144).
8. *Ibid.*, p. 239 (H194–195).
9. Johan Huizinga, *Homo Ludens*, Beacon Press, (Boston, 1950), p. 26.
10. George Santayana, *The Sense of Beauty*, Dover, (New York, 1955), p. 18. Also Howard S. Slusher, *Man, Sport and Existence: A Critical Analysis*, Lea and Febiger, (Philadelphia, 1967), Ch. IV.
11. Soren Kierkegaard, "The Subjective Thinker" from *Concluding Unscientific Postscript* in *A Kierkegaard Anthology*, ed. Robert Bretall, Modern Library, (New York, 1946), p. 226.
12. Soren Kierkegaard, *The Concept of Dread*, trans. Walter Lowrie, Princeton Univ. Press, (Princeton, 1967), p. 116.
13. The Deer Park episode in the *Concluding Unscientific Postscript* indicates the seriousness with which Kierkegaard regarded daily life in the light of faith.
14. *The Concept of Dread*, p. 118.
15. "Diapsalmata" from *Either/Or* in *A Kierkegaard Anthology*, p. 35
16. John Updike's *Rabbit Run* is one of a number of works whose theme is that of the ex-athlete disillusioned with life because of the ambiguity he finds in it.
17. Eugen Fink, "The Oasis of Happiness: Toward an Ontology of Play," in *Game, Play, Literature*, ed. Jacques Ehrmann, Beacon Press, (Boston, 1968), p. 19.
18. Fink, p. 21.
19. Slusher, p. 11.
20. *Ibid.*, pp. 37 and 63ff.

An Analysis of the Futural Modality of Sport*

WILLIAM J. MORGAN

I propose in the present analysis to exact an account of what I take to be the distinctive futural character of sport. Following Heidegger's lead that the manner in which man temporalizes his time out of the future determines the complexion of the various types of Being he assumes,[1] the major thesis to be entertained in the investigation is that the origin and development of the way of Being indigenous to sport is based in an esoteric (non-everyday) projection of the future. In defense of this thesis, the futural dimension of sport will be contrasted with the futural dimension of the pre-competitive condition of sport nominally referred to as training.

The Futural Character of Training

Training, for the present analysis, will be defined as a process of making ready for a determinate end which it actively seeks to bring about. Conceived in this sense, its phenomenal character aligns itself with that activity generally referred to as making-plans. That is, training as a pre-condition of sport, and thus neither a necessary nor sufficient condition of sport proper, is founded in a project-act domain whose directed activity draws its significance rather immediately from the end sought. In light of this cursory characterization, the claim will be advanced that the phenomenal realm of training is at bottom grounded in the rather determinate way the athlete temporalizes his time out of the future, i.e., in an explicit futural reckoning which

*From *Man and World: An International Philosophical Review*, 9 (Dec., 1976), 418–434.

serves as the abiding clue for the regulation of his activities in this realm. The focal point of this futural reckoning is, of course, the postulated future not-yet province of sport. In the formulation of this thesis, we are following Dauenhauer's lead stated in a more general way with respect to the activity of making plans:

> Making plans [of which training is ascertained to be a determinate instance] is developing a self-proposed, free course of action, . . . to achieve some desired state; it is located in the individual's "future perfect lived time."[2]

Training, therefore, takes its direction from a non-thematic postulation of the future not-yet state of sport, as that projection which circumscribes the legitimate horizon of training in which its function as a process of making-ready is defined. In this futural orientation of training, time is essentially understood and interpreted as a time-for something. With this in mind, as the analysis unfolds it will attempt to show that the sense in which the athlete "has" time as a time-for something underlies the purposive character of training and further reveals its temporal nature as commensurate to the manner in which one "has" time at work.

In the pre-competitive mode of training, then, the athlete explicitly assigns himself time according to the structure time-for, and as such, projects his time in an essentially empty way. Time is experienced as empty in this fashion in a two-fold sense. First of all, in the more provisional sense, the formulation of a specific proposal for training is rooted in a futural projection which is to be filled in, given content, in a corresponding actualization of the proposal. Secondly, and more fundamentally, the subsequent actualization of the proposed projects of training does not nor in principle cannot stand as the veritable fulfillment of these proposals. This conclusion forces itself upon us in cognizance of the ultimate futural aim of training as grounded in the disparate temporal horizon of sport. Consequently, the instrumental nature of the futural reckoning peculiar to training, as that which points beyond its own temporal orbit for fulfillment, is in virtue of its ownmost temporal character a fundamental instance of empty time. This designation of the future time-for structure of training conforms with Heidegger's denomination of the inauthentic future as a form of "awaiting" which the translators, Macquarrie and Robinson, have suggested more closely approximates the expression ". . . being prepared to reckon with that which one awaits."[3]

Now it will be argued that the empty way in which man projects his future in training, a projection which has a linear structure in that it points beyond itself to sport as its not-yet terminus, underlies the manipulative posture he assumes in his dealings with the objects that comprise the equipmental complex —a complex that includes not only the implements of a specific sport form but as well one's self (in this case the body being the locus of this manipulative stance) and one's fellow athletic participants—of the particular sport he is engaged in. In the instrumental horizon generated by this specific futuralization of one's possibilities then, man's involvement with the items of his equipmental complex is predicated on securing some determinate end thereby reducing all these objects to the simple status of use-objects. As a result, an endless means-end schema is set in motion whereby every projected end becomes, in turn, a means designed to appropriate some further end *ad infinitum*. Consequently, every possibility fastened upon in training is understood and interpreted as a partial one that points to some elusive whole in virtue of the empty manner in which it looks to the future for direction.

Moreover, since training points to a future state which intentionally exceeds the borders of its own temporal ambit, it is best characterized as an open-ended activity calling only for a tentative decision and commitment in accord with its projection of an open future. In this manner of temporalizing the future,

the self disperses itself over a myriad of possibilities deciding only as to their provisional adequacy and never their final actualization. This is so because the final actualization of these possibilities initially considered in an experimental way in training is based on a decision that thrusts the athlete forward into the disparate realm of sport. It is, then, an activity which remains "still under consideration" as long as its phenomenal character stands intact, that is, unsullied by any decision to situate one's training in the past.[4]

Hence, the athlete's manipulation of the objects of his concern in training springs from the specific manner in which these objects are gathered into the instrumental purview provided by his futural temporalization of time. Thus, as a way of having time, it is rooted in an inauthentic projection of the future which determines the temporal complexion of the athlete's activity in such a way that his possibilities for Being are construed exclusively in instrumental terms, that is, only in terms of his success or failure in dealing with a particular object of his concern. This form of temporality is thus constituted in a forgetting of one's self, of one's creative possibilities for Being as an athlete, in order to sustain its preoccupation with the objects that make up its discrete equipmental milieu. It is precisely this condition of forgetting one's more fundamental possibilities for Being, Heidegger avers, that grounds man's daily involvement in the world in the mode of work:

> Letting something be involved is constituted in such a manner, indeed, that the making-present which arises from this, makes possible the characteristic absorption of concern in its equipmental world . . . a specific kind of forgetting is essential for the temporality that is constitutive for letting something be involved. The self must forget itself if, lost in the world of equipment, it is to be able "actually" to go to work and manipulate something.[5]

By way of a summary, then, it can be said that the veritable link between training and sport consists in the recognition that the directed activity of training is based in a futural projection whose realization and consequent fulfillment rest in the disparate temporal horizon of sport. Hence, the direct significance of training, that which distinguishes it from the other insipid activities of everyday life, lies in its specific function as a process of making one ready for the exigencies of sport proper. This requires, therefore, that the futural orientation of training be kept in sight as the legitimate locus of this activity. Training, then, must be recognized for what it essentially is, a precondition of sport which allows the athlete to meaningfully structure his activities in a non-arbitrary way in planning for the future time of sport.

The Futural Character of Sport Proper

Sport, as intimated by our previous remarks, is born of the decision to locate one's training in the past. This decision itself, however, springs from a futural projection on the basis of which man qua athlete catapults himself into the discrete temporal arena of sport. Hence, it is through this specific projection of the future that the temporal domain of sport is circumscribed and thus marked off from the temporal ken of training. The thesis that presents itself for immediate inspection, therefore, is that sport is grounded in a distinctive (non-everyday) projection of the future. In the attempt to validate this thesis, we will be pressed into an account of the essential features of sport's futural ecstasis, those lineaments which distinguish it from the futural character of training.

The first thing to be noted in this regard is that sport has its origin in a non-instrumental projection of the future. As such, it phenomenally manifests itself as a self-contained temporal domain which points only to its own temporal ambit in keeping with its particular projection of the future. In contradistinction to training then, fulfillment in sport is specifically a function of one's direct involvement in this medium and, therefore, not contingent upon its intersection with other phenomenal spheres. Hence, the futural projection peculiar to sport, as that which posits and seals off the self-contained phenomenal sphere of sport, precludes any attempt to adjudicate one's participation in sport in terms of a means-end relationship which takes the form of a futurally founded concern for the so-called broader concerns of life. This does not mean, of course, that sport is a human enterprise of limited concern but only that the type of concern it exhibits—as a reflection of its discrete manner of projecting the future—differs from that common to the everyday world.

Of course, in training one can speak of fulfillment in purely formal terms as a bringing to concretion the vague expectation(s) embodied in a proposed course of action through a subsequent actualization. Such talk of fulfillment, however, has at best only a facile formal meaning in that any bringing to pass of a future expectation in training is necessarily incomplete owing to its total subservence to the projected future goal of training, the posited not-yet province of sport. Sport then, unlike training, offers man an opportunity to be a whole being by creating its own fulfilled totality, a self-constituted plenum which does not infinitely disperse itself by indeterminately pointing beyond itself. And it is a genuine whole we speak of here, inasmuch as sport entails a commitment and expression of man's whole being. Indeed, it is this aspect of the futural dimension of sport that undergirds the frequent allusion to sport as that human endeavor, in a fragmented world, which offers man an opportunity to be a complete or whole being.

Hence, as the underlying projective dimension of sport, the future discloses itself as the expansive element of sport, as that temporal ecstasis which opens up a disparate realm of Being and, therewith, a unique way of confronting one's possibilities for Being. Sport thus originates in a futurally constituted distancing movement from the everyday world whose direct result is the establishment of a world unto itself. It accomplishes this result by mediating man's immediate absorption in the objects of his daily milieu thereby diverting him from his ordinary stance towards the world.[6] Thus, on the basis of this futural divertissement,[7] a temporal transposition of the everyday world is evinced in which man's calculative view of the world and his instrumental valuation of it is displaced in favor of an open disposability towards one's possibilities, possibilities which otherwise would not be available to him, and an intrinsic regard for them.

It is in and through this futural projection, then, that an ephemeral mastery of the everyday world is achieved in the name of sport; a mastery accomplished not by providing a representation of the everyday world, nor by securing some sort of mystic flight into the "other worldly," but by staking out a temporally unique way of standing in the world in a creative summons of Being. In this way, the inexorable grip our everyday way of Being exercises over our understanding of our various possibilities for Being is broken thereby altering, in a fundamental way, our vision of the world and our comportment in that world.[8] Thus, in virtue of this futural projection, man qua athlete is able to secure a genuine dwelling place in the world, one which is to be distinguished from the multitudinous positions we drift into and out of in daily life as dictated by our mindless absorption in the sundry affairs of everyday existence.

As we have argued, then, sport is based in a futural distancing movement that partitions sport off from the mart of ordinary life. However, the futural expansive element of sport includes within itself a limiting movement. And it is by means of this limiting phase that the opening forged by the expansive dimension of sport is circumscribed thus closing off and completing man's severance of his ties to an everyday mode of Being. The projection of the future indigenous to sport, then, is a closed one, that is, an opening of possibilities and a staking of the limits in which and by which these possibilities are to be realized. Hence, this limiting or closing movement is not a separate temporal moment but the necessary accompaniment of the horizon-opening projection of the future intrinsic to sport. As such, the limits introduced by the closing element of sport's futural projection are not of an external origin—as is the case in everyday life in which man is thrown into a dependent relation on the entities of the world he must deal with 'in-order-to' survive[9]—but arise directly out of this projection of a distinctive way of Being. In sport, then, man becomes the "thrower" of his own possibilities for Being by founding a world grounded not in necessity—our - being - thrown - into - the - world - unto-our-death—but in possibility—our free expression of our temporal self-being out of the future.[10]

Thus, the projection of a closed future in sport suspends the dispersal of the self in its daily mode of comportment and thereby opens up a unique way of standing in the world. In this sense, the future provides the direction for the athlete's projective extension of his self-being by overturning the equivalence of all possibilities characteristic of an everyday type of Being—the consequent effect of such an equivalence is that man is pushed and pulled pell-mell in many directions none of which are an issue for its Being because they are bound up with its forgetful deflection of itself in the immediate objects of its concern —and by disclosing possibilities for Being which are of direct issue for the athlete because they are self-constituted. It is not the case, therefore, that sport lacks direction and is purposeless, but, on the contrary, its direction and purpose are intrinsic to itself as secured by the athlete's projection of a self-enclosed temporal sphere. The future thus serves as the normative guide of the athlete's protentional disclosure of his Being in sport. Sartre provides further insight on this point:

> This position which I quickly assume on the court has meaning only through the movement which I shall make immediately afterward with my racket in order to return the ball over the net. But I am not obeying the "clear representation" of the future motion nor the "firm will" to accomplish it. . . . It is the future motion which, without being thematically posited, hovers in the background of the positions I adopt, so as to clarify them, to link them, and to modify them . . . each position has meaning only through that future state.[11]

Unlike training then, sport is not an open-ended activity calling only for a tentative commitment. Quite the contrary, the enclosed projection of the future in sport closes off as well the superficial commitment that ensues from the disposition that there is always more time to dicker with possible courses of action. In training, on the other hand, the athlete necessarily holds himself back from committing his whole being to a particular possibility owing to the fact that the open-ended future of training always grants him more time to experiment yet further with possible modes of response. In sport this condition of holding-oneself-back is averted by positing a self-contained temporal medium which demands a timely response precisely because it offers no guarantee of a future reckoning or rectification. Hence, the oft-cited resolute character of the commitment displayed in sport is at bottom rooted in the distinctive way in which sport is temporalized out of the future.

In his projection of a closed future in sport, the athlete's temporalization of time out of the future reveals itself as finite, that is, conscious of a self-imposed limit which it cannot legitimately transgress and within which its particular mode of Being transpires. However, the finite temporal nature of sport is experienced in a yet more fundamental way. That is to say, the finite status of the future element of sport lies not only in its projection of an enclosed phenomenal domain but as well in the indeterminacy which flows from this projection. This indeterminacy stems from the fact that the athlete's projection of his future possibilities includes within itself the possibility of its not-being, in other words, that the possibilities he projects and opens himself to may not be realized. Moreover, because these future possibilities are self-chosen and self-constituted, the finite character of the future assumes a resolute complexion; such that, the realization (being) or non-realization (not-being) of these future possibilities is of utmost concern for the athlete's Being. In this fashion, athletic participation takes on a measure of risk not commonly found in other human endeavors which strikes at the inner core of the self-being of the athlete. Slusher speaks further to this point:

> . . . sport provides for actualization through self-extension. . . . Man cannot count on status or social position or previously achieved excellence. He is never granted tenure. He accepts and thrives on the endless chain of uncertainty. To this end, he is a man who seeks freedom to express his humanity.[12]

The finite constitution of sport's futural ecstasis further distinguishes this activity from fantasy in which the self experiences itself, relates to itself, as pure possibility. The realm of fantasy is the realm of the "merely possible." And it is the realm of the "merely possible" owing exclusively to its surfeited projection of the future. Thus, in fantasy one's possibilities are the product of an excessive abstract futuralization whereupon the self loses itself in its fantastic projection of the future. It is for this reason that fantasy is best characterized as a "never-dwelling-anywhere" which because it projects itself "everywhere" is truly "nowhere." As Kierkegaard writes:

> . . . if possibility outruns necessity, the self runs away from itself. . . . The self becomes an abstract possibility. . . . Possibility then appears to the self ever greater and greater, more and more things become possible because nothing becomes actual . . . this is precisely when the abyss has swallowed up the self. . . . What the self lacks is surely reality.[13]

As we have attempted to show then, the futural enclosing-expanding dimension of sport founds the distinctive manner in which man qua athlete resolutely grasps his possibilities for Being. Indeed, the future manifests itself as the transcendental ground which allows the athlete to project "ahead-of-itself," and to live his life in the vision generated by his ability to be "ahead-of-itself." Hence, "the possible corresponds precisely to the future. For freedom the possibility is the future."[14] Following this line of argument, it will be suggested, in more definitive terms, that the discrete way in which man qua athlete futuralizes his time underlies the dynamic nature of the competitive zeal unique to sport. It will thus be argued that the competitive strife of sport is to be distinguished from the mundane competitive urges of everyday life precisely in relation to its distinctive temporality which temporalizes itself authentically out of the future.

As suggested by our previous remarks, the futural ecstasis of sport—including its central competitive element—is not the product of a contrived instrumental reckoning, but rather is characterized most fundamentally as a throwing of oneself towards one's possibilities in keeping with the sheer lived spontaneity of sport. Indeed, the competitive motif of sport itself demands such a going towards one's possibilities in response to the Being of sport "for-the-sake-of-which" the athlete commits himself in resolute participation. As Hyland writes in a phenomenological description of his involvement in sport:

> As I played, I played always *towards* [emphasis mine] what was to be next, not any definite shot or act, but toward any possibility that the game—and I—would realize. Thus I did not . . . pause and calculate my next move, I played, and my play was the game and what was to be the game.[15]

The authentic futural directionality of sport does not, however, preclude the fact that various remnants of time-reckoning do indeed filter into the phenomenal context of sport, principally in the form of strategy. What in fact the future character of sport does rule out, however, is that such instances of time reckoning can assume other than a subordinate role in sport, occupying at most an incidental and fleeting function, and, therefore, must ultimately give way to a temporalization of the future proffered in response to the exigencies of the competitive struggle itself.

If, however, time reckoning looms as the dominant element in the agonistic struggle of sport, such that one does not go towards its possibilities but instrumentally reckons with them in a variety of ways, then the result is an inauthentic transformation of the fundamental temporal spirit of sport which carries the predicate sport in this instance only in a vacuous nominal manner. Consequently, such instances of time reckoning can be said to impinge upon the genuine temporal constitution of sport, and, if they become the pre-eminent concern of the athlete, succeed in reducing the creative striving interior to athletic competition to a work-based circumspective deliberation of one's possibilities, a process which underscores our everyday dealings in the world. This inauthentic temporal metamorphosis of sport is felicitously conveyed in Roger

Bannister's reflections on his premature attempt to crack the barrier of the four-minute mile by running a completely planned race with his friends providing the necessary pace in this venture: "My feeling as I look back is one of great relief that I did not run a four-minute mile under such artificial circumstances."[16]

Hence, the competitive strife of sport, here construed in a manner which belies its more fashionable everyday signification, is based in the individual's resolute projection of the future, as that temporal ecstasis which grounds the authentic tenor of the sportive engagement and thus allows for one being genuinely carried away in the very momentum of the competition. Drawing this point of argument out yet further, it is argued that the athlete's resolute projection of his temporality certifies as well the authentic character of one's being-with-others in the agonistic struggle of sport. Following Heidegger's clue that: ". . . only by authentically Being-their-selves in resoluteness can people authentically be with one another,"[17] it is similarly claimed that one's genuine testimony with the significant others in sport emanates from the individual athlete's resolute decision to "take" and "have" his time in a veritable fashion. In lieu of such a resolute futuralization of one's possibilities, one's athletic colleagues are treated as mere objects to be considered only insofar as they can be manipulated to ensure the securement of one's own futurally reckoned goal. Bannister's comments are again instructive in this regard as they focus specifically on an astronomic form of time reckoning and the corresponding response to the significant others of sport which follows rather immediately from this explicit manner of assigning oneself time:

> . . . the time taken in a race depends on the way in which it happens to be run . . . if the time is the real object of the race [time here obviously refers to world-time specifically in the sense of a temporal measurement], other competitors must be ignored, unless they cooperate wittingly or unwittingly in the time schedule.[18]

On the other hand, in an authentic open response to one's future, a possibility for being-with-others resolutely is documented in the competitive element of sport which takes the form of what Heidegger calls "letting-be," that mode of response in relation to Being which constitutes the essence of what it means to be resolute in one's existence.[19] We must now subject this claim to further critical scrutiny.

For Heidegger, the easily misunderstood notion of "letting-be" does not signify any semblance of passive indifference but, on the contrary, indicates a quite significant way to be in the world, of being open and fully responsive to Being. As he remarks:

> We usually talk of "letting-be" when, for instance, we stand off from some undertaking we have planned. . . . The phrase we are now using, namely the "letting-be" of what is, does not, however, refer to indifference and neglect, but to the very opposite of them. To let something be is in fact to have something to do with it . . . "letting be" expresses itself to what-is-as-such and brings all behavior into the open. "Letting-be," i.e., freedom, is in its own self "exposing."[20]

"Letting-be," then, represents the innermost expression of our freedom to be as we are, and thus to respond to other beings as they essentially are in themselves. "Letting-be" springs from the self's ontological potentiality to "stand out from" and to "stand forth in" Being. This potentiality is grounded in our ecstatical mode of Being and, therefore, takes its cue from the self's futural transportation out of itself into the clearing of Being. Thus in sport, in letting our future be in a resolute projection of our potentiality for Being, we, in turn, let the other's future be and in this way testify with each other in the struggle of competition. Hence, together in a resolute grasp of our temporality out of the future, mundane time reckoning yields to a creative temporal expression in such a manner that the decisiveness of one's involvement is in no way mollified but enhanced. Indeed, it is in this authentic prolepsis of the future that we are thrown forward together in the momentum of the event itself. At the risk of redundancy, Bannister's remarkable insights into the nature of sport once more warrant quotation, this time in connection with his commentary on his great duel with the champion Australian miler John Landy in the British Empire Games of 1954:

> His boldness forced me to abandon my time schedule and lose myself completely in the struggle itself. After this experience I felt that I could never be interested again in record-breaking without the thrill of competitive struggle.[21]

In one respect, the foregoing analysis can be construed as an attempt to phenomenologically ferret out the fulfilled temporal horizon of sport from the empty temporal structure of our everyday way of Being. As part and parcel of this analytic endeavor, the project-act sphere of training as a determinate instance of an everyday time reckoning was distinguished from the temporal province of sport. And, in consonance with our major thesis, it was argued that what distinguishes the temporal horizon of sport from that of training, and for that matter everyday life, is the distinctive way in which it temporalizes itself out of the future. In closing, then, we would be remiss if we failed to point out that the distinctive futural character of sport may ultimately allow us to claim, from Heidegger's philosophic vantage point at any rate, an ennobling place for sport in the general scheme of things. That is to say, the "letting-be" quality of man's involvement in sport, a quality which owes its form and substance to sport's particular way of futuralizing its possibilities, suggests a possible kinship between sport and the other esteemed humanistic endeavors of life—most notably the fine arts and philosophy; for there is sufficient grounds, particularly in Heidegger's later philosophy, for distinguishing the activity of the artist and philosopher from the everyday man on the basis that in the former instance man lets beings be as they are in themselves and in the latter case beings are viewed exclusively as instruments of man's circumspective deliberation.[22]

NOTES

1. In following this lead, we are expressing as well a fundamental allegiance to Heidegger's pivotal distinction between human temporality—that form of time peculiar to the finite existing self which is characterized by the fact that it temporalizes itself out of the future in an integral temporal unity—and world-time—that form of objective time which marks the successive occurrence of things and events in the world and is characterized by its sequential nature which follows a specified genetic order emanating from the past through the present and into the future. In the present analysis, of course, our focus will be restricted to the former notion, that of human time.

2. Bernard P. Dauenhauer, "Making Plans and Lived Time," *Southern Journal of Philosophy*, VII (Spring, 1969), p. 83. As one might gather from our quotation of Dauenhauer's comments, the present investigation of training will focus exclusively on the individual athlete as a planner and subsequent doer. As such, neither the role of the coach, nor the collective making-plans specifically entailed in training for team sports, will be considered in this analysis.

3. Martin Heidegger, *Being and Time*, trans. by John Macquarrie and Edward Robinson (New York: Harper and Row, 1962), p. 386.

4. This feature of the futural character of training is common to all instances of making-plans. As Dauenhauer avers: "Since making plans is an activity which is engaged in for the future, the plan is, as such, still open to being altered, discarded or adopted. . . . all the elements of the plan are tentative." Bernard P. Dauenhauer, "Making Plans and Lived Time," p. 85.

5. Martin Heidegger, *Being and Time*, p. 405. As Hannah Arendt adroitly points out, the central issue raised by the adoption of a work-like stance towards the world is the generalization that flows directly from this stance: namely, the absolutization and exultation of work as man's highest possibility: "The issue at stake is, . . ., not instrumentality . . . as such, but rather the generalization of the [work] experience in which usefulness and utility are established as the ultimate standards for life and the world of men. This generalization is inherent in the activity of *homo faber*." Hannah Arendt, *The Human Condition* (Chicago: Univ. of Chicago Press, 1969), p. 157.

6. In this sense, it is akin to art. As Keyes writes: "If myth and experience are allowed to speak, what matters about art is that it can give us a temporary discontinuity from our ordinary way of looking at the world." C.. D. Keyes, "Art and Temporality," *Research in Phenomenology*, 1 (1971), p. 64.

7. An oblique insight into the futural distancing character of sport can be gleaned from a cursory consultation of its etymological meaning. As Keating tells us in this vein: " 'Sport', . . . is an abbreviation of the Middle English desport or disport, themselves derivative of the old French *desporter*, which literally meant to carry away from work." James Keating, "Sportsmanship as a Moral Category," *Ethics*, LXXV (October, 1964), p. 27. In conjunction with this point, we have merely argued that this "movement away from work" intrinsic to sport has its foundation in the specific manner in which man qua athlete temporalizes his time out of the future. What is interesting to note here, however, is the interpretation lexicographers have attached to this root meaning of sport. As Keating again relates: "Following this lead [the literal root meaning of sport] Webster and other lexicographers indicate that, diversion, recreation, and pastime are essential to sport. It is that which diverts and makes mirth, a pastime," p. 27. The intimation added here, one that on our view covers over the original sense of diversion suggested by its etymological root meaning, is that the diversion essential to

sport is of a mundane sort, i.e., that sport is merely a capricious interlude from the more serious business of work. What is more, accompanying this alleged shift in the etymological meaning of sport is a corresponding shift in the understanding of its temporal structure as indicated by the employment of the notion 'pastime.' Now to experience something as a 'pastime' is to experience that thing or event in its unadulterated emptiness as it passes away in the transient flow of world-time. As Gadamer points out, the view of time ". . . as something present by its emptiness . . . is connoted in part by the German expression . . . Zeitvertreib (pastime)." Hans-Georg Gadamer, "Concerning Empty and Ful-Filled [sic] Time," Southern Journal of Philosophy, VIII (Winter, 1970), p. 344. Thus, two conditions must be satisfied to fully certify the experience of sport as a 'pastime.' First of all, a leveling-off of the discrete temporal character of sport must occur in which the temporal distance that separates sport from the ordinary world is bridged thereby reducing sport to the status of an everyday time reckoning, and thus, on our account, a work-like manner of "having" time. The second condition that must be met, that condition which strips away the pretension to serious conduct that masks the empty foundation of our everyday manner of assigning ourself time, is the concomitant move which issues from the leveling-off of the temporal nature of sport: namely, the subordination of sport to the major complex of activities that collectively make up the fabric of daily life. As Horkheimer's following remarks attest, both of these conditions are implicitly fulfilled in the popular conception of sport as an instrument of ordinary life—a view which requires as an irreducible minimum a corresponding instrumental conception of sport's futural character —which is to be afforded meaning only as it serves to sustain and enhance the conduct of our daily lives: "It has often been said that sport should not become an aim but should remain an instrument . . . as long as it is only an instrument, and consciously recognized as such, it may be viewed . . . just as a pastime." Max Horkheimer, "New Patterns in Social Relations," in International Research in Sport and Physical Education, ed. by Ernst Jokl and E. Simon (Springfield, Illinois: Charles C Thomas, 1964), pp. 184–85.

8. The consequent effect of this altered vision of the world, a vision which has its origin in sport's futural anticipation of a unique domain of Being, is what Sartre refers to as a "diminishing of the reality of the real (ordinary) world," a diminishing based on the realization of a new way to-be-in-the-world which transcends the narrow boundaries of everyday existence. As he writes: ". . . play [Sartre regards sport as a form of play thus offering no apparent distinction between these two concepts] as contrasted with the spirit of seriousness appears to be the least possessive attitude; it strips the real of its reality. The serious attitude [in contrast to the sportive attitude] involves starting from the world and attributing more reality to the world than to oneself; at the very least the serious man confers reality on himself to the degree to which he belongs to the world." Jean-Paul Sartre, Being and Nothingness, trans. by Hazel Barnes (New York: Washington Square Press, 1972), p. 740. It is further worth noting that this relativizing of the "real" world effected by sport's futural ecstasis suggests a possible relation between the temporal structure of sport and that of music, generally considered by most scholars to be the purest prototype of the temporal arts, as indicated by Keyes' following remarks: "Music is a purely non-existent state of affairs made real in the presentation. But to make an otherwise non-existent state of affairs into a concrete presentation is to make the world of actual experience appear more relative as a result. Music is the reversal of priorities that makes the non-existent concrete through a sheer act of anticipation and, as long as we are under its control, makes the real world seem less absolute." C. D. Keyes, "Art and Temporality," p. 70.

9. As Heidegger states: "In existing, [Dasein] has been thrown, and as something thrown, it has been delivered over to entities which it needs 'in order to' be able to be as it is." Martin Heidegger, Being and Time, p. 416.

10. As Netzky has argued elsewhere: ". . . in most cases necessity is the ground of human freedom; in [sport] freedom is the ground of necessity." Ralph Netzky, "Sartre's Ontology Reappraised: Playful Freedom," Philosophy Today, XVIII (Summer, 1974), p. 126. It should be further noted in this regard that at this juncture our analysis departs in a major way from its Heideggerian foundation which locates the authentic character of temporality in Dasein's futural anticipation of death. As Heidegger maintains: "The more authentically Dasein resolves—and this means that in anticipating death it understands itself unambiguously in terms of its ownmost distinctive possibility—the more unequivocally does it choose and find the possibility of its existence, . . . only by the [futural] anticipation of death is every accidental and 'provisional' possibility driven out. Only Being-free for death gives Dasein its goal outright and pushes existence into its finitude." Martin Heidegger, Being and Time, p. 98. As Abbagnano has cogently argued, however, this conception of man's authentic projection of his future possibilities actually entails the negation of the very notion of human possibility. In this vein, he argues that from Heideg-

ger's espoused vantage point: ". . . the only possible choice for man is to live for death, and in the face of this, other choices are fictitious and improper. This response . . . implies the possibility of a choice; but this possibility is, in effect, a necessity because there is only one possible choice. It is easy to see how, from this viewpoint, the problematic nature of existence is inverted to its contrary, that is, to necessity. The only authentic possibility of existing is the impossibility of existing. Now impossibility is necessity [necessity considered in its negative form], and if existence has a problematic nature, then it cannot be reduced to an impossibility. . . . [In this way then] existence as possibility is negated in the very act of its acknowledgment." Nicola, Abbagnano, *Critical Existentialism,* trans. by Nino Langiulli (New York: Doubleday Co., 1969), p. 44. Thus, in light of Abbagnano's compelling rejoinder, and stemming from our analysis of sport which in a tacit manner has countered Heidegger's absolutization of being disposed towards death as the only bonafide mode of authentic existence by showing another manner in which Dasein exists authentically in lieu of this disposition, the present investigation has studiously avoided this aspect of Heidegger's theory of temporality. It is worth mentioning, however, that Heidegger himself appears to offer an amendment of this equation of authentic existence and death in his later works when he suggests a connection between resolute human response and the notion of "letting-be." Because this apparent connection will directly occupy our attention in the subsequent analysis, however, it will suffice for the present to merely mention this point saving further development for the ensuing analysis.

11. Jean-Paul Sartre, *Being and Nothingness,* p. 181.
12. Howard Slusher, *Man, Sport, and Existence: A Critical Analysis,* (Philadelphia: Lea and Febiger, 1967), p. 82.
13. Søren Kierkegaard, *Fear and Trembling and The Sickness Unto Death,* trans. by Walter Lowrie (Princeton, New Jersey: Princeton Univ. Press, 1969), p. 169.
14. Søren Kierkegaard, *The Concept of Dread,* trans. by Walter Lowrie (New Jersey: Princeton Univ. Press, 1973), p. 82.
15. Drew Hyland, "Athletics and Angst: Reflections on the Philosophical Relevance of Play," in *Sport and the Body: A Philosophical Symposium,* ed. by Ellen Gerber (Philadelphia: Lea & Febiger, 1972), p. 90.
16. Roger Bannister, *The Four Minute Mile* (New York: Dodd, Mead and Co., 1958), pp. 195–96.
17. Martin Heidegger, *Being and Time,* p. 344.
18. Roger Bannister, *The Four Minute Mile,* pp. 186–87.
19. Heidegger brings this connection between resolve and "letting-be" to light in his work, *An Introduction to Metaphysics,* where he states that: "Re-solve is no mere decision to act, but the crucial beginning of action that anticipates and reaches through all action. . . . the essence of resolve lies in the opening, the coming-out-of-cover of human being-there into the clearing of being . . . its relation to being is one of letting-be." Martin Heidegger, *An Introduction to Metaphysics,* trans. by Ralph Manheim (New York: Doubleday Co., 1961), p. 17. What is particularly interesting about this concatenation of resolve and "letting-be" is that it suggests a possible line of rapproachment between Heidegger's early and later work concerning the Dasein side of the pivotal Dasein-*Sein* relationship. That is, it suggests that Heidegger's later denomination of Dasein as a shepherd or guardian of Being—an appellation regarded by many as an indication of a fundamental shift in Heidegger's thinking regarding the role played by Dasein in the revelation of Being—requires, as does his earlier conception of Dasein, that in order for Dasein to carry out this special function it must become its own 'there,' something which it can do only by resolutely grasping its possibilities for Being. This resolute response, then, is the requisite condition of letting-something-be (a point which comes clean in his further elaboration of this latter notion), of being fully open to the call of Being. Starbuck crystallizes this point for us in his following account of sport which gives us a brief inkling, though somewhat obliquely, of the decisive element embodied in an open stance towards the world: "An athlete . . . sometimes awakens suddenly to an understanding of the fine points of the game and to a real enjoyment of it, . . . If he keeps on engaging in sport, there may come a day when all at once the game plays itself through him—when he loses himself in some great contest. In the same way, a musician may suddenly reach a point at which pleasure in the technique of the art entirely falls away, and in some moment of inspiration he becomes the instrument through which music flows." Starbuck, *Psychology of Religion.* As quoted by William James, *The Varieties of Religious Experience* (New York: Collier Books, 1970), p. 172.
20. Martin Heidegger, "On the Essence of Truth," in *Existence and Being,* ed. by Werner Brock (Chicago: Henry Pegenery Co., 1968), pp. 305–07.
21. Roger Bannister, *The Four Minute Mile,* p. 242.
22. Further corroboration of this point is supplied by James Churchill in the adjoining remarks to his translation of Heidegger's first Kant work, *Kant and the Problem of Metaphysics* (Bloomington: Indiana Univ. Press,

1972), p. 236, ftn. 17. In this vein, Churchill relates that: "The notion of letting-be adumbrated in *Sein und Zeit* . . ., later becomes an important factor in Heidegger's conception of what distinguishes the activity of the artist from that of the ordinary man. Although never clearly stated as such, this conception seems to be that the artist differs from the ordinary man who looks upon essents [beings] only as objects having value for him as tools, etc., in that the artist lets the essent [being] be what it is in itself. . . . There is also a suggestion in Heidegger that the activity of the thinker (the true philosopher) is not unlike that of the artist in that the thinker 'lets Being be'."

Man and Sport*

KEITH ALGOZIN

Paul Weiss answers his question about man's fascination with athletic events in terms of our concern for excellence: "Unlike other beings we men have the ability to appreciate the excellent. We desire to achieve it. We want to share in it." The athlete, consciously or not, desires to achieve bodily excellence, and spectators of the game participate in the athlete's achievement: "In the athlete all can catch a glimpse of what one might be were one also to operate at the limit of bodily capacity." "The athlete is matched here by the thinker, the artist, and the religious man. Without loss of their individuality they too instantiate man in splendid form, which the rest of us accept as an idealized portrait of ourselves. But the athlete shows us, as they do not, what we ideally are as bodies."

Weiss's account of the game seems to me to invite a still fuller characterization of what it is about this event that rivets men's attention and calls forth their passionate emotional involvement. In this paper I will begin by sketching Weiss's account of the game and then I will go on to suggest those ingredients which are perhaps implied in Weiss's account but which seem to me to deserve more explicit stress.

I

For Weiss the model of the athletic display of bodily excellence is the Olympic Games. Men and women of all nations have trained their bodies to challenge the resistances of

*From *Philosophy Today*, Carthagena Station, Celina, Ohio 45822 (Fall, 1976), 190–195.

space and time with the speed, endurance, strength, accuracy and coordination prescribed by the various particular sports. Each nation is a team of athletes, a single body whose members strain to function at the outermost limits of their specialized capacities. The nations contest in the Games for the prize of being judged by impartial witnesses to represent human bodily excellence. A particular sport is the rules which keep a particular contest fair and at the outermost limits of man's bodily capacity in a particular situation. It is also the historical record of man's bodily achievement under these trying conditions. Thus, all sports taken together may be said to represent the form of the human body, both the self-definition it has so far achieved and the rules by which this effort to define itself by outdoing itself is to continue. In the Games the contesting athletes instantiate this event of human bodily self-definition; they represent the human body challenging itself to surpass itself. The record-setting victor of the Game instantiates human bodily excellence on behalf of all nations: all stand united and completed in the public display of that bodily excellence which all have helped reveal, which all now know they cherish, and which all now vicariously share: "By representing us the athlete makes all of us be vicariously completed men. We cannot but be pleased by what such a representative man achieves." To be sure, the athlete cannot claim to represent the full nobility of human being; he represents only the bodily substrate of those higher, spiritual values which are instantiated in the spiritual leaders of civilized mankind and whose enactment by all men would be the crowning unification of nations. For this reason men in pursuit of excellence need neither engage in athletics nor even enjoy the Games. But in the Games all men can find a facet of the perfection they seek as men, and one which reflects in its way their higher aspiration: "By participating in a public game with others, the athlete makes an intimately related whole with them. The more the players act together, despite competition, to produce a common game, the closer is the bond uniting them all. Athletes make more vital that harmonization of men which religious men suppose God's presence in the world entails."

I have tried here to suggest the philosophical scope of Weiss's theory of sport for this can serve as a measure of any attempt to contribute further to our philosophical understanding of the widespread fascination with athletic events. As Weiss suggests, a plausible philosophical account of this phenomenon must relate it to man's basic concern for fulfillment. Sport is philosophically relevant because it does in fact attract men of all times and cultures; the wide-spread attraction of sport is the philosopher's clue that there is operative here, in some fashion, the most basic tendency of human nature. And a genuinely philosophical account of sport must therefore clarify what this activity is and must be simply because it is a human activity reflective of human nature itself. It must tie sport into the whole round of human endeavor by means of some principle which relates sport to everything else that men strive to be and do. Now when Weiss views the game in this philosophical light he sees it as an instance of man's universal endeavor to discover and to be what he is. Better: for Weiss the game is but one instance of man actually being what he is, namely, the communal discovery of what he is. While those involved in the game are focusing upon bodily excellence, the philosopher sees that what binds all elements of the game into a whole and relates that whole to all other human endeavor is the event of communal self-revelation itself. Thus, sport is seen to reflect human nature itself, and such a vision is the goal of a philosophical account. An alternative philosophical account of the game (which Weiss spars with throughout his book) highlights the factor of competition and the fanatical enthusiasm of those whose deepest concern is for the victory, not of impersonal human excellence, but of their own side over the other: sport as but one instance of men's basic concern to subjugate one another, a socially acceptable outlet for aggression, a training ground for war. Both of these accounts of sport agree that the game is an occasion for some specifically human fulfillment, and both can argue their case without appealing to what those who are involved in sport say they find fascinating about the game. For only one who sees the game in the light of the whole of human endeavor can judge what it is that is really going on here.

While I would agree that a philosophical account of the fascination of the game cannot rest its case upon a poll of sports enthusiasts, I discern in myself and others some agreement as to why the game is exciting, an agreement which rests upon a common experience which may at first seem trivial but which may urge us to reflect upon the fascination of the game from a yet broader perspective. This broader perspective would not so much settle the issue between these two rival views of sport as it would complement them both. It would abstract from their disagreement over what particular goal men seek by nature and focus attention upon the assumption they share, that man is primarily a being that seeks to enact goals. The common experience that persuades me to occupy this middle ground between these opposed theories of the game is simply that of the excitement that is engendered by a close contest. The suspense of a close contest grips and excites us, but what is remarkable about this excitement is its independence from our concern with either bodily excellence or subjugation: while it may heighten because the contest is between the world's best athletes, it may be present also during a close contest between the world's worst; and while it may heighten when we are committed to one side over the other, it can occur too when the contest is close and we do not really care who wins. In short, when we speak of a good game we are often referring neither to how it is being played nor to who is winning but simply to the fact that it is close.

Excitement over the closeness of the game stands somewhere between the enthusiasm of the biased fan and the enthusiasm of Weiss's impartial spectator of bodily excellence. This excitement refers, I believe, to something which is at the core of our fascination with the game but which both of these opposed views must treat as relatively accidental, namely, its vivid display of utterly effective action. Both of these views are prevented from appreciating fully men's fascination with athletic events because their attempt to explain sport in terms of one particular human goal as opposed to another leads them to neglect the display here of what all human beings, regardless of their particular goals and by virtue of their very situation as human beings, must find pleasing: "unalienated action," action which is both fully illuminated with knowledge of the difference between victory and defeat and utterly effective because reverberating for good or ill throughout its world. What game is played, what victory and defeat are taken to mean, may well be personally or culturally relative, but there remains —especially at the climax of the game—that which can be the object of universal fascination—the display of unalienated action. In the following remarks I will try to place our fascination with the close game in the context of our human aspiration for unalienated action.

II

We humans exist by nature beyond our animal issue of merely staying alive; we search for that proper way of life which connects our accidental being to the substance of the world. It is our privilege, apparently, to know that something is at stake in the world, that there is a difference between good and evil; and it is our despair not to know what this difference is, or, when we feel we know it, to be powerless to enact it. In the paralysis of doubt, indecision and powerlessness we are on the periphery of things, outside of the garden looking in, and aware of our nakedness. To be sure, we are always dressed up to some extent in our language, in the revelations uttered by generations of men upon discovering what we are to be and do in various situations. In a language the basic units of meaning are the model actions of good conquering evil which are our customs and institutions, and to live within a language is to be guided daily by such models. In the light of such a model we see everything in our situation as it really is: this or that resistance or assistance to the good we supremely value. And if, in addition, we have the power to enact these immediate, absolute, final judgments upon our situation, our action is unalienated: we trip the lever which effectively transforms our situation of unfulfillment into one of fulfillment. Here, in the midst of unalienated action (e.g., doing everything appropriate to romantic love, driving a car, managing affairs of state) we are on top of the world, moving spontaneously from within our immediate perception of challenges and tools, keeping alive that order of things to which we are committed. Yet in the midst of our daily lives we often find ourselves estranged: we sense that what we can effectively bring about in the world is ultimately worthless. This estrangement occurs when we find that our attempts to bring about what is supremely good are ineffective. It occurs too when we no longer know what it is supremely good to be, do, and bring about in the world, when, consequently, everything in our world, including ourselves, appears ambiguous because we do not know precisely what is really at stake in our lives. In either case our action is alienated for we suspect that what we are doing is trivial. And we experience here our human aspiration toward that action by which we would engage, as spontaneously and effectively as we drive our cars or eat our meals, in the issue that is ultimately at stake in our lives. In such unalienated action we would be shaping our lives in terms of that meaning which defines our relationship to the essence of the world; we would be god-like actors who effectively order our world to conform to our idea of its truth; we would ourselves be the model of being human in the world. It is against this background of our human aspiration for unalienated action that I believe we may best appreciate our fascination with the close game.

The game carries to completion that mastery of our situation which we all glimpse in our daily lives but which often eludes us. In this connection it should be stressed that the world of the game is a real world: the players, who are trying throughout to keep their victory alive, are not actors following a script but men responding on their own to the challenges of contingent events. Thus the game can be a microcosmic display of what we feel we ourselves are going through when we are keeping alive the bonds of a family, remaining faithful in crises to a friendship, meeting challenges of a profession. But the game is an unreal world: it rests upon the arbitrary two-dimensional decision that in this delimited setting we will be dedicated solely to this definition of victory. The result of this decision is a single context of action, horizontally delimited from beginning to end and ruled vertically throughout by a hierarchy of unquestioned values. Especially important here are the sharp, unequivocal definitions of victory and defeat and the elimination of all skeptical questioning as to whether such victory is supremely worth-while. When more important matters break in upon the game, trivializing it, its spell is broken. To enter the world of the game is to leave behind that dimension of ourselves which can doubt and belittle all values and is to live within a closed system of action whose every present moment is both fully illuminated by a well-defined supreme value and transparently related to every other moment in the whole. Precisely such a closed, translucent system is necessary if there is to be a display of unalienated action.

At every moment of the game the athlete is at the center of this translucent system, acting spontaneously from within his immediate apprehension of what everything in his world truly is and requires in the light of the whole. At his disposal are the supreme value he is to realize, the unambiguous facts of his situation, and his practiced capacity to counter obvious resistances with obvious tools. He is the picture of action flowing smoothly from final judgments and decisions of conscience in appropriate response to the changing situation. (This illusion of conscious judgment and decision is heightened by slow-motion reruns of his action coupled with commentary on what was presumably going through his mind.) The delightful opportunity this spectacle affords those who know the intricacies of the game should not be underestimated. We men crave to pass final judgments upon things and often enough we make fools of ourselves by doing so, but in the midst of the translucent game we are in that delightful situation of being able to estimate with some accuracy the ultimate worth of actions and of men.

Finally, in addition to being unalienated in the sense of being fully illuminated with the knowledge of victory and defeat, the athlete's action is unalienated in the sense of being decisively effective in settling the issue at stake in this world. What is at stake, what victory in the game means to us—whether the triumph of bodily excellence or of ourselves over the other—is not as important here as the fact that an entire world is seen to be at stake, suspended between equally possible alternative completions and awaiting the decisive action that will settle its fate. At the center of this world the athlete is performing at every moment—especially at the climax of the game when all see that either victory or defeat might be the last word about this world—that utterly effective, world-reverberating action which, so unlike our own futile stabbing about, decides the fate of the world. At this moment it is as though the athlete is an extension of ourselves: we stretch in suspense toward knowing the outcome of the world and find in him the decisive action that settles the issue. Thus our dislike of chance outcomes and

ties, and thus too our effort to pin-point the turning-point of the game. Man is the being to whom it can appear that the world is at stake, and games are ultimately symbols of the serious religious business of world-transfiguration and salvation. This feature of any game permits us to imagine that even the most minor contest is a world championship with everything riding on its outcome. It permits too wide-spread hero-worship of the athlete who has been at the absolute center of things performing the paradigmatic heroic action.

But from this perspective on athletic events as symbolic of world-salvation we should not be led to identify fascination with the game with the will to escape the real world: the game as an illusory world, like that of drunkenness or drugs, where defeated man can have the meaning and power denied him in the real world. No doubt the game can serve as the occasion for escape from reality, but it can just as well serve to display and confirm the lives of those men who are creatively engaged in unalienated action in the important social and political dimensions of any culture.

Are we then to view the fascination with the game as essentially human self-worship: the game as the image of human self-salvation, man playing God? I think not. I have located our fascination with the athletic game at the intersection of our human suspense about the outcome of the world and our human aspiration toward the unalienated action which decides the issue. Suspense is a broad category of fundamentally human experience which occurs whenever we are in doubt about an outcome. And, of course, doubtful outcomes are of the very stuff of our lives. We are the being who can surround any beginning with the open space of many possible alternative endings. We are in suspense during a joke, a roll of the dice, a sentence, our inquiry into a crime or the universe, a prayer to God, and, in general, from one moment to the next. But in the midst of our suspense we look always to that decisive operation of the essence of our situation which we believe will properly complete what has begun, and even when we believe that this essence of things is no human action whatever we think that some way of properly being ourselves is essentially bound up with its operation: the dice player's superstitious rituals, the penitent's good deeds or properly prayerful attitude, the scientist's appropriate attitude of impartial openness to the truth, etc. etc. In short, in our suspense we look always to some unalienated agency which is the essential truth of the situation, and we feel that there is something we are to appropriately be or do, some unalienated action we are to perform, in order to be properly attuned to this essential truth of things. Whatever agency is thought to be operative in the universe, unalienated action is the primary human concern, and I have contended only that because the athletic game is a vivid, concretely physical display of unalienated action itself, it can be an object of fascination for all men. In closing it should be noted that we have gone no distance in resolving the issue between Paul Weiss and his opponent as to whether athletic competition is essentially men's dialogical revelation of bodily excellence or an instance of their will to power. The question, whether communication or tyranny is the unalienated action given to men to perform lies subsequent to the general fascination with unalienated action itself, which can draw both groups to the game.

Limits of the Life-Order: Sport*

KARL JASPERS

The self-preservative impulse as a form of vitality finds scope for itself in sport; and as a vestige of the satisfaction of immediate life, finds scope for itself in discipline, versatility, adroitness. Through bodily activities subjected to the control of the will, energy and courage are sustained, and the individual seeking contact with nature draws nearer to the elemental forces of the universe.

Sport as a mass-phenomenon, organised on compulsory lines as a game played according to rule, provides an outlet for impulses which would otherwise endanger the apparatus. By occupying their leisure, it keeps the masses quiet. It is the will to *vitality*, in the form of movement in the fresh air and sun, that leads to this communal enjoyment of life; it has no contemplative relationship to nature as a cipher to be elucidated, and it makes an end of fruitful solitude. The exercise of the combative instinct or of the desire to excel in sport demands the utmost skill, each competitor wishing to establish his superiority over the others. For those animated by this impulse, the all-important thing is to make a record. Publicity and applause are essential. The necessity of observing the rules of the games establishes an obedience to good form, thanks to which in the actual struggle of life rules are likewise observed which facilitate social intercourse.

The venturesome doings of individuals show forth what is unattainable by the masses, but

* From *Man in the Modern Age*. Translated by Eden and Cedar Paul. Garden City, New York: Doubleday, 1957. Reprinted with permission of Routledge & Kegan Paul Ltd.

what the masses admire as heroism and feel they would themselves like to do if they could. Such exemplars stake their lives as mountain-climbers, swimmers, aviators, and boxers. These, too, are victims, at the sight of whose achievements the masses are enthused, alarmed and gratified, being inspired all the while with the secret hope that they themselves, perhaps, may become enabled to do extraordinary things.

A collaborating factor in promoting a delight in sport may, however, be that which, in classical Rome, unquestionably helped to attract crowds to the gladiatorial shows, namely the pleasure that is felt in witnessing the danger and destruction of persons remote from the spectator's own lot. In like manner the savagery of the crowd is also manifested in a fondness for reading detective stories, a feverish interest in the reports of criminal trials, an inclination towards the absurd and the primitive and the obscure. In the clarity of rational thought, where everything is known or unquestionably knowable, where destiny has ceased to prevail and only chance remains, where (despite all activity) the whole becomes insufferably tedious and absolutely stripped of mystery—there stirs among those who no longer believe themselves to have a destiny establishing ties between themselves and the darkness, the human urge towards the alluring contemplation of eccentric possibilities. The apparatus sees to it that this urge shall be gratified.

Even so, the activities of modern man in

sport are not made fully comprehensible through an understanding of what such mass-instincts as the aforesaid can make out of sport. Looming above sport as an organised enterprise wherein the human being forced into the labour mechanism seeks nothing more than an equivalent for his immediate self-preservative impulse, we discern, we feel, in the sport movement, something that is nevertheless great. Sport is not only play and the making of records; it is likewise a soaring and a refreshment. To-day it imposes its demands on every one. Even a life that is over-sophisticated gives itself up to sport under stress of natural impulse. Some, indeed, compare the sport of contemporary human beings with that of classical days. In those times, however, sport was, as it were, an indirect participation of the extraordinary man in his divine origin; and of this there is no longer any thought to-day. But even contemporary human beings wish to express themselves in one way or another, and sport becomes a philosophy. They rise in revolt against being cabined, cribbed, confined; and they seek relief in sport, though it lacks transcendent substantiality. Still, it contains the aforesaid soaring element—unconsciously willed, though without communal content—as a defiance to the petrified present. The human body is demanding its own rights in an epoch when the apparatus is pitilessly annihilating one human being after another. Modern sport, therefore, is enveloped in an aura which, though the respective historical origins differ, makes it in some ways akin to the sport of the antique world. Contemporary man, when engaged in sport, does not indeed become a Hellene, but at the same time he is not a mere fanatic of sport. We see him when he is engaged in sport as a man who, strapped in the strait-waistcoat of life, in continuous peril as if engaged in active warfare, is nevertheless not crushed by his almost intolerable lot, but strikes a blow in his own behalf, stands erect to cast his spear.

But even though sport imposes one of the limits upon the rationalised life-order, through sport alone man cannot win to freedom. Not merely by keeping his body fit, by soaring upward in vital courage, and by being careful to 'play the game', can he overcome the danger of losing his self.

Man Alone*

WILLIAM A. HARPER

Of late it has become increasingly difficult for man to become aware of his unique existence. He is constantly being categorized, functionalized, labeled, and numbered. He is a passive witness to the demise of his own uniqueness and to the extinction of his own being. Man is handing over his personal identity in exchange for the comfort and security afforded him in the Heideggerian *they*. It is this notion of personal identity with which I am here concerned, a notion that can be likened to asking the question: "Who am I, really?" It is the intention of this article to demonstrate that because the asking of the question "Who am I?" presupposes *that I am*, it is first necessary to become aware of my existence (that I am) before I can consider answering the proposed question of personal identity. And it will be suggested that man's relative aloneness in sport can provide an opportunity for seizing upon the awareness of one's own unique existence.

The surrendering of one's self can be no better explicated than by reference to the "official dossier" as characterized by Marcel,[4] in which the essence of a human being is reduced to a few pages of paper: pages indicating his name, his address, his financial standing, his vocation, and his physical characteristics:

The point here is not only to recognize that the human, all too human, powers that make up my life no longer sustain any practical distinction

* From *Quest*, XII (May, 1969), 57-60.

between myself and the abstract individual all of whose "particulars" can be contained on the few sheets of an official dossier, but that this strange reduction of a personality to an official identity must have an inevitable repercussion on the way I am forced to grasp myself. . . . What does a creature who is thus pushed about from pillar to post, ticketed, docketed, labeled, become, for himself and in himself?[4:36]

The submerging of the individual identity attains an even more crucial position in the metaphysics of Heidegger,[2] where I (*Dasein*) am absorbed and hiding in the everyday world of the *they*. *Dasein* is captive in the everyday through the phenomena of idle talk, curiosity, and ambiguity whereby I tend to seek anonymity in holding the public values and championing the everyday knowledge:

In utilizing public means of transport and in making use of information services such as the newspaper, every Other is like the next. This Being-with-one-another dissolves one's own Dasein completely into the kind of being of the "Others," in such a way, indeed, that the Others, as distinguishable and explicit, vanish more and more. In this inconspicuousness and unascertainability, the real dictatorship of the "they" is unfolded. We take pleasure and enjoy ourselves as *they* (man) take pleasure; we read, see, and judge about literature and art as *they* see and judge; likewise we shrink back from the "great mass" as *they* shrink back; we find "shocking" what *they* find shocking.[2:164]

The I is lost in the averageness of the *they*, in the publicness of the Other. And this public-

125

ness controls the way in which everything (both the world and I) is interpreted; it is never wrong. For Heidegger, "everyone is the other, and no one is himself."

And still another voice adding support to the case for the "surrendering of self" and the difficulty in maintaining one's personal identity, is that of Jean-Paul Sartre.[3] The everyday man, according to Sartre, who is in a state of self-deception (bad faith) by public demand, abandons his own unique individuality in fulfilling a particular function:

Let us consider the waiter in a cafe. His movement is quick and forward, a little too precise, a little too rapid. He comes toward the patrons with a step a little too quick. He bends forward a little too eagerly; his voice, his eyes express an interest a little too solicitous for the order of the customer. Finally there he returns, trying to imitate in his walk the inflexible stiffness of some kind of automaton while carrying his tray with the recklessness of a tight-rope walker by putting it in a perpetually unstable, perpetually unbroken equilibrium which he perpetually reestablishes by a light movement of the arm and hand. All his behavior seems to us a game. He applies himself to chaining his movements as if they were mechanisms, the one regulating the other; his gesture and even his voice seem to be mechanisms; he gives himself the quickness and pitiless rapidity of things. He is playing; he is amusing himself. But what is he playing? We need not watch long before we can explain it: he is playing *at being* a waiter in a cafe.[3:255-256]

For Sartre, society (Heidegger's *they*) demands that he fulfill his function and that he limit himself to his function. Self-deception is maintained when man is not what he is.

Since the common denominator in the three aforementioned descriptions of the abrogation of the self is a state of being whereby man is as others wish him to be, it must now be relatively apparent that to seek an answer to the question "Who am I, really?" is a project guided by uncertainty, ambiguity, and mystery. The man who seeks an answer is condemned to struggle, sentenced to tentativeness. And yet the search goes on. Men want to know. Therefore, it would seem that the initial undertaking is by far the most crucial: man must *become aware* of his unique existence (that he is). Man must realize *that he is* before he can attempt an understanding of *who he is*. And it is in a state of aloneness, a state of solitary presence within-one's-self, that one may realize his uniqueness. Being alone is not dependent upon physical isolation. I can be "with others" while locked in a closet, and I can be with myself in a room full of people.

Being alone is, in a sense, a oneness; a singularity; a unity within one's self. And in being aware of this whole or total state one can truly understand *that he is*.

Man is alone in sport. When he is actively involved, his personal success or failure depends solely upon him. The man in sport cannot shirk being alone; he cannot defer this state in preference for a public substitution. His only choice is to play or not to play. If he chooses the former, he is condemned to solitude. However, an awareness of this single state is by no means guaranteed. True, the realization of his isolation belongs only to the participating man himself, but this awareness is not a cognitive, predetermined choice. The feeling is not easy to come by. Many times this revealing understanding comes about when a man does not fulfill his expected potential, an experience more than merely isolating:

For Manager Brown, getting along is making do with the material at hand—of which the best is schizophrenic Snoopy, who sometimes imagines he is an alligator but steals second base like a lion. A second worthy principle is tolerance. It is horrible, sure, to see easy fly balls muffed, but horribler yet to muff them yourself.[7:46-51]

Only those who are less than perfect in the athletic endeavor can understand what it means to drop a fly ball, miss an easy lay-up, double fault on set point, or pull a six-inch birdie putt. The experience is indeed individualizing.

Many other times it may be the acceptance of personal responsibility which opens one up to knowing that he is. And it is the *awareness* of this personal responsibility which characterizes the man who really knows he is alone in the sport experience. In his aloneness the obligation to himself distinguishes his sport experience from the "other" determined experiences of the everyday world. And it is this reliance upon his own special capabilities and potentials, and not the public panaceas, that allows the sport participant to realize his unique individuality. In an awareness of his personal responsibility, Rick Barry, a professional basketball player, says the following:

"There are a lot of guys who work hard at defense, they play you close and they make you work for every shot. But it all comes down to whether you can put them in or not. In the final analysis, it is not them stopping you but *you* missing it." He kept talking in the second person, but as he went on and expanded, the "you" seemed to contract more and more from the general to the personal.[1:82-85]

In short, the occasion of this awareness may be any immediate happening. It may be the loneliness of the cross-country bicyclist; the suffering of the long distance runner; the pain and agony of the mile runner; the physical beating taken by the boxer; or the frequent "hits" received by participants in contact sports. It may also be the elation in winning; the deep despair of losing; the nervous tension and excitement before a competition; the fear of an opponent; the battle against nature; the freedom of movement; or the frightening realization of one's mortality that comes in facing death:

Auto racers, they defy death. I stare it right in the face. I believe we were born dead. I did not ask to be put on earth. I have accepted the fact that dying is a part of living.[5:60-70]

Evel Knievel, the motorcycle jumper who plans to jump the Grand Canyon on a jet propelled bike, went on to say, "My thing is a serious thing. . . . I'm awful nervous . . . [but] I'm really doing what I'm doing."

The occasions are many; the feeling is real. It is for man himself, in the end, to realize himself as man, to shake himself loose from his death grip on the averageness of the everyday, and to *be*. In the aloneness of sport man is potentially able to realize that he is— that he is unique—that there is no other person like him in the world. He is, and that in itself is important. One must imagine that Don Schollander, captain of the Yale swimming team and winner of four gold medals in the 1964 Olympics, has loosened his grip on publicness, when, in rejecting functionalization, he describes well the task before each man:

I don't call myself a swimmer at all. I'm a person who happens to swim. . . . Before you decide how you want to live your life, you must look at yourself and *attempt* to know yourself. I look at myself as a person who is trying to develop as an individual. It's been important to me throughout my life to be much more than a student, to be much more than an athlete, to be much more than anything.[6:24-34]

Whether he is hurling a javelin, soaring off a ski-jump, performing a double back flip off a diving board, or screaming towards earth in a free fall sky dive, man is alone. He is beyond the world of public determinations; of official identities; of functions; of self-deceptions and of everydayness. And in the solitary state of oneness, man can meet himself. Whether he meets a friend or a complete stranger, he very suddenly knows *that he is*.

REFERENCES

1. Deford, Frank. "Razor-cut Idol of San Francisco," *Sports Illustrated*, February 13, 1967, 32-35.
2. Heidegger, Martin. *Being and Time*, translated by J. Macquairre and E. Robinson. New York: Harper and Brothers, 1962.
3. Kaufmann, Walter. *Existentialism from Dostoevsky to Sartre*. Cleveland: World Publishing Co., 1956.
4. Marcel, Gabriel. *The Mystery of Being*: Volume I, *Reflection and Mystery*. Chicago: Henry Regnery and Co., 1950.
5. Rogin, Gilbert. "He's Not a Bird, He's Not a Plane," *Sports Illustrated*, February 5, 1968, 60-70.
6. Rogin, Gilbert. "Is Schollander a Swimmer?," *Sports Illustrated*, April 1, 1968, 24-34.
7. Schulz, Charles. "The Woes of a Peanut Manager," *Sports Illustrated*, June 20, 1966, 46-51.

Identity, Relation and Sport*

ELLEN W. GERBER

I

Psychiatrists, sociologists and educators, in particular, have noted the phenomenon of sport as being a part of every culture that has ever existed. At one time or another participants have included every age group from children to the aged, and every stratum of people within a society. The attempts to explore the reasons for this phenomenon have led to the development of a whole set of Freudian symbols connected to sport; to theories concerning the diversion of the Darwinian-designated instincts for survival to competition on the field of play; to the idea of sport as preparation for life; and to the concept that sport is a way for man to demonstrate his ability to control his environment. Each of these approaches appears to have validity as it is applied to different people at different times. This article seeks to explore another possible dimension as answer to the questions of why people participate in sport—what satisfaction they gain from it, what meaning it has for them.

This approach may be expressed by the following hypothesis: When people are engaged in the act of competing in a sport they are essentially engaged in a dialogue between themselves and the other players. The relationship of the players to each other is basically an I-Thou relationship, thus making sport a medium for self-definition and the creation of man's essential being (or being of essence).

The ontological question has been studied by philosophers since the beginning of philosophical thought, but new questions focusing on the differences between the being of existence, the primeval life force, and the being of essence—man as the sum total of his individual experiences—have been the focus of thinkers in the mid-twentieth century. The crucial relevance of this question was not to the philosophers alone, but to the artists, poets, dramatists, theologians, novelists, and readers as well. Exploration of the question became loosely systematized into the formal philosophy of existentialism, but writers who did not necessarily consider themselves existentialists explored the nuances of the problem in tangential ways. Among these was the philosopher-theologian Martin Buber.

Buber's concern was with existential meaning, particularly how and where man finds meaning and how this relates to the development of his own being. William Barrett, author of *Irrational Man*, a study in existential philosophy, commented:

Buber is one of the few thinkers who has succeeded in the desperate modern search for roots, a fact with which his work continuously impresses us. . . . At first glance his contribution would seem to be the slenderest of all the Existentialists, to be summed up in the title of his most moving book, *I and Thou*. . . . But this one thought—that meaning in life happens in the area between person and person in that situation of contact when one says *I* to the other's *Thou*—is worth a lifetime's digging.[1:16-17]

* From *Quest*, VIII (May, 1967), 90-97.

Unlike Sartre, Buber believed that man is not doomed to live alone and alienated, finding himself only in a confrontation with his own non-Being. In *I and Thou* he theorizes that man finds himself, man becomes, man is, only in relation to his Thou. Through relation, through the encounter of the I with the Thou, through the dialogue, man finds himself, his meaning and his roots.

As Buber discussed and explored this concept of relation he indicated that unfortunately it is the exception, rather than the rule in man's life. Man is more likely to meet man not as a Thou, but as an It. It is more likely that he will experience another than that he will stand in relation to him.

Man travels over the surface of things and experiences them. He extracts knowledge about their constitution from them: he wins an experience from them. He experiences what belongs to the things.[8:5]

Man meeting an It is not an unimportant happening. As man grows in his ability to experience and to use, he transmits this knowledge from generation to generation, so that in each succeeding culture the world of objects and the manipulation of Its becomes more extensive. But (and this is the dilemma of the whole cybercultural revolution), the development of the real man, the essential man, striving for meaningful life, can occur only through the I-Thou relation.

All things have within them the disposition to be Thous, however briefly, however rarely. In fact Buber emphasizes that only God never becomes an It. Man, animals, natural objects, inanimate objects, all move in and out of true relation with each other, move from the I-It stand to the I-Thou, to the I-It, living the I-Thou encounter sometimes briefly, sometimes lengthily.

But when one that is alive arises out of things, and becomes a being in relation to me, joined to me by its nearness and its speech, for how short a time is it nothing to me but Thou! It is not the relation that grows feeble, but the actuality of its immediacy.[8:98-99]

The value, the tremendous importance of the I-Thou encounter, is that ". . . Without *It* man cannot live. But he who lives with *It* alone is not a man."[3:34] Man finds himself and defines himself, not by his experience with "Its," but by his relationships with "Thous." "That essence of man which is special to him can be directly known only in a living relation."[6:205]

II

The I-Thou relationship is the dialogue between man and man. "I-Thou is the primary word of relation. It is characterized by mutuality, directness, presentness, intensity and ineffability."[8:57] An examination of the attributes of this special relationship as they may occur when playing a sport, follows in this article. Any sport might be used in demonstration, for the basic structure of competition to score points against opposition within defined areas and under defined rules, is present in all sports where players compete connectedly.* From among the possibilities, tennis doubles was selected because it is a sport played by both men and women; is the same game for both; is sometimes played by both at the same time; and has the situation of having both opponents and teammate.

The level of competition is an important factor affecting the entire discussion, because the extent of the individual's involvement is crucial to the whole subject of relation. It is assumed that the degree of involvement will depend upon what is at stake to the individual participant at the moment of the game, and this may range from one end of a continuum to another. Hidden psychological need for status or overt desire for a high grade could make a simple class contest a very important event to a student. The important point is that the potential for relationship exists and the degree to which it occurs is dependent upon the player's level of involvement.

Mutuality. The meaning of the word "mutuality," perhaps the most crucial of all the words describing relation, is the most difficult to comprehend. Buber considers that man lives in a two-fold world, in accordance with his two-fold attitude. In the one world man is an object among objects, perceiving and experiencing the qualities of things and events around him; in the other world man lives as an authentic being—the world lives neither within him (as the idealists would say) nor outside of him (as the realists would say)—but rather they take their stand in mutual relation to each

* This arbitrarily excludes sports where players compete separately, such as weight lifting, or field events, but it is acknowledged that it might be possible to uncover the elements of an I-Thou relationship in these sports also—especially with regard to man and his implement. However, in the last of Buber's books, *The Knowledge of Man,*[4] he deliberately attempts to distinguish the *I-Thou* as a dialogue between man and man, excluding the relationship between man and objects in nature that had been included in earlier writings.

other. "Only when a structure of being is independently over against a living being (*Seiende*), an independent, opposite, does a world exist."[4:61]

The implications of mutuality make the point particularly crucial. It must be asked: "*Who* is this I, this man, who can take his stand in relation?" This is the basic question of Being that existentialism is so concerned with.

This human being is not *He,* or *She,* bounded from every other *He* or *She,* a specific point in space and time within the net of the world; nor is he a nature able to be experienced and described, a loose bundle of named qualities. But with no neighbour, and the whole in himself, he is *Thou* and fills the heavens.[8:8]

He is "whole in himself"; he is independent, therefore, for dependency cannot exist concurrently with wholeness; and he accepts the wholeness, independence and authenticity of the Thou. When two beings take their stand in mutual relation to the other each chooses and is chosen, and in so doing affirms and is affirmed.

But the speaker does not merely perceive the one who is present to him in this way; he receives him as his partner, and that means that he confirms this other being, so far as it is for him to confirm.[4,p.85]

Whether the players in a tennis match perceive each other as objects or take their stand in mutual relation to each other, can now be considered. The ball is put into play and the four players move about the court:

But what is it that motivates my* movements? It is you—both my opponents and my teammate; it is not a quality of you, not your strength, or beauty, or known skill that I consider and move in response to. Rather it is you as a totality. I quite literally move in relation to you. My own movement is at once a response and an instigation. During the course of play there is no thought, no examination, no experiencing, but simply the response of my being to that of yours, and vice-versa. Before play, or after play, or perhaps during a pause, this mutuality slips away and the object "I" very much evaluates the object "you." I may consider your ability to place your fore-

* The choice was made to use first person when demonstrating the I-Thou relationship situationally. It is believed that this will make clearer the realities of the dialogue by enabling the reader to enter the situation in a more personal way.

hand; the relative strength of your backhand; your short serve; your tired physical condition; your sense of humor; your sportsmanship—I can examine any one of a number of qualities in this "it." My partner is better than I and we carefully consider this as we arrange ourselves on the court; your service is stronger and we decide that you shall serve our first game, but when play begins, or resumes, these examinations, these considerations melt away and we play with a wholeness of self that cannot be taken apart. Your grace or lack of it goes unnoticed; I see you, but I do not look at you. I summon the totality of my powers; in the deepest recesses of my being I know that your presence is there. I send the ball across—the ball that is now part of me because it too has stood in relation to my effective power—and you step forth to meet this ball that is part of our mutual relation. And in the act of my sending the ball across I affirm your presence. And in the act of meeting it and returning it, you affirm my presence. We stand in mutual relation to each other.

Directness. There are two connotations to the word "direct" when used in connection with relation. The first is that:

No system of ideas, no foreknowledge, and no fancy intervene between *I* and *Thou.* . . . No aim, no lust, and no anticipation intervene between *I* and *Thou.* . . . Every means is an obstacle. Only when every means has collapsed does the meeting come about.[8:11-12]

And the second is that "In face of the directness of the relation everything indirect becomes irrelevant."[3:12]

In the first instance Buber expresses an essential phenomenological approach. In the light of the I-Thou there is nothing but the real, the essential *I* and the essential *Thou,* uncluttered by the distortions that man habitually places upon objects as he looks at them in terms of how he may use them or what they can mean and do for him. When one meets a *Thou* directly there is no use, no need, no plan, no temporizing and therefore, no distortion. In the words of Paul: "For now we see in a glass darkly, but then face to face. Now I know in part; then I shall understand fully, even as I have been fully understood."[10:I Cor.13:12]

Probably nowhere more than in a sport situation is this concept clearly demonstrated. The naked clarity of self-distortion superimposed upon the other stands out in this type of action situation where all judgments are acted upon and returned with immediate results.

In our tennis game I am continually confronted with the fact that you are where you are, rather than where I might have thought you to be. I can place the ball down the alley and score a point if you truly cannot get to the ball; however, if I theoretically believe you cannot get there, and you do, you can return the ball. The evidence is always there. There are many times though when the habit of manipulation becomes too strong and I will try to play the shots as they come to me, and also to manipulate your future shots—perhaps by forcing you to set-up a ball to me. In these instances, when I am playing my own game *and* yours, I fall back into an I-It relationship.

The second instance is also demonstrated with especial clarity in the context of sports. My concern, my relation, on the tennis court is with the others, with the balls, and with the racquet. I must face all of these directly—and if I do so the world drops away, becomes irrelevant. When the game is over and the directness slips into indirectness, there is the sudden realization that it's late; that I have an aching blister on my hand; that I am hot and thirsty; that my partner did not play well, etc. In the face of direct relation all these became irrelevant. In direct relation I accept all that is around me as it is and respond as I am. In sport this is greatly facilitated by the constant pattern of action and response that in its immediacy exposes illusion.

Presentness. "The real filled present exists only in so far as actual presentness, meeting, and relation exist."[3:12] When Buber talks of the "real filled present" he distinguishes between the use of the word present in ordinary concepts of time, and the word present (perhaps it should have a capital P) that signifies the illuminated now, when both past and future come together. T. S. Eliot, the poet, expressed this perfectly when he said:

At the still point of the turning world. Neither flesh nor fleshless; Neither from nor towards; at the still point, there the dance is, But neither arrest nor movement. And do not call it fixity, Where past and future are gathered. . . .[7:119]

Presentness is a condition of relation, but relation is also a condition of presentness. To Buber, "True beings are lived in the present, the life of objects is in the past."[3:13] "Its" and things find meaning only in the completed action, or the examined quality, because only afterward can they be related to other things which are useful and have meaning. But the men in dialogue find their meaning *within*

the encounter, *within* the relation, and thus know the "real filled present."

As I face the others in our tennis game, the past and the future coalesce into the present moment. Whatever you mean to me, you mean now, at this moment, because our actions recognize the reality of each other. From this recognition comes our meaning, and from this meaning comes our recognition. The present moment is affirmed in your movement of response to me, in your act of sending the ball—of sending yourself to me, in my act of receiving, and in my partner's racing to be by my side at the net. There is no past and no future to be considered; in our relation is presentness.

Intensity. What is meant when one speaks of a human being as intense, or a human relationship as an intense relationship? In the mechanical world degrees of heat can be measured, but in the human world there is no such gauge. Instead, intensity refers to degree of involvement. In an I-Thou relationship the involvement of the individual must be total and undivided. "Every real relation with a being or life in the world is exclusive. Its *Thou* is freed, step forth, is single, and confronts you."[3:78] "What then do we know of *Thou?*—Just everything. For we know nothing isolated about it any more."[3:11] When one speaks of degree of involvement in the context of intensity it does not mean that the whole person is involved to greater or lesser degree, but that more and more of the person is involved, concentration and perceptions are more singly focused, until finally *all* of the person's powers are involved, and then it can be said that there is total involvement and intensity.

When I enter into our game of tennis I am more fully I than just before we have begun. The difference lies here: as I play—run, swing, lunge, push myself to limits of physical giving and endurance—I am involving that part of me which is only rarely called forth, the strength and swiftness of my body. You call this forth from me—you demand the response that involves *all* my powers. If I am to really play, really compete, the only way in which I can respond is with total involvement. I have to gather together all my forces and expend them totally in the single swinging thrust of hitting the ball. Sometimes I do not; sometimes you do not ask for all of me; sometimes the demand is not there and I can return the ball, or not return it, with only partial involvement—with no intensity. But other times in the magic of a well placed shot you ask me for everything. And in that moment there is a heightened, very real intensity between us.

Ineffability. Ineffability is the summing up characteristic of relation; all the other factors are inherent in the meaning of the term. With utterance, directness and intensity and presentness would fall away, for the demands of speech call forth examination, which in turn sends one back into the past and breaks up unity; it sets up barriers between people as they strive to understand the meaning of the utterances. For a relationship to be ineffable does not mean that it must be silent, though in such a relationship much silent communication takes place, but it means that it must be silent about itself.

As my partner and I move up and down the court together we do not need to discuss where we are or should be—we are simply there together, moving in concert. As I hit the ball and cause you to respond by bringing your whole being to its meeting, there is no speech between us or even within us singly. The meaning of the dialogue between us would be changed by speech; it would be destroyed by analysis—as indeed it does become when later we talk of "why" and "when" and "how." At that time we may argue, accuse, reject, criticize, suggest. But earlier, in the silence of our dialogue, there was only acceptance. Relation is ineffable.

III

"And in all the seriousness of truth, hear this: without *It* man cannot live. But he who lives with *It* alone is not a man."[3:34] Man finds himself and defines himself, not by his experiences with "Its," but by his relationships with "Thous." The I-Thou relationship is characterized by being mutual, direct, present, intense, and ineffable. When the kind of relationship that exists between the players in a game of tennis is examined, it is evident that it exhibits the characteristics of an I-Thou relationship. It must be understood that this does not happen every moment of every game, but rather it does happen, or can happen, in the circumstances described. The importance of this may be suggested by the final quotation:

But the *I* that steps out of the relational event into separation and consciousness of separation, does not lose its reality. Its sharing is preserved in it in a living way. In other words, as is said of the supreme relation and may be used of all, "the seed remains in it."[3:68]

The nature of the game, and of sports in general, is such that this kind of relationship tends to occur. Thus, through the medium of the game man approaches his fellow players as *Thous,* and finds meaning in his own *I.*

REFERENCES

1. Barrett, William. *Irrational Man.* New York: Doubleday Anchor Books Edition, 1962.
2. Buber, Martin. *Between Man and Man.* New York: Macmillan Paperbacks Edition, 1965.
3. ————. *I and Thou.* New York: Charles Scribner's Sons, 1923.
4. ————. *The Knowledge of Man.* New York: Harper Torchbooks Edition, 1965.
5. ————. *The Way of Man.* Pennsylvania: Pendle Hill Pamphlet 106.
6. ————. *Two Types of Faith.* New York: Harper Torchbooks Edition, 1961.
7. Eliot, Thomas Stearns. *The Complete Poems and Plays, 1909-1950.* New York: Harcourt, Brace and Company, 1952.
8. Friedman, Maurice S. *Martin Buber: The Life of Dialogue.* New York: Harper Torchbooks Edition, 1960.
9. Howe, Reuel L. *The Miracle of Dialogue.* Connecticut: The Seabury Press, 1963.
10. *New Testament,* Revised Standard Version I Corinthians 13:12.

Competition and Friendship [1][*]

DREW A. HYLAND

I would suppose that nearly everyone who has participated in competitive sports, from sand-lot games through the more organized level of high school and college teams to professional athletics, has had one version or another of the following two experiences. On the one hand, we have experienced that situation in which our competitive play breaks down into alienation. This can of course take on a variety of forms and degrees of intensity. It can be as mild as a slight feeling of irritation when we feel that our opponent has hit us, or perhaps hit a ball *at* us, harder than he or she needed to. Or it can be the stronger and more pervasive feeling which some of us have that we "do better" in competitive sports when we are angry at our opponents, that somehow this spurs us on so that we "really want to win." It can show itself at those times when we hurt someone in competitive play, yet instead of feeling apologetic or at least sympathetic towards our injured opponent, we find ourselves exhilarated. At its extreme form within the context of sports, the game actually degenerates into fisticuffs. In all such cases as these, we have that co-presence of competition and alienation which is so common that it has led some to see a causal relation: competition *causes* alienation. Anyone who has never experienced one form or another of alienation in their competitive play has had an extraordinarily fortunate—not to say sheltered—sporting experience. But there is a second kind of competitive experience which most of us have also

had, one very different from the latter. I refer to that experience of competitive sport in which our relation to our opponent can be that mode of positive encounter which deepens into a form of friendship. Many of our closest friends are people whom we "get to know" in competitive situations. For many of us, playing sports with someone is a way of preserving and deepening an established friendship. Sometimes we can even say that "I never play harder than against my friend," yet even this greater intensity enhances rather than diminishes the positive strength of the relationship. I note with interest that there is less disposition to attribute a causal relation here between competition and friendship; we are rarely informed that competition causes friendship. Still, anyone who has never experienced this sort of friendship in competitive play has had an extraordinarily unfortunate—not to say perverse—sporting experience.

Now the point of these remarks is to enable me to establish what I take to be an apparently obvious but strangely controversial beginning: the empirical news is that both alienation and friendship sometimes accompany competition. This raises a set of questions upon which I should like to reflect in this paper. First, can we speak of a causal relation between either competition and alienation or competition and friendship? If neither, what then is the nature of their respective relations? If both, how can competition be causally tied to such apparently opposite phenomena as alienation and friendship? For that matter, is the direction of the causal relation reversed,

*From *Journal of the Philosophy of Sport,* V (Fall, 1978), 27–37.

that is, do either alienation or friendship *cause* competition?[2] It is important to reiterate that despite the empirical presence of both alienation and friendship in the competition of play, there is and has been a strong tendency to associate competition closely with alienation, and to regard friendship as in tension not just with alienation but with competition itself. Because the relation between competition and friendship is less obvious and perhaps less prevalent, I shall focus on that relation in this paper, though I hope my remarks will be germane to a reflection on the relation of competition and alienation as well.

A second sort of question raised by the co-presence of friendship and alienation in competitive play is this; since both do sometimes occur in play, it would seem to follow that our competitive play ever and again *risks* alienation. (Can we say as well that it risks friendship?) What is the broader significance of this risk-taking element in our competitive play?

I wish to make it clear immediately that these questions are by no means peculiar to the play situation. The relation of competition and alienation, competition and friendship, competition and risk-taking, these are issues of human being itself. At the same time, as I have argued elsewhere, (8: p. 87) the play situation, by its natural intensity and its—sometimes arbitrary—delimitation in space, time, and purpose, can make certain themes more visible than in our ongoing everyday lives. To be sure, play and playful competition can without doubt be engaged in for their own sake; that is compatible with my conviction that the foundational issues of play are not limited to play itself. For this reason, a good part of this paper may seem to wander far from the explicit issue of play. But if I am successful, I will be able to show the intimacy between play and human being by showing how they shed light on *each other*. Let me begin with the following considerations.

The view has been stated by many an armchair philosopher that human beings are "by nature" competitive, by which is usually meant that in one way or another, whether in our business dealings, or our creative projects, our play, or our love affairs, the "competitive instinct" will eventually show itself. Moreover, this thesis, when it is set out with care, seems usually to be coupled with a second thesis about the natural *alienation* of human beings. Thus Hobbes speaks of the "state of nature" as a "war of all against all," (6:pp. 87, 106) and Hegel, in his famous account of the development of self-consciousness in the *Phenom-enology of Spirit,* speaks of a primordial "fight to the death" arising out of the desire for recognition (4:pp. 113–114). In perhaps its most popular version, Marx, who does *not* accept the teaching that human being is *by nature* competitive and alienated, still preserves such a close connection between the two that he argues that the removal of competition—through the overcoming of capitalism —will bring about the abolition of alienation (10:pp. 131, 155 et al.).

On the other hand, there is another thesis about human being, usually associated with romanticism, that argues that human beings are by nature friendly, or loving, that only the perversions of society or history bring about the rise of competition or alienation.[3] Significantly, the view that human beings are naturally friendly is usually contrasted to the view that we are by nature competitive.

Perhaps I can now reformulate the guiding themes of this paper at a more fundamental level. Is it the case that there is a necessary connection between human being as competitive and alienation? Or is there a conception of human being which would allow that we be, in a sense, both *by nature* competitive and *by nature* given to friendship? I wish to entertain the thesis that there is indeed such a conception, and moreover, that human play is just the theatre where that complex nature gets most visibly manifested. But the sense of human nature in which competition and friendship are not merely compatible, but closely connected, needs some working out.

Let me begin by delineating two conceptions of the individual which, once again, are usually taken as in tension if not utterly opposed. I shall call them respectively the monadic and the relational. Briefly, the spokesmen for the monadic conception of the individual argue that human being is—or at least should be—an autonomous, self-reliant monad, whose essence, literally whose being, is intrinsic. To be sure, such individuals will enter into relations with others; this is not a view which argues that becoming a hermit is the *telos* of human existence. But such relationships as people enter will not on this view be literally essential to their nature. Our relations with others may please us, trouble us, amuse or bore us. But they will not make us what we are. As three well-known versions of this view of the individual, I would mention the position presented in Adam Smith's foundational work on capitalism, the *Wealth of Nations* (14:passim, esp. pp. 14, 423, 651), Friedrich Nietzsche's ideal of the *Übermensch,* for whom friendships arise not as a "need" but as a free gift of the "overfulness" of that autonomous individual (11:pp. 168, 173–174, 190, 273), and finally, the individual as presented in the works of Henry David Thoreau, a self-reliant being capable of living as a "world unto himself."[4] Let me emphasize that the spokesmen for this conception present it as desirable, sometimes even as an ideal; and indeed, most of us do experience this sense of autonomy as a positive one. Conversely, we often are troubled when we feel our relations with others to be what we disparagingly call "dependency relationships." Let it suffice to say that this model of the individual has a long, a complex, and we can even say a noble history in our tradition; but no more so than the second conception of which I spoke earlier, that of the relational individual.

According to the spokesmen for the relational individual, we are relational by nature. We are what we are and who we are, positively or negatively, in terms of the name and nature of our relations with others. For example, at the level of social role definition, if I am a father, husband, teacher, and athlete, these definitive roles all refer to modes of relations with others. I want to emphasize that the difference between this view and the former does not depend on whether or not we do relate to others, but on how essential those relations are to our being. As examples of well-known versions of the relational conception of the individual, I would cite the Aristotelian definition of human being as "the political animal" (2:1253a), its Marxian reformulation as "species being" (10:p. 127 et al), and the standpoint of the existentialist thinker, Martin Buber, who begins his famous book, *I And Thou*, with the teaching that,

> "There is no I taken by itself, but only the I of the primary word I-thou and the I of the primary word I-it." (3:p. 4)

As in the case of the monadic individual, so here, the adherents to this view in nearly all cases *affirm it*, see it not only as the natural way for humans to be but as desirable and something to be perpetuated. Indeed, the appeal of participatory involvements, from team sports to nationalism, would hardly be understandable if the conception of the individual as relational did not contain some truth.

The study of the histories of these two viewpoints, the ebb and flow of their dominance, and the efforts to reconcile them would shed considerable light on the development of our tradition. Our purpose here is a more limited one, for which the above sketch will hopefully suffice. We need to ask the relationship, if any, between these conceptions of the individual on the one hand and on the other the themes of competition, alienation, and friendship which are central to the present reflection. I would submit the following thesis, that the conception of the individual as monadic typically and most easily develops an understanding of human being in which competition is present and tends toward alienation, whereas the relational view more easily develops a version of natural friendship, either as original or as a goal. It is not difficult to cite as *prima facie* evidence for these associations some of the previous examples. There is a clear relation between the monadic conception of the individual and the competition of capitalism for Adam Smith, who in order to claim that some *good* will emerge from this situation is forced to the somewhat desperate expedient of the "invisible hand" (14:p. 423). Nietzsche, who clearly argues for the monadic view, accepts and even affirms alienation as part of the life of genuinely creative individuals (11:pp. 168, 190). Again, Marx draws a clear connection between the abolition of alienation under capitalism and the fulfillment of the relational ideal of species being (10: p. 155). Finally, the connection between the relational view and a natural tendency to friendship can be seen in Buber's fundamental thesis that the I-thou relation is the highest possibility for human being (3:passim). If this is plausible, then we must note immediately that the oppositional character of our subject seems to have been deepened. Natural competition and alienation seem grounded in a conception of the individual as monadic, natural friendship in the individual as relational, and these two conceptions seem themselves in fundamental opposition.

But the greatest minds of many a generation have been unsatisfied with this initial opposition. Because both have their appeal, because most of us when we reflect about it want to consider ourselves both monadic, with its connotations of autonomy and authenticity, and relational, with its connotations of community and participation, efforts have been made again and again to argue that the opposition is not irreconcilable, that human being is both monadic *and* relational, a position whose attractiveness is mitigated only by the recognition that it is easier said than justified. Still, numerous efforts at reconciliation of the two positions have been made, and I wish to appeal briefly to one of the most famous, again only with sufficient depth to enable us to relate it to our guiding theme. The position I shall outline might be associated with the Socrates of the Platonic dialogues.

According to the Platonic Socrates in the *Symposium,* the human soul is decisively characterized by eros (love).[5] We are erotic in our very being. Eros, in turn, is characterized by three fundamental aspects. On the one hand, it is incompleteness, partiality. Erotic beings are beings who, in their being, are incomplete, who are not whole. Second, eros is the experience of, or in its highest instances the explicit recognition of, this incompleteness. Erotic beings experience their incompleteness and the most self-conscious of them recognize it as such. Thirdly, consequent upon the first two aspects, eros is the striving to overcome experienced incompleteness, the striving for the attainment of wholeness out of partiality. Erotic beings, then, are incomplete, experience that incompleteness, and strive to overcome it. This, according to Socrates, is the basic structure of what we call our "love affairs," to be sure, but in fact we use the term "love" to refer to only one of its instances. *All* situations in which we strive to overcome experienced incompleteness, whether of sexuality, of political power, of wealth, of creativity, or of wisdom, all are testimony to our erotic nature. In short, we are erotic through and through.

Now it is not difficult to see how this view attempts to hold that we are both relational and monadic. On the one hand, as incomplete, we are not autonomous; we do not contain the ingredients of completeness within ourselves. We *are* a relation to others—to all other things but especially to other humans—in so far as we see in those others the possibility of fulfillment. I am what I am in terms of the way I experience my eros; my relations with others are the ways in which I seek wholeness. Thus, to use earlier examples, if I am a father, husband, teacher, and athlete, these all testify to ways in which I have experienced incompleteness and strived to overcome it; they are the ways in which I manifest my eros.

On the other hand, my experience of incompleteness, my choice of the ways I shall strive to overcome it, make me what I am as a unique individual. To paraphrase Martin Heidegger's remarks about Dasein, eros is "in each case mine" (5:p. 68). Part of the much discussed striving for "identity" could be construed as the effort to get clear for ourselves about our *own* eros, about our *own* experience of incompleteness and how we will choose to

strive after fulfillment. In this sense, to again borrow phraseology from Heidegger, eros is indeed "our ownmost possibility, nonrelational, certain and as such indefinite, not to be outstripped" (5:p. 303 et al). In short, our eros makes us each what we are, as individuals, and as such unique. To now put these two points together, we could say that our eros *individualizes* us—makes us each the unique indivdiuals that we are—but it individualizes us *as* relational beings. The beings that get individualized by their eros are relational beings.

To repeat, I have outlined the above sketch of the Socratic understanding of human being only in order to enable us to pursue our theme somewhat further. Hopefully, we are now in a position to ask, if indeed the monadic and relational conceptions of the individual are not irreconcilable, if there is a sense in which human being can be both, what does this suggest about the relationship between competition and alienation on the one hand, which we earlier associated with the monadic individual, and friendship on the other, which we connected most fundamentally with relational individuality? Evidently, it suggests a closer relation than at first appeared. The problem is to work it out adequately.

In order to do so, it will be necessary for me briefly to review two positions I have developed in earlier publications (7:p. 36–49). There I have tried, first, to develop an adequate characterization of what I have called the stance of play, the orientation or mode of comportment we take toward the world and toward other people when we play. I have called that stance "responsive openness." Let me explain as briefly as possible. When we play, whether that play be skiing, tennis, checkers, fishing, or playing house, it seems to me on the one hand that we are more aware of things, more open to possibilities than we are in typically nonplayful situations. To take an obvious example, the person skiing is more aware, more open to, the quality of the snow, the placement of trees, the movements of other people, than is the person, even the same person, slogging through the snow on the way to work. At the same time, the stance of play cannot simply be openness, for as such it could be mere passivity, and play is usually —though not always—considered an active phenomenon. In addition to openness, the player must also be responsive to what he or she is open to; one must be capable of responding with one's mind and body to that with which our openness presents us. Thus again the skier does not merely "take in" the snow, trees, and other people but responds to them with the activity of his or her mind and body. Although these qualities are usually present to some degree in all conscious experience, I find them heightened in situations which we regard as play, and so I have characterized the stance of play as responsive openness.[6] Moreover, this stance can easily be related to the characterization of human being as erotic. Because we are incomplete, because, as I earlier put it, we do not contain the ingredients of completeness within ourselves, we must look to others—to things in the world and to other people—for what fulfillment can be ours. This means, of course, that we must be open to others, aware of their presence, their nature, their possible relation to us. At the same time, again, we cannot merely be open but must respond to that openness, a response which constitutes our erotic effort to seek fulfillment. In this sense, responsive openness is seen to be literally a natural stance, a stance founded in our nature as erotic beings. And so from this standpoint, play as responsive openness can be seen—and recommended —as natural to human being, as one of the most fundamental ways in which we come to be as human.

Second, I have argued (7:p. 44 ff) that there is a close kinship between play as responsive openness and the Socratic conception of philosophy as a stance of questioning, or as Socrates regularly puts it, of aporia. Let me again explain briefly. Philosophy, as the love of wisdom, is an explicit, self-conscious manifestation of our erotic nature. As lovers of wisdom, philosophers are distinguished from wise beings (who, suggests Socrates, would have to be gods) (13:203e–204a) by a lack of wisdom, but are distinguished from the non-philosophers by their having experienced and recognized that lack and the desirability of overcoming it. Now, if, *per impossible*, someone were wise, if, that is, one were capable of giving a comprehensive and consistent account of the whole, the proper mode of discourse for the expression of this wisdom would of course be assertion. The wise person would assert the truth. But according to Socrates, philosophers are not in this position. The proper mode of *philosophic* discourse must be one true to the philosophers' situation as *lacking* wisdom but striving for it. That appropriate mode of speech, indeed the appropriate stance toward the world, is one of questioning, a stance for which Socrates himself becomes famous through the Platonic dialogues. For questioning, the stance of questioning, testifies at once to a lack of wisdom —otherwise we would not need to ask questions—yet at the same time to a striving for it —that is why we question. But one could equally well say, questioning testifies at once to an *openness* to things, yet at the same time to a responsiveness toward what we question openly. The Socratic interrogative stance, or aporia, is thus the philosophic manifestation of responsive openness, which is why several times in the Platonic dialogues philosophy is associated with the highest forms of play (12:276c.d).

To summarize briefly the points needed to develop our theme; it has been suggested, first, that play is characterized by a stance toward our world of responsive openness; second, that this stance is itself founded in the nature of human being as erotic; third, that philosophy is also a manifestation of our erotic nature; fourth, that the appropriate Socratic philosophic stance is one of questioning; and finally, that questioning itself exhibits the stance of responsive openness, and so of play, in the highest degree.

We are now prepared to relate what has been said to the possible reconciliation of competition and friendship. Let us begin with competition. Consider first the original meaning of the word. *Com-petitio* means "to question together, to strive together." Immediately we see that according to the original meaning of the word, competition is in no way necessarily connected to alienation; instead, it is easily tied to the possibility of friendship. It is a questioning of each other *together*, a striving *together*, presumably so that each participant achieves a level of excellence that could not have been achieved alone, without the mutual striving, without the competition. We find the same sense in the related word "con-test," a testing together, where again the notion of togetherness suggests a cooperation which points much more naturally to friendship than to alienation (cf. 9:pp. 23–30). There are, of course, related words which do suggest the elements of alienation. Perhaps the most obvious is "opposition," in which we *posit* ourselves *against* the other, a characterization which clearly makes space for alienation. It is as if the elemental words developed for our play situation indicate the possibility both of alienation and of friendship as naturally tied to play. For our purposes, what we need to emphasize is that competition in its root meaning suggests an affinity more with friendship than with alienation.

Now of course, etymological meanings, though instructive, hardly would be sufficient alone to establish this philosophic point. But there are at least two other considerations which suggest that the connection between competition, questioning, and friendly cooperation is no etymological accident. First, I would remind you of what we could call the existential evidence adduced at the beginning of this paper. From time to time, friendship does arise and is even deepened within the context of competition. To be sure, this establishes no causal relation, but it does testify clearly to the compatibility of the two, and establishes at least the possibility of a closer connection. It is clearly commensurate, for example, with the older conception of friendship as a "demand relationship," wherein friends, far from "not hassling" each other or letting each other "do their own thing," exhibit their friendship through the constant if implicit demand that each be the best that he or she can be. Competition manifestly can be a mode of this form of friendship. Second, the considerations earlier proposed about the relation between eros, responsive openness, play, philosophy, and questioning offer, I believe, a kind of ontological evidence, or perhaps better, an ontological framework within which we can understand that and how competition and friendship, though not necessarily in a causal relation, are nevertheless intimately connected. Competition, as a questioning or striving together, is grounded in our eros, our sense of incompleteness and striving for fulfillment. Here, however, the sense in which that fulfillment is enhanced by and with others is made explicit. In competing with others, our chances for fulfillment are seen as occurring within a framework of positive involvement with, a cooperation with or a friendship with, others. Far from being opposed, competition and friendship are seen to be founded together in our natures as erotic.

At the beginning of this paper, I asked after the relation between competition and friendship, competition and alienation. I specifically wondered whether that relationship was causal. The gist of these reflections is to incline me to answer, no. Competition *causes*, in the sense of efficient causality, neither friendship nor alienation, nor vice-versa. That is not the accurate statement of the relation. Nor is it adequate merely to say they are compatible, that competition is occasionally accompanied by friendship (or alienation). I have argued in my development of the Platonic standpoint that the relationship is more intimate than

that, that both are founded together in our nature as erotic. Let me now try to specify that relation. What I am pointing toward, I believe, is a *teleological* relation between competition and friendship. That is, I am saying that competition, as a striving or questioning together towards excellence, *in so far as it most adequately fulfills its possibilities*, does so as a mode of friendship. To state it differently, the apotheosis or highest version of competition is as friendship. Moreover, like all good teleologists, I hold the *highest* possibility to be the truly *natural* situation, in the light of which other manifestations of competition, specifically that of alienation, are to be judged defective. According, then, to my teleological account of competitive play, all competitive play which fails to attain its highest possibility, that of friendship, must be understood as a "deficient mode" of play. This could even be interpreted as implying an ethical injunction: we *ought* to strive at all times to let our competitive play be a mode of friendship.

Now of course, this happy state of affairs can and does break down all too regularly. Our "competition," we could now say, devolves into "opposition," and we experience the common co-presence of alienation and play. Why does such alienation occur? There are no doubt myriad reasons, ranging from the personal psychology of the individual participants, even our moods and what has happened to us before we play, to social convention (it is obviously more acceptable to have fights in hockey games than in basketball games; indeed, one sometimes gets the feeling it is socially expected), to the *Zeitgeist*, the tenor of the times. The point of the preceding remarks is to establish that it is not *natural* that competition lead to alienation; we need not accept it as "part of what competition is," and thus by accepting it implicitly affirm its presence, warrant its perpetuation. Still, to repeat, and by way of assuring you that I am not playing the ostrich with my head in the sand, alienation does occur regularly in competition. It is part of the risk we take when we play competitively, and this leads us to the second of the questions we raised at the outset of this paper, the question of the risk-taking element in competitive play.

Usually, the risk-taking that is taken as thematic in discussions of play is the risk of physical injury and even, as in sports such as car racing, deep sea diving, and rock-climbing, the risk of death (cf. 1:Pages 203–205). To this can be added the psychological risk involved in the possibility of losing, and the effect that might have on our egos. I want now to add to that the risk that is present in nearly all instances of competitive play, the risk that what begins as friendly encounter will end in alienation. Why do we humans, who, we are sometimes told, seek nothing so much as security and self-preservation, for whom insecurity is supposedly one of the most distressing of psychological states, why should we regularly and freely choose to enter into situations—nearly all our play—in which the aforementioned variety of risks are so obviously present? You can no doubt now predict my proposed answer. It is because of our eros.

In competition, wherein we strive together to become more than and better than we are, we question each other together. In so doing, *we call each other and call ourselves into question.* One aspect of our status as erotic is the constant sense of dissatisfaction we have with ourselves in so far as we experience ourselves as incomplete. This dissatisfaction at the sense of lack, this negativity in ourselves, spurs us on to become more than we are. In this way, we constantly hold ourselves open to question. In turn, this calling into question of ourselves, I believe, is at the heart of our willingness, indeed our enthusiasm, to embark upon risk-taking projects, our play foremost among them. We freely choose to take risks because we sense, sometimes consciously, sometimes unreflectively, that risk-taking is a way of engaging in that calling into question of ourselves by which we become what we can become, by which we exhibit our erotic nature. In taking risks, as we sometimes say, we "put ourselves on the line;" risk-full situations *individualize* us, they offer occasions in which we find out who we are in the midst of becoming who we are.[7]

So by way of a brief conclusion we can join together the two sets of questions with which I began this paper. Because of the greater sense of immediacy, of intensity, of immersion that often accompanies play, our playful encounters with others often involve greater, or at least more obvious risks than in other situations. One of the most powerful of such risks is the risk that our play will degenerate into alienation. However, as my latter remarks suggest, this risk is not likely to disappear, for it is part of the very appeal of competitive play, a literally natural consequence of our erotic nature. As erotic beings who play, we will take these risks, and therefore, since a risk without occasional failure soon ceases to be such a risk, we will occasionally find our play infected with alienation. But the first part of my paper has been intended to support my conviction that we need not and should not find such alienation natural, something to be accepted. Alienation in our competitive play is in every case a failure of the *telos* of competition, and indirectly of our very natures as erotic. Both in its origins and in its goal, its *archē* and its *telos,* competitive play should be one of those occasions where our encounters, intense, immediate, total, are those of friendship, in which we attain to a fulfillment, however momentary, together. A simple conclusion perhaps, a sentiment most of us would like to believe in the face of all too regular evidence to the contrary. The issue this paper has addressed is, can it be grounded in human nature?

NOTES

1. An earlier version of this paper was presented at the R. Tait McKenzie Symposium On Sport, University of Tennessee, May 4, 1978.
2. Marx, to take an important example from outside the sporting domain, is profoundly ambiguous on the direction of the causal link between competition and alienation (10:Page 131). My use of "alienation" in this essay is close to Marx's third and fourth senses of alienation developed in the same work: alienation from our "species being" and so from our fellow humans (10:Pages 127, 129).
3. A view perhaps most easily associated with the writings of Rousseau, but pervasive today in both "liberal" and "radical" analyses of society.
4. Perhaps most obviously set out in his famous *Walden* (15:pp. 15–235).
5. (13). See especially the entire speeches of Aristophanes and Socrates, 189b–193d, and 199c–212c.
6. (7). See the "Palinode" for a discussion of difficulties (7:pp. 46–49).
7. See 4:p. 240. We can of course call ourselves into question and take risks alone, as well as with others (cf. 9:pp. 23–31).

Bibliography

1. Alvarez, A. "I Like To Risk My Life," in *Sport And The Body: A Philosophical Symposium,* edited by Ellen Gerber, Philadelphia, Lea and Febiger, 1972.
2. Aristotle, *Politics,* in *Introduction to Aristotle,* edited by R. McKeon, New York, Modern Library, 1947.
3. Buber, Martin, *I And Thou,* translated by R. G. Smith, New York, Charles Scribners Sons, 1958.
4. Hegel, G. W. F., *The Phenomenology of Spirit,* translated by A. V. Miller, Oxford, Clarendon Press, 1977.

5. Heidegger, Martin, *Being And Time,* translated by Macquarrie and Robinson, New York, Harper and Row, 1962.
6. Hobbes, Thomas, *Leviathan,* New York, Bobbs-Merrill, 1958.
7. Hyland, Drew, " 'And That Is The Best Part of Us' Human Being And Play" in *Journal Of The Philosophy Of Sport,* Volume IV, 1977.
8. Hyland, Drew, "Athletics And Angst: Reflections On the Philosophical Relevance of Play," in *Sport And The Body: A Philosophical Symposium,* edited by Ellen Gerber, Philadelphia, Lea & Febiger, 1972.
9. Kretchmar, Scott, "From Test to Contest: An Analysis Of Two Kinds Of Counterpoint In Sport," in *Journal Of The Philosophy Of Sport,* Volume II, 1975.
10. Marx, Karl, *Economic And Philosophic Manuscripts of 1844,* in *Karl Marx: Early Writings,* translated and edited by T. B. Bottomore, New York, McGraw-Hill, 1963.
11. Nietzsche, Friedrich, *Thus Spoke Zarathustra,* in *The Portable Nietzsche,* edited by W. Kaufmann, New York, Viking Press, 1954.
12. Plato, *Phaedrus* in *Platonis Opera,* edited by John Burnet, Oxford, Clarendon Press, 1960, Volume II
13. Plato, *Symposium,* in *Platonis Opera,* edited by John Burnet, Oxford, Clarendon Press, 1960, Volume II.
14. Smith, Adam, *The Wealth of Nations,* New York, Modern Library, 1937.
15. Thoreau, H. D., *Walden And On The Duty Of Civil Disobedience,* New York, Collier, 1962.

BIBLIOGRAPHY ON SPORT AND METAPHYSICAL SPECULATIONS

Ahrabi—Fard, Iradge. "Implications of the Original Teachings of Islam for Physical Education and Sport." Unpublished Doctor's dissertation, University of Minnesota, 1974.

Algozin, Keith. "Man and Sport." *Philosophy Today*, xx (Fall, 1976), 190-195.

Axelos, Kostas. "Planetary Interlude." *Game, Play, Literature*. Edited by Jacques Ehrmann. Boston: Beacon Press, 1971.

Banks, Gary C. "The Philosophy of Friedrich Nietzsche as a Foundation for Physical Education." Unpublished Master's thesis, University of Wisconsin, 1966.

Bouet, Michel. "The Function of Sport in Human Relations." *International Review of Sport Sociology*, 1 (1966), 137-140.

Byrum, Charles S. "Philosophy as Play." *Man and World: An International Philosophical Review*, 8 (August, 1975), 315-326.

Byrum, Steven. "The Concept of Child's Play in Nietzsche's 'of The Three Metamorphoses.'" *Kinesis*, 6 (Spring, 1974), 127-135.

Caillois, Roger. *Man, Play, and Games*. Translated by Meyer Barash. New York: Free Press of Glencoe, 1961.

Cherry, Christopher. "Games and the World." *Philosophy*, (Jan., 1976), 57-61.

Coe, George Albert. "A Philosophy of Play." *Religious Education*, LI (May-June, 1956), 220-222.

Coutts, Curtis A. "Freedom in Sport." *Quest*, X (May, 1968), 68-71.

Cox, Harvey. "Faith as Play" in *The Feast of Fools: A Theological Essay on Festivity and Fantasy*. Cambridge: Harvard University Press, 1969.

Druckman, A. "Sport as a Human Dimension." Unpublished paper presented at the National Convention of the American Association of Health, Physical Education and Recreation, Anaheim, California, March, 1974.

Ehrmann, Jacques, Ed. *Game, Play, Literature*. Boston: Beacon Press, 1971. (First published 1968: Yale French Studies.)

Elena, Lugo. "Jose Ortega y Gasset's Sportive Sense of Life: His Philosophy of Man." Unpublished Doctor's dissertation, Georgetown University, 1969.

Esposito, Joseph L. "Play and Possibility." *Philosophy Today*, XVIII (Summer 1974), 137-146.

Fink, Eugen. "The Ontology of Play." *Philosophy Today*, 4 (Summer, 1960), 95-110.

Fink, Eugen. "The Ontology of Play." *Philosophy Today*, XVIII (Summer, 1974), 147-161.

Fraleigh, Sandra H. "Man Creates Dance." *Quest*, XXIII (Jan., 1975), 20-27.

Fraleigh, Warren P. "On Weiss on Records and on the Significance of Athletic Records." *The Philosophy of Sport: A Collection of Original Essays*. Edited by Robert G. Osterhoudt. Illinois: Charles C Thomas, 1973.

————. "Some Meanings of the Human Experience of Freedom and Necessity in Sport." *The Philosophy of Sport: A Collection of Original Essays*. Edited by Robert G. Osterhoudt. Illinois: Charles C Thomas, 1973.

————. "Sport—Purpose." *Journal of the Philosophy of Sport*, II (Fall, 1975), 74-82.

————. "The Moving 'I'." *The Philosophy of Sport: A Collection of Original Essays*. Edited by Robert G. Osterhoudt. Illinois: Charles C Thomas, 1973.

Fredrick, Mary Margaret. "Naturalism: The Philosophy of Jean Jacques Rousseau and Its Implication for American Physical Education." Unpublished EdD. dissertation, Springfield College, 1961.

Frobel, Friedrich. *Pedagogics of the Kindergarten*. Translated by Josephine Jarvis. New York: D. Appleton and Company, 1900.

Garrett, Roland. "The Metaphysics of Baseball." *Philosophy Today*, XX (Fall, 1976), 209-226.

Gebauer, G. "The Logic of Action and Construction of the World—Contribution to the Theory of Sport." *Sport in the Modern World—Chances and Problems*. Edited by Ommo Grupe, Dietrich Kurz and Johannes Teipel. New York: Springer-Verlag, 1973.

Genasci, James E. and Klissouras, Vasillis. "The Delphic Spirit in Sports." *Journal of Health, Physical Education, and Recreation*, 37 (February, 1966), 43-45.

Gerber, Ellen W. "Identity, Relation and Sport." *Quest*, VIII (May, 1967), 90-97.

Gregg, Jearald Rex. "A Philosophical Analysis of the Sports Experience and the Role of Athletics in the Schools." Unpublished Ed.D. dissertation, University of Southern California, 1971.

Harper, William A. "Man Alone." *Quest, XII* (May, 1969), 57-60.

————. "Human Revolt: A Phenomenological Description." Unpublished Ph.D. dissertation, University of Southern California, 1971.

————. "Taking and Giving in Sport." Unpublished essay presented at the Symposium on the Philosophy of Sport, Brockport, New York, February 10-12, 1972.

Herald, Childe [Thomas Hornsby Ferril]. "Freud and Football." *Reader in Comparative Religion: An Anthropological Approach*. Second Edition. Edited by William A. Lessa and Evon Z. Vogt. New York: Harper & Row, 1965.

Herman, Daniel J. "Mechanism and The Athlete." *Journal of the Philosophy of Sport*, II (September, 1975), 102-110.

Herrigel, Eugen. *Zen in the Art of Archery*. Translated by R. G. C. Hull. New York: McGraw-Hill, 1964. (First published 1960, New York: Pantheon Books.)

Hinman, Lawrence M. "Nietzsche's Philosophy of Play." *Philosophy Today*, XVIII (Summer, 1974), 106-124.

————. "On Work and Play: Overcoming a Dichotomy." *Man and World: An International*

Philosophical Review, 8 (August—1975), 327-346.

Hoffman, Shirl J. "The Athletae Dei: Missing the Meaning of Sport." *Journal of the Philosophy of Sport*, III (September, 1976) 42-51.

Horkheimer, Max. "New Patterns in Social Relations." *International Research in Sport and Physical Education*. Edited by E. Jokl and E. Simon. Illinois: Charles C Thomas, 1964.

Huizinga, Johan. *Homo Ludens*. London: Routledge & Kegan Paul, 1950.

Hyland, Drew. "Athletics and Angst: Reflections on the Philosophical Relevance of Play," Unpublished paper, 1970.

————. "And That is The Best Part of Us: Human Being and Play." *The Journal of the Philosophy of Sport*, IV (Fall, 1977), 36-49.

Jaspers, Karl. "Sport" in *Man in the Modern Age*. Translated by Eden and Cedar Paul. Garden City, New York: Doubleday, 1957.

Jolivet, Regis. "Work, Play, Contemplation." Translated by Sister M. Delphine. *Philosophy Today*, V (Summer, 1961), 114-120.

Keating, James W. "Sartre on Sport and Play." Unpublished paper presented at annual convention of the American Association for Health, Physical Education, and Recreation, Chicago, Illinois, March, 1966.

Kleinman, Seymour. "The Nature of a Self and Its Relation to an 'Other' In Sport." *Journal of the Philosophy of Sport*, II (September, 1975), 45-50.

Krell, David Farrell. "Towards an Ontology of Play." *Research in Phenomenology*, II (Oct., 1972), 63-93.

Kretchmar, Robert Scott. "A Phenomenological Analysis of the Other in Sport." Unpublished Ph.D. dissertation, University of Southern California, 1971.

————. "From Test to Contest: An Analysis of Two Kinds of Counterpoint in Sport." *Journal of the Philosophy of Sport*, II (Sept., 1975), 23-30.

————. "Meeting the Opposition: Buber's 'Will' and 'Grace' in Sport." *Quest*, XXIV (Summer, 1975), 19-27.

————. "Ontological Possibilities: Sport as Play." *The Philosophy of Sport: A Collection of Original Essays*. Edited by Robert G. Osterhoudt. Illinois: Charles C Thomas, 1973.

————. "Phenomenology of Sport." *Sport in the Modern World—Chances and Problems*. Edited by Ommo Grupe, Dietrich Kurz and Johonnes Teipel, New York, Springer-Verlag, 1973.

Kretchmar, R. Scott and Harper, William A. "Why Does Man Play?" *Journal of Health, Physical Education, and Recreation*, 40 (March, 1969), 57-58.

Kuntz, Paul Grimley. "Paul Weiss: What is a Philosophy of Sports?" *Philosophy Today*, XX (Fall, 1976), 170-189.

Lawton, Philip. "Sports and the American Spirit: Michael Novak's Theology of Culture." *Philosophy Today*, XX (Fall, 1976), 196-208.

Lenk, Hans. "Herculean 'Myth' Aspects of Athletics." *Journal of the Philosophy of Sport*, III (September, 1976), 11-21.

McLuhan, Marshall. "Games" in *Understanding Media: The Extensions of Man*. New York: A Signet book, 1964.

McMurtry, John. "The Illusions of a Football Fan: A Reply to Michalos." *The Journal of the Philosophy of Sport*, IV (Fall, 1977), 11-14.

Mead, George H. "Play, the Game, and the Generalized Other" in *Mind, Self and Society from the Standpoint of a Social Behaviorist*. Edited by Charles W. Morris. Illinois: University of Chicago Press, 1959.

Meier, K. "Authenticity and Sport: A conceptual Analysis." Unpublished Ph.D. dissertation, University of Illinois, 1975.

————. "The Kinship of the Rope and the Loving Struggle: A Philosophic Analysis of Communication in Mountain Climbing." *Journal of the Philosophy of Sport*, III (September, 1976), 52-61.

Metheny, Eleanor. *Movement and Meaning*. New York: McGraw-Hill, 1968.

Michalos, Alex C. "The Unreality and Moral Superiority of Football." *Journal of the Philosophy of Sport*, III (September, 1976), 22-24.

Morgan, William J. "An Analysis of the Futural Modality of Sport." *Man and World: An International Philosophical Review*, 9 (Dec., 1976), 418-434.

————. "On the Path Towards An Ontology of Sport." *Journal of the Philosophy of Sport*, III (September, 1976), 25-34.

————. "Sport and Temporality: An Ontological Analysis." Unpublished Ph.D. dissertation, University of Minnesota, 1975.

Moser, S. Ansatzpunkte einer philosophischen Analysedes Sports. In: id., Philosophie un Gegenwart, 193 sqq. Meisenham, 1960.

Netzky, Ralph. "Playful Freedom: Sartre's Ontology Re-appraised." *Philosophy Today*, XVIII, (Summer, 1974), 125-136.

Neale, Robert E. *In Praise of Play*. New York: Harper & Row, 1969.

Novak, Michael. *The Joy of Sports: End Zones, Bases, Baskets, Balls, and the Consecration of the American Spirit*. New York: Basic Books, 1976.

Orringer, Nelson Robert. "Sport and Festival: A Study of Ludic Theory in Ortega y Gasset." Unpublished Ph.D. dissertation, Brown University, 1969.

Roochnik, David L. "Play and Sport." *Journal of the Philosophy of Sport*, II (September, 1975), 36-44.

Rossi, Ernest Lawrence. "Game and Growth: Two Dimensions of our Psychotherapeutic Zeitgeist." *Journal of Humanistic Psychology*, 7 (Fall, 1967), 139-154.

Sadler, William A., Jr. "Play: A Basic Human Structure Involving Love and Freedom." *Review of Existential Psychology and Psychiatry*, 6 (Fall, 1966), 237-245.

————. "Creative Existence: Play as a Pathway

to Personal Freedom and Community." *Humanitas*, V (Spring, 1969), 57-79.

Sartre, Jean-Paul. "Doing and Having" in *Being and Nothingness*. Translated by Hazel E. Barnes. New York: Philosophical Library, 1956.

Schacht, Richard L. "On Weiss On Records, Athletic Activity and the Athlete." *The Philosophy of Sport: A Collection of Original Essays*. Edited by Robert G. Osterhoudt. Illinois: Charles C Thomas, 1973.

"She I, or the Meaning of the Ceremony of Archery." In Woody, Thomas, *Life and Education in Early Societies*. New York: The Macmillan Co., 1959. (Reprinted from Muller, F. M., Eds. *The Sacred Books of the East*. Volume XXVIII Oxford: Clarendon Press, 1879-1910.)

Slovenko, Ralph and Knight, James A., Eds. *Motivations in Play, Games and Sports*. Illinois: Charles C. Thomas, 1967.

Slusher, H. S. "Existential Humanism and Sport." *Sport in the Modern World—Chances and Problems*. Edited by Ommo Grupe, Dietrich Kurz and Johonnes Teipel. New York: Springer-Verlag, 1973.

———. "Sport and Existence: An Analysis of Being." Unpublished paper presented at the History and Philosophy Section of the American Association for Health, Physical Education, and Recreation, Chicago, Illinois, March 21, 1966.

———. *Man, Sport and Existence*. Philadelphia: Lea & Febiger, 1967.

Stokes, Adrian. "Psycho-Analytic Reflections on the Development of Ball Games. Particularly Cricket." *International Journal of Psychoanalysis*, 37 (1956), 185-192.

———. "The Development of Ball Games." *Motivations in Play, Games and Sport*. Edited by Ralph Slovenko and James A. Knight. Illinois: Charles C Thomas, 1967.

Stone, Roselyn E. "Assumptions About the Nature of Human Movement." *The Philosophy of Sport: A Collection of Original Essays*. Edited

by Robert G. Osterhoudt. Illinois: Charles C Thomas, 1973.

Suits, Bernard. "The Elements of Sport." *The Philosophy of Sport: A Collection of Original Essays*. Edited by Robert G. Osterhoudt. Illinois: Charles C Thomas, 1973.

———. "Words on Play." *The Journal of the Philosophy of Sport*, IV (Fall, 1977), 117-131.

Thomson, Patricia. "Ontological Truth in the Game of Golf." Unpublished Ph.D. dissertation, University of Southern California, 1967.

Van Den Berg, J. H. "The Human Body and the Significance of Human Movement." *Psychoanalysis and Existential Philosophy*. Edited by Hendrik M. Ruitenbeck. New York: E. P. Dutton, 1962.

Wachholz, William H. "The Nature of Man and the Nature of Competition in Sport and Athletics." Unpublished Master's thesis, University of Minnesota, 1974.

Walsh, John Henry. "A Fundamental Ontology of Play and Leisure." Unpublished Ph.D. dissertation, Georgetown University, 1968.

Weiss, Paul. "Records and the Man." *The Philosophy of Sport: A Collection of Original Essays*. Edited by Robert G. Osterhoudt. Illinois: Charles C Thomas, 1973.

———. *Sport: A Philosophic Inquiry*, Carbondale: Southern Illinois University Press, 1969.

———"Stratagems and Competition." Unpublished essay presented at the Inaugural Meeting of the Philosophic Society for the Study of Sport, Boston, Massachusetts, Dec. 28, 1972.

Wertz, Spencer K. "Zen, Yoga, and Sports: Eastern Philosophy for Western Athletes." *The Journal of the Philosophy of Sport*, IV (Fall, 1977), 68-82.

Zeigler, Earle F. "In Sport, As In All of Life, Man Should be Comprehensible to Man." *Journal of the Philosophy of Sport*, III (September, 1976), 121-126.

SECTION III

The Body and Being

Thinkers who believe that humans are unified beings, integrated wholes, nevertheless often resort to dualistic terminology. Thus one often reads that a human is composed of mind, body and spirit, or that there are physical and mental aspects of a human's functioning. For example, the early physical educators in America assumed their role to be the fostering of body development to parallel the mental development occurring in academic classes. Luther Halsey Gulick conceived of the symbol of the inverted triangle, the spirit upheld by mind and body, encircled to represent unity. Jessee Feiring Williams insisted that all activities taught should have mental and spiritual values, as well as physical benefits.

These beliefs have been reflective of the ideas advanced by philosophers who have wrestled with the problem of defining the relationships between body, mind and soul. The question of the relative value of each dimension is also inherent in the problem, and opinions range from those who accord greatest importance to the soul, to those who think that mind is the essential quality of humanness. Few philosophers have contended that the body has greatest value, though the seventeenth century sense empiricists did establish the importance of the body to the person's ability to know. In so doing, they clearly rejected the earlier idealistic rationalism, based upon Descartes' assertion that he is not a bodily person, but a thinking person who knows through pure "intellection" and not through sensation.

Descartes' position is similar to, but more extreme than, the influential description of the body-soul relationship* detailed in Plato's *Phaedo*. In the excerpt presented on later pages, Plato clearly indicates a separation of the body and soul, and a denigration of the kinds of knowledges available from the senses. In fact, his attitude towards the body is quite negative, a position doubtless derived from his personal struggles with bodily passions coupled with his intense belief in the values of harmony, balance and moderation. (Plato's negative opinions about the body should not be confused with his positive approach to sport, a position clearly delineated in The *Republic* and The *Laws*.) Descartes extends the concept of the dualism of mind and body to the point where he states that "we clearly perceive mind, that is, thinking substance, without body, that is to say, extended substance . . .; and conversely, body without mind . . ."† In the selection included in this book, Rene Descartes examines the relation between mind and body.

A whole body of philosophical literature has been created in modern times which continues

*Plato's use of the term soul is to be taken as having the broad connotations of spirit and mind— the enduring, essential quality of the individual.
†From the "Second Replies to Objections" as quoted in T. V. Smith and Marjorie Grene, *Philosophers Speak for Themselves* (Chicago Press, 1957), p. 124. However, in a persuasive discussion Stuart F. Spicker demonstrated that Descartes' position was really not as extreme as appears. He concluded that Descartes himself would have rejected what has come to be known as Cartesian dualism. See *The Philosophy of the Body* (Chicago: Quadrangle Books, 1970), pp. 8–18.

145

in the tradition of Cartesian dualism. Seeking to clarify the relationship of mind and body, a branch of philosophy known as "philosophy of mind" has evolved. Because the primary stress is on mind, works of these philosophers have not been included in this book, but some of the more pertinent articles have been listed in the bibliography.

The most interesting approaches to the study of the body have been those made by contemporary phenomenologists. They have completely broken from the dualistic Cartesian thinking and have, instead, worked from the point of view that the body is the primary self. In other words, the body is not an instrument of the mind, nor is it connected to it; it is not a vehicle for directed sensation, nor is it a devilish antagonist to the spirit. The body is you; you are your body. Your body is your mode of being-in-the-world. The body as object—to be perceived, studied, analyzed by self or others—is a different mode of being, called by Sartre being-for-others. The selection by Calvin O. Schrag describes the general parameters of the phenomenologist's approach to a consideration of the body. The short excerpts from Jean-Paul Sartre and Gabriel Marcel both illuminate the dimensions of the two approaches to the body: as self and as object.

Strangely, those who have been interested in sport and/or physical education, have shown little interest in the philosophy of the body. They have treated the body as an object to be trained, trimmed, studied in a laboratory, or made a cause célèbre. In the first quarter of the twentieth century when the physical educators became satisfied with the idea of unity of mind and body, they ceased to speculate about it in any meaningful way. The articles in this book by Kaelin, Kleinman, Gerber, Weiss, and Meier represent an important portion of the literature devoted to a philosophical study of the body in the context of physical activity.

What are the connections between sport and the body? What can be learned about oneself, and what experiences of being-in-the-body can occur in the sport experience? What affects these experiences? How does the experience of self differ if the body is trained and if it is untrained? What can be learned by studying the body as an object and determining such factors as its strength and agility? What effect does it have on the sport experience if the body is treated as an object? How much does deliberate concentration and/or reflection about the body contribute to the experience of the body in sport? Is it important

to know the limitations of the body? If so, why?

Numerous books and articles have been published on the philosophy of the body. One of the best is a collection of readings edited by Stuart F. Spiker (1970). *Humanitas,* II (Spring, 1966) is a publication devoted entirely to "The Human Body." A number of its articles, however, fall into the psychological realm, particularly the area of "body image." Although the subject of body image is important and has captured the interest of many physical educators as well as psychologists, it was not included in this book because it really is tangential to a study of the philosophy of the body. Sarano's book (1966) is most interesting and Zaner (1964) presents a beautiful and comprehensive study of the phenomenology of the body.

Some of the significant articles on the radical reality (i.e., the roots or grounds of reality) include Hengstenberg (1963), Kwant (1966) and Jonas (1965). Books on existential phenomenology, such as Luijpen and Dondeyne (1960) usually include one or more chapters on the body.

Studies which examine the body in dynamic moving environments such as sport, include Belaief's essay (1977)—which characterizes sport as a positive bodily confrontation with the demonic—Meier's article (1975)—which develops the implications of Merleau-Ponty's conception of the body for sport—and Hammer's work (1973) which views sport as a bodily expression of the ego. Of interest here, also, are Van Den Berg's work (1962), and the articles by Beets (1964) and Wenkart (1963).

Some of the analytic writings about the body which might be of interest include Long (1964), Kohler (1960) and Shaffer (1965). Volume II of the Minnesota Series is an important collection in this area (Feigl, Maxwell and Scriven, 1958). *Body and Mind,* subtitled "A History and Defense of Animism," an early work by McDougall which was reprinted in 1961, includes an insightful historical account of its subject.

The philosophy of the body is a fascinating subject. It is one that those who are interested in sport and/or physical education would find highly relevant. Thus far the focus from people with such interests has been primarily on the body-for-others—in other words, the body as object. Some persons have been interested in the dysfunctional body, and some have focused their attention on the relation between body image and personality. However, a concern crucial to sport is the body as being-in-the-world—or the body as subject. A particularly important area for research is the possible difference experienced by the lived body in a sport situation, as opposed to a situation which is not marked by physical effort. It would also be significant to know the difference between experiences in various sports demanding different modes of body action; for example, the body as attacker (as a tackler in football) may provide a different experience of self than the body as strategic and skillful stroker (as in tennis). The body experience in different media also bears examination—in the air, in the water and on land. Finally, the differences between the body acting alone as opposed to acting in concert with others might be analyzed. The challenge to those who wish to undertake such studies definitely includes the development of philosophical techniques which reliably attempt the most difficult task of analyzing someone's subjective experience. Most likely this will involve a detailed study of the philosophy of phenomenology which has deliberately attempted to develop methods for just this purpose.

The Separation of Body and Soul*

PLATO

Do we believe death to be anything?

We do, replied Simmias.

And do we not believe it to be the separation of the soul from the body? Does not death mean that the body comes to exist by itself, separated from the soul, and that the soul exists by herself, separated from the body? What is death but that?

It is that, he said.

Now consider, my good friend, if you and I are agreed on another point which I think will help us to understand the question better. Do you think that a philosopher will care very much about what are called pleasures, such as the pleasures of eating and drinking?

Certainly not, Socrates, said Simmias.

Or about the pleasures of sexual passion? Indeed, no.

And, do you think that he holds the remaining cares of the body in high esteem? Will he think much of getting fine clothes, and sandals, and other bodily adornments, or will he despise them, except so far as he is absolutely forced to meddle with them?

The real philosopher, I think, will despise them, he replied.

In short, said he, you think that his studies are not concerned with the body? He stands aloof from it, as far as he can, and turns toward the soul?

* From Plato: *Phaedo*, translated by F. J. Church, copyright © 1951, by The Liberal Arts Press, Inc., reprinted by permission of the publisher, The Bobbs-Merrill Company, Inc.

I do.

Well, then, in these matters, first, is it clear that the philosopher releases his soul from communion with the body, so far as he can, beyond all other men?

It is.

And does not the world think, Simmias, if a man has no pleasure in such things, and does not take his share in them, his life is not worth living? Do not they hold that he who thinks nothing of bodily pleasures is almost as good as dead?

Indeed you are right.

But what about the actual acquisition of wisdom? If the body is taken as a companion in the search for wisdom, is it a hindrance or not? For example, do sight and hearing convey any real truth to men? Are not the very poets forever telling us that we neither hear nor see anything accurately? But if these senses of the body are not accurate or clear, the others will hardly be so, for they are all less perfect than these, are they not?

Yes, I think so, certainly, he said.

Then when does the soul attain truth? he asked. We see that, as often as she seeks to investigate anything in company with the body, the body leads her astray.

True.

Is it not by reasoning, if at all, that any real truth becomes manifest to her?

Yes.

And she reasons best, I suppose, when none of the senses, whether hearing, or sight, or pain, or pleasure, harasses her; when she has dismissed the body, and released herself as far as she can from all intercourse or contact with it, and so, coming to be as much alone with herself as is possible, strives after real truth.

That is so.

And here too the soul of the philosopher very greatly despises the body, and flies from it, and seeks to be alone by herself, does she not?

Clearly.

And what do you say to the next point, Simmias? Do we say that there is such a thing as absolute justice, or not?

Indeed we do.

And absolute beauty, and absolute good?

Of course.

Have you ever seen any of them with your eyes?

Indeed I have not, he replied.

Did you ever grasp them with any bodily sense? I am speaking of all absolutes, whether size, or health, or strength; in a word, of the essence of real being of everything. Is the very truth of things contemplated by the body? Is it not rather the case that the man who prepares himself most carefully to apprehend by his intellect the essence of each thing which he examines will come nearest to the knowledge of it?

Certainly.

And will not a man attain to this pure thought most completely if he goes to each thing, as far as he can, with his mind alone, taking neither sight nor any other sense along with his reason in the process of thought, to be an encumbrance? In every case he will pursue pure and absolute being, with his pure intellect alone. He will be set free as far as possible from the eye and the ear and, in short, from the whole body, because intercourse with the body troubles the soul, and hinders her from gaining truth and wisdom. Is it not he who will attain the knowledge of real being, if any man will?

Your words are admirably true, Socrates, said Simmias.

. . . .

Let us assume then, he said, if you will, that there are two kinds of existence, the one visible, the other invisible.

Yes, he said.

And the invisible is unchanging, while the visible is always changing.

Yes, he said again.

Are not we men made up of body and soul?

There is nothing else, he replied.

And which of these kinds of existence should we say that the body is most like, and most akin to?

The visible, he replied; that is quite obvious.

And the soul? Is that visible or invisible?

It is visible to man, Socrates, he said.

But we mean by visible and invisible, visible and invisible to man; do we not?

Yes; that is what we mean.

Then what do we say of the soul? Is it visible or not visible?

It is not visible.

Then is it invisible?

Yes.

Then the soul is more like the invisible than the body; and the body is like the visible.

That is necessarily so, Socrates.

Have we not also said that, when the soul employs the body in any inquiry, and makes use of sight, or hearing, or any other sense— for inquiry with the body means inquiry with the senses—she is dragged away by it to the things which never remain the same, and wanders about blindly, and becomes confused and dizzy, like a drunken man, from dealing with things that are ever changing?

Certainly.

But when she investigates any question by herself, she goes away to the pure, and eternal, and immortal, and unchangeable, to which she is akin, and so she comes to be ever with it, as soon as she is by herself, and can be so; and then she rests from her wanderings and dwells with it unchangingly; for she is dealing with what is unchanging. And is not this state of the soul called wisdom?

Indeed, Socrates, you speak well and truly, he replied.

Which kind of existence do you think from our former and our present arguments that the soul is more like and more akin to?

I think, Socrates, he replied, that after this inquiry the very dullest man would agree that the soul is infinitely more like the unchangeable than the changeable.

And the body?

That is like the changeable.

Consider the matter in yet another way. When the soul and the body are united, nature ordains the one to be a slave and to be ruled, and the other to be master and to rule. Tell me once again, which do you think is like the divine, and which is like the mortal? Do you not think that the divine naturally rules and has authority, and that the mortal naturally is ruled and is a slave?

I do.

Then which is the soul like?

That is quite plain, Socrates. The soul is like the divine, and the body is like the mortal.

Now tell me, Cebes, is the result of all that we have said that the soul is most like the divine, and the immortal, and the intelligible, and the uniform, and the indissoluble, and the unchangeable; while the body is most like the human, and the mortal, and the unintelligible, and the multiform, and the dissoluble, and the changeable? Have we any other argument to show that this is not so, my dear Cebes?

We have not.

The Real Distinction Between the Mind and Body of Man*

RENÉ DESCARTES

First, since I know that all the things I conceive clearly and distinctly can be produced by God exactly as I conceive them, it is sufficient that I can clearly and distinctly conceive one thing apart from another to be certain that the one is distinct or different from the other. For they can be made to exist separately, at least by the omnipotence of God, and we are obliged to consider them different no matter what power produces this separation. From the very fact that I know with certainty that I exist, and that I find that absolutely nothing else belongs necessarily to my nature or essence except that I am a thinking being, I readily conclude that my essence consists solely in being a body which thinks or a substance whose whole essence or nature is only to think. And although perhaps, or rather certainly, as I will soon show, I have a body with which I am very closely united, nevertheless, since on the one hand I have a clear and distinct idea of myself in so far as I am only a thinking and not an extended being, and since on the other hand I have a distinct idea of body in so far as it is only an extended being which does not think, it is certain that this "I"—that is to say, my soul, by virtue of which I am what I am—is entirely and truly distinct from my body and that it can be or exist without it.

Furthermore, I find in myself various faculties of thinking which each have their own particular characteristics and are distinct from myself. For example, I find in myself the faculties of imagination and of perception, without which I might no doubt conceive of myself, clearly and distinctly, as a whole being; but I could not, conversely, conceive of those faculties without me, that is to say, without an intelligent substance to which they are attached or in which they inhere. For in our notion of them or, to use the scholastic vocabulary, in their formal concept, they embrace some type of intellection. From all this I reach the conception that these faculties are distinct from me as shapes, movements, and other modes or accidents of objects are distinct from the very objects that sustain them.

I also recognize in myself some other faculties, such as the power of changing location, of assuming various postures, and other similar ones; which cannot be conceived without some substance in which they inhere, any more than the preceding ones, and which therefore cannot exist without such a substance. But it is quite evident that these faculties, if it is true that they exist, must inhere in some corporeal or extended substance, and not in an intelligent substance, since their clear and distinct concept does actually involve some sort of extension, but no sort of intelligence whatsoever.

* From René Descartes: *Meditations on First Philosophy*, translated by Laurence J. Lafleur, copyright © 1951, 1960, by The Liberal Arts Press, Inc., reprinted by permission of the publisher, The Bobbs-Merrill Company, Inc.

Furthermore, I cannot doubt that there is in me a certain passive faculty of perceiving, that is, of receiving and recognizing the ideas of sensible objects; but it would be valueless to me, and I could in no way use it if there were not also in me, or in something else, another active faculty capable of forming and producing these ideas. But this active faculty cannot be in me, in so far as I am a thinking being, since it does not at all presuppose my intelligence and also since those ideas often occur to me without my contributing to them in any way, and even frequently against my will. Thus it must necessarily exist in some substance different from myself, in which all the reality that exists objectively in the ideas produced by this faculty is formally or eminently contained, as I have said before. This substance is either a body— that is, a corporeal nature—in which is formally and actually contained all that which is contained objectively and by representation in these ideas; or else it is God himself, or some other creation more noble than the body, in which all this is eminently contained.

. . . .

To begin this examination, I first take notice here that there is a great difference between the mind and the body, in that the body, from its nature, is always divisible and the mind is completely indivisible. For in reality, when I consider the mind—that is, when I consider myself in so far as I am only a thinking being— I cannot distinguish any parts, but I recognize and conceive very clearly that I am a thing which is absolutely unitary and entire. And although the whole mind seems to be united with the whole body, nevertheless when a foot or an arm or some other part of the body is amputated, I recognize quite well that nothing has been lost to my mind on that account. Nor can the faculties of willing, perceiving, understanding, and so forth be any more properly called parts of the mind, for it is one and the same mind which as a complete unit wills, perceives, and understands, and so forth. But just the contrary is the case with corporeal or extended objects, for I cannot imagine any, however small they might be, which my mind does not very easily divide into several parts, and I consequently recognize these objects to be divisible. This alone would suffice to show me that the mind or soul of man is altogether different from the body, if I did not already know it sufficiently well for other reasons.

I also take notice that the mind does not receive impressions from all parts of the body directly, but only from the brain, or perhaps even from one of its smallest parts—the one, namely, where the senses in common have their seat. This makes the mind feel the same thing whenever it is in the same condition, even though the other parts of the body can be differently arranged, as is proved by an infinity of experiments which it is not necessary to describe here.

I furthermore notice that the nature of the body is such that no one of its parts can be moved by another part some little distance away without its being possible for it to be moved in the same way by any one of the intermediate parts, even when the more distant part does not act. For example, in the cord A B C D which is thoroughly stretched, if we pull and move the last part D, the first part A will not be moved in any different manner from that in which it could also be moved if we pulled one of the middle parts B or C, while the last part D remained motionless. And in the same way, when I feel pain in my foot, physics teaches me that this sensation is communicated by means of nerves distributed through the foot. When these nerves are pulled in the foot, being stretched like cords from there to the brain, they likewise pull at the same time the internal part of the brain from which they come and where they terminate, and there produce a certain movement which nature has arranged to make my mind feel pain as though that pain were in my foot. But because these nerves must pass through the leg, the thigh, the loins, the back, and neck, in order to extend from the foot to the brain, it can happen that even when the nerve endings in the foot are not stimulated, but only some of the intermediate parts located in the loins or the neck, precisely the same movements are nevertheless produced in the brain that could be produced there by a wound received in the foot, as a result of which it necessarily follows that the mind feels the same pain in the foot as though the foot had been wounded. And we must make the same judgment about all our other sense perceptions.

Finally, I notice that since each one of the movements that occurs in the part of the brain from which the mind receives impressions directly can only produce in the mind a single sensation, we cannot desire or imagine any better arrangement than that this movement should cause the mind to feel that sensation, of all sensations the movement is capable of causing, which is most effectively and frequently useful for the preservation of the human body when it is in full health. But experience shows us that all the sensations which nature has given us are such as I have just stated, and therefore there is nothing in their nature which does not show the power and the goodness of the God who has produced them.

Thus, for example, when the nerves of the foot are stimulated violently and more than is usual, their movement, passing through the marrow of the backbone up to the interior of the brain, produces there an impression upon the mind which makes the mind feel something—namely, pain as though in the foot—by which the mind is warned and stimulated to do whatever it can to remove the cause, taking it to be very dangerous and harmful to the foot.

It is true that God could establish the nature of man in such a way that this same brain event would make the mind feel something quite different; for example, it might cause the movement to be felt as though it were in the brain, or in the foot, or else in some other intermediate location between the foot and the brain, or finally it might produce any other feeling that can exist; but none of those would have contributed so well to the preservation of the body as that which it does produce.

In the same way, when we need to drink, there results a certain dryness in the throat which affects its nerves and, by means of them, the interior of the brain. This brain event makes the mind feel the sensation of thirst, because under those conditions there is nothing more useful to us than to know that we need to drink for the conservation of our health. And similar reasoning applies to other sensations.

From this it is entirely manifest that, despite the supreme goodness of God, the nature of man, in so far as he is composed of mind and body, cannot escape being sometimes faulty and deceptive. For if there is some cause which produces, not in the foot, but in some other part of the nerve which is stretched from the foot to the brain, or even in the brain itself, the same effect which ordinarily occurs when the foot is injured, we will feel pain as though it were in the foot, and we will naturally be deceived by the sensation. The reason for this is that the same brain event can cause only a single sensation in the mind; and this sensation being much more frequently produced by a cause which wounds the foot than by another acting in a different location, it is much more reasonable that it should always convey to the

mind a pain in the foot rather than one in any other part of the body. And if it happens that sometimes the dryness of the throat does not come in the usual manner from the fact that drinking is necessary for the health of the body, but from some quite contrary cause, as in the case of those afflicted with dropsy, nevertheless it is much better that we should be deceived in that instance than if, on the contrary, we were always deceived when the body was in health; and similarly for the other sensations.

And certainly this consideration is very useful to me, not only so that I can recognize all the errors to which my nature is subject, but also so that I may avoid them or correct them more easily. For knowing that each of my senses conveys truth to me more often than falsehood concerning whatever is useful or harmful to the body, and being almost always able to use several of them to examine the same object, and being in addition able to use my memory to bind and join together present information with what is past, and being able to use my understanding, which has already discovered all the causes of my errors, I should no longer fear to encounter falsity in the objects which are most commonly represented to me by my senses.

And I should reject all the doubts of these last few days as exaggerated and ridiculous, particularly that very general uncertainty about sleep, which I could not distinguish from waking life. For now I find in them a very notable difference, in that our memory can never bind and join our dreams together one with another and all with the course of our lives, as it habitually joins together what happens to us when we are awake. And so, in effect, if someone suddenly appeared to me when I was awake and afterward disappeared in the same way, as do images that I see in my sleep, so that I could not determine where he came from or where he went, it would not be without reason that I would consider it a ghost or a phantom produced in my brain and similar to those produced there when I sleep, rather than truly a man.

But when I perceive objects in such a way that I distinctly recognize both the place from which they come and the place where they are, as well as the time when they appear to me; and when, without any hiatus, I can relate my perception of them with all the rest of my life, I am entirely certain that I perceive them wakefully and not in sleep. And I should not in any way doubt the truth of these things if, having made use of all my senses, my memory, and my understanding, to examine them, nothing is reported to me by any of them which is inconsistent with what is reported by the others. For, from the fact that God is not a deceiver, it necessarily follows that in this manner I am not deceived.

But because the exigencies of action frequently oblige us to make decisions and do not always allow us the leisure to examine these things with sufficient care, we must admit that human life is very often subject to error in particular matters; and we must in the end recognize the infirmity and weakness of our nature.

The Lived Body as a Phenomenological Datum*

CALVIN O. SCHRAG

Phenomenology, as a methodological principle, designates a disciplined attempt at a descriptive analysis and interpretive explication of the data of immediate experience. Husserl's formula *Zu den Sachen Selbst!* has become normative for all phenomenological enquiry. Heidegger, Scheler, Sartre, Merleau-Ponty, and others, have taken over Husserl's formula and applied it to various regions of man's lived experience. The differences among the phenomenologists are due primarily to variegated applications of the phenomenological method rather than to disputes concerning the nature of the phenomenological principle itself. My present task is not that of a historical examination of the similarities and differences between the different phenomenologists. Such an undertaking would indeed be helpful toward a further clarification of what is meant by phenomenology as a philosophical method, but the pursuit of this task would lead us too far afield. The specific purpose of this essay is that of developing a phenomenological analysis of the lived body. The phrase "the lived body" denotes a structure of human subjectivity. It indicates the experience of my body as it is disclosed to me in my immediate involvements and concerns. Sartre, Marcel, and Merleau-Ponty have given studied attention to the phenomenon of the lived body; but their descriptions are often fragmentary and singularly impoverished on rather decisive issues. Heideg-

* From *The Modern Schoolman*, XXXIX, (March, 1962), 203-218.

ger, on the other hand, has virtually nothing to say about the body. His *Dasein* appears to be a disembodied *Existenz* who moves about in his world of care in an abstracted unawareness of his bodily engagements and orientations. As Hegel, in his *Science of Logic,* had viciously abstracted reason from its context in man's lived historical existence, so it would seem that Heidegger comes perilously close to abstracting *Existenz* from its concrete bodily involvement. What is sorely needed as a corrective to the Heideggerian's neglect of the body is another Feuerbach to call us to an awareness of the bodily dimension of human existence, and another Nietzsche to remind us that life is lost in the moment that man no longer remains faithful to the earth.

In the following discussion I will seek to analyze and describe the datum of the lived body as it evinces a fourfold expression: (1) the lived body as self-referential, (2) the lived body in reference to other, (3) the lived body and human space, and (4) the lived body and human time.

I. THE LIVED BODY AS SELF-REFERENTIAL

I experience my body as uniquely and peculiarly my own. My body is so intimately related to what and who I am that the experience of selfness is indissolubly linked with the existential projects which radiate from my body as it is actually lived. My body is immediately experienced and initially disclosed as my concrete mode of orientation in a world of practical and personal concerns. The phenomenon in question is *my* body as *concretely lived*. The body as immediately apprehended is not a corporeal substance which is in some way attached to, or united with, another substance, variously called in the tradition a "soul," "mind," or "self." The body thus conceptualized is a later abstraction and objectivization, which is phenomenologically eviscerated and epistemologically problematic. I experience my body first as a complex of life-movements which are indistinguishable from my experience of selfness. My primordial experience is one of engagement in a world of concrete projects—projects which receive their significance through my body as the locus of concern. The distinctions between soul and body, or mind and body, as they have been formulated in the tradition (particularly by Descartes), are reified and objectivized distinctions, foreign to man's experience as it is immediately lived. Thus, the body as *concretely lived* must be consistently contrasted with the body as *objectively known*. The body as objectively known is a proper datum to be sure, but it is a scientific datum for the investigations of the anatomical and physiological sciences. The body as objectively known is a corporeal entity, properly defined as a complex of brain waves, neural pathways, endocrinal discharges, and muscular fibres. This is the body as it exists for the physiologist and the physician. But this is not the body which I experience in my lived concreteness and which I apprehend as being indelibly and uniquely my own. The body as an item for the special sciences, in which all data necessarily are objectivized, is an abstracted and general body which applies to everyone but characterizes no one in particular. It becomes a body conceptualized in its objectivized mode of being-for-another. No one can "know" his pituitary gland or his cerebral cortex as it is known objectively by the brain surgeon. To be sure, I can infer from my knowledge of cadavers that I have the same anatomical structures and the same physiological functions as have other bodies; but this is a level of knowledge in abstraction from the experience of my body as concretely lived.

The lived body, I have suggested, signifies a mode of orientation rather than a conceptualized entity. This mode of orientation is part and parcel of man's preobjective world. Merleau-Ponty has made the notion of a preobjective world central not only to his phenomenology of perception, but to his philosophy as such.[1] Being in the world, as a primordial experience, is a global structure of interrelating practical projects and not a conceptualization of a world schematized through the objectivizing categories of substance, quantity, and abstract quality. The world is initially disclosed as an instrumental world in which tools are accessible for the realization of my practical concerns, and a social world in which I already find myself concretely related to other selves. A putty knife, in the primitive and subjective experience of my world, is a utensil with which I seal the window pane to keep out the wintry draft. The putty knife *as object*, although still the same putty knife, is a thematized and conceptualized entity to which I attach certain abstract qualities of weight, shape, and solidity. The former movement discloses my preobjective world; the later is a construction of my objective world. Now it is in this preobjective world that the lived body makes its appearance. Preobjectively understood, the lived body is always related to an environment and social horizon, but in this relational complex it always appears as that which refers to itself as the locus of this relatedness. The lived body is self-referential.

It is through the orientation of my lived body that the personal meanings of my preobjective being in the world are disclosed, established, and broadened. The hand plays a privileged role in this disclosure and creation of meanings in my world orientations. It is through the use of my hand that I project meanings by pointing and touching, by writing and counting, by striking and stroking, by giving and taking. It is through the use of the hand that I create new worlds and refashion the old. The hand makes man a creator. Clocks and microscopes are works of the hand which express man's creativity and his power over the given. The lived body creates meanings by refashioning that which is simply given. Man becomes a maker of tools and a creator of values through the use of his hand. So also

[1] See particularly *Phénoménologie de la perception* (Paris: Gallimard, 1945), Part I, "Le Monde Perçu," and Part II, "L'Etre-pour-soi et l'être-au-monde." Also pertinent to the topic is his book *La Structure du comportement* (Paris: Presses Universitaires, 1953), especially Chap. 3: "L'Ordre physique, l'ordre vital, l'ordre humain." Gabriel Marcel points to the same phenomenon when he speaks of the world being initially presented as a confused and global experience: "What is given to me beyond all possible doubt is the confused and global experience of the world inasmuch as it is existent" (*Metaphysical Journal* [Chicago: Henry Regnery Co., 1952], p. 322).

it is through the use of my hand that the personal meanings in my relations with others are established and expressed. In the handshake and in the gesture, complexes of meaning are at once created and revealed. Karl Jaspers in his illuminating discussion of the hand in *Von der Wahrheit* has concretely defined man as that being who makes use of his hands. Man is *homo faber* as well as *homo sapiens*. It is this existential quality which differentiates man from the animal. An animal is bound to its environment and must accommodate itself to it; man modifies his environment through the use of his hand, which determines the application and use of his thought. One of the fateful errors of philosophy, continues Jaspers, is the vicious separation of doing and thinking. All activity involving the use of the hand already discloses thought as inextricably intertwined with the activity, and it is through the activities of the hand (*Handtätigkeiten*) that the activities of thought (*Denktätigkeiten*) are explicated.[2] The body in its lived concreteness expresses a concomitant upsurge of thought and activity through which I both grasp and shape the meaning of my incarnated being-in-the-world.

The self-referential quality of the lived body is most directly disclosed in my experience of my body as that which individualizes me. The body confers upon me my existential identity. The tradition was right in viewing the body as a principle of individuation but erred in objectivizing the individuating principle as an abstract *materia signata quantitate* which individuates the particular by somehow uniting with form. Particularly in the Aristotelian tradition does individuation remain abstract and objective, with the result that individuation never *individualizes*. Only when I apprehend my body in the particularity of its lived concreteness is it disclosed as a factor of individuation. The body individuates me in that it signifies the projects which are peculiarly my own—my hand grasping the pen with which I write, my head nodding to the person with whom I converse, my anticipation of the death which I alone must die. Sartre has clearly expressed this notion in stating that the body "represents the individualization of my engagement in the world."[3] I apprehend myself as

being marked off from other selves, and from objects and things, in the moment that I apprehend my lived body in its concrete involvements, referring to projects that are peculiarly and uniquely my own.

The lived body is not a *something*, objective and external to the self, which when attached to the self individuates it and marks it off from other selves. This external view of the body transforms it into an objectively conceptualized material substance. But on the level of the preobjective experience of the body as mine no such material substance can be found. Marcel elucidates this when he writes: "In the fact of *my body* there is something which transcends what can be called its materiality, something which cannot be reduced to any of its objective qualities."[4] Further clarification on the distinction between the objective and the preobjective understanding of the body is forthcoming in Marcel's distinction between "having" and "being." Viewed as an objective determinant of individuation, the body is understood as something that the self *has*. The self has a body analogous to the way in which the courthouse has a goldplated dome. The body, in such a view, is adventitious or external to the self. On the other hand, the body preobjectively understood as the *lived body* is not something which I *have*; rather it signifies who I *am*. I *am my body* or *I exist as body*. Immediate experience testifies to the fact that the body is not something which I possess and consequently use in one way or another as an instrument or a utensil. As formulated by Marcel: "I do not *make use of* my body, I *am* my body. In other words, there is something in me that denies the implication that is to be found in the purely instrumentalist notion of the body that my body is external to myself."[5] I am not related to my body in an external way. It is not a possession which I have and use. The lived body makes use of instruments and utensils in its world orientations, but the body is not itself an instrument. The body is myself in my lived concreteness. It is *who I am*, and indicates the *manner in which I am*. The lived body refers to my personal manner of existing, and the meanings attached to this manner of existing, in a world in which I experience presence.

II. THE LIVED BODY IN REFERENCE TO OTHERS

My body is lived in an existential immediacy and is apprehended as uniquely my own. But

[2] "Wie sehr alles Tun mit der Hand schon ein Denken in sich schliesst, ist daran zu bemerken, dass Denktätigkeiten durch Handtätigkeiten ausgedrückt werden" (*Von der Wahrheit* [München: Piper, 1947], p. 329).

[3] Sartre, *Being and Nothingness*, trans. Hazel Barnes (New York, Philosophical Lib.), p. 310.

[4] Marcel, *Metaphysical Journal*, p. 315.

[5] *Ibid.*, p. 333.

my body is also lived in such a manner that it is apprehended by the other. The lived body is not an isolated phenomenon. It is intentionally related to a world—a world which emerges in one's preobjective experience as a phenomenon in which various regions of concern are manifested. A most fundamental region of concern in one's primordial experience of being in the world is the region of interacting and interdependent selves. I apprehend my body in a communal context in which other selves are disclosed as already being there. This communal context adds another aspect to the experience of my body in its lived concreteness. A phenomenological analysis and description of this communal aspect will disclose a structure of experience in which there are two separable moments of awareness—the body of the other as known by me and the reapprehension of my body as known by the other. The experience of my body as mine is always coextensive with my experience of the body of the other and the consequent reappraisal of myself as existing in the world of the other. These two moments of consciousness can and must be separated for purposes of analysis, but it must not be forgotten that in man's immediate experience they are simultaneously given. The postanalytic fallacy, in which there is a reification and separation of analyzed components read out of a situation of prior relatedness, must be judiciously avoided. The engagements of the lived body always proceed within a self-other correlation. I seek to realize the projects of my lived body through a continuing encounter with the body of the other. The other is disclosed as part of my situation. His body is a factor in my world. It arises in my world either as an obstacle to be overcome (a coefficient of adversity, as Sartre would say), or as an instrument which I can use (coefficient of utility), or as an occasion for authentic communication and mutual fulfillment (the possibility of the latter would seem to be denied by Sartre). In any case, I must reckon with the incarnated other. I must assume some kind of existential attitude toward him.

After being thrust into the presence of the other I seek to apprehend his lived body as I seek to apprehend my own. Now what kind of knowledge is rendered possible through my encounter with the other? Quite clearly, I can never "know" the body of the other as he lives it. The interior of the projects of the other never becomes fully transparent to me. The movements of his body and the projects which they intend are always in some sense

clothed with opaqueness and mystery. To be sure, I can describe empirically some of the obvious characteristics relative to his pigmentation, bone structure, eye color, texture of the hair, and the like; but in the specification of all these empirical determinants one can hardly attest that the lived body of the other has been comprehended. There is, however, a reality element which is disclosed in my encounter with the lived body of the other. His body is revealed as a unity of life movements which expresses a world orientation of its own. The body of the other constitutes *his* project of being in the world. I cannot penetrate this project as lived by the other, but I can apprehend and describe the project as it exists for me. In this apprehension I always apprehend a totality. Sartre makes this point when he says that the body of the other "appears within the limits of the situation as a synthetic totality of life and action."[6] There is the simple corporeal unity of arms, legs, thorax, and head disclosed as a living complex. We never experience the arm or the foot or the eyes of the other in isolation. To experience them thus would be to experience them as lifeless appendages or parts of a material composite but not as expressions of a living unity. We perceive the other as kicking his leg, raising his arm, squinting his eyes. In each of these perceptions a project or a complex of products of the other as a living whole becomes apparent. We find a negative testimony of this *Gestalt* character in the perceptual shock which occurs when one sees staring eyes which are not localized in a head, or fingers severed from a hand. Sartre in *Being and Nothingness* reminds us of the horror which we feel when we see an arm which looks as if it did not belong to any body, and perceive a hand (when the arm is concealed) crawling like a spider up the side of a doorway.[7] All these instances point to a structural life-unity which characterizes the lived body of the other as it is apprehended by me.

In my encounter with the lived body of the other there is thus the structural moment of the other as known by me. But equally a part of the situation of encounter is the structural moment of the reapprehension of my lived body as known by the other. When I emerge in the world I find that I am already looked at. My body is perceived by the other and exists for the other. The other, in formulating and executing his projects, sucks me into the orbit of his concerns and transforms me into

[6] *Being and Nothingness*, p. 346.
[7] *Ibid.*

an item for his world. I then reapprehend myself in the mode of being apprehended by the other. I become aware that the other has a certain image of my lived body and makes an appraisal of it, either tacit or explicit. I can take over this image and appraisal made by the other and seek to shape my life in accordance with them. I can also reject the formulated images and appraisals, and seek means of changing them or seek to affirm my individuality and my freedom in spite of them. In any case, whatever my particular response may be, my life and action are defined in reference to the other. The other is inescapable. He constitutes an irreducible element in my world orientations. He is responsible for my situation being one in which I stand before the other—in fear, anger, shame, and love. It is only in the presence of the other that I can experience these existential moods. These are revelatory moods, in the guise of preobjective intentional disclosures, which reveal my lived body as a body viewed and appraised by the other.

We have seen that the lived body in reference to the other involves at the same time an apprehension of the other and a being apprehended by the other. This structure of intersubjectivity or being with the other exhibits two possible existential qualifications—alienation and communication. I alienate myself from the other either by objectivizing his lived body and thus transforming it into an object or a thing, or by apprehending it solely as an instrument which I can use and manipulate for my own private ends. I thus deprive his lived body of its life quality—that is, its unique existential freedom—by dissolving his world of projects. Indeed, I seek to remove the other as lived body by transforming him into material for my self-actualization. But this can never fully succeed because I confront resistance through the counter projects of the other. I do not constitute the other; I encounter him. And in my encounter with the other I not only apprehend the other, but I experience myself as apprehended by the other. The other seeks to absorb me into his world of projects and divest me of my subjectivity, just as I seek to render him into an item for my projects. Alienation is the dialectical movement of perceiving and being perceived, acting and being acted upon, using and being used. Sartre has formulated an engaging elucidation of this dialectical movement in his chapter "The Look" in *Being and Nothingness*. The other decentralizes my world through his look and divests me of my freedom by transforming

me into a "being as object" or a "being as seen by another." The "fall" of man for Sartre comes about through the emergence of the other.[8] Sartre's dialectical analysis and description of the resistance of the other in the movement of alienation or estrangement seems to draw heavily from the insights of Hegel's teaching on the "unhappy consciousness" and the master-servant polarity. The master, which is self-consciousness striving for purity, actualizes himself by transforming the other into a servant. The master exercises his power over his servant by demanding various services. Thus the servant is dependent upon the master. But in the moment that the servant becomes conscious of himself as servant he drives toward independence and elevates himself above the status of a servant. Only through the servant can the master enjoy the services which are provided. The master now becomes dependent upon the servant. This is the structure of dialectical movement toward the unhappy or alienated consciousness.

All the movements of the lived body in its intersubjective field express various forms of alienation or estrangement. There is, however, another existential quality, equally important, which defines the relations of selves. This is the drive toward communion. It is on this point that Sartre's analysis remains singularly impoverished. Alienation, for Sartre, plays the trump card. Jaspers, Marcel, and Merleau-Ponty, on the other hand, have made the theme of communion central to their philosophies and thus established a counter-thrust to the alienating egocentrism of Sartre's existentialism. Marcel has formulated a doctrine of intersubjectivity in which the other can be encountered as a nonobjectivized presence. Communion is made possible only when the other is acknowledged as a subject with whom I experience a copresence in such a manner that our individual freedoms are mutually acknowledged. Communion involves communication. If I am to exist in communion with the other I must be able to communicate the meanings which are disclosed in the projects of my immediate concerns. The lived body

---

[8] *Ibid.*, p. 263. Cf. p. 267: "Thus being-seen constitutes me as a defenseless being for a freedom which is not my freedom. It is in this sense that we can consider ourselves as 'slaves' insofar as we appear to the Other. But this slavery is not a historical result—capable of being surmounted—of a *life* in the abstract form of consciousness. I am a slave to the degree that my being is dependent at the center of a freedom which is not mine and which is the very condition of my being."

plays a significant role in this communication of meanings. The projects of my lived body are intrinsically communicative. My lived body is an *act of communication*. This is to say more than to say that the body is simply a vehicle of communication. To speak of the body as a vehicle is already to externalize it and make it adventitious to the communication process itself. Merleau-Ponty has described the body as "expression and speech" in one of the chapters in his book *Phénoménologie de la perception*.[9] I convey meanings to the other through the gestures and movements which constitute my body as a living synthetic unity. The smile and the frown, the wink and the stare, the caress and the kiss, the handshake and the slap, are all modes of speech which disclose meanings in the world of my concrete lived experience. Merleau-Ponty elucidates this point when he refers to speech as a gesture which intends or signifies a world ("la parole est un geste et sa signification un monde").[10] Speech is a mode of orientation through which one discloses to others the world of one's projects. The gesture-complex of the lived body is an example of speech thus understood. Ordinary language gives clear evidence of such an apprehension of the lived body: "he speaks with his hands"; "her eyes reveal her inmost feelings;" "he uses the language of love." All these phrases bear testimony to a lived body as expression and speech. Any phenomenology of experience, which seeks to remain true to the data as they show themselves, will need to give disciplined attention to this form of communication.

III. THE LIVED BODY AND HUMAN SPACE

Spatiality is an existential quality of the lived body. The concept of space, in both the history of philosophy and the history of science, has fallen heir (or victim) to widely differing interpretations. Some have argued that space is infinite; others have argued that it is finite. Some have maintained it is absolute; others have maintained that it is relative. Some have asserted that it is to be identified with matter; others have persuasively denied its materiality. It becomes evident upon investigation that such arguments pro and con presuppose space to be some kind of externally observable entity or state which can be objectively defined. It may indeed be that Kant

has demonstrated in his transcendental dialectic once and for all that space as a unifying condition in one's objective view of the cosmos remains for ever unknowable. In any case, the spatiality which qualifies the lived body is not an objective space. It is *human space*, or what Merleau-Ponty has appropriately called "espace orienté." The space in which I live and in which I apprehend my lived body is articulated in and through my practical and personal projects, and as such must be consistently contrasted with the quantitative and measurable space which defines my objective world as an extensive continuum. Mathematical space, as an instance of quantifiable space, is properly defined as an abstract extensive continuum constituting a region of points. Whether this space is Euclidean or non-Euclidean, three-dimensional or multi-dimensional, is at this point irrelevant. The point which is relevant is that mathematical space is isotropic —that is, all the dimensions have the same value—and it is precisely this which makes it measurable in terms of spatial co-ordinates. Human or oriented space, which qualifies the lived body, is what Henri Ellenberger has called "anisotropic," having dimensions of different specific values and thus being contrasted with the abstract space of mathematics. The dimensions (or what might preferably be called "directions") of oriented space take on different values relative to the situation in which the lived body actualizes its projects. Merleau-Ponty has contributed the distinction between "spatiality of position" (*spatialité de position*) and "spatiality of situations" (*spatialité de situation*). The former characterizes the abstract space of mathematics, the latter the concrete oriented space of the lived body.[11]

Human space has three directional axes. The primary axis is the horizontal axis of front and back, or before and behind. In this primary axis the existentially proximate direction is that of frontward or forward. For the most part I spatialize my world in a forward direction. I face the table on which I write; I face the mountain which I must surmount; I face the person to whom I speak. In each of these projects an existential distance is already disclosed. The table is near when it is accessible for the writing of my book; it is too far away when it makes difficult the task of writing, producing a coefficient of adversity. Utensils become most readily accessible on the horizontal axis of front and back; and the concrete movements of my body, such as actualizing a proj-

---

[9] See Part I, Chap. 6: "Le Corps comme expression et la parole."

[10] *Phénoménologie de la perception*, p. 214.

[11] *Ibid.*, p. 116.

ect by walking, proceed for the most part on this axis. But there is also the directional axis of right and left. The hammer with which I pound the tack is to my left. Its place in my field of concerns is not some abstract locus geometrically defined relative to an extensive continuum of points, but rather that place where it belongs so as to be accessible for the realization of my project. It is near when it is in its right place—within reach—and thus can be spatially distinguished from other utensils, which, although metrically nearer, are existentially remote from the lived body. For example, at the same time that I reach for the hammer there may be a garden spade to my right which is six inches closer to me than the hammer. But the garden spade, in the context of my situation, remains exterior to my projects and thus existentially remote. Human space, and the value of its directions, varies with the situation. Human space is anisotropic. It is indissolubly linked with the projects of human concern. A proper phenomenological use of language, therefore, would refer to the body not as something which is *in* space but rather as a field of concern which *lives* its space.

The third directional axis is the vertical axis of up and down. I also live my space in the upward and downward direction. In standing up and sitting down, in raising and lowering my arm, in perceiving what is above and what is below, I express a concrete movement along this vertical axis. These various directional axes disclose themselves through the concrete movements of the lived body. The task of phenomenology is that of describing the phenomena as they show or disclose themselves. Hence any phenomenology which seeks to return to the data of immediate experience must pay due attention to the reality of human or oriented space. Ellenberger states the case clearly when he writes: "We know that the horizon and the celestial dome are not scientific concepts; but for our daily experience and for phenomenology, they are very important entities."[12]

IV. THE LIVED BODY AND HUMAN TIME

Phenomenology discloses not only the spatiality of the lived body but also its temporality. These two phenomena are disclosed simultaneously in the fundamental project of the body as a living synthetic unity. The concrete movements of the body always occur within a correlated complex of lived space and lived time. My body is immediately and preobjec-

tively revealed as coming from a past and moving into a future. Just as there is a spatial directionality, so also there is a temporal directionality. I will describe this temporal directionality in terms of a retentional protentional axis (categories already used by Husserl). The lived body is qualified by its past, indicating a retentional mode. My lived body is constituted by that which I have been. Hence my body *is* its past. To speak of the body as *having* a past is to externalize the past and violently abstract the body from its concrete temporalization. The past which qualifies the lived body is never left behind so long as the body exists. My past projects and the environmental and social complex in which these projects were defined are continuing determinants of my lived body. To be sure, my environmental and social world are no longer objectively present, but they remain *subjectively real*. The past is still a living reality, and it is lost in the moment that it is objectivized as a series of discrete nows which have somehow "passed by" and become divested of reality. The lived body is not an objectivized instant within an objectively measured time. The categories of quantitative or objectively measured time are inapplicable to the lived time of human experience. Human time is qualitatively unique. Quantitative time is an abstracted and objectivized time, which transforms the temporal unity into an infinite succession of nows correlated with geometrical points. Quantitative time co-ordinates time and space by postulating an abstract spatio-temporal continuum. Human time, or the time of immediate experience, remains concealed so long as time is understood as a succession of abstracted nows which precede each other in an objective order of coming to be and passing away. Quantitative time severs the past from

[12] R. May, E. Angel, and H. Ellenberger (eds.), *Existence: A New Dimension in Psychiatry and Psychology* (New York: Basic Books, 1958), p. 110. It is interesting to note that Ludwig Binswanger has made extended use of the phenomenological concept of oriented space in his existential psychotherapy. In its psychological expression oriented space becomes what he calls "attuned space" (*gestimmter Raum*), space conditioned by one's emotions and feelings. Space thus becomes allied with a psychological mood. One's mood determines space as being full or empty, expanding or constricting. For example, love is "space-binding" in that it produces a feeling of nearness to the beloved, even though the metrical distance may be great. Happiness expands attuned space, sorrow constricts it, and despair makes it empty (*ibid.*, pp. 110 ff.).

the future and both from the present. Human time has a past which is still present and a future which is already present. The directions of time are integrated in a synthetic unity of the body as concretely lived. Only for the anatomical biologist and the physiologist does the body become a lifeless object which somehow rests within an order of objective time. The lived body has time within itself. It does not *occur in time;* it *exists as time.* All of its projects or orientations are permeated with temporality. This temporality has both a retentional and a protentional direction. The lived body is temporalized retentionally in that at every moment it is a synthetic unity of its past projects, which includes its past environmental and social influences. This is what Heidegger and Sartre have called the *facticity* of human existence; that is, existence as qualified by pastness. But human existence is also qualified by futurity. The lived body is temporalized protentionally as well as retentionally. It is this protentional directionality which constantly reopens my past and keeps it from being solidified into a series of objectivized nows. It rescues my past from the determinism of an empirical necessity. In any given moment I can remember my past lived body as a burden—as an occasion for regret or remorse.[13] But this past, for human time, is not irrevocably closed or finally fixed. It can be translated into an existential possibility through the acknowledgment of futurity. The past can be retrieved and changed through the adoption of a new attitude toward it. That which weighs upon me as a burden can be transformed into a burden to be overcome—into a creative possi-

[13] Minkowski has differentiated regret and remorse in terms of different retentional values. The zone of remorse is the zone of the immediate past. The zone of the regretted is the zone of the mediate past. Finally, there is the zone of the obsolete which corresponds to the remote past. See his book *Le Temps vécu* (Paris: D'Artre, 1933).

bility. The memory of my lived body as a body whose projects have been limited by a withered arm can be translated into a future possibility of reappraisal.

The phenomenon of the lived body thus shows itself in immediate experience as a body qualified by temporality—qualified retentionally in that it is a body which has already become that which it is, defined by itself, its environment and other selves; but also it is qualified protentionally in that it is a body which has not yet lived out its projects. It is protended into a future and confronted with the task of appraising the meaning of its past as this past is translated into possibility. In this protentional directionality a final limit to the projects of the lived body is disclosed. This limit is death or the total dissolution of my being in the world. The unity of the lived body as a synthetic whole is achieved only when this final limit is interiorized and taken up in the present projects of the existing subject. Heidegger has elucidated this in his existential concept of *Sein-zum-Tode,* which means that death is a mode of existence qualifying man's being as soon as he is and so long as he is. (However, it is not clear in what sense death, in the Heideggerian analysis, has a bodily reference.) Death is not simply an empirical factuality apprehended only in the instant. This would comically place death outside experience insofar as when it would occur the lived body would no longer be there. Death is a mode of existence which involves the task of assuming some kind of existential attitude toward one's final limit. Death can become the occasion for cowardly retreat, poetic melancholy, martyrdom or dying for a cause, or resolute and courageous acceptance of it as the irrevocable limit of existence. The final meaning of the lived body as a synthetic unity of past and future is thus achieved in the taking over of one's death as the final possibility of the body. Death itself is interiorized and translated into subjectivity.

The Body*

JEAN-PAUL SARTRE

The problem of the body and its relations with consciousness is often obscured by the fact that while the body is from the start posited as a certain *thing* having its own laws and capable of being defined from outside, consciousness is then reached by the type of inner intuition which is peculiar to it. Actually if after grasping "my" consciousness in its absolute interiority and by a series of reflective acts, I then seek to unite it with a certain living object composed of a nervous system, a brain, glands, digestive, respiratory, and circulatory organs whose very matter is capable of being analyzed chemically into atoms of hydrogen, carbon, nitrogen, phosphorus, etc., then I am going to encounter insurmountable difficulties. But these difficulties all stem from the fact that I try to unite my consciousness not with *my* body but with the body *of others*. In fact the body which I have just described is not *my* body such as it is *for* me. I have never seen and never shall see my brain nor my endocrine glands. But because I who am a man have seen the cadavers of men dissected, because I have read articles on physiology, I conclude that my body is constituted exactly like all those which have been shown to me on the dissection table or of which I have seen colored drawings in books. Of course the physicians who have taken care of me, the surgeons who have operated on me, have been able to have

* Reprinted by permission of Philosophical Library, Inc. from *Being and Nothingness* by Jean-Paul Sartre, translated by Hazel E. Barnes, © Copyright, 1956, by Philosophical Library, Inc., New York.

direct experience with the body which I myself do not know. I do not disagree with them, I do not claim that I lack a brain, a heart, or a stomach. But it is most important to choose the *order* of our bits of knowledge. So far as the physicians have had any experience with my body, it was with my body *in the midst of the world* and as it is for others. My body as it is *for me* does not appear to me in the midst of the world. Of course during a radioscopy I was able to see the picture of my vertebrae on a screen, but I was outside in the midst of the world. I was apprehending a wholly constituted object as a *this* among other *thises*, and it was only by a reasoning process that I referred it back to being *mine*; it was much more my *property* than my being.

It is true that I see and touch my legs and my hands. Moreover nothing prevents me from imagining an arrangement of the sense organs such that a living being could see one of his eyes while the eye which was seen was directing its glance upon the world. But it is to be noted that in this case again I am the *Other* in relation to my eye. I apprehend it as a sense organ constituted in the world in a particular way, but I can not "see the seeing;" that is, I can not apprehend it in the process of revealing an aspect of the world to me. Either it is a thing among other things, or else it is that by which things are revealed to me. But it can not be both at the same time. Similarly I see my hand touching objects, but do not *know* it in its act of touching them. This is the fundamental reason why that famous "sensation of effort" of Maine de Biran does not really exist. For my hand reveals to me the resistance of objects, their hardness or softness, but not *itself*. Thus I see my hand only in the way that I see this inkwell. I unfold a distance between it and me, and this distance comes to integrate itself in the distances which I establish among all the objects of the world. When a doctor takes my wounded leg and looks at it while I, half raised up on my bed, watch him do it, there is no essential difference between the visual perception which I have of the doctor's body and that which I have of my own leg. Better yet, they are distinguished only as different structures of a single global perception; there is no essential difference between the doctor's perception of my leg and my own present perception of it. Of course when I touch my leg with my finger, I realize that my leg is touched. But this phenomenon of double sensation is not essential: cold, a shot of morphine, can make it disappear. This shows that we are dealing with two essentially different orders of reality. To touch and to be touched, to feel that one is touching and to feel that one is touched—these are two species of phenomena which it is useless to try to reunite by the term "double sensation." In fact they are radically distinct, and they exist on two incommunicable levels. Moreover when I touch my leg or when I see it, I surpass it toward my own possibilities. It is, for example, in order to pull on my trousers or to change a dressing on my wound. Of course I can at the same time arrange my leg in such a way that I can more conveniently "work" on it. But this does not change the fact that I transcend it toward the pure possibility of "curing myself" and that consequently I am present to it without its *being me* and without my *being it*. What I cause to exist here is the *thing* "leg;" it is not the leg as the *possibility which I am* of walking, running, or of playing football.

Thus to the extent that my body indicates my possibilities in the world, seeing my body or touching it is to transform these possibilities of mine into dead-possibilities. This metamorphosis must necessarily involve a complete *thisness* with regard to the body as a living possibility of running, of dancing, etc. Of course, the discovery of my body as an object is indeed a revelation of its being. But the being which is thus revealed to me is its *being-for-others*. That this confusion may lead to absurdities can be clearly seen in connection with the famous problem of "inverted vision."

We know the question posed by the physiologists: "How can we set upright the objects which are painted upside down on our retina?" We know as well the answer of the philosophers: "There is no problem. An object is upright or inverted in relation to the rest of the universe. To perceive the whole universe inverted means nothing, for it would have to be inverted in relation to something." But what particularly interests us is the origin of this false problem. It is the fact that people have wanted to link *my* consciousness of objects to the body of the Other. Here are the candle, the crystalline lens, the inverted image on the screen of the retina. But to be exact, the retina enters here into a physical system; it is a *screen* and only that; the crystalline lens is a *lens* and only a lens; both are homogeneous in their being with the candle which completes the system. Therefore we have deliberately chosen the physical point of view—i.e., the point of view of the outside, of exteriority —in order to study the problem of vision; we have considered a dead eye in the midst of the visible world in order to account for the visibility of this world. Consequently, how can we be surprised later when consciousness, which is absolute interiority, refuses to allow itself to be bound to this object? The relations which I establish between the Other's body and the external object are *really* existing relations, but they have for their being the being of the for-others; they suppose a center of intra-mundane flow in which knowledge is a *magic* property of space, "action at a distance." From the start they are placed in the perspective of the Other-as-object.

If then we wish to reflect on the nature of the body, it is necessary to establish an order of our reflections which conforms to the order of being: we can not continue to confuse the ontological levels, and we must in succession examine the body first as being-for-itself and then as being-for-others. And in order to avoid such absurdities as "inverted vision," we must keep constantly in mind the idea that since these two aspects of the body are on different and incommunicable levels of being, they can not be reduced to one another. Being-for-itself must be wholly body and it must be wholly consciousness; it can not be *united* with a body. Similarly being-for-others is wholly body; there are no "psychic phenomena" there to be united with the body. There is nothing *behind* the body. But the body is wholly "psychic."

If I am my Body*

GABRIEL MARCEL

October 24th, 1920

I am not at all sure about the soundness of the observations I made yesterday. This is the point I thought I had reached: if *I am my body* only means "my body is an object of actual interest for me" we have nothing that can confer on my body a real priority in relation to other objects. This is not so if "my body" is regarded as the necessary condition for an object to become a datum for my attention. But in that case the attention which is brought to bear on my body presupposes the exercise of this mediating element which itself falls outside the realm of the knowable. Only by an arbitrary step of the mind as in (*b*) can I identify the body-as-object with the body-as-mediator.

But what are we to think of the idea of a primary instrument of the attention (whether or not it coincides with what I habitually call my body)? From what I pointed out yesterday it emerges that no idea of a mediating principle by which the attention can be exercised is possible for me. But is that which can in no way be an object for me by that very fact incapable of being an object for anyone? Can we not conceive a type of organic structure and optics of the intellect that are different from ours so that from their standpoint the problem would collapse?

We must first of all delve deeper into the nature of the instrumental relation. Funda-

* From *Metaphysical Journal*. Translated by Bernard Wall. Chicago: Henry Regnery Company, Publishers, 1952.

mentally it seems to me that every instrument is a means of extending or of strengthening a "power" that we possess. This is just as true as regards a spade as regards a microphone. To say that these powers themselves are instruments would be merely playing with words; for we would need to determine what these powers themselves really prolong. There must always be some community of nature between the instrument and the instrumentalist. But if I look on my body as my instrument am I not yielding to a sort of unconscious illusion by which I give back to the soul the very powers which are merely prolonged by the mechanical dispositions to which I have reduced my body? It must be noted, moreover, that if I deny that the body is entirely thinkable, I am contesting that it can be treated as an instrument, since an instrument is essentially that of which an idea is possible, indeed that which is only possible through this idea of it.

Under such conditions the initial question changes its appearance. When I insisted on the necessity of a mediation for the attention to be concentrated on any object, had I not the impression that I was speaking of an instrument? And on the other hand when I said that, strictly speaking, I could not form an idea of that mediation, was I not implicitly denying that it was an instrument? I appear to be involved in a whole network of contradictions. All this should be taken up in detail.

If I think of my body as instrument I thereby attribute to the soul, whose tool it is, the potentialities which are actualised by means of this instrument. Nor is that all. I furthermore convert the soul into a body and in that way become involved in regression without end. To suppose on the other hand that I can become anything whatever, that is to say, that I can identify myself with anything whatever, by the minimum act of attention implied by an elementary sensation without the intervention of *any mediation whatsoever,* is to undermine the very foundations of spiritual life and pulverise the mind into purely successive acts. But I can no longer conceive this mediation as being of an instrumental order. I will therefore call it "sympathetic mediation." Is the idea of such mediation possible for an intelligence that is different from ours? Once again we need to make a roundabout approach. Instrumental mediation and sympathetic mediation seem to be bound up together and even unthinkable apart. But what exactly does their bond imply?

All that I can say from the standpoint which I have so far attained is that telepathy, for example, is doubtless only a particular case of a general mode of mediation which is alone capable of making instrumental mediation possible. But obviously we will not get an inch nearer the solution of the problem I have stated by interposing an unknown occult body between spiritual activity and the visible body. Moreover, the expression "spiritual activity" does not satisfy me. Things must be considered on a higher level. To say that the attention cannot be exercised directly on an object is to refuse to regard the attention as an independent reality. Could we not say that attention is always attention to self and inversely that there is only self where there is attention? Besides it is quite clear that to pay attention to something is always to pay attention to oneself as a feeling being. Yet we need to grasp that this *self* still *falls short* of all objectivity. Here we come back to the criticism that I made earlier of formalistic doctrine of the ego (as object that has nothing objective about it, that is neither a *what* nor a *who*).

I am unable to appear to myself otherwise than as an attentive activity bound up with a certain *"this"* on which it is exercised and without which it would not be itself. But have I not said that no idea of this *"this"* is possible? Whereas must it not at every moment be a given *such,* that is to say, must it not be determined? (I would not like to insist here on the problem regarding time that we will come up against soon enough). The *this* of which I am speaking is not an object, but the absolute condition for any object whatever to be given to me as datum. I wonder whether I would be betraying the thought I am trying to "bring to birth" at this moment if I said that there is no attention save where there is at the same time a certain fundamental way of feeling that cannot in any way be converted into an object, that is in no way reduced to the Kantian *I think* (since this is not a universal form) and without which the personality is annihilated. To sum up, this fundamental sensation is confounded with attention to self (the self being no more than absolute immediacy treated as mediation).

But we must grasp clearly that this *Urgefühl* can in no way be felt, precisely because it is fundamental. For it could only be so in function of other sensations—but by that very fact it would lose its priority. But is it not conceivable that for other beings placed on another plane, this fundamental quality can on the contrary be felt? . . .

When I re-read the bulk of the foregoing reflections I think I can see a "hole" in my argument. Can I not be reproached for having taken as a sort of self-evident postulate that this fundamental quality cannot be identified with my body? Whereas I am really unable to identify the object and the condition of objectivisation.

Nor are we at the end of our difficulties. If my body is not to be identified with this mediating quality, how does it happen that my body appears to me as being *more* than an object amongst other objects? I think the answer is that for sympathetic mediation to take place, there must also be instrumental mediation. Hence, for there to be a medium there must also be a knowable instrument—i.e., a body.

The kind of antinomy involved in all this is essentially bound up with the very nature of personal life, because were all instrumental mediation lacking, we would be in the realm of pure diversity, of that which cannot be grasped.

Being in the Body*

EUGENE F. KAELIN

Il n'y a pas d'autre manière de le comprendre que de le regarder, mais alors il dit tout ce qu'il veut dire. Sa signification est la trace d'une existence, lisible et compréhénsible pour une autre existence. — Maurice Merleau-Ponty, *La Phénoménologie de la perception*, p. 371.

I

One of the funniest lines ever written by a philosopher is found in the life of Plotinus, by his respectful student, Porphyry. In translation it reads, "Plotinus, the philosopher, our contemporary, seemed ashamed to be in the body." Porphyry himself, I would presume, had no difficulty understanding this sentence, and anyone familiar with the context of Plotinus' philosophy would, after some study, be able to give a reasonable interpretation of it. I once tried to do so to a group of students, and their immediate reaction to my explication was a raucous belly laugh. That was how I discovered the sentence is funny. The students grasped immediately something which I had not yet understood, and concerning which I should like to come to an understanding today. After all, why do people listen to philosophers or read their books, and sometimes pay them magnificent sums of money, if it is not in the hope that the philosophers in question will be of some help in the attempt to solve the problems of everyday life?

Philosophical beliefs usually turn up in any

* From National Association for Physical Education of College Women. *Report of the Ruby Anniversary Workshop*. Interlochen, Michigan, 1964.

organized attempt to control and direct human behavior, and when they do, it is in disguise as unexamined presuppositions about the nature of human beings, the ends it is good or possible for them to achieve, and the available means for achieving them. Since they are in disguise and unexamined, such beliefs which are also erroneous can do much harm. Starting out as attitudes on the part of teachers, for example, they become ingrained as habits within the responsive patterns of students, who as usual suffer most from the errors of their teachers. I do not know whether it is more difficult to shuck off a bad habit or to take on a good one. Each learning process, however, is difficult in its own way, so the strain of each may be incommensurate with that of the other. Nevertheless, habitual actions are engaged in without thought, and may continue in spite of thought, whereas the difficulty of initiating the habit we know to be good demands reflection upon the goodness of the proposed manner of behaving, as well as upon the means available for inducing it in ourselves or others. It is not enough to repeat the classical dictum, *mens sana in corpore sano;* we must come to know what these words mean in the conduct of our lives. Critical reflection on such ideals as this is, and has always been, the concern of philosophical inquiry.

Unfortunately, however, it is not always clear whose problems the philosopher is trying to solve. Plotinus, for example, seems to have had some problems of his own: where was he when he was not in the body? and what was it

167

like to be there? The answer to one of these questions is funny-ha-ha; to the other, only funny-odd. I do not propose to tell you which is which, for that would be to give away my game before it is time to do so. Perhaps the best I can do is to put the two questions back into their original form by asking, Who was Plotinus? And one answer to that question is "the philosopher who seemed ashamed to be in the body," a man, obviously who was confused as to who and where he was. The life and the biography of such a man eminently qualify for being both funny-odd and funny-ha-ha.

People interested in, and dedicated to, educational theory and practice are well situated to understand the oddity and the humor of Porphyry's words concerning Plotinus' feelings in the body. But perhaps it should be said, in order to escape the predicaments of Plotinus and his student, that your own interests as members of the National Association for Physical Education of College Women are better described as "the theory of educational practice and the practice of educational theory." Certainly we do not want to pursue a theory for its own sake. If it is to be any good at all, a theory must stem from, and result in improved, practice. Moreover, the theory and practice of physical culture for women, if qualified as anything but educational, might be interpreted to invite pleasantries which on this occasion would be out of place, if not in direct violation of taste. When I was a school boy—my mother always referred to me as a "college man"—the dandies of the day called the coeds who elected physical education as their major, "sweat socks," to distinguish them from their masculine counterparts, called by another name. By any other name, each would have smelled as sweet; or perhaps, as in Chinese cuisine, it would be better here to introduce the notion of the sweet and sour.

As you can see, the pendulum of my thought has returned full swing, back to the physics of the matter at hand. If Plotinus' idealism allowed him to separate mind from matter, or soul from body, and to find his ideals only in the realm of mind or soul, the realists among you have sometimes been criticized by your humanistic colleagues for acting as if the bodies you are training had no minds at all. You would be hard put, if pushed, to indicate any ideal or aim of your activities outside the development of motor skills. You will be shocked, I hope, to hear that the rationale of your own educational postures is equally as funny—odd and ha ha—as those of your ideal-

istic opponents. In what follows I hope to make this clear and to suggest one way of removing the oddity and the humor continuously associated with the concept of physical education.

As a start, my major contention is: minds and bodies, like theories and practice, cannot be separated from the context of direct human involvement in the processes of life. Neither are they substances, capable of being weighed in a balance or precisely measured by any instrument of quantitative analysis. Any insistence upon quantitative precision at this stage of our inquiry would merely serve to falsify our result, which should be an adequate conception of mind and body, of mind-body, as a relational system coming into existence and passing away in a single, indeterminate environment I shall here refer to as a phenomenal field. Much of this work has already been performed by philosophers and psychologists on the continent of Europe, and I shall be making almost exclusive use of two studies by Maurice Merleau-Ponty, the only French existentialist who was also a reputed academic philosopher.

These studies, *La Structure du comportement* and *La Phénoménologie de la perception*, have recently been translated, and there already exists a running commentary on their contents.[1] I shall select only those parts of Merleau-Ponty's philosophy that are relevant to my thesis. The business of philosophy is the criticism of an on-going social institution; when this job is not done, by a philosopher or someone else, none of our social behavior is minded or intelligent in the fullest sense of the word, that is, fully self-conscious. You will see then that I am not posing as a scientist, who must record, hypothesize, and predict; that is the work which must follow what I am about to do. As a philosopher, my present task is to evaluate, and what I shall be evaluating is the adequacy of the concepts used by scientists and educators in their descriptions and direction of the educational process. If you did not think such a project is possible, you would not have invited a philosopher to address your convention, and if I did not think it possible, I should not have accepted your kind invitation to be here.

II

When asked to justify the theory and practice of physical education, teachers have sometimes responded with ideas of great generality and widespread social approval. Physical education has been said to "teach character," or to "develop leadership potential," or to make its adepts "better citizens, in a democratic sort of way." The trouble with such answers as these is that no one, not even those who offer them as justification for their educational policies, believes them. No one believes them because no one can.

We cannot teach character to our athletes while insisting that they win at all costs or by turning them into underpaid professionals. Leadership in any field other than athletics has little to do with physical strength, endurance, or skill—President Franklin D. Roosevelt led this country admirably for more than twelve years from the restricted confines of a wheel chair. Better citizens need more qualities than teammanship. To work with others in pursuit of a common goal is precisely that quality instilled in the fanatical German populace by a power-mad dictator. The essence of democracy is another habit—that of considering in concert the desirability of a proposed common goal and maintaining respect for those who cannot acquiesce in the choice to pursue one goal rather than another.

Each of these so-called justifications of physical education is conceived from an external point of view, and each is grafted onto the actual practice of education in virtue of an extraneous, albeit tangential, relationship to the development of the human personality by physical means. One might as well argue, within the restricted framework of physical education for women, that the end of our educational program is the development of more physically fit wives and mothers. If this is truly the case, then perhaps we have been working on the wrong sets of muscles.

The corrective to these abortive attempts to justify physical education is a return to the phenomena of our physical existence. We cannot, like Plotinus, continue to feel ashamed to be in the body; we cannot, like some physical educators, continue to cover over our shame by espousing the ideals of mind, character, or social utility as justifications of our interest in educating the body. It is true, of course, that in some sense we are aiming to educate the "whole person" and not just the body or the mind, but if this is so, we must, in order to convince our skeptical opponents, be able to show how the intrinsic development of the human personality follows naturally from what we do to it in our efforts to educate it. In other words, if we are to break down the false separation of minded activity from bodily activity, we must show the continuity of physical responses and intelligent responses to the set of

stimuli playing upon the human personality by virtue of its relationship to an environment—physical, biological, and social—in which goals are first perceived, evaluated, and pursued in the business of continued life. And this is another description of what I have previously referred to as the "phenomenal field" of human existence.

Education of whatever sort must take place within this field, and its purpose is the enrichment of the lives of the individuals capable of this kind of existence. Education must start with individuals at a level of development where they are found; they are to be led out of their narrow pre-occupation with self; they are to be put in a position to conceive and to build a newer environment of ever receding horizons, always working with what is given and, within the limits of possibility, changing what is given into what is desirable, the significant into something more significant because it is more satisfying, and, not least, the personal creation of men. The range of education therefore covers the full extent of human expression: from seeking an object at a distance, to feeling ashamed to be in the body; from the facts man constructs by his habit of seeing, to the values he conceives—and with luck turns into new facts—by his habit of feeling anything at all.

Existentialist philosophers refer to this enlargement of the horizons of human experience as "transcendence," and if education is to mean anything at all, it should help man transcend the limits placed upon his development by the raw facts of nature. He can do this, I am convinced, because within the structures of his experience, or existence if you prefer, he is capable of taking on a second nature; he can and does develop habits of conduct we loosely refer to as intelligent, meaning thereby a comparative or superlative degree of adaptability to the conditions of an environment. The term being compared is, I suggest, "significant," a delightfully ambiguous word used to qualify any fact possessing a meaning to some organism for its continued life process, or transcendence. I need only add here that significance is not properly speaking something we "understand"; it is, however, always, whether understood or not, something which we feel and with respect to which we must act. Since perception of significance starts with the body, and the body must be oriented to perform an action, it is no mystery why education must start with the body. Any further development of experience will likewise have reference to the body in that further significance will be constituted by other, varying ways in which the body may comport itself.

Continuity between body and mind is thus one of the facts of human existence. The question arises, however, as to the best manner of expounding this relationship, and here we have a choice. Phenomenological (or existential) philosophers are fond of saying that we can take the "natural attitude," or the "phenomenological." We can assume the guise of physical or natural scientists, abstracting completely from our own feelings or values, and describe in total objectivity what takes place in the area of our concern; then, relating this area to others, we will eventually have described everything that is true of the natural world, including the artifacts of men, moving from quality, to fact, to law, and finally to the law of laws or nature itself. The difficulty that goes along with this attitude is not merely one of knowing where and how to find our facts or of achieving the degree of objectivity necessary to describe the facts as they happen independently of our own deliberate intervention; our frustration goes much deeper than this. It is of a theoretical sort in that the natural attitude itself dissimulates the nature of the enterprise we should be investigating every time man and his behavior are the subject of investigation. In matters of education, we cannot be "objective" in the sense that our own values would make no difference for the outcome of our inquiry; our own values are part and parcel of the very process of education, and to abstract from them is to emasculate the experience it is our business to inculcate in our subjects (even if they are women).

The alternative to the natural attitude is the phenomenological. According to the latter, a phenomenon appears when a given subject is undergoing some kind of experience, which of course may later be described. An art critic, for example, allows the experience of a work of art to take place; he allows the work to engage his attention as completely as it might. In a very real sense, the work must happen first, and then it may be described according to the manner in which it has controlled the critic's experience. Edmund Husserl, who invented the method, called this technique "pure description." In order for it to work, the subject must "bracket the world," that is, suspend belief in the reality of the real, physical world and hold in check the propensity to appeal to facts or laws of the sciences describing the real world. Our belief in a real world, and our appeals to the physical conditions of having an experience of it, are merely two ways of prej-

udicing the experience we should be describing. Instead of recounting what has happened in the phenomenal occurrence, we appeal to what should have happened according to known or supposed scientific prescriptions. To proceed phenomenologically, then, we let ourselves go to the experience and, in a moment of reflection, describe what has happened to us as it has occurred. As a sculptor friend of mine once wrote, men were lovers long before they became gynecologists, and all the results of the most sophisticated kind of gynecology has had no bearing at all upon their capacity as lovers.[2] On the contrary, the abstractions of the gynecologist may very well have impeded that capacity. To get out of such a predicament, our scientist friend must reassume the phenomenological attitude.

This is what Martin Heidegger meant, in *What is Metaphysics?* when he snidely remarked that if you ask a scientific question you are likely to get a scientific answer. The pejorative he intended has never been understood by many Anglo-American philosophers who have been seduced by the scientism of our own age. The fact of the matter is that education is not a science at all, not even an applied science; it is an art, one of the useful arts, which, of course, may well use the technological results of any science, but which does so in the pursuit of a specified human value. To show that the phenomenological attitude is a necessary part of a viable educational procedure, I shall in what follows describe the human body first in "natural" and then in "phenomenological" terms. My guide is, again, Merleau-Ponty.

III

Within the natural attitude, the body can be considered in its most simple form as a purely physical entity. As physical, the body possesses mass and occupies space and its matter is convertible into energy. Mass is the constant we know relatively as weight, which, like the space the body occupies, can achieve enormous and unhealthy proportions. The function of the mind is to keep this from occurring; of themselves, bodies can only continue to occupy space, each part related to every other part contiguously and coextensively. Like stones, chairs and tables, and marble statues, the human body has a contour and is bounded into a shape which cuts its figure into "objective" space, the three dimensional container of all physical existents; like stones and chairs, the human body, if it were nothing but physical, could not move unless it were moved by another thing. Plato was so struck with this last thought that he used it to establish both the existence and the immortality of the soul.[3] After all, the human body does move, and not necessarily by the action of another physical thing. Whence, the soul. The soul is not moved by another thing, so is self-moving. What is self-moving must be eternal, so the soul will never die, even when it has left the body and given it over to rot.

In our own day of psychological enlightenment we should be shocked to hear stories of the body and soul. Or would we? We often declare our passion "body and soul," but for what purpose is never clear. Like Socrates, who could not resist the physical charms of the young Phaedrus, we begin to discourse upon the soul whenever the body begins to feel uncomfortable at the sight of our beloved. And should we fail to communicate we could even use the same myth as that invented by Socrates to explain our misadventure: the wise charioteer and the good steed always find it difficult to control the evil but powerful steed rearing its ugly head. This was the reason Plotinus felt ashamed to be in the body, but legend has it that he succeeded in getting out of his body at least seven times in his career. To show that the myths of the ancients have not really been surpassed in our own time I need only refer to those instructors of dance who teach their students to express themselves, that is, to feel something and then to make the movements that will convey that feeling to a sympathetic audience.

Feeling, movement, feeling; what could be simpler—and more misguided? It should suffice to point out that self-expression and artistic expression are different concepts, that whereas the latter is always the former, the former only rarely attains to the latter. I am expressing myself now, as I write these words; I could do the same by scratching the back of my head, yelling at my wife, or shooting my mother-in-law. Each of these acts would be mine, but hardly a work of art. Walking across the street, kicking a ball, or dancing each engage roughly the same muscular structures of the human body; each may be preceded by an intention of the mind; all, if continued long enough, are capable of producing another feeling—extreme fatigue. The lesson to be learned is that the feeling I have before or after moving my body is not the feeling embodied in a dance.

Can we say, for this reason, that the feelings of the dance are unfelt and merely symbolized by the movements of the dancers, the patterns of which correspond to patterns of sentience, as Suzanne Langer does?[4] If so, we must explain how the dance which is seen by an audience becomes translated into kinesthetic reactions, and how these present a feeling to be understood. Better, it would seem, to show that the feelings expressed in a dance *are* the movements of a body, felt in the first instance and only then by the dancers as they move, and by an audience which perceives the forms of the movements themselves. Such feelings are objective, or at least intersubjective, and can be described in terms of the spatial and temporal coordinates necessary to define the force expended by the body in movement. Let us then forget the romantic notion of expression for the moment and adopt the language of movement considered as spatial and temporal forms.

The dancer works with the body as instrument, creating a dance *in* space and time, the two ultimate realities of everything physical. Given a space and a time, we could calculate the force necessary to move from here to there; or given the force, the direction, and the destination, we could calculate the time, etc. This, I am told, is the way dance is taught in many institutions, and there is only one thing wrong with the approach: the dancer's body is not a billiard ball rolling down a polished inclined plane, nor is it freely falling from the leaning tower of Pisa. We shall see later that it is not even an instrument, for who would be using the instrument? the soul? the mind? or another body? And the space through which it moves, and the time it consumes? Are these given before the dance, before the body moves? Or, on the contrary, does the body, by moving, create a unique space and a unique time in creating the dance? We must be led to think so, lest we continue to be misled by our concepts of the soul as feeler of feelings to be expressed, and thus as mover of the body; of an instrument without instrumentalist; of space and time without life; and of consciousness without the body, whether in pride or shame. Of course, all this can be avoided; we have only to insist that the only person to come into contact with the human body as a physical object is an undertaker. And only that profession is interested in embalming and burying its objects.

To move from physics to physiology is an interesting step. The phenomenon of movement no longer plagues us, the soul is dispatched to limbo or some other place, and the mind is explicable in terms of the reflex arc or conditioned reflexes.

The reflex arc poses a simple model: stimulus-organism-response, the incoming (afferent) nervous impulses transmitted to the central nervous system where connections are made and transferred into effective action of the body by means of the out-going (efferent) paths. Stimuli, it is supposed, can be controlled and overt behavior can be observed, and measured. Lights, sounds, and pressures can be increased or decreased, reactions noted, and thresholds established. With all this scientific precision, what could go wrong? What, indeed, except the precision itself? Our figures may be exact, but what do they represent? Are stimuli the causes of responses? If so, they should have the same effect at least upon the same subject. But they don't. Even discounting fatigue, reactions to the "same" stimulus differ when that stimulus is presented along with another stimulus of the same kind. There seems to be no absolute significance to any given form of stimulation.

Aestheticians have known this for a long time: an identical red presented contiguously with an equally intense and saturated green is seen as a space tension, and no longer as a red plus the green. And what are we to make of the connections in the central nervous system? Are they made there as in a switchboard, a dialing system, or a transformer? All the mechanical models used to explain the arc of the reflex system fail to account for the fact that each species and each subject, to some extent at least, interpret what is to count for them as a stimulus. The attempt to construct complex patterns of behavior in terms of additive functions of simpler reflex connections is to reduce the rhythm of life to the hygienic conditions of a laboratory, where all the selection of stimuli is made by the experimenting animal, the psychologist himself. Under these conditions the experimental animal always comes off as sick, pathologically related to an unreal environment. But we have made a gain: in the physicist's universe, you will recall, he was pronounced dead and ready for burial.

The learning of complex behavioral patterns by the conditioning of responses takes away some of the pathology, even if it introduces some theoretical problems of its own. One of Pavlov's dogs, you may remember, exhibited what Pavlov himself referred to as the "freedom reflex,"[5] an expression he used to cover the case where an observed response was a rejection, on the part of an overstimulated dog, of the whole experimental situation. How human of the dog, and how cynical (or canine) of the little boy who, if not allowed to pitch, picks up his ball and goes home!

Conditioning allows for the transference of a response proper for one stimulus to another. It can and does take place under conditions of control and in the ordinary life processes of living beings working out solutions of problems by trial and error. The transference of reactions to different stimuli allows the physiologist further to suppose a general law of irradiation, according to which any reaction whatever might follow upon any given stimulus—whence, the superiority of the conditioning process over the simple connections of the reflex arc.

But whence, too, comes the necessity to suppose some kind of limit on irradiation? If, in the life of lower animals, anything can become a stimulus to any kind of response theoretically, then there must be some further law operative in order to explain the specific responses of some species. A toad, for example, will not snap at anything but a moving prey and will continue to do so even if it butts its head against an invisible screen. It will even overcome any inhibition one would expect from having successfully nipped off a piece of moving paper and go on to other trials following this error. Obviously, then, excitation, conditioning, and/or inhibition do not successfully explain all the learning behavior of animals even of a lower order, even though experimenters have succeeded in conditioning reflexes of animals having no cortex, such as fish.

Enough has been said, perhaps, to understand that the doctrine of conditioned reflexes is not "scientific," in any but an extended sense of the term. Since one might always appeal to the law of conditioning to explain any positive results, and to that of conditioned inhibition to explain any negative, the theory is unassailable; but this means that it can be neither confirmed nor disconfirmed. Moreover, since the term "physiological fact" properly speaking is used for the observed processes of the nervous system, the so-called "laws of conditioning, irradiation, and inhibition" are not physiological facts in the same sense. They are theoretical concepts supposed by the experimenter to exist, and then imposed upon the facts of observed behavior.

Rightfully speaking, then, physiological laws are facts of the observer's symbolic behavioral reactions. How otherwise to explain the continued pursuit of many errors in the behavior of experimental animals? or the fixation of one successful trial as the reflex response to a given experimental situation? As in the simple reflex-arc behavior, the character of the stimulus is after all determined by what is meaningful to the organism being tested. This is why the toad continues on its merry way in spite of our efforts to condition his behavior. Some stimuli, moreover, seem to change character. Animals have been noted to react positively to two negative (inhibitory) stimuli when they are presented simultaneously. He who would count on a double, or reinforced inhibition is sadly mistaken. All behavioral responses are *forms* of behavior, and all are occasioned by *forms* of stimuli which are detached from the environmental situation by the animal responding. This evaluation of a situation by an organism is of another order than the physiological and leads us forward to descriptions purely psychological. At this stage, even if the reflexes are gone, Mehitabel could still sing in her characteristic manner, "What-thehell, archie, *toujours gai;* there's a dance in the old dame yet."

The psychology of formal behavioral structures was pushed to its highest development in the work of the gestaltists. It is tempting to indicate that the failures of physiological explanation of perception, even in lower animal orders, stemmed from the inherent difficulty of describing the full nature of a complex physical stimulus. There seems to be no way of compounding simple stimuli. If colors in juxtaposition appear as spaces, and two inhibiting stimuli presented simultaneously fail to inhibit response because when presented as a whole they constitute a qualitatively different sort of stimulus, the least perceptible element in human perception is contrast, a most elementary kind of formal relationship. No contrast, no light—and we are in the dark of night, where, Hegel has pronounced, all cows are black.

The gestaltists concluded that all reactions are to forms, defined as a complex stimulus having a character different from any of its components in isolation. A change in any one of the components radically changes the total quality of the stimulus, whereas total transposition of the complex into another which maintains the relative values of the components fails to change the character of the whole: a change in key does not destroy the unity of a melody. There seems moreover to be no physical explanation of this phenomenon. The structure of any stimulus can be known only through the structure of responses to it. Hence, any attempt to explain the structure of a given response by reference to the structures of the stimulus is obviously an explanatory circle. Whatever description can be given to structured responses must therefore be phenomenological in character: the experience must first

be had, and then described as it has occurred.

Whether the behavioral forms are "syncretic," that is determined by the "rhythm of the organism's life" and tied to a specific characteristic of its environment, as in the spider's reaction to a vibration of its web; or whether they are "mutable," that is transferable from one situation to another, as in conditioned reflexes; or, finally, whether they are truly "symbolic" and capable of expression in the absence of any correlative stimulus—these responses take place within the organism in reaction to the things and other organisms found in its environment. The relationship between organism and environment thus defines the field in which phenomena make their appearance.

I shall maintain that walking across the street, playing a game, or creating a dance are merely continuous modifications of the phenomenal field. The modification is achieved by abstraction from "assigned" significance to "conventional" significance, and from there to "auto-significance." I shall not maintain, however, that only humans dance; if my account is correct, if I have not been misled by Merleau-Ponty, only those organisms dance which are capable of responding in symbolic forms.

. . . .

V

In order to show in what manner the human species transcends any limitation set upon it by the conditions of its physical and even biological environment by creating for itself a cultural and social environment, I shall once more follow the lead of Merleau-Ponty, whose metaphysics is sometimes called a "philosophical anthropology," centered around the notion of continuity. Educators have always pursued continuity in theory and practice out of fidelity to experience which exhibits a continuous gradation between lower and higher animals and, within the behavioral patterns of the higher, between the life of the organism and the processes of art. Theory and practice cannot be separated because art and life cannot be separated. Art and life cannot be separated because, in living, certain organisms have achieved an order of response of unique significance, an order of response no longer dedicated to the sheer purpose of continued life, but to that of enriching life by suffusing existence with human qualities—those which only a man can feel, only a man express. All this, to be sure, is already well known; what is not so well known is that man has achieved the heights of expression, not because he has a mind, but because he has learned to use his body in significant ways and in an increasing order of complexity. Whether physical or mental, conduct is intelligent when it is ordered to an end.

Consideration of the kinds of ends a man can intend will afford a means of measuring the degree of significance our species may import into its life. In a word, the more significance man achieves, the more intelligent is his behavior. If it is the purpose of education to inculcate the higher, more significant behavioral patterns of human conduct, it cannot pursue this end by derogating the less significant or by supposing that the higher have no relation to the lower. Indeed, a closer inspection of human existence reveals a continuity between man and nature, between mind and bodily response. Each higher order of response is the "mind" with respect to those responses of lower order immediately surpassed. The creation of a human, cultural environment is a product of a body having transformed its signals into symbols, but the signalizing responses are themselves mind with respect to the reflex behavior of immediate response, and reflex behavior is mind with respect to the action and reaction of the physical body within the system of universal gravitation.

We must learn to trace the ascent of man from corpse to living thing and from signalizer to symbolizer much in the same way as Plato and Plotinus envisaged the ascent of the soul. Their most grievous error seems to have been the supposition that the soul continues to ascend when it has lost contact with the body. It matters little that the one imagined the ascent to be directed toward the Good, while the other saw the process as a return to the One. These notions are themselves symbols for the highest ideals of mankind, and ironically, understandable only in terms of the continuity between matter and life and expression.

For all his intelligence, and no matter how absent-minded, man cannot lose contact with his body. These very words call up imagery of infancy, in which the organism is notoriously incapable of controlling either end of its anatomy. The child's sucking reflex fails to lose its significance in adulthood and even gains for having been transported into the ceremony of love. Muscular contraction and expansion, along with the action and reaction between foot and pavement, permit locomotion to both children and adults. But even our locomotion may achieve an added significance, as when

we send our young ladies to finishing schools to "learn how to walk"—that is, in style or with grace. The grossest kind of coquette does nothing basically different. She may slink, swing, jiggle, or bounce; every movement of her body added to the strict necessity of getting from here to there announces the advent of art. Engaged in one kind of activity, the walker holds out a promise of still another, richer and more rewarding for signalizing an intent not bound to the limits of our physical space. Those actions which are so bound, the syncretic forms of human response, are usually taken for granted. We all know how to walk, or have learned to, and so forget the triumph of our infancy when we first stood erect, pulling ourselves up on a chair or our mother's knee. An injury or a virus may well cause us to have to relearn.

But even walking is not our first encounter with space. That occurred when we first saw an object, at a distance or near, a rattle or a hand, both our own, and what a joy to touch! Seeing, reaching, touching; consummation; the thing was ours, wedded to our corporeal structure. Our physical education, it can be supposed, began with the synchronization of these formal perceptual responses. A figure on a ground relative to me; a perceived space tension, coordination of muscle and movement; a kinesthetic trajectory toward that fascinating object, contact and caress; the object yields over its form.

Thus, the bodily schema at this very low order of organization already contains three coordinated structures: visual reaction, anticipated tactile consummation, and kinesthetic synthesis of the body in motion. In a higher order, each of these may become symbolic of the other; here each is linked to the other by the necessity of life. The significance of the syncretic responses, then, are assigned, either by the structure of the organism or the nature of the environment. As the spider will approach anything that sets up a vibrating motion of its web in search of a fly, a child is attracted to what it sees. What it can see, of course, depends upon the objects in its environment, those making their appearance in its phenomenal field. How it propels itself toward the object depends upon the structure of its anatomy. Imagine, if you can, the woman capable of throwing an overhand fast ball; she can't. But she can learn to walk in the most seductive of manners, throwing the most insidious kind of curve.

When she does, her responses have already left the realm of the syncretic and entered the mutable. Freed from the necessity of getting from there to here, she has room to play with her own responses. Her game is conventional, and its end is arbitrarily set up for a purpose of her own. In making this move, she has performed a kinesthetic abstraction. Since the end (or significance) is no longer strictly dictated by the limits of her own structure or that of her environment, she has abstracted the movements for the sake of what they represent or suggest. Seeing her at a distance, I can note her style visually, kinesthetically, or in the other manner; but if I should do that, I will be playing her game, since that is what she intends.

Organized sports, again, are not basically different from this mode of significance. A terrain is set up arbitrarily; goals and movements ordered to the achievement or frustration of attaining the goals within the conventional terrain are likewise regulated by arbitrary decision. Just as above, where some affairs can be illicit, some pitches are illegal and some blows, foul. Since the achievement of the goal measures the significance of the act, all niceties of movement over and above those necessary to achieve the goal are for the form. A pitcher winds up to prepare his muscles for the delivery of his pitch; his goal is to throw the ball past the batter—preferably in the strike zone; his follow-through is for balance and power or break—all action intending an object. Yet some pitchers have style, and others lack form. Warren Spahn's overhand left-handed delivery and Robin Roberts' fluid side-arm right-handed motion are prodigies of human grace; both cases are not unakin to the slower motion grace of a cat stalking a bird.

A further abstraction puts all the significance of the movement into this characteristic of the kinesthetic-visual phenomenon. Diving, skiing, skating, and the like are judged for excellence in form, the figure of the body moving through space as a dynamic configuration. And at this level of abstraction (from locomotion) we are at the approaches of fine art. All that remains for the sport to become art is the symbolic response to the kinesthetic form, that is, for the visual form to call out the kinesthetic feeling. When this occurs, movement is dance. The significance at this last level of locomotor abstraction is created by the movements themselves, by the dancer in motion. It is for this reason that I have referred to the rhythms of dance as "auto-significant." The dance means only itself.

A last point may be made by comparing this scheme to the dance theory of Suzanne K. Langer. For her, too, the dance is symbolic of a pattern of sentience. The symbolism is explained by the dancer's activity of abstracting physical movements, describable in terms of space, time, and force, into a dynamic image of virtual power, which appears only to the attentive consciousness. Her theory runs aground, however, since the pattern of feeling cannot be ascribed to any one person, either to the dancer who composes the image or the audience who perceives its structure. If the feeling is not felt, it is said to be "understood," both by the dancer and his audience.

This theoretical appeal to the understanding of the dancer poses all the old problems of mind and body that have been the bane of philosophy and psychology since the inception of each. Her model for the explanation of mental behavior—a transformer—is as mechanical and as inadequate as the switchboard of the physiologists. To suggest that a dancer first understands a feeling, and then translates it into kinesthetic imagery, is to suggest that a dancer dances before dancing. Since the counters (she says "elements") of the dance medium are movements, the dancer must already have made the movements in order to have gained his or her "idea." Outside of the notion of a locomotor motif, which can be taken from any ordinary life situation and which must be developed in context as an element of the total dance image, the word "idea" has no application in the dance art—unless it be a reference to the finished dance itself. But this must be perceived to be believed. Like her model for the mind, her model for creative communication via works of art is seriously defective. The dancer communicates through her finished product, and she can "understand" its "import" only by making the movements presenting the image of a virtual power.

The same kinds of shortcomings are apparent on the other side of the communication process. If the dancer makes the dance kinesthetically, the audience must take in the dance visually. The "form" of a figure skater or water skier fails to fulfill all the requirements of balletic expression because the athlete is perceived visually, and only visually. The configuration of the athlete's motion outlines a dynamic image in physical space; it may even achieve the status of a virtual power; but the connection between what we see and the feeling expressed remains a theoretical surd. What Mrs. Langer lacked in order to have achieved the most significant interpretation of the dance is a working concept of the bodily schema, of a body which "understands" before a mind has had the time to function.

It is not uncommon for dancers to respond to the question, "How does this dance feel?" by making an appropriate balletic gesture. It feels like this. They are not inviting us to make an overt expression of our own physical bodies in order to understand what "this" means. And they don't have to. We see how the dance feels because the feeling is the global kinesthetic image, a modification of the dancer's bodily schema, and when we respond visually our bodily schemata undergo a similar kinesthetic modification. This is possible because within the bodily schema seeing and feeling and moving are correlative structures of a single system, of a single human existence in transcendence:

> Vision and movement are specific manners of relating ourselves to objects; and if, by all these experiences, a unique function is expressed, it is the unfolding of an existence which does not suppress the radical diversity of its contents. For, it relates whatever contents it has not by

placing them under the strict control of an "I think" (that such and such must be the case), but by orienting them towards the intersensorial unity of a "world."[6]

And this is how, by modifying her world, the dancer succeeds in modifying mine, for as long as I attend to her dance I am inhabiting her world. All the significance of the dance is to be found in this experience.

REFERENCES NOTES

1. Kaelin, E. F., *An Existentialist Aesthetic* (Madison: University of Wisconsin Press, 1962).
2. Steppat, Leo, commenting on "The University and the Creative Arts," by McNeil Lowry, *Arts in Society* (II, 1963, no. 3, p. 35).
3. This account is culled from the *Phaedrus*.
4. Langer, Suzanne K. *Feeling and Form* (New York: Charles Scribner's Sons, 1953, *passim*).
5. Cited in Merleau-Ponty, *La Structure du comportement* (Paris: Presses Universitaires de France, 1942), p. 134.
6. Merleau-Ponty (*ibid.*, p. 160, translation by author).

The Significance of Human Movement: A Phenomenological Approach*

SEYMOUR KLEINMAN

It is rather ironic that those activities which are most intimately concerned with body are precisely the ones which physical educators choose to ignore or pay only a minimal amount of attention to. Those activities which explore movement with great scope and depth appear to be studiously avoided. For a long period of time gymnastics was almost a dirty word in this profession. And the discipline which encompasses all aspects of movement, the dance, is almost completely alienated from physical education. In men's physical education, dance is practically nonexistent. It appears that in our pursuit of and subservience to game and sport, the body almost acts as an obstacle which must be overcome in order that the ends of sport and games be achieved. We have come to regard the body as a thing to be dealt with rather than as an existent presence or mode of being. The body and its movement is viewed as the means to attain the ends of a game. We seek neither significance nor meaning to human movement. The game has become the thing. We have become uneasy about body and movement. Witness our testy attitude toward the emphasis on fitness and our embrace of the impersonal scientific analysis of human activity. We have divorced the body from experience and we do not attempt to understand it as it operates in the life world.

* From National Association for Physical Education of College Women. *Report of the Ruby Anniversary Workshop.* Interlochen, Michigan, 1964.

Rather, we attempt to explain it as a physiological organism. We don't look at it as it is but as we conceptualize it scientifically.

To understand one's body as one lives with it is foreign to us, but not to the phenomenologist. For the phenomenologist, to understand the body is to understand its existential being in the world. This is different from viewing the body as an object for study the way one would study a thing. Merleau-Ponty held that such a view of the body is a secondary meaning of bodily being. He wanted to penetrate into a primordial meaning of the human body. Probably the best and most widely noted illustration of this is Jean-Paul Sartre's description of the three dimensions of the human body. An understanding and awareness of these dimensions will help us understand from whence human movement derives its significance. I will use Sarte's example as described by Van Den Berg in an essay from the book *Psychoanalysis and Existential Philosophy.*[1]

A mountaineer about to set out to achieve a difficult peak makes careful plans and pays careful attention to things like his ropes, his shoes, his pitons, and other items of equipment. He concerns himself with the preparation of his body for the task. He is cognizant and actively aware of his body. However, as soon as he begins the climb, all these thoughts vanish. "He no longer thinks of his shoes to which a short time ago he gave such great attention; he forgets the stick that supports him while he climbs . . . he 'ignores his body' which he trained for days beforehand. . . . For only by forgetting, in a certain sense, his body, will he be able to devote himself to the laborious task that has to be performed." What remains, what *is*, is only the mountain. He is absorbed in it, his thoughts are completely given to it. And it is *because* he forgets his body that the body can realize itself as a living body. "The body is realized as *landscape*"; its length is demonstrated by the difficulties which must be faced from hand hold to hand hold. "Fatigue shows itself first as the changed aspect of the landscape, as the changed physiognomy of the objects." The rocks, the snow-fields, the summit appear more hostile.

"The qualities of the body: its measurements, its efficiency and vulnerability can only become apparent when the body itself is forgotten, passed over in silence for the landscape." *It is only the behavior, the act, the movement that explains the body.* In this dimension the landscape is where the significance lies. It is to the landscape that the movement is directed and there in the landscape is where the movement is furnished with significance. Knowing one's body is not revealed by scientific analysis or observation. We just do not come to know our bodies in this way. Wolff discovered that on the average only one out of ten persons can recognize his hand when shown a series of photographs which includes a likeness of his own hand. And yet in fact we *do* know our bodies. It "is that which is most our *own* of all conceivable things, which is least opposed to us, least foreign and so, least antagonistic."[2]

"The second dimension of the body comes into being under the eyes of his fellow man. In the first dimension, remember, the mountaineer in order to accomplish his task transcended his body, 'passed beyond' it in silence." The only change introduced into the second dimension is that the mountaineer unknown to him is being watched by another. The viewer in this dimension concentrates on the very thing that the climber has transcended. He sees the boots, the movements, the bruises. He sees the *body*. The viewer's landscape is centered in this moving body—this object. That which holds least significance to the climber contains the most significance for the hidden viewer. It is this recognition of another as a functioning organism which makes anatomical and physiological analysis possible. And it has been with this dissectable thing—the body— that psychology has been until recently solely concerned. Also physical education has been

content to limit its study of movement to this dimension. We have embraced physiological and anatomical analysis with such vigor and tenacity that it has become the only dimension of being in the world which we recognize. We regard man as a moving organismic thing—an object, capable of being completely understood by means of stimulus-response conditioning, laws of learning, transfer of training, and neurological brain wave analysis. But I shall return to this point later.

The third dimension of the body comes into being when the mountaineer becomes aware that he is being watched. For Sartre, this dimension of being is destructive. It destroys the "passing beyond." The climber becomes annoyed, uncomfortable. He feels vulnerable and defenseless. He miscalculates, he stumbles, he becomes ashamed. For Sartre, the look of the other always results in alienation. Van Den Berg disagrees. "Sartre's look is the look from behind, the malicious look of an unknown person. There is (on the other hand) the look of understanding, of sympathy, of friendship, of love. It may impart a happiness far exceeding in value any solipsistic satisfaction."

The significance of the movements on this dimension lies *in the look*. The somewhere where the movements take place also lies in the look. Under the gaze of the other, whether it be one of approval or disapproval, my body, my movements, my being is out there at the gaze, at the look. This dimension has great meaning and implication for teachers.

Now it is important to note that only one of these three dimensions of being attributes and suggests significance to movement as we physical educators generally regard it. Our profession's approach to movement has been by means of the mechanical, the kinesiological, the physiological, and the anatomical. The psychologically and sociologically oriented people in our field who attempt to study and predict cultural patterns and behavior strive to operate on this same kind of scientific level. During the course of experimentation and observation the individual comes to be regarded as an organism capable of being manipulated. He becomes a thing or an object in the eyes of the other. Analysis and explanation of human movement results but not real understanding.

To the phenomenologist, to understand the body is to see the body not in terms of kinesiological analysis but in the awareness and meaning of movement. It's to be open to gestures and action; it's the grasping of being and acting and living in one's world. Thus movement becomes significant not by a knowledge about the body but through an awareness of the self—a much more accurate term.

What are the implications of this view for physical education? From the phenomenological view it becomes the purpose of the physical educator to develop, encourage, and nurture this awareness of and openness to self—this understanding of self.

I suggest that this will not be accomplished if we continue to equate physical education with sports and games. Games provide satisfactions and fulfill a need to play and compete, but I contend that it is not the function of physical education to take as its responsibility the teaching and playing of games, especially when there is so much more that can be done in the way of enhancing fulfillment and realization through movement.

Thus the objectives of physical education become the following:

1. To develop an awareness of bodily being in the world.
2. To gain understanding of self and consciousness.
3. To grasp the significations of movements.
4. To become sensitive of one's encounters and acts.
5. To discover the heretofore hidden perspectives of acts and uncover the deeper meaning of one's being as it explores movement experiences.
6. To enable one, ultimately, to create on his own an experience through movement which culminates in meaningful, purposeful realization of the self.

This last I feel is the stage of true freedom, ultimate existence, and being. Its result is the attainment of the truly, independent spirit, and this should be the goal of all education.

Needless to say this is not the purpose or function of sports and games. Nor should it be! I am not here to deprecate games. But somehow back in its earlier days this profession reacted against the stultifying discipline of gymnastics and equated play with democracy and freedom. Our readiness to accept and encourage the concept of sport and physical education as being one and the same has brought us to this present state of uneasiness and dissatisfaction—a profession in search of a discipline. Nothing could be more shattering to a dedicated group of people such as we have in this field. It has resulted in a fantastic race to justify our existence and gain respectability by publishing nonbooks, nonarticles, and *non*sensical data by the score. This attempt to convert a field such as ours which operates on a human experiential level into a science would be absurd were it not so tragically close to being accomplished. Physical education is an art, not a science. In our attempts to exhaustively analyze movement, exercise, fatigue, and the like we have moved farther and farther away from the experience as it is acted out— as it *actually* occurs.

This flight to science for respectability has turned many of our best people toward research in this area. But might I point out that whatever these people do in the sciences, be they behavioral or physical, they are not doing physical education. If they study muscle fatigue, they are doing physiology. If they study mechanics of movement, they are doing physics. If they study behavior, they are doing psychology. If they study games and sports, they are doing sociology. But these fields are disciplines in their own right. They are certainly not the discipline of physical education. In fact, I don't believe this profession knows that it means to *do* physical education.

How does one go about *doing* physical education? It is, I believe, our job to deal with the experience of movement, and it is our role to make this movement experience as highly significant as possible. The student must "enter into" the movement as completely as possible. And I am convinced that no other area in our field fills this need as successfully as the dance. Dance points toward this objective specifically and directly. The interesting thing about this is that most of the dancers and choreographers don't intellectualize and verbalize the experience to death. They just do it and it comes. The objective is attained in the experiencing of it.

Dance is the most demanding of all movement activities. It requires almost complete submissiveness to an iron discipline. And teachers of dance aren't known usually for the democratic spirit that exudes from their studio. Yet despite all of the "wrong" educational techniques the results are astonishing. Out of this experience emerges, not a slave, but a truly free individual—one who has such knowledge and command of his body that he is capable of experiencing movement at its highest and most significant level.

Although all participants in a dance may be performing exactly the same movements, the individual, if he is truly engaged in the act, knows nothing of others. He is completely absorbed in his landscape. He is acting only as *he* can act. He is deriving meaning and significance only in the way *he* is capable. He is aware of his movements as a creative art. It almost doesn't matter that he didn't design the move. He brings to it what he has to offer and what emerges is a noble experience, an enriching experience, a rewarding experience. Even the gaze of the other is transcended at this point. The audience becomes part of the landscape too. The spectators gain their rewards by what they as individuals bring to the experience.

Of course, all this happens if these movements—the dance—are good. So much of dance is extraordinarily poor. On these occasions both audience and dancers suffer. But dance, even when it fails, is by its nature concerned with significant movement.

Of the three dimensions of being outlined in this paper, those two, the first and third, which are most intimately related to physical education still await investigation and description. This is most unfortunate because it is here, in the phenomenological realm, where most of the work needs to be done. Gaining greater sensitivity and awareness of landscapes and their importance in contributing to significant movement is a task with which physical education must become intricately involved.

"Existence as a giver of meaning, manifests itself in all human phenomena, in the gestures of our hands, the mimicry of our face, the smile of the child, the creation of the artist, speech and work. . . The body is this power of expression. It gives rise to meaning; it makes meaning arise on different levels. . . ."[3] My contention is that for physical education the goal should be meaning and significance on the highest level of existence. I don't believe this can be achieved by a physical education as we know it today. Games and sports by their inherent nature do little toward achieving this goal at best and, in fact, often do much to keep us from it.

REFERENCES NOTES

1. J. H. Van Den Berg, "The Human Body and the Significance of Human Movement," *Psychoanalysis and Existential Philosophy*, H. M. Ruitenbeek, editor (F. P. Dutton & Co., New York, 1962, pp. 90-129).
2. F. J. J. Buytendijk, *General Theory of Human Carriage and Movement* (Utrecht, Spectrum, 1948).
3. R. C. Kwant, *The Phenomenological Philosophy of Merleau-Ponty* (Duquesne University Press, Pittsburgh, Pa., 1963, p. 57).

My Body, My Self

ELLEN W. GERBER

When I was in mid-adolescence, I read William Butler Yeats' poem "Sailing to Byzantium" (1952, pp. 191–192) in which he decries his lot as a creature of nature, born to rot and die. Like Yeats, I yearned to be a "monument of unageing intellect," a golden nightingale singing through eternity to the lords and ladies of Byzantium. Many years later, when my Puritan heritage was finally overcome and I could enjoy my hedonistic appreciation of the flesh, I published a poem of my own (1966, p. 57) in which I renounced the concept of the "disembodied intellect," and concluded that "those who know the burning/ Moment of the living flesh/Cannot be tricked . . . Those who choose to claim/The meaning of the being whole/Touch upon their immortality/In the living moment of the present."

It is probably impertinent of me to begin a paper with these personal comments, but somehow I see the evolution of my own understanding as a microcosm of the ambivalence with which most, if not all, of us have faced the concept of the body. Because each of us has a body—and is a body—the matter is a uniquely personal one. But it is also a matter of professional concern for those whose work requires them to deal with others in a context that focuses on bodies in physical activity. Therefore, this paper will discuss ways in which one views one's body, focusing particularly on one's body as oneself. The topic will also be dealt with in terms of the relationship between sex and embodiment and, finally, in terms of the body-self in physical activity.

THE CONCEPT OF THE BODY AS SELF

Fundamentally, there are three ways of viewing one's own body. (This is the position taken by Sartre [1956] and aptly translated into viewing movement experiences by Van Den Berg [1962] and Kleinman [1964].) Note that no value accrues to any of the three perspectives. Each dimension is part of living and it is probably essential that each person experience himself/herself at every conceivable level. If there is any valuing to be done, it will have to relate to the notion of proportion or to the valuing of the effects of viewing ourselves from each different perspective.

The first mode, most distant from the personal, is seeing one's body through the eyes of others. For example, the adolescent is particularly concerned with how others—especially the opposite sex—perceive his/her body. Thus there is an endless round of considerations which stem from thoughts such as: "If I develop bulging muscles will he (she) think me unattractive (attractive)." From this perspective, not only does one's body exist as an object for self, but as an object for others. One's personal sense of one's body is subordinated to assumptions of what others think of the body. Instead of looking at one's body directly, one sees it as it is reflected in the lens of another's eyes.

The second perspective entails the viewing of one's body as if it was an object apart from oneself, a thing among things—an entity whose qualities can be quantified and modified. For example, one looks in the mirror and says: "There's a fat slob." Or, one says: "I've got to work on this leg till it can lift 50 pounds." Every time one stands back and reflects on or considers the qualities of something or someone, one is objectifying it. "Abstractive reflexion deprives the body of its dimension of subjectivity and constitutes it as an object beside others in the world" (Duhrssen, 1956, p. 32). As the philosopher Martin Buber (1923) pointed out, one is relating in an I–It manner. The I–It or objective mode of relation is fundamental to all of our behavior because it is through this process that we gather data. In order to function one needs to know facts. One needs to know how heavy an object is before one attempts to lift it or throw it because that knowledge is essential to selecting the appropriate amount of effort. One needs to know facts about other individuals in order to relate to them. One needs to know what are their capacities before one invites them to join in an intended action. Thus it is with one's body.

In order to function appropriately there are many objective facts about one's body which it is essential to know with a fair degree of accuracy. Strength? Level of endurance? Conformance of shape to that of others? Size in relation to objects such as a chair? Every time one seeks to answer these questions, every time one reflects about one's body or examines it critically in a manner designed to provide information, one is treating one's body as an object in the environment.

Similarly, every time one separates the consideration of the body per se from other elements of one's own being, such as when one talks of mind, body and spirit, for example, or even physical and cognitive functioning, one is objectifying the body. And, needless to add, every time one treats the body, giving consideration to "it" only, as in medicine or training, one is perceiving it as an object in the environment. As with one's relationships with other persons and things, this I–It perspective of the body is the one utilized most of the time.

The third dimension of the body is the body as subject, the body as the radical root of personal reality—in short, the body as self. The philosopher Marcel (1952) explicated two phrases which symbolize the distinction between the objective and subjective modes of viewing the body. In the objective mode, a person says: "I have a body." In the subjective mode, the person says: "I am my body." In other words, subjectively speaking, my body is myself. "My body is *who I am*. I exist in the world as embodied." (Schrag, 1969, p. 131) "My body . . . *is* my consciousness . . . its concrete position in the world." (Duhrssen, 1956, p. 31)

In order to represent this concept, Schrag (1969) used the term "the lived body." Zaner (1966) called it "the radical reality of the human body." Sartre (1956) referred to "the being-for-itself." The point of these terms is that the philosophers attempted to discuss the body, the physical being, in terms which indicate that it is the experiencing manifestation of self. Recall that in Yeats' poem the poet was glorifying intelligent acts, represented by the golden nightingale singing, as separate from the physical being located in nature. The body was a vessel—an annoying one at that because of its tendency to ultimately rot—for the "unageing intellect." The "lived body," however, has no such distinctions. The concept of the lived body incorporates the notion that the human being in order to have thought, to act intelligently or consciously, must have experiences. These experiences never occur in a disembodied manner. No experience takes place without one's physical presence. Each person is in the world as an embodied presence. The body is the manifestation of self in the world. Each of us is an "embodied experiencer" (Schrag, 1969). That is what Marcel means when he says: "I am my body."

Most people are familiar with Descartes famous expression: "*Cogito ergo sum*," "I think, therefore I am." The phenomenologist might modify that to "I am, therefore I think." The phenomenologist—so-called because he/she is dealing with the being, the phenomenon, itself—recognizes that it is one's embodied or physical presence in the world that allows one to have the experience of being. "It is by virtue of his/her embodiment that the experiencer is exposed to the world" (Schrag, 1969, p. 133).

Conversely, it is by virtue of his/her embodiment—through sense experiences—that the world is exposed to the individual. Since one is always present as one's body, it is as one's body that one can experience the world—perceive it, touch it, inspect it, hold it. As a body-self one comes to know the world and as a body-self one interacts with the world, lives the world. Thus, through one's lived body the world is opened to self. But, that also implies that one's interaction with the world is bounded by one's lived body and its capacities. One can never directly experience the world in ways which go beyond the powers of one's lived body. People can never experience the world as a bird does, in free flight. People can never experience the world from two perspectives simultaneously. "I am constantly 'here' and not 'there'. . . ." (de Waelhens, 1967, p. 159). One's view is always from where one stands—a matter which has profound philosophical implications, for not only can one never stand or be embodied in two places simultaneously, but no one else can ever simultaneously experience the world from where one stands. A change in position, a lapse in time, ensures that no one else can ever have another's exact experience of the world. Thus one's personal embodiment is central to his/her experience of the world. One's experience of the world is central to the being one is. "I must, fatefully, 'be and do' as embodied by this body which at once determines and is determined by myself—for it is 'animated' by me and I 'embodied' by it" (Zaner, 1966, p. 85).

EMBODIED FEMALE— EMBODIED MALE

One of the interesting questions which, to my knowledge, phenomenologists have not attempted to answer, is "does a different experience follow if one is embodied in the world female vis-à-vis male?" This question is central to contemporary society's concerns about the relative and changing roles of women and men, and also affects decisions about men and women, boys and girls in sport.

Let us be clear about the meaning of the question itself. If one answers, "yes, because I am embodied female I inevitably must experience the world in a manner different from males," then one is suggesting that there is a common core of experience of the world which *all* females share by virtue of their female embodiment and which *no* males experience because of their male embodiment—and vice-versa, of course. This common experience would have to pervade each sex, and be present in each and every culture throughout time and in all places. Such a notion strains credulity. As is true of true-false tests, if the words "all," "always," or "never" appear in the sentence it must be false.

On the other hand, responsible and thoughtful scholars have pointed out that "a scientific attitude itself requires, if not actually the belief, then at least recognition of the possibility that as universal a distinction—through virtually all forms of life, through aeons of evolution—as that of sex cannot be simply a limited, 'functionally-specific' difference, affecting only

reproduction in a narrow sense and completely independent of the rest of our feeling and behavior; that it must, particularly in as complex a creature as [hu]man[s], be associated with subtle and far-ranging differences, from the level of biological functioning to that of personality and mental organization." (Ruderman, 1971, p. 50) In other words, Ruderman claims that it is also straining credulity to believe that such a pervasive phenomenon as the anatomical distinction between females and males could have no significance in terms of human personality organization. Note that both positions rely on logic rather than empirical data to support their hypotheses. There is no other choice, for at the moment, like the existence of God, the proposition defies either proof or disproof. This issue could be discussed from several angles but it shall be addressed only in terms of the phenomenon of the lived body, the radical root of being.

Every characteristic of one's embodiment affects one's interaction with the world and its inhabitants and therefore affects one's being. Once a house was set up in such proportion as to allow adults strolling through it to view the world as small children inevitably must. It was a powerful way to illustrate the part size plays in shaping one's interaction with the environment. Size is important not only in direct terms, such as a short person having to look up to a tall person, but also indirectly in proportion to the variance one experiences in relation to one's peers. As Gulliver found in his travels, it is quite strange and upsetting to be a relative giant in a world of tiny Lilliputians. Similarly, to be missing a limb, or to be deprived of some ability to perceive things sensually, e.g. loss of hearing, or to be uncommonly beautiful or handsome, or even to have a head of flaming red hair, inevitably affects one's interaction with the environment. Thus the shape or form of one's embodiment affects his/her being.

But how and to what extent? Is there a common experience shared by all those who are tall or all who are short? Is it inevitable that all very short men have a Napoleon complex? Are all beautiful women vain about their bodies? Obviously not. Why? Because concomitant with the inevitability of the effect of embodiment is the inevitability of the modifying effect of social context and by other attributes which people possess. While Gulliver felt queer among the Lilliputians, there is no evidence to suggest that he felt different while at home. A very tall man who plays basketball for a living is possibly much more comfortable with his height than a similarly endowed man who teaches first grade. A beautiful and brilliant woman surely interacts differently with the world than a beautiful and dull woman. The characteristics of one's specific embodiment have the *potential* to affect one, but the way in which they influence one's experiences, and thus oneself, depends upon the social milieu in which one interacts. Furthermore, this process has a cumulative effect. As each experience affects personhood, one's being, one's sense of self, the embodied self is modified and thus reacts differently to a later experience than would have been the case before such modification.

If that process is extended to the anatomical sexual aspects of embodiment, then it can be concluded that being embodied male or female is a fact that has the potential to affect our beings. But this potential effect also is modified by the contexts in which people function and the other attributes which individuals possess. If one accepts this logic, then the mere fact of being female or being male is not sufficient to insure a commonality of experience among all members of the same sex, which is absent from all members of the opposite sex. Too many factors both intrinsic to the individual and specific to the environment intervene to contaminate the purity of the sex-differentiated experience.

For example, persons embodied female have the capacity to bear children. According to some scholars, this means that this capacity is fundamental to the female presentation of self in the world. Some think females inevitably will be more protective of their beings because of this potential to reproduce life and that this concern will be reflected in their bodily attitude or bearing. Such an assumption does not account for females too young to be aware of their reproductive capacities, too old to care, or too opposed to the idea to ever intend to exercise that function. Similarly, some scholars suggest that the tens of thousands of times that a male experiences the tumescence-detumescence cycle has an inevitable effect on his experience. However, no one has suggested what that effect might be. If recent research such as that engendered by Masters and Johnson is valid, then the male and female experience of sex in much the same in its effect on the individual. It appears that an attempt to locate a commonality of experience shared by all members within a sex is unlikely to be successful.

Thus logic leads to the conclusion that being embodied female or male does not neces-sitate a particular or sex-differentiated experience of the lived being. No inherent or inevitable sensations or understandings or reactions will arise because one experiences the world embodied female or male, as the case may be.

Yet, this proposition must be modified somewhat because interaction with the world is, like all interaction, twofold. To varying degrees, people modify their environment, and environments modify people. As stated earlier, one mode of viewing the body is seeing it through the eyes of others. As well as being oneself and looking at oneself, one sees self in reaction to the eyes of others. From birth onwards one is presented to the world with a sexual identification. John Money (1973), probably one of the country's leading experts on sexual identification, concluded ". . . that there is no primary genetic or other innate mechanism to preordain the masculinity or femininity of psychosexual differentiation. . . . In fact, the expected norm of reaction may be completely reversed by factors that come into play after birth" (pp. 18–19). According to Money, sexual identification becomes permanently imprinted and indelible in the first few years after birth, chiefly because of a sexual assignment made by *others* on the basis of the appearance of the external genitalia. This assignment, which is a reaction to the form of one's embodiment, then becomes a powerful influence in determining psychosocial behavior. In other words, as one thrusts self into the environment in bodily form, other people within that environment react to one's appearance in sex-differentiated ways. The extent to which this occurs has been documented profusely in numerous studies.

The cumulative effect, therefore, is that the sex of one's embodiment *does* cause a different experience of the lived being. But, because the reaction of one's environment is social, and not biological, it is less binding and less predictable. It will vary over time, cultures, particular geographical locales, or specific family or social situations. Therefore, there is no pervasive experience of being female or male, but only a statistical probability that the form of one's embodiment *may* affect one's behavior. But the ways in which one is affected are uncertain, modifiable and, most important, leave one free to transcend them.

MY BODY, MYSELF IN PHYSICAL ACTIVITY

Throughout most of recorded history, athletes and physical educators in roles such as paidotribes, teachers, trainers, coaches, have dealt with the body as an object. This has been true both with reference to their own bodies and those of others. The focus of interest and inquiry has been on questions and problems associated with physical health and training and conditioning and not on the body as a source of identity. Despite twentieth century attempts at renouncing dualism, now as earlier the basic question has been what to do *to* the body to make it stronger, more flexible, resilient, capable of generating more power, running faster, and so forth. A passage from a second century dialogue of Lucien, in which Socrates and Anacharsis supposedly are conversing, epitomizes this point:

> As to their bodies—for that is what you were especially eager to hear about—we train them as follows. When, as I said, they are no longer soft and wholly strengthless, we strip them, and think it best to begin by habituating them to the weather, making them used to the several seasons, so as not to be distressed by the heat or give in to the cold. Then we rub them with olive oil and supple them in order that they may be more elastic, for since we believe that leather, when softened by oil, is harder to break and far more durable, lifeless as it is, it would be extraordinary if we should not think that the living body would be put in better condition by the oil (Robinson, 1955, p. 69).

The willingness of professionals in an educational setting to sponsor and applaud sports in which men injure, mutilate and occasionally kill each other, is further evidence that many people believe the body to be *merely* an object, a thing among things. To be willing to harm the body of another in order to win a sporting contest—and by this is meant not only illegal acts but entering contests such as boxing and perhaps tackle football which require the player to physically attack his opponent—is only conceivable if the opponent's body is but a thing to be conquered and not a person to be encountered. In fact, techniques are devised to ensure the social separation of opponents in order to help prevent the development of feeling for the other as a person. It is easier to smash a body than a person. Furthermore, it is easier to smash one's own body, to ignore the pain and injuries, to press it beyond fatigue, to strain it to almost impossible levels of performance, if one separates oneself from one's body.

Central to the perception of body as self is the notion of oneness, the experiencing of self as a totality without reference to parts. To achieve this, one cannot be conscious of elements of acts, but rather one must have a sense almost of thoughtlessness—i.e. without contemplation—driving towards an *inner* goal. For the athlete the goal must be or become internalized or personalized, because to reach for an external goal requires thought or a certain degree of conscious direction. Roger Bannister's recollection of his experience as he neared the completion of the first four minute mile exemplifies this point. Although his terminology appears dualistic, the sense of his remarks is a remarkable portrayal of the lived body. Bannister (1966) wrote:

> I was relaxing so much that my mind seemed almost detached from my body. There was no strain. I barely noticed the half-mile . . . Three hundred yards from the finish, I had a moment of mixed joy and anguish, when my mind took over. It raced well ahead of my body and drew my body compellingly forward. I felt that the moment of a lifetime had come. There was no pain, only a great unity of movement and aim. The world seemed to stand still, or did not exist. The only reality was the next two hundred yards of track under my feet. The tape meant finality—extinction perhaps. I felt at that moment that it was my chance to do one thing supremely well. I drove on, impelled by a combination of fear and pride. The air I breathed filled me with the spirit of the track where I had run my fire race. . . . My body had long since exhausted all its energy, but it went on running just the same. . . . The arms of the world were waiting to receive me if only I reached the tape without slackening my speed. If I faltered, there would be no arms to hold me; and the world would be a cold, forbidding place because I had been so close. I leapt at the tape like a man taking his last spring to save himself from the chasm that threatens to engulf him (p. 659).

Experiencing the body as self is in some way to apprehend one's environment, to learn new things, to have a physical encounter with the world. Of course it is true that all human thoughts and acts are in some way dependent upon a sense experience. However, some acts, such as those which occur in sport and dance, elicit a more intense awareness of one's body. It is a well-accepted part of the definition of sport used by those who study it academically that the outcome must, in part, depend upon physical skill. That is, one can differentiate board games, for example, from field or court games. What this implies is that within the sport experience the awareness of the power of self as manifested through acts of physical skill is heightened. Thus his/her body is important to the athlete, not only because as the instrument or tool its ability to function is important to the outcome, but because it is the athlete's self which is on the line. If the game is lost, it is not the body which failed to perform sufficiently well, but the person who was less good than the opponent.

All too often, however, that understanding is avoided. The athlete is taught that it is a matter of endless repetitions until acts are almost reflexive (i.e. no judgement involved), of weight, how much meat there is on the hoof, how high it is piled, how many units of energy can be generated from gatorade or steak, how many units are dissipated by sex, how many hours of sleep, how many pulls on the weights, are needed to add up to a winner. These calculations are probably necessary —but when made to the exclusion of all the personal considerations, the athlete also begins to perceive himself/herself as a slab of meat. Under such conditions it is difficult to feel personal responsibility for the contest.

The appreciation of the athlete as a being who is putting his/her self on the line is limited. This is the central point made by Alan Sillitoe in his book, later a movie, called *The Loneliness of the Long-Distance Runner* The runner refused to complete and win his race, halting near the finish line, because he understood that it was his self that was being corrupted; his body was being used to achieve someone else's goal.

The experience of the body as self is crucial to the individual's self-identification. It relates to the experiencing of self as a strong, skilled person who is able to accomplish certain physical tasks with a high degree of excellence. To be able to feel good about one's physical performance is to be able to feel good about oneself—and the converse is also true.

The last point to be made concerns the female and male experience of the body in physical activity. It has been assumed by many people that there is a sex-differentiated experience of the body and therefore of physical activity. It is believed that males enjoy physical contact and that females do not, or that females experience a certain aesthetic pleasure that males do not enjoy. As stated earlier, there is really no basis for this assumption except in the enactment of the self-fulfilling prophecy. That is, women and men, boys and girls have been socialized into believing, accepting and desiring different types of experiences. Then statisticians have confirmed that

the differences exist! (Though the research on this is really too scanty and questionable to claim even a statistical relationship.) In being guided by this idea, theorists have largely ignored those who fall on the other side of the predictions. Males have been discouraged from choosing activities such as ballet and other dance forms and even sports such as badminton which do not appear to provide an overt experience of bodily aggressiveness and force. People like to see males use their bodies powerfully because it is believed that males should be powerful and aggressive. Conversely, women have been discouraged from participating in activities such as football, ice hockey, and long distance running because these sports *do* provide an overt experience of bodily aggressiveness and force and people do not believe that women should be powerful and aggressive.

Men and women live themselves in their bodies. The importance of having good bodily experiences which enhance self is equally necessary to both sexes, despite Paul Weiss' (1969) incredible assumption that women are naturally one with their bodies, while men have to learn to master theirs (p. 217). Physical activities have the potential to provide opportunities for heightened experiences of the physical self and therefore provide an important dimension of experience. Thus it is essential that all males and females be provided with equal opportunity to risk themselves by putting their bodies in some danger, to test themselves by striving for achievement, to behave aggressively, competitively, gracefully, and skillfully in all types of physical action which is available.

SUMMARY

There is an objective dimension to one's body and if one is to function efficiently one needs to understand and learn the boundaries of his/her capacities. There is a dimension of one's body which exists in terms of others' perceptions of it. And there is a subjective dimension to one's body which is synonymous with one's being-in-the-world. One's existence, one's location in the environment is corporeal, embodied. Thus, the actions of one's body are the actions of oneself.

Being embodied male or female does not necessitate a particular or sex-differentiated experience of one's lived being. But others' perceptions of one's embodiment are so pervasive that in an uncertain and modifiable way, the form of one's embodiment may in fact affect one's behavior and experience of self.

Sport experiences can elicit an intense awareness of one's body. In this context it is essential to have positive experiences of one's strength and skill and thus of oneself. This necessity extends in like manner to both sexes. Each individual can "know the burning/ Moment of the living flesh/ . . . Choose to claim/The meaning of the being whole."

BIBLIOGRAPHY

Bannister, Roger. "The Four-Minute Mile." *The Realm of Sport*. Edited by Herbert Warren Wind. New York: Simon and Schuster, 1966.

Buber, Martin. *I and Thou*. Trans. by Ronald Gregor Smith. New York: Charles Scribner's Sons, 1923.

Duhrssen, Alfred. "The Self and the Body." *Review of Metaphysics*, 10 (September, 1956), 28–34.

Gerber, Ellen W. "Can We Let the Body Burn?" *Quest*, VII (December, 1966), 57.

Keen, Sam. "We do not *have* bodies, we *are* our bodies." *Psychology Today*, 7 (September, 1973), 65–73, 98.

Kleinman, Seymour. "The Significance of Human Movement: A Phenomenological Approach." National Association for Physical Education of College Women. *Report of the Ruby Anniversary Workshop*, Interlochen, Michigan, 1964. (Reprinted in Gerber, *Sport and the Body*.)

Marcel, Gabriel. *Metaphysical Journal*. Translated by Bernard Wall. Chicago: Henry Regnery, 1952.

Money, John. "Developmental Differentiation of Femininity and Masculinity Compared." *Sexism: Scientific Debates*. Edited by Clarice Stasz Stoll. Reading, Mass.: Addison-Wesley, 1973.

Robinson, Rachel Sargent. *Sources for the History of Greek Athletics*. Ohio: By the author, 439 Ludlow Avenue, Cincinnati, Ohio, 1955.

Ruderman, Florence A. "Sex Differences: Biological, Cultural, Societal Implications." *The Other Half. Roads to Women's Equality*. Edited by Cynthia Fuchs Epstein and William J. Goode. Englewood Cliffs, N.J.: Prentice-Hall, 1971.

Sartre, Jean-Paul. *Being and Nothingness*. Trans. by Hazel E. Barnes. New York: Philosophical Library, 1956.

Schrag, Calvin O. "The Embodied Experiencer" in *Experience and Being. Prolegomena to a Future Ontology*. Evanston: Northwestern University Press, 1969.

Sillitoe, Alan. *The Loneliness of the Long-Distance Runner*. New York: Knopf, 1960.

Van Den Berg, J. H. "The Human Body and the Significance of Human Movement." *Psychoanalysis and Existential Philosophy*. Edited by Hendrik M. Ruitenbeck. New York: E. P. Dutton, 1962.

Waelhens, Alphonse de. "The Phenomenology of the Body." Trans. by Mary Ellen and N. Lawrence. *Readings in Existential Phenomenology*. Edited by Nathaniel Lawrence and Daniel O'Connor. New Jersey: Prentice-Hall, 1967. (Excerpt reprinted in Gerber, *Sport and the Body*.)

Weiss, Paul. *Sport: A Philosophic Inquiry*. Carbondale: Southern Illinois University Press, 1969.

Yeats, William Butler. *The Collected Poems*. New York: Macmillan, 1952.

Zaner, Richard M. "The Radical Reality of the Human Body." *Humanitas*, II (Spring, 1966), 73–87.

The Challenge of the Body[*]

PAUL WEISS

We men live bodily here and now. This is as true of the most ecstatic of us as it is of the most flat-footed and mundane. No matter what we contemplate or how passive we make ourselves be, we continue to function in a plurality of bodily ways. Whatever our mental state, throughout our lives our hearts beat, our blood courses through our arteries, our lungs expand and contract. Our bodies grow and decay unsupervised, and, in that sense, uncontrolled. Only a man intoxicated with a Cartesian, or similar, idea that he is to be identified with his mind will deny that he is a body too.

Some, with the brilliant Merleau-Ponty, think that man's body is unique, not to be compared with the bodies of other living beings. Most men, instead, follow Darwin and view the human body as a minor variant on the kind of body that primates have. Today a number are reviving La Mettrie's idea that the human body is only a machine. They, and sometimes some of the others, occasionally claim that a man is nothing more than a body. Since they have at least mind enough to think there is nothing more than a body, I have no mind to follow them. The body is, of course, a precondition for the exercise of some, and perhaps even all, mental functions. This fact is sufficient to make it desirable to cultivate the body, and to consider the body seriously in any attempt at understanding the nature of

man, without requiring us to suppose a man is only a body.

Everyone lives at least part of the time as a body. Occasionally our minds are idle, sometimes we sleep; we can spend much time in just eating and drinking. Though no one is merely a body, every one of us can be lost in his body for a time. Sooner or later, however, the minds in most of us awaken and we stray to the edges of reflection.

Even a dedicated sybarite has flashes of self-consciousness. Like the rest of us, he sometimes remembers and expects. He, too, looks to what lies beyond the here and now, and even beyond the whole world of bodily experience, to take account of ideals, if only to dismiss them. And sometimes, with poets and religious men, he deliberately detaches himself from his body and tries for a while to have a non-bodily career, occupied with fancies, myths, and transmundane beings.

He who gives himself to the life of the mind acknowledges as limits only what, if anything, is found to be beyond the reach of thought. But no one can totally identify himself with his mind. Bodily demands are imperious; the body's presence intrudes on consciousness. A man may escape the thrall of his body for a while, crush his desires, or focus on what is eternal, but sooner or later his body will show that it will not be gainsaid. It has needs and makes demands which must be met.

The life of thought proceeds at a different pace and pursues a different set of ends than that which concerns the life of the body. Each

[*] From *Sport: A Philosophic Inquiry* by Paul Weiss. Copyright © 1969 by Southern Illinois University Press. Reprinted by permission of Southern Illinois University Press.

exhibits in a special shape what man can possibly be and do. Neither is replaceable, though the full use of either at a given time precludes the full use of the other; a career devoted to one alone is possible to only half a man.

The body is voluminous, spread out in space. Through it we express tendencies, appetites, impulses, reactions, and responses. The mind, in contrast, is a tissue of implications, beliefs, hopes, anticipations, and doubts. It has no size, and cannot, therefore, be identified with a brain. But the two, body and mind, are not distinct substances, closed off from one another. They are linked by the emotions.

Emotions are at once bodily and mental, inchoate unifications of mind and body. A controlled expression of the emotions drains them of their confusion at the same time that it intensifies the unity which they provide for the mind and the body. That is why emotions should not be allowed to come forth unchecked and unguided. Because art and sport involve a controlled expression of emotions, making it possible for minds and bodies to be harmonized clearly and intensely, they offer excellent agencies for unifying man.

Never in full possession of their bodies, men are always more than they bodily reveal themselves to be. Their bodies can only partly reflect what they are; the fullest bodily life exhibits them as less than they can be and less than they ought to be. This remains true even when the mind is put at the service of the body. A more independent and freer exercise of the mind is desirable, for the controlled expression of the emotions is then given a greater role, thereby making possible the production of a more complete man.

These remarks summarize a vast literature, bypass discussions centuries old, and hide perhaps as much as they make evident. Our minds are mysteries. The interplay of mind with body is more a matter of supposition and speculation than of solid fact, unimpeachably evidenced. But if we stop here to make sure that all will be persuaded about that which all believe, we will lose our chosen topic. This is not the place to give full attention to the nature of the mind or the emotions, and the way they can and should relate to one another or to the body. Perhaps, though, enough has been said to make what follows not be as dogmatic as it may at first sound.

At the very beginning of life the mind's course is determined by what the body does and what it encounters. Soon the imagination, aided by language, the consciousness of error, self-awareness, and the unsatifactoriness of what is available, begins to operate. The mind then turns, sometimes hesitantly but occasionally boldly, to topics which may have little relevance to what the body then needs, to what it may encounter, or to the ends it should serve.

One cannot live a life solely of the mind for very long. Its exercise is brought suddenly to a halt when the unsupervised body becomes mired in difficulty. To restrain, redirect, and protect the body, the mind must be forced back into the service of that body. But now it need no longer wait on bodily prompting. By itself it has learned a good deal about ideals, abstract categories, and logical consequences. Some of that knowledge it can now use to point the way the body ought to go. A mathematical notion will help clarify how this is done.

Mathematicians speak of a "vector" as a quantity having a direction and magnitude. The term has been adapted by astronomers and biologists for more special uses. I follow their lead and treat the bodily relevant mind as a vector, reaching from the present toward a future prospect. Normally that mind terminates at a bodily pertinent prospect, an objective for the body to be realized in subsequent bodily action. The mind in this way provides the body with a controlling future.

Far down in the scale of living beings, bodies are comparatively simple, but they still thrust vectorally, albeit not consciously, toward the future. What they do is triggered in good part by occurrences that are relevant to their welfare. As we go up the scale the bodies become more and more complex, and some impulses arise without any bearing on external occurrences. And some of the occurrences that elicit responses may do so at the wrong time and in the wrong way, leading the individual into disaster and maybe death.

Were there any completely unsupervised, complex bodies their health would be most precarious and their life span very short. Fortunately, the higher organisms embody an intelligence, at service to their bodies. Without effort, though, none embodies as much intelligence as it can.

The human body, like all others, on one side is part of an external world. It too is to be understood in terms of what the world offers and insists upon. To be fully a master of its body, a being must make it act in consonance with what that body not only tends to, but what it should, do. This is an accomplishment possible only to men. Only they can envisage what is really good for the body to be and to produce. Only men can impose minds on bodies. Those minds have many grades and functions, running from attention to commitment. Man uses his mind to dictate what the body is to do.

Literally, "attention" means "a stretching out" (of the mind). Since this implies a consciousness, he who is attentive evidently has a vectorial, conscious mind. By directing itself at bodily relevant prospects, that mind makes certain places and objects into attended referents for that body. Desire, intention, and commitment, as we shall see, build on this base.

The athlete comes to accept his body as himself. This requires him to give up, for the time being, any attempt to allow his mind to dwell on objectives that are not germane to what his body is, what it needs, and what it can or ought to do. But that to which he consciously attends is not always that which his body is prepared to realize. It becomes a prepared body only after he has learned how to make it function in accord with what he has in mind. Normally, he does this by habituating his body to go through a series of acts which, he has learned, will eventuate in the realization of the prospect to which he attends. Training—of which therapy is a special instance—is the art of correcting a disequilibrium between mind and body either by altering the vector, or, more usually, by adjusting the way in which the body functions until the body follows the route that the vector provides.

To function properly as a body, it is necessary for the athlete to correct the vectorial thrust, or to alter the body so that it realizes the prospect at which the vector terminates. Correction of the vectorial thrust is one with a change in attitude and aim, themselves presupposing some change in what the mind does. Alteration of the body demands a change in the bodily organization and activity. Both changes are involved at the very beginning of the process of making an athlete. To ignore the need to undergo these changes is to remain with a disaccord of body and mind, of present and future. It is to allow the body to react to what occurs, or to allow the mind to follow its own bent, without regard for what the body is to do. Most of us exhibit the disaccord too frequently in the first of these ways. It is a characteristic defect of the intellectual; in his occupation with the life of thought, he leaves his body insufficiently supervised and directed.

The correction of the direction of the vectorial thrust is promoted by the awareness of the inadequacy of a project, an appreciation of other goals, and a temptation to change. Men usually make this correction after listening to authorities. Coaches, teachers, and models help them to change their course so that they have an object of attention which they will bodily realize.

. . . .

A training program's central purpose is to make men well trained. By making them go through various moves and acts many times its aim is to get their bodies to function in accord with what those bodies are expected to do. Training helps them to be their bodies, to accept their bodies as themselves. It makes those bodies habituated in the performance of moves and acts while enabling them to function harmoniously and efficiently, and thereby be in a position to realize the projects at which the vectorial minds terminate.

Some men do not train. Their bodies proceed from beginning to end, often without needing to be redirected in the course of it. Eventually, it is hoped, he who trains by mastering distinct moves will reach this state too, though it is a question whether he will then ever do more than blur the checking points that his moves provided.

. . . .

No one is completely ripened, incapable of being improved through training. Whether young or old, all must learn not to yield to the body, not to allow its reactions and responses to determine what will be done. The body is to be accepted, but only as subject to conditions which make it function in ways and to a degree that it would not were it left to itself. He who refuses to do this is self-indulgent, almost at the opposite pole from the self-disciplined and controlled athlete. Men do not play well persistently unless they are well trained.

A man who is content to be successful in the perpetual adventure of withstanding or overcoming the world he encounters is hard to distinguish from a well-functioning animal. A man should do more. He should use his mind to quicken and guide his body. He should make his body a locus of rights and duties, and a source of acts, desirable and effective. Only if he so structures and directs this body will he have a body that is used and not merely worked upon by what is external to it. Only he who expresses his emotions through such a possessed and structured body can become well-unified and not be undone by what he feels.

Most men, a good portion of the time, are in control of their bodies. What they do part of the time, without much thought or concentration, the athlete does both persistently and purposively. It is tempting, therefore, to say that for the athlete the body has an exclusive role, in contrast with the intellectual for whom it serves only as a place in which, and perhaps as an avenue through which, he expresses what he has independently discovered. But no athlete lives entirely in his body, any more than a thinker has only thoughts that are entirely unrelated to what is going on somewhere in the physical world.

Athlete and thinker differ in the attention they give to improving their bodies and their bodies' performance. The former, but not the latter, pushes himself toward the state where he so accepts his body that he cannot, without difficulty, distinguish himself from it. Mind and body are united by both. In neither case are mind and body related as are hand and glove. Their connection is more like that of fingers to one another. They presuppose a self just as the fingers presuppose a hand.

. . . .

An athlete makes use of his good condition to vitalize moves and acts under restrictive rules, both in practice sessions and in actual contests and games. He prepares himself primarily to be ready to discover in the course of a genuine struggle how good he is in comparison with others. Until he meets that test, although he is fulfilled as well-trained, he is still unfulfilled as an athlete.

The good coach makes a preparation be more than an exercise and less than a game. He understands that the body offers a challenge to one who would achieve excellence through bodily acts, and that it must be structured, habituated, and controlled by the object of a vectorial mind. This makes it possible for him to see to it that his athletes are in fine condition, and that this condition enables them to perform well. No preparation can, of course, guarantee a fine performance. The circumstances may be untoward, or the athlete may be out of sorts at the time.

The art of training and coaching is the satisfying and dissatisfying of athletes at one and the same time. It is also part of the art of making men. That art comes to completion when the athlete makes himself be not merely a fine body, but a body in rule-governed, well-controlled action. Athletics is mind displayed in a body well made, set in particular situations, involved in struggles, and performing in games.

Embodiment, Sport, and Meaning*

KLAUS V. MEIER

As even a cursory glance at the history of philosophy attests, the significant task of elucidating and resolving the problem of the interdependence of mind and body presents a plethora of intriguing and intricate difficulties. Indeed, David Hume (6:pp. 76–77) asserted that there is no "principle in all nature more mysterious than the union of soul with body, by which a supposed spiritual substance acquires such an influence over a material one that the most refined thought is able to actuate the grossest matter."

The recent literature in the philosophy of sport has addressed itself, in part, to anthropological inquiries investigating the nature and structure of man. Specifically, the question of the relationship of mind and body and its applicability to, or manifestation in, sport has been actively pursued (1; 7; 12; 17; 22:pp. 33–42; 24:pp. 37–57). Unfortunately, philosophical research efforts concerned with the problem of embodiment and sport have often produced expositions replete with imprecise statements, contestable assertions and, at times, unsupported or simply erroneous conclusions. Thus, it appears appropriate to investigate anew the basis of contemporary perceptions of the ontological structure of man and, subsequently, to clarify some of the essential components of man's engagement in sport in relation to the formulated parameters.

*This essay is a significantly revised statement and discussion of the substance of theses advanced in "Cartesian and Phenomenological Anthropology: The Radical Shift and Its Meaning for Sport," *Journal of the Philosophy of Sport*, 2 (1975), 51–73.

The systematic theory of the relationship between the human body and the human mind developed by René Descartes provided philosophy with a conception of man with which it has struggled for more than three centuries. It is, therefore, necessary to scrutinize, in a limited manner, the labours and achievements of this renowned philosopher. Following the investigation of Descartes, the phenomenological anthropology of Maurice Merleau-Ponty will be delineated, including his significant criticism of Cartesian and ensuing mechanistic anthropologies, to provide a contemporary philosophical alternative for the resolution of the mind-body problem. Finally, the significance of the radical shift in the characterization of the nature of man will be analyzed specifically in relation to man's engagement in sport. At this stage it will be necessary to criticize certain philosophy of sport expositions deemed to be inadequate in light of the analysis conducted within this study and, also, to provide an orientation perceived to be more efficacious.

I

Descartes sought to develop a foundation for science that would avoid the presuppositions and inadequacies of Scholasticism and possess the rigorous certainty of mathematics. He contended that only through an extension of mathematical procedures to the investigation of things in the natural world could clear, certain, and final knowledge be attained.

Following careful and extensive deliberations utilizing, among other procedures and techniques, the process of "radical doubt" and the doctrine of "clear and distinct ideas," Descartes concluded that man is composed of two distinct substances—body and mind (or soul, to utilize Descartes' term)—the essential attributes of which differ radically. The body is viewed as an unthinking, extended, material substance; the mind is a thinking, unextended, immaterial substance. The body is an unconscious machine, as mechanical as a watch (3:p. 116), conforming to the unwavering and rigid laws of nature; the mind (the true "essence" of man) is a conscious and free substance possessing no qualities of extension and, therefore, not susceptible to, or dominated by, the mechanical laws of nature. The two substances are thus perceived to be totally distinct and independent.

The postulation of such an extreme bifurcation of mind and body, of course, elicits immediate difficulties. Despite the apparent impossibility of any interaction between two such dissimilar, demarcated, and mutually exclusive substances, open reflection on lived human experiences indicates that perhaps the distinction is not absolute. Although occasional, specific human activities may be performed unconsciously and mechanically, through reflex action for example, selected components of conscious perception and awareness, such as sensations of pain and sound, appetites of hunger and thirst, and the elicitation of emotions and passions, challenge significantly the dualistic structure through the implication of an intimate union between mind and body. Numerous other occasions attesting to, at least, a "quasi-substantial" union of the mind and body may be readily forwarded. In some sense, for example, it is surely legitimate to assert that the mind possesses the ability to suppress or re-direct sensual appetites. Also, particular mental states such as excitement or elation appear to manifest noticeable changes in the cardio-respiratory system and in the degree of intensity of the performance of physical activities.

Descartes, of course, was cognizant of experiences of the aforementioned nature; in the "Sixth Meditation" he claimed that they were the result of "certain confused modes of thought which are produced by the union and apparent intermingling of mind and body" (3:p. 192). To explain consciously directed or volitional action, Descartes acknowledged further that the body deviates from its mechanical procedures of performance at "the direction of the will," which in turn depends on the mind (3:p. 195). Such occurrences can only be intelligibly comprehended through the

acknowledgment of some form of structural intercourse or unity of composition.

The admission that the mind consciously influences the motions of the body, and conversely is affected by its physiological states or activities, clearly demonstrates the basic difficulty of Cartesian dualism: namely, how can an extended, material substance be influenced by a spiritual substance that has no extension and, therefore, no spatial location for interaction? In other words, how can radically distinct substances form a substantial union?

In an attempt to respond to this difficulty, Descartes stated that the mind is indeed connected to the body, however, the nature of this interaction is, at the very least, obfuscated. Attuned to the necessity for the explication of mind-body interaction and fully aware of the constraints of his ontological edifice, Descartes couched his response in such nonspecific and imprecise terms as "occasion" or "spontaneous occurrence." Nonetheless, despite the utilization of, at times, deft linguistic manipulations, the essential difficulty remained unshaken.

Descartes attempted to solve the problem by asserting that the interaction of the mind and body is limited to one central location. Although the soul radiates throughout and "is in each member of the body," it exercises its functions most particularly in one specific part —the pineal gland, the apparent convergent or terminal of all nerve systems, situated in the midst of the brain (3:pp. 293, 345). Through its diverse manipulations in the pineal gland, the soul was postulated to regulate and thrust forth "animal spirits," (subtle and exquisitely refined parts of the blood, flowing to and from the brain through the arteries and nerves almost like "air or wind"), to direct the movements of the body's limbs (3:p. 333).

The choice of the pineal gland as the locus of the elusive connection and incarnation of the substantial union of body and mind, wherein the mind can exercise control of the body's movements and conversely be affected by the "animal spirits" agitated by physiological change, was certainly ingenuous, if not accurate. However, it was also "regarded as signally unfortunate" (5:p. 144) even in Descartes' own day. The reason for this reaction, of course, was that the introduction of "animal spirits," even of a highly rarified and special nature, was simply a matter of procrastination. The frustrating question of how there can be interaction between a substance that is purely spiritual and a substance that is purely material remained to be answered. The pineal gland, rather than providing a solution, appears to be simply an attempt at a "metaphysical tour de force."

Nonetheless, the influence of Descartes' philosophy was enormous. Enamoured by the thrust, mode, and content of Descartes' writings on the nature of man, a significant number of his contemporaries and followers forwarded many concepts and theories based largely on his work. The ideal of a purely mechanistic doctrine of physiology, with its view of the 'body-machine' working under the strict dictates of mechanical laws, was accorded considerable support in the European scientific community and has guided scientists since the seventeenth century.

The influence of mechanistic physiology on the contemporary understanding of man in sport is vast and will be discussed shortly; however, it is first necessary to delineate briefly a substantively different conception of the nature of man.

II

The problem of relating mind and body in the manner attempted by Descartes may be artificially created. It is extremely difficult, if not logically precluded, to meaningfully synthesize two elements or substances which are asserted to be of such radically diverse, distinct, and discontinuous natures into one functioning, complex entity. However, the attempt itself to promulgate a conception of man rent thusly asunder may be the source of fundamental error. If the postulated bifurcation is perceived to be the major dilemma, the problem may be approached in an entirely different manner. Rather than forwarding and championing an inherent dualistic conception, a monistic approach which accounts for both consciousness and embodiment may be noticeably more productive.

Maurice Merleau-Ponty (13; 14; 15; 16) dedicated his abbreviated philosophic career, to a considerable extent, to resolving the Cartesian problem of how man can experience himself as incarnate through a rigorous and adroit phenomenological analysis of man's 'being-in-the-world' and the nature of his corporeality.

Existential phenomenology in general, and the works of Merleau-Ponty specifically, are based on the tenet that "the most decisive trait of human consciousness, coloring all its manifestations, is that it is an *embodied* consciousness" (11:p. 10). Existence furnishes the point of departure. Man's contingencies, his finiteness, and his 'being-in-the-world' as a

subject are, thus, perceived as the starting points. Consequently, the Cartesian categories are opposed as presupposing too little and offering misdirection.

Man is viewed as an incarnate subject, a unity not union of physical, biological, and psychological events all participating in dialectical relationships. The motions and activities of the 'lived-body' are not distinct from consciousness; rather, consciousness is deeply embodied in them. Merleau-Ponty perceived man as a 'body-subject' or incarnate consciousness—a being in the world concerned with his unfolding in the world. The existence of a disembodied, separate, or distinct mind is emphatically denied. For him, body and mind are simply limiting notions of the 'body-subject' which is a single entity or reality neither simply mental nor merely corporeal, but both, simultaneously.

Any delineation depicting man as being solely an intellectual interiority (the mind), or the simple seat of sensations (the extended body), or even a union of these types of being is rejected. Phenomenologists repeatedly assert that the human body is not a mere thing or object subject to the inclinations of the mind, rather, it is a subject in itself, deriving its subjectivity from itself. "To say that the soul acts on the body is wrongly to suppose a univocal notion of the body and to add to it a second force which accounts for the rational significance of certain conducts" (13:p. 202).

Similarly to Gabriel Marcel, Merleau-Ponty raised significant questions concerning the appropriateness of such statements as "I have a body" or "I use my body." He emphasized the peculiarity and inappropriateness of conceiving of one's body as an object or implement. "The body is more than a commodious instrument that I could do without: my body is myself, the man who I am" (20:p. 49). The manner in which man lives his body from the inside presents a sharply different perception than the objective body which is externally observed through the delimited scope of the anatomical and physiological sciences. The 'lived-body' is not an object which man possesses, rather it *is* man and man *is* his body. Man's mode of insertion into the world is the body; it is his foundation in existence. It is "the constantly moving and constantly irrevocable manner in which I insert myself in reality" (23:p. 164). Therefore, it may be seen that "being a body" is a radically different characterization than "having a body" or "using a body."

However, there is a specific sense in which

man does indeed "use" his body as an instrument, but certainly not in the same sense as he uses, for example, a hammer or a chair (26:p. 81). Since consciousness and the body may be described as inexorably inseparable— that is, consciousness is primordially embodied in the world—the body is man's means of perception of, and action upon, objects and the world. The body is not simply another object in the world, rather it is "an anchorage in the world"; it is man's mode of communication and interaction with it.

Thus, the rigid Cartesian structure of the mind-subject as a totally distinct and superior substance somehow controlling the inferior body-object is perceived to be erroneous and replaced by a structure deemed more appropriate.

It must be noted at this point that the investigation of an incarnate consciousness, projecting itself in the world and fully immersed in its perceptions and experiences, necessarily elicits ambiguity. No longer can the account of man and reality be delineated with total lucidity.

> I have no means of knowing the human body other than that of living it, which means taking up on my own account the drama which is being played out in it, and losing myself in it. I am my body, at least wholly to the extent that I possess experience, and yet at the same time my body is as it were a "natural" subject, a provisional sketch of my total being. Thus experience of one's own body runs counter to the reflective procedure which detaches subject and object from each other, and which gives us only the thought about the body, or the body as an idea, and not the experience of the body or the body in reality. (14:pp.198–99)

Ambiguity, rather than lucidity, is an integral component of the manifestation and essence of human existence. The numerous, diverse perceptions and meanings of embodiment; the lived experience of "the chiaroscuro of the body" (10:p. 46); and the open dialogue with the sensible world—are precisely the occurrences which must be investigated and not rejected because they violate arbitrary Cartesian doctrines of "clear and distinct" ideas. Human existence, due to the distinct nature of incarnate consciousness, is obfuscated and, therefore, ambiguity arising in its investigation is simply an indication that the analysis has not departed from reality or succumbed to artificial distortion or inappropriate reduction.

An analysis of man's incarnation reveals that man is an opaque and partially concealed 'body-subject' without clear and precise points of demarcation for the various aspects of his being; he is a unity of physical, biological, and psychological relationships necessarily interrelated and only meaningfully investigated when analyzed as a whole.

Man's 'being-in-the-world' is given a viewpoint only through his body. The body is "the seat or rather the very actuality of the phenomenon of expression" (14:p. 235); it is the locus of a dialectical relationship with the world and the fabric into which all objects are woven; and, finally, it is the center of openness, intentionality, and meaning-producing acts.

> The body is our general medium for having a world. Sometimes it is restricted to the actions necessary for the conservation of life, and accordingly it posits around us a biological world; at other times, elaborating upon these primary actions and moving from their literal to a figurative meaning, it manifests through them a core of new significance: this is true of motor habits such as dancing and sport. Sometimes, finally, the meaning aimed at cannot be achieved by the body's natural means; it must then build itself an instrument, and it projects thereby around itself a cultural world (14:p. 146).

Through his corporeality man is provided with a foundation in, and is open to, the world. Meaning arises, is created, and is constituted by the interaction of the 'body-subject' and the world through the body's power of expression. Man, dwelling in a world of fluctuating perspectives, possesses the possibility of unfolding diverse projects of personal import —in the laugh of a child, a gesture of a hand, the work of an artist, or the movement of an athlete, meaning is manifested.

Thus, in summary, the phenomenological analysis of man depicts him in a radically different manner than the inadequate and deceptive Cartesian dualistic structure which "portrays man as ontologically schizophrenic" (4:p. 156). Rather than stripping him of his existential character and delineating him as composed of two diverse and discrete substances, man is characterized as embodied consciousness—the distinction between the subjective and objective poles is blurred in the experience of the lived, meaning-bestowing body. Man is acknowledged as an open and engaged being dwelling in the world, capable of developing personal meaning in the process of actively manifesting himself.

III

It would appear to be most logical to assume that, of the multitudinous realms of human enterprise, the particular areas of the philosophy of sport and theories of physical education would be the most enlightened in regard to the nature of man's corporeality and, therefore, predisposed to advocate and actively support an image of man consummate with the phenomenological analysis of the 'lived-body.'

However, such an assumption would be most imprudent. The philosophy of sport is replete, both in theory and practice, with implicit and explicit restatements and affirmations of Cartesian dualism, despite occasional assertions to the contrary. The flight to the respectability and acceptability of the natural scientific framework and the appropriation of stimulus-response and behaviouristic schema are much in evidence, with the ensuing result that man's incarnate being is more often objectified and reduced, than expressed or celebrated.

Paul Weiss (24), for example, in one of the first two philosophical treatises to investigate sport in considerable detail, stated that the fundamental task facing the athlete is that of eliminating the dissonance and disequilibrium between mind and body by struggling toward unification and harmony. According to Weiss (24:pp. 221, 218, 41), although he "starts with a separated mind and body," "the athlete becomes one with his body through practice," and "comes to accept the body as himself."

A very brief delineation of Weiss' conception of man will clarify the preceding statements and those which follow. In a manner similar to Descartes, Weiss divided man into two diverse substances—an extended, "voluminous" body characterized by "tendencies, appetites, impulses, reactions, and responses" and an unextended, immaterial mind, "a tissue of implications, beliefs, hopes, anticipations, and doubts." He asserted further that the two substances are linked by the emotions which are at once "bodily and mental, inchoate unifications of mind and body" (24:p. 38).

Much akin to Descartes' supposition of the pineal gland as the locus of the interaction between mind and body, recourse to the emotions (the nature of which remains largely unspecified), elicits and amplifies, rather than diminishes difficulties. Weiss stated further that the emotions require control, and to supply this regulating force he professed the existence of a "self" (24:p. 54). Unfortunately,

he declined the opportunity to elaborate and clarify the intriguing distinctions and relationships among mind, body, emotions and self. The inevitable result is a rather bewildering and confusing portrait of man in general and the athlete in particular.

Of specific interest to the present discussion is Weiss' extensive and active support of a hierarchical, dualistic conception of man. He strongly and repeatedly emphasized the power of mind over body throughout his analysis of the athlete and his body. Weiss (24:pp. 41, 46) declared that an athlete, on his journey toward the attainment of excellence in sport, engages in a rigorous training program designed "to correct" or "to alter the body" by means of "adjusting the way in which the body functions," until it proceeds in accord with the mind's expectations; "man uses his mind to dictate what the body is to do."

> Whether young or old, all must learn not to yield to the body, not to allow its reactions and responses to determine what will be done. The body is to be accepted, but only as subject to conditions which make it function in ways and to a degree that it would not were it left to itself (24:pp. 53–54).

The dualistic structure immediately evident in the preceding statements is reinforced continuously in Weiss' analysis: the mind uses, alters, directs, controls, restrains, restructures, disciplines and conquers the body (24:pp. 40, 217). The precise and pointed terminology clearly demonstrates that, for Weiss, the athlete utilizes the body as an object; he must subdue and control his corporeal aspects. This orientation obviously depicts the athlete as "possessing" a body rather than fully "being" a body.

In much of modern sport theory and practice, the human body is compeltely reified and reduced to the status of an object to be altered and manipulated or an obstacle to be surmounted. To utilize Sarano's (20:p. 63) suggestive metaphor, the body is often perceived as an entity which "must be bridled as a restive mount." Thus, in preparation for athletic endeavours the body is drilled, trimmed, strengthened, quickened and otherwise trained to improve its fitness and functioning and often handled as an instrument or utensil to be appropriately directed and mastered.

In accord with such an orientation, the anatomical, kinesiological, bio-mechanical, and physiological sciences are intensely and tenaciously pursued and granted almost exclusive sanction to scrutinize, analyze, and manipulate man's corporeal nature and his participation in sport. As a result, the athlete is often regarded as "capable of being completely understood by means of stimulus-response conditioning, laws of learning, transfer of training, and neurological brain wave analysis" (9:p. 176).

However, as the phenomenology of the body demonstrated, objective approaches are inadequate and inappropriate to fully comprehend the nature of man's embodied being. The 'body-subject' not only is sensed, but also does the sensing. The body perceived totally as an object is, in a legitimate sense, drained of its humanity; it is a dead body devoid of its vivifying, expressive and intentional abilities and qualities.

The rejection of Cartesian concepts and dichotomies permits man to rescue the objectified, maligned, and mistreated body to attain an increasing awareness of the depth and richness of his 'lived-body' and to approach it as a diverse and dynamic reality. Rather than continued repetition and support of discrete, hierarchical notions of mind-body interaction, it appears to be substantially more fruitful to transcend such limiting orientations. If reductive approaches are altered and mental-physical polarities are eliminated, it is possible to accord the physical attributes of man due respect as integral facets of his nature and, subsequently, to rejoice in the total aspects of the conscious body. Consequently, instead of perceiving human action as depersonalized movement largely, if not totally, comprehensible through external quantification, the unfortunate manner in which much of sport is currently viewed, such activities may be openly apprehended as configurations inscribed with shapes and qualities expressive of the texture of the being of the participant.

Man is anchored and centered in the world through his body which provides him with an oriented focus for action and projection. "Nothing is more expressive than the human body, our hands and fingers, our dancing feet, our eyes, our voice in joy and sorrow" (17:p. 114). It is through the power and gestures of the 'lived-body,' fully and openly engaged in dialogue with the world, that man discloses, establishes, and broadens the personal meanings of his existence. Moments of "intense realness" available in sport provide opportunities for the unfolding of new insights and the restructuring of previous perceptions. During instances of total immersion and dynamic individuation man unfolds his powers, becomes

aware of his capabilities and his limitations, develops forms of self-expression, and affirms himself.

In addition, it should also be noted that "the body is the vehicle of an indefinite number of symbolic systems" (16:p. 9). Consequently, sport, as a vibrant form of human endeavor capable of manifesting and transmitting affective states and meanings, may be viewed both as a symbolic medium and as a potentially artistic enterprise capable of releasing and celebrating the creative subjectivity of the participant.

Thus, it may be seen that the open and aware athlete apprehends and experiences his body neither solely as an object or an instrument to be manipulated nor externally as others view him, but rather, as a multi-faceted being totally, uniquely, and indelibly an embodied consciousness. The comportment of the body is the manner in which man exists for himself and sport permits him to attain acute insight into the depth and mettle of his existence. Further, sport affords the athlete the opportunity not only to become aware of his incarnation, but it also "multiplies, extends, consolidates, and confirms this insertion" (20:p. 154), through engagement in the world in the form of projects which express his individual being.

In conclusion, it may be asserted that if the radical philosophical shift from Cartesian to phenomenological conceptions of the nature of man is acknowledged and accepted, the distinctive potentialities of man's participation in sport may be vigorously and profitably explored. Rather than concentrating solely on the objectified, treadmill image of sport, predominantly centered upon the development and attainment of physical strength, motor skills, and technical efficiency, it appears to be legitimate, fruitful, and imperative to focus upon the full range of dynamic, lived experiences available therein.

Through free, creative, and meaning-bestowing movement experiences, man becomes cognizant of the limits and potentials of his existence. His actions in sport represent, express, and affirm his capabilities, intentionality and mode of being. In short, sport may be characterized and extolled as the celebration of man as an open and expressive embodied being.

BIBLIOGRAPHY

1. Abe, Shinobu. "Interdependence of Body and Mind as Related to Sport and Physical Education." Essay presented at the Annual

Meeting of the Philosophic Society for the Study of Sport at the University of Western Ontario, London, Canada, November 16, 1974.

2. Barral, Mary Rose. *Merleau-Ponty: The Role of the Body Subject in Interpersonal Relations*. Pittsburgh: Duquesne University Press, 1965.

3. Descartes, René. *The Philosophical Works of Descartes*. Vol. One. Translated and edited by E. S. Haldane and G. R. T. Ross. Cambridge, England: Cambridge University Press, 1967.

4. Dillon, M. C. "Sartre on the Phenomenal Body and Merleau-Ponty's Critique." *Journal of the British Society for Phenomenology*, 5 (1974), 144–158.

5. Hocking, William Earnest. *Types of Philosophy*. Third Edition. New York: Charles Scribner's Sons, 1959.

6. Hume, David. *An Inquiry Concerning Human Understanding*. Edited by Charles W. Hendel. New York: The Liberal Arts Press, 1955.

7. Kaelin, Eugene F. "Being in the Body." *Sport and the Body: A Philosophical Symposium*. Edited by Ellen Gerber. Philadelphia: Lea and Febiger, 1972.

8. Kapp, R. O. "Living and Lifeless Machines." *British Journal of the Philosophy of Science*, 5 (1954), 91–103.

9. Kleinman, Seymour. "The Significance of Human Movement: A Phenomenological Approach." *Sport and the Body: A Philosophical Symposium*. Edited by Ellen Gerber. Philadelphia: Lea and Febiger, 1972.

10. Kwant, Remy. *The Phenomenological Philosophy of Merleau-Ponty*. Pittsburgh: Duquesne University Press, 1963.

11. Lawrence, N. and O'Connor, D. (Eds.). *Readings in Existential Phenomenology*. Englewood Cliffs, New Jersey: Prentice-Hall, 1967.

12. Meier, Klaus V. "The Pineal Gland, 'Mu,' and the 'Body-Subject': Critical Reflections on the Interdependence of Mind and Body." Essay presented at the Annual Meeting of the Philosophic Society for the Study of Sport at the University of Western Ontario, London, Canada, November 16, 1974.

13. Merleau-Ponty, Maurice. *The Structure of Behaviour*. Translated by A. L. Fisher. Boston: Beacon Press, 1963.

14. ———. *The Phenomenology of Perception*. Translated by Colin Smith. London: Routledge and Kegan Paul, 1962.

15. ———. *The Primacy of Perception and Other Essays*. Edited by James M. Edie. Northwestern University Press, 1969.

16. ———. *Themes from the Lectures at the College de France 1952–1960*. Translated by John O'Neill. Evanston, Illinois: Northwestern University Press, 1970.

17. O'Neill, John. "The Spectacle of the Body." *Journal of the Philosophy of Sport*, 1 (1974), 110–122.

18. Pirenne, M. H. "Descartes and the Body-Mind Problem in Physiology." *British Journal of the Philosophy of Science*, 1 (1950), 43–59.

19. Ryle, Gilbert. *The Concept of Mind*. Harmondsworth, England: Penguin Books Ltd., 1966.

20. Sarano, Jacques. *The Meaning of the Body*. Translated by James H. Farley. Philadelphia: The Westminster Press, 1966.

21. Schrag, Cavlin O. "The Lived Body as a Phenomenological Datum." *Sport and the Body: A Philosophical Symposium*. Edited by Ellen Gerber. Philadelphia: Lea and Febiger, 1972.

22. Slusher, Howard S. *Man, Sport and Existence*. Philadelphia: Lea and Febiger, 1967.

23. de Waelhens, Alphonse. "The Phenomenology of the Body." *Readings in Existential Phenomenology*. Edited by N. Lawrence and D. O'Conner. Englewood Cliffs, New Jersey: Prentice-Hall, 1967.

24. Weiss, Paul. *Sport: A Philosophic Inquiry*. Carbondale, Illinois: Southern Illinois University Press, 1969.

25. Zaner, Richard M. *The Problem of Embodiment: Some Contributions to a Phenomenology of the Body*. The Hague: Martinus Nijhoff, 1964.

26. ———. "The Radical Reality of the Human Body." *Humanitas*, 2 (1966), 73–87.

BIBLIOGRAPHY ON THE BODY AND BEING

Aristotle. "De Anima." Translated by J. A. Smith. *Introduction to Aristotle*. Edited by Richard McKeon. The Modern Library. New York: Random House, 1947.

Barral, Mary Rose. "Merleau-Ponty: The Role of the Body in Interpersonal Relations." Unpublished Ph.D. dissertation, Fordham University, 1963.

Beets, N[icholas]. "The Experience of the Body in Sport." *International Research in Sport and Physical Education*. Edited by E. Jokl and E. Simon. Illinois: Charles C Thomas, 1964.

——. "Historical Actuality and Bodily Experience." *Humanitas*, II (Spring, 1966), 15–28.

Belaief, Lynn. "Meanings of the Body." *The Journal of the Philosophy of Sport*, IV (Fall, 1977), 50–68.

Broekhoff, Jan. "Physical Education and the Reification of the Human Body." Gymnasion, IX (Summer, 1972), 4–11. Also published in *Proceedings of the Second Canadian Symposium on the History of Sport and Physical Education*, University of Windsor, Windsor, Ontario, Canada, May 1–3, 1972.

Chryssafis, Jean E. "Aristotle on Physical Education." *Journal of Health and Physical Education*, 1 (January; February; September, 1930), 3–8, 50; 14–17, 46–47; 14–17, 54–53.

Cornman, James W. "The Identity of Mind and Body." *Journal of Philosophy*, LIX (August, 1962), 486–492.

Descartes, René. "Of the Existence of Corporeal Things and of the Real Distinction Between the Mind and Body of Man" in *Meditations on First Philosophy*. Translated by Laurence J. Lafler. The Library of Liberal Arts. New York: Bobbs-Merrill, 1960.

Doherty, J. Kenneth. "Holism in Training for Sports." *Anthology of Contemporary Readings*. Edited by Howard S. Slusher and Aileene S. Lockhart. Iowa: Wm. C. Brown, 1966.

Duhrssen, Alfred. "The Self and The Body." *Review of Metaphysics*, 10 (September, 1956), 28–34.

Fairs, John R. "The Influence of Plato and Platonism on the Development of Physical Education in Western Culture." *Quest*, IX (December, 1968), 14–23.

Feigl, H., Maxwell, G. and Scriven, M., Eds. *Concepts, Theories, and the Mind-Body Problem*. Minnesota Studies in the Philosophy of Science, Vol. II. Minneapolis: University of Minnesota Press, 1958.

Fraleigh, Warren P. "A Christian Concept of the Body-Soul Relation and the Structure of Human Movement Experiences." Unpublished paper, 1968.

Gerger, Rudolph J., S. J. "Marcel's Phenomenology of the Human Body." *International Philosophical Quarterly*, IV (September, 1964), 443–463.

Hammer, J. "Bodily Experience of the Ego in Sports." *Sport in the Modern World—Chances and Problems*. Edited by Ommo Grupe, Dietrich Kurz and Johannes Teipel. New York: Springer-Verlag, 1973.

Hengstenberg, Hans-Eduard. "Phenomenology and Metaphysics of the Human Body." *International Philosophical Quarterly*, 3 (May, 1963), 165–200.

Holbrook, Lenoa. "A Teleological Concept of the Physical Qualities of Man." *Quest*, I (December, 1963), 13–17.

Hook, Sidney, Ed. *Dimensions of Mind*. New York: Collier Books, 1961.

Horne, Herman H. "The Principle Underlying Modern Physical Education [body-mind unity]." American Physical Education Review, XV (June, 1910), 433–439.

Jonas, Hans. "Life, Death, and the Body in the Theory of Being." *Review of Metaphysics*, 19 (September, 1965), 3–23.

Kaelin, Eugene F. "Being in the Body." National Association for Physical Education of College Women. *Report of the Ruby Anniversary Workshop*. Interlochen, Michigan, 1964.

Keen, Sam. "Sing the Body Electric." *Psychology Today*, 4 (October, 1970), 56–58, 88.

——. "We do not have bodies, we are our bodies." *Psychology Today*, 7 (September, 1973), 65–73, 98.

Kelly, Darlene Alice. "Phenomena of the Self-Experienced Body." Unpublished Ph.D. dissertation, University of Southern California, 1970.

Kennedy, John F. "The Soft American" in *Background Readings for Physical Education*. Edited by Ann Paterson and Edmund C. Hallberg. New York: Holt, Rinehart and Winston, 1965.

Kleinman, Seymour. "The Significance of Human Movement: A Phenomenological Approach." National Association for Physical Education of College Women. *Report of the Ruby Anniversary Workshop*. Interlochen, Michigan, 1964.

——. "Will the Real Plato Stand Up?" *Quest*, XIV (June, 1970), 73–75.

Kohler, Wolfgang. "The Mind-Body Problem." *Dimensions of Mind*. Edited by Sidney Hook. New York: Collier Books, 1961.

Kwant, Remy. "The Human Body as the Self-Awareness of Being." *Humanitas*, II (Spring, 1966), 43–62.

Long, Douglas C. "The Philosophical Concept of a Human Body." *Philosophical Review*, 73 (July, 1964), 321–337.

Luijpen, William A. "The Body as Intermediary" in *Existential Phenomenology*. Pittsburgh: Duquesne University Press, 1960.

McDougall, William. *Body and Mind*. Boston: Beacon Press, 1961. (First published London: Methuen, 1911).

Marcel, Gabriel. *Metaphysical Journal*. Translated by Bernard Wall. Chicago: Henry Regnery, 1952.

Meier, Klaus V. "Cartesian and Phenomenological Anthropology: The Radical Shift and Its Meaning for Sport." *Journal of the Philosophy of Sport,* II (September, 1975), 51–73.

Nietzsche, Friedrich. "The Despisers of the Body" in *Thus Spake Zarathustra.* Translated by Thomas Common. The Modern Library. New York: Random House, n.d.

O'Neil, John. "The Spectacle of the Body." *Journal of the Philosophy of Sport,* 1 (September, 1974), 110–122.

Peursen, C. A. Van. *Body, Soul, Spirit: A Survey of the Body-Mind Problem.* Translated by Hubert H. Hoskins. London: Oxford University Press, 1966.

Plato, *Phaedo.* Translated by F. J. Church. New York: The Liberal Arts Press, 1951.

Sarano, Jacques. *The Meaning of the Body.* Translated by James H. Farley. Philadelphia: Westminster Press, 1966.

Sartre, Jean-Paul. "The Body" in *Being and Nothingness.* Translated by Hazel E. Barnes. New York: Philosophical Library, 1956.

Schrag, Calvin O. "The Lived Body as a Phenomenological Datum." *Modern Schoolman,* XXXIX (March, 1962), 203–218.

———. "The Embodied Experiencer" in *Experience and Being. Prolegomena to a Future Ontology.* Evanston: Northwestern University Press, 1969.

Shaffer, Jerome A. "Recent Work on the Mind-Body Problem." *American Philosophical Quarterly,* 2 (April, 1965), 81–104.

———. "Persons and Their Bodies." *Philosophical Review,* XXV (January, 1966), 59–77.

Shvartz, Esar. "Nietzsche: A Philosopher of Fitness." *Quest,* VIII (May, 1967), 83–89.

Spicker, Stuart F., Ed. *The Philosophy of the Body.* Chicago: Quadrangle Books, 1970.

Staley, Steward C. "The Body-Soul Concept" in *The Curriculum in Sports (Physical Education).* Illinois: Stripes Publishing Company. 1940.

Van Den Berg, J. H. "The Human Body and the Significance of Human Movement." *Psychoanalysis and Existential Philosophy.* Edited by Hendrik M. Ruitenbeck. New York: E. P. Dutton, 1962.

Waelhens, Alphonse de. "The Phenomenology of the Body." Translated by Mary Ellen and N. Lawrence. Readings in *Existential Phenomenology.* Edited by Nathaniel Lawrence and Daniel O'Connor. New Jersey: Prentice-Hall, 1967.

Weiss, Paul. *Nature and Man.* New York: Henry Holt, 1947.

———. *Sport: A Philosophic Inquiry.* Carbondale: Southern Illinois University Press. 1969.

Wenkart, Simon. "The Meaning of Sports for Contemporary Man." *Journal of Existential Psychiatry,* 3 (Spring, 1963), 397–404.

———. "Sports and Contemporary Man." *Motivations in Play, Games and Sports.* Edited by Ralph Slovenko and James A. Knight. Illinois: Charles C Thomas, 1967.

Zaner, Richard M. *The Problem of Embodiment. Some Contributions to a Phenomenology of the Body.* The Hague: Martinus Nijhoff, 1964.

———. "The Radical Reality of the Human Body." *Humanitas,* II (Spring, 1966), 73–87.

SECTION IV

Sport as a Meaningful Experience

An examination of the sport experience depends, first of all, upon an understanding of the term "experience." Experience as a subject lies in the philosophical realm of epistemology because ultimately all questions of truth or confirmation of knowledge relate to experience. It is one of the more complicated philosophical problems because it deals with the mysterious relationship between subject and object. In what manner does the experiencer experience the experienced? What is the nature of that experience? It is generally assumed by contemporary philosophers that "Experience is not restricted to so-called sense experience. There is . . . experience of relations, meanings, values, other minds, social and cultural phenomena. Any kind of cognitive contact with particular data is an occasion for genuine experience."[1] In the articles which follow, the authors have explored many of these different kinds of experiences. However, they could not (as philosophers cannot) really define satisfactorily the way in which this happens—the connections between the external object of experience and the subjective knowing.

There are generally accepted universal characteristics of experience, which are, as summarized by Farber:[2] (1) experience is temporal in character, (2) has elements of organic, physical and cultural relatedness, (3) involves the past, present and future, (4) has a space-

time locus, (5) is always experience of some object or phenomenon, and (6) is of various types, such as perceptual, imaginative and conceptual.

Acceptance of the universality of the characteristics of experience, does not imply acceptance of the universality of each experience. In fact, it should be understood that each experience is peculiar to the experiencer. Individuals do not have identical perceptions, nor do they process their perceptions to the same conclusions. In other words, there is no such thing as a universal experience and, hence, no possibility of saying that the meanings inherent in an experience are universal. It can only be said that there are similar meanings experienced by different people. Theoretically, data could be gathered to support hypotheses relating to the high incidence of similarity of certain meanings occurring in the sport experience.

It is a general characteristic of the articles which attempt to describe the meaning of the sport experience, that they assume a certain universality of meaning. Although this, in some way, oversteps the bounds of philosophical precept, there is nevertheless some justification for believing in the similarity of meaning derived by many sport participants. Large numbers of books and articles written by sports participants, descriptive of their experiences, give evidence of similarity. However, there is also a certain homogeneity of condition among these writers who recount their own sport experiences, despite their diversified sport activities. Most are people who have great involvement in their sport, have invested much of

[1] Herbert Spiegelberg, "Toward a Phenomenology of Experience," *American Philosophical Quarterly*, I (October, 1964), 327.

[2] Marvin Farber, *Basic Issues of Philosophy* (New York: Harper & Row, 1968), pp. 121-122.

themselves in terms of time and effort, have attained a high level of skill, and have both the ability and desire to verbalize their experiences. Researchers who have attempted to generalize about the sport experience seem to have written primarily about people who fit the above description.

It is only recently that philosophers of sport have turned their attention to the question: Why do people play? In their article, R. Scott Kretchmar and William A. Harper set the question in historical context by showing that research relating to humans and play essentially ignores this question. Furthermore, there has been an assumption that the action of playing has been rationally motivated and that this conscious motivation is somehow inherent in the activity. Although they do not attempt really to explore answers to their question, the authors' perspective sets the stage for the articles which follow.

In " 'Great Moments in Sport:' The One and the Many," White undertakes an examination of the constitutive features of the so-termed 'great moments' in sport. In his analysis, he identifies two conditions or elements that must be present in order to predicate the adjective "great" of the various moments of sporting performance: (1) a superior athletic performance, and (2) the presence of a special bond between the athlete and the audience whereby both communally share in the excellence engendered by superlative athletic performances. Kurt Riezler's article deals with one of the factors affecting the meaning of the sport experience: the player's attitude. The extensiveness of the experience is directly related to whether a person "merely plays" or plays in such a manner that the "merely" is negated and an "ultimate horizon" of human life and the world is affirmed. The articles by George Santayana, J. Kenneth Doherty, and Eleanor Metheny, each using somewhat different emphases, examine the subjective meanings potentially derived from the sport experience. Each seems to assume that because sport demands a certain fullness of commitment and extended effort from its participants, it, in turn, extends to them a meaningful experience. Jan Progen offers a unique analysis of the sport experience as it occurs in a natural, non-competitive setting. Contrary to the point of view expressed by the above essays, Pieper argues that play is at bottom a meaningless act. The final selection from J. B. Priestley, gives a flash of insight into the meaning of the spectator's sport experience.

Asking "Why do I play?" leads to questions about the potential similarity of meanings for any given particular sport population. For instance, are the meanings to be found in competitive sport different from those associated with non-competitive sport? Does the natural sport experience differ in meaning from the game-type experience? What external conditions affect the meaning of the sport experience? Can one have a meaningful sport experience in a physical education class? Does the teacher or coach have any role to play in enhancing or inhibiting the meaningfulness of the sport experience? What personal variables affect the experience? In what sense does the spectator add to or detract from the meaning of sport?

Attempts to analyze the meaningfulness of the sport experience have not been numerous. McMurty (1977) advances the causal thesis that sport not only reflects the extant meanings of the general social order but sustains and reinforces such meanings. Sadler (1977) speculates about the possibility of using sport, practiced in a playful and creative way, as a mechanism to overcome the alienation of young people in the modern era. Hoffman (1976) explores the theological meanings the modern day christian athlete finds in sport and, in turn, shows up some of the shortcomings of the attempt to integrate christian theology within the context of sport. Bouet (1973) analyzes the meaning of high performance sport and develops its implications for mass sport. Franke (1973) critically examines the wide array of social meanings commonly attributed to sport and concludes that such attempts are doomed to failure because sport has its own peculiar system of signs, as specified by the rules, which cannot be properly understood by sign systems derived from non-sporting contexts. Weiss (1969) offers some original ideas concerning the human significance of sport in a chapter titled, "The Attraction of Athletics." Bouet (1968) locates the meaning of sport in terms of the self's endeavor to overcome the obstacles found therein. Metheny's *Movement and Meaning* (1968) comprises a systematic examination of the meaning of three movement forms: sport, dance and exercise. Slusher's book, *Man, Sport and Existence 1967*, also treats this topic in a systematic manner. *Motivation in Play, Games and Sport* (1967), edited by Slovenko and Knight, contains many essays which address the meaning topic with respect to sport. Amsler (1958) considers the meaning of sport with regard to its transcendent aspirations. And Ortega y Gasset (1955) speaks somewhat grandly of sport as one of the primal sources of meaning in modern life.

In general, writers have attempted to isolate one or more factors inherent in the sport experience which they have assumed engender meaning to the participant. Hout's discussion (1970) of the peak experience is a good example of this. Rupp (1958), in a paean to winning, assumes the inherent meaningfulness of victory, of success. Desmonde (1952) explores the meaning of a sport, the bullfight, as a religious ritual. In fact, numerous writers have examined the meaningfulness of play as a spiritual experience, including particularly Miller (1970), Rahner (1967) and Huizinga (1950).

Several articles offer theories which involve basic beliefs about the nature of man and the meaningfulness inherent in the satisfying of basic drives or needs. Lionel Tiger (1969) sees in sport the satisfaction of the need to engage in the hunting pattern, developed in man through evolution. Furlong (1969), Klausner (1968) and others contributing to his book, delineate the phenomenon of sport as a medium for stress-seeking through risk-taking. Neale (1969) sets forth an original theory of play as the absence of the usual inner conflict which results from man's need to discharge energy and to design experience. Lorenz (1966), assuming man's basic aggressive nature, singles out the cathartic effect of sport. Beisser (1961) discusses at length the "psychodynamics" or psychological meanings in sport.

And finally, McMurty (1971), Scott (1971), and Davis (1936) present some interesting comments relating to negative meanings potentially accruing from sport.

Researchers will find this aspect of sport philosophy a fruitful area of study. It would be interesting to explore the various kinds of experiences to see which are particularly relevant to sport. A model of various types of sport experiences could be developed to account for types of experience and levels or varieties of sport situations. This would make it possible to study the meaningfulness of sport in more diverse conditions than hitherto has been done. For such studies, available sources of data include the verbalized sport experience of individuals or groups (perhaps a class or team), as gained through interviews or published accounts such as are found in numerous autobiographies of sports figures. Certain kinds of experiences can also be analyzed from data collected by observation of the sporting event—either by being there, watching a telecast, or studying films. However, the latter two sources of data are contaminated by the cameraman's selectivity and judgments based, perhaps, on criteria irrelevant to the study. The methods of phenomenology seem particularly appropriate to an analysis of the meaning of the sport experience. Techniques of description or reduction are meant to provide rigorous tools for precisely this kind of analysis: the universalization of the subjective experience. Logically, the researcher's own sport experience will provide the primary data for this type of analysis.

Those interested in examining the meaningfulness of the sport experience, will find such analysis lends itself to a variety of nonverbal expressive forms. One's own statement of meaning can be conveyed through choreography of movement, through pictures, films, tapes, and verbal forms such as poetry and descriptive statements. Hopefully, attempts to understand the meaning of one's own experience will enhance the experience itself.

Why Does Man Play?*

R. SCOTT KRETCHMAR
WILLIAM A. HARPER

Why do you play? Is it for health, fun, or social relationship? Are you satisfied with these answers? Are there other possibilities? Do these reasons accurately explain your presence in sport? Why *do* you play?

Health, fun, and social contact, among other factors, are utilized by many as short but sufficient solutions to the question of "why I play." It is difficult to find individuals who do not have logical explanations for an activity; it seems that nearly everybody knows why he plays.

Historically, play (the term, for the purpose of this paper includes the traditional activities within sport and dance while eliminating the nonactivity games such as chess or cards) precedes any formalized teaching. It precedes compilation of a body of knowledge which might constitute a discipline. Children play. Aboriginal tribesmen play. Animals play. And they all play without any sophisticated notions of *why* they should. Play is a more primary category than play *for* education, than play *for* health and fitness, than play *for* social acquaintances.

Individually, the physical education professional person generally encounters the intrigue of play prior to coming to any decision to pursue a career in the field. Much of the fervor which is at times apparent in the actions of the teacher usually stems from an exciting en-

* From American Association for Health, Physical Education, and Recreation: *Journal of Health, Physical Education, and Recreation,* 40 (March, 1969), 57-58.

counter, either past or present, with some form of play. The instructor knows this enjoyment to be a part of his own history, and he often continues to recreate the actual engagement of sport or dance throughout his active life.

Empirically, most of the research in physical education relates to play—how one can participate with greater skill or for a longer time; how one can train better and learn faster; or how one can play more safely. It seems then, that play is the cornerstone of the profession, of the professional man, and of the field's scientific research. Play precedes all of the superstructure which develops around it.

Given the significance of play for the field and the number of statements which purport to describe this relationship between man, play, and the profession, it is a curious fact that so little attention is *now* directed toward this issue. It is paradoxical that physical education, based on play should house several scientific and humanistic branches which at this time seem to consider themselves self-sufficient, intellectual disciplines apart from ties with actual activity. It seems that the end of research—an understanding of play in all of its parameters, both scientific and humanistic—has been forgotten and the means have become a new goal. Statistics are exciting; scientific research is a challenge; philosophical and historical study command a compelling interest. Yet the priority, play, remains forgotten in the background. Play, which initiated the profession, lies buried under mounds of research and academic discussion. It remains the victim of its own children. Is the issue of the relationship between man and play dead?

But perhaps the question of demise is premature. Many of the traditional answers or "solutions" appear inadequate. Many physical educators begin their theorizing with two assumptions, that one can logically deduce "ought" statements from "is" descriptions and that man is rational. The discipline's philosophers articulate the various benefits which accrue to man through participation. They argue for the goals of increased longevity, safety, greater vigor, and increased opportunity for social interaction, among countless others. Both on scientific and sociological grounds the arguments for these objectives carry some weight, though they certainly lack verification.

For the purpose of this paper, let us assume that they are, in toto, true. It may be said these idealisms do occur in play. But it is the subsequent utilization of these "facts" which leads the theoreticians astray. From the fact that various goals *are* realized, they progress to the proposition that goals *should* be achieved and, further, to the notion that man will work actively toward these objectives once he is convinced of the validity of the proposition. It is these latter two extensions of logic which place the rationale for play on tenuous ground.

These difficulties can be clarified by means of examples. An instructor may lecture on the dangers of sky diving in an effort to discourage participation by any of his pupils. He begins with several statements of fact: (1) sky diving has a relatively high mortality rate and (2) man does not search out situations in which he has a great chance of dying. Given the fact that every student is a man, the teacher believes he is justified in concluding that the student *should not* sky dive. However, the instructor, when he initiates his argument with descriptive statements (the "is" facts), can conclude only in that same mood. There are no grounds for his leap from an "is" *description* to an "ought" *prescription*. The theoretician cannot logically state:

1. All men who do not want to die do not sky dive.
2. John is a man who does not want to die.

Therefore:

3. John *should not* sky dive.

All he is justified in stating is:

1. All men who do not want to die do not sky dive.
2. John is a man who does not want to die.

Therefore:

3. John *does not* sky dive.

The physical educators, then, have many facts relative to the outcome or benefits of play. They incorrectly suggest that mere availability of the facts leads to valid conclusions concerning why man *should* play. Given the various facts of play, such as fitness, health, vigor, and community, the instructors suggest that the student *should* play for these ends. What these instructors assume with such argumentation is that these entities are, in themselves, universal values. Fitness is not only a *value*, but equally, a *necessity!* Man should become fit! But common sense rebels against this reasoning. An object can remain a "good" without any obligation to achieve it. Fitness can intellectually be recognized as a value without deciding it is necessary for oneself.

It is clear then, that one who attempts to describe man's contact with play on logical grounds has major difficulties. For his account to be valid he must assume that the values of health, fitness, and vigor carry with them their own command for action. But even if one could agree on the values of play, it would still not be clear why man *should* strive for these ends.

It might be objected, at this point, that man does and must make value judgments, whether they be logical or not. In this light, all of the foregoing discussion becomes a wasted intellectual exercise. Who cares if a value judgment lies behind much of the profession's theory? Physical education is willing to stand behind its claims of value!

It might be maintained, then, that the instructor has no difficulty convincing the student of a specific "good." For example, a teacher may argue for the value of fitness, and the student may accept his discussion. The student intellectually agrees to the proposition that fitness is a worthy value and that his subsequent actions should reflect that conviction. The student has complete knowledge of the connections between fitness and play and has no qualms in accepting the value of the former.

However, is it not paradoxical that man, with some consistency, acts contrary to knowledge and commitment? Many people acknowledge the value of fitness while maintaining a sedentary existence. Many people who value their lives and who know that smoking may shorten the expected life span continue to smoke. Evidence shows that man often acts irrationally. Even the most disciplined individuals do inexplicably act against reason or the knowledge suggesting a singular mode of behavior.

The rationalists want to make play the result of consciously accepted goals and understandings. Though play may be a result in isolated situations, though an individual may initiate activity on rationalist grounds (i.e., "it is good for me"), he may continue to play in ignorance of benefits and in spite of potential detrimental effects.

Perhaps man intuits that play is somehow an irrational activity. He often plays for no good reason, yet he cannot, it seems, let himself live with this fact. Play becomes acceptable when man can explain his activity on rational grounds. The rational is superimposed upon the irrational. The absurd is made to conform to the reasonable. Does one not hide behind the rational facade because he fears, as an academician, the indeterminate, the unpredictable? Is it not more comfortable to have the ready answer and finite reply for the interrogator? But does not this disposition restrict the search for answers to a predetermined arena, that of the rational? By limiting the range of the quest does one not presuppose the nature of the answer, that it must be logical? What if the truth were to fall outside of this realm?

Clearly, it has been suggested that the solution does supersede the rational cause-and-effect motif. Man's intrigue and persistent relationship with play cannot be sufficiently explained through a rationalist method. Health, fitness, strength, relaxation, and other objectives probably accrue from play, but to suggest that these *explain* man's presence in play seems unfounded. To propose that man is in sport because he should be, or that he participates as a result of knowledge of and commitment to a value, vastly oversimplifies the situation. Man is in sport or dance on grounds independent of the practical or rational.

It was once asked what would happen to play if it were shown to have absolutely no beneficial results. Would play terminate? Once its useful ends were negated would its captivating effect on man likewise end? It is contended that play would not cease. It would, in fact, continue as before, perhaps with even more success because of its less artificial place in man's life.

The riddle of "why I play" has no simple answer. Man plays before he asks the question. He plays while continually ignoring the question. He plays in spite of known detrimental effects. Play and man seem bound together with reason or without it.

To explain the relationship between the phenomena of man and play on rational, cause-and-effect grounds is to render both man and play lifeless. The problem of "why I play" is equal and related to the incredible complexity of man. Man plays for many reasons, he plays for no reason at all. Man cannot be given an input of reasons and be expected to produce consistent, mechanical behavior. Man will act with spontaneity, irrationality, and abandon. The lived reality of this union between man and play defies all attempts to reduce it to a rationally explicable understanding.

Great Moments in Sport: The One and the Many*

DAVID A. WHITE

Sport contains experiences which for participant and spectator alike are frequently unique in their intensity. In this respect, sport is comparable to other human activities. Love and art also generate experiences which may in fact equal or surpass the intensity of sport. Even so, the claim that sport is at least as intense in its own way as other types of experience seems defensible. Two general problems must be faced if one deems a philosophical defense of this phenomenon worthwhile. The first problem is basically descriptive and enjoins the philosopher to describe the intensity of these experiences through that vision or insight which allows the transcription of actual full-blooded experiences into language amenable to reasoned evaluation. The second problem is basically conceptual and involves precision in drawing distinctions which preserve the essential components of sport's intensity while separating out elements common to sport and other intense activities. Each of these problems is difficult in different ways, and each is equally vital to an adequate philosophical account of sport. But the following remarks are generally restricted to the first problem, that of incisive description. The justification for this restriction, if justification be required, is that we must have a descriptive awareness of an activity before we attempt to distinguish conceptually one activity from another.

* From *The Journal of The Philosophy of Sport*, II (Sept., 1972), 124-132.

I

There is little philosophical history with respect to sport to serve as a guideline for terminology and distinctions which will serve either of these ends. An existing vocabulary could be adopted and the ensuing analyses would not be vitiated just by the decision to adopt that vocabulary. After all, those who have labored philosophically include many of the finest minds mankind has produced. The results of their toil—from the Greeks to the existentialists—need not necessarily lead us astray when applied to new investigative areas. But philosophizing on a relatively untouched subject suggests that relatively untouched means are to be used, at least to stimulate inquiry. Thus, a certain methodological openness should surround efforts to philosophize about sport, not perhaps to the point where, e.g., descriptions are larded with the earthy expletives mouthed by the athlete in action, but to the extent that the philosophical language employed be, a least initially, as fresh and different as the experiences themselves.

With this openness in view, I have selected as a heuristic device one of the slogans from the parlance which enlivens sport, parlance fostered and enhanced by the news media and echoed in the discussions of fans when they argue sports from the spectator's perspective. Such language is not always mere jargon, mere trite and unthinking verbal responses built upon highly formalized and predictable structures. At times, its evocations are flecked with that embedded insight which moves many professional philosophers to consider "ordinary language" as the controlling paradigm for all language (although the language they scrutinize professionally is rarely that of the athletic arena). Consider an example illustrating the point in a straightforward and interesting manner. In the late 1960's, sports commentators began to designate especially skilled athletes, whether amateur or professional, as "super stars." Prior to this shift, those so skilled were simply called "stars." Why the change in terminology? Perhaps the term "star" had simply worn out as the indicator for those participants distinguished by ability from the mere "regulars," the athletic rank and file. The shift would then be merely an insignificant verbal variation, principally in service to that constant quest for novelty which apparently is a necessary feature in popular culture.

As noted, this is the simple and evident explanation, but there is another which is more provocative. This more provocative explanation is based on the premise that reasons for the shift can be specified which cut deeper than the mere juggling of terms for the sake of the role linguistic novelty plays in the parlance of sports commentary. In this case, the reason is that the change in parlance is a directional hint of a change in what the parlance is about. The fact that skilled athletes are described as super stars rather than as stars might be an indication that those athletes who now excel in a certain sport are better than those athletes who excelled in the same sport in the past (when the only appellation required to set them off was the term "star"). This suggestion in turn raises the more general question concerning whether athletes are constantly improving, so that future performances will be even more proficient than present performances. And following the same line to its ultimate end, one wonders whether the relation between man and nature is such that there are limits which will not be surpassed, e.g., the rate of speed for the dash events in track. If so, how will the attainment, or even the approximation, of such limits affect that pursuit of athletic excellence measured by recording these speeds?

Such questions are both interesting and relevant to the philosophy of sport. They are also too complex to be addressed here. All I want to suggest is the ready intimacy between the popular language found in the casual description of sport and the theoretically problematic dimensions also present in these activities. It should be noted that investigation of the above set of problems need not be triggered solely by stylistic alterations in the language of sports commentators. Even a superficial awareness of sports lore indicates that records in, say, track and swimming have and are continually improving, from which isolated fact the questions raised may naturally flow. The point is not that the linguistic contrivances of sports jargon *alone* reveal interesting and important philosophical problems, but that it is helpful to pay heed to the availability of such parlance, since (for whatever internal reasons) its twists and turns may well point the way to these problems more directly and with more vivacity than other less humble approaches.

The particular slogan I do want to investigate is the frequently used phrase "great moments in sport." This phrase occurs in annual summaries of the key events in the world of sports and also with reference to those especially intense events in the biography of athletes when their performances have ranked far above the routine—stellar, in a word. Now it is worth noting at the outset that such great moments are not the sole property of those who experience these moments by instigating them. For the spectators at athletic events may participate in those factors which make a given moment great for the athlete himself. The principal goal of this paper is to sketch the experience of a great moment from the perspective of the participating athlete. But the nature of this perspective is such that, as we shall see, the presence of the crowd plays a vital role in determining the factors constituting both the greatness of a great moment and the peculiar temporality of such moments.

II

If scrutinized sympathetically, the popular language of sport suggests important philosophical problems. But this fact by itself does not illuminate the directions that should be taken to clarify the issues arising from such language. A hint for at least one relevant direction may be obtained by addressing two leading questions to the general sense of the phrase "great moments in sport." For example, does the fact that the great moments of one athlete (or one team) frequently occur before an audience of many spectators bear on the constitution of these moments as great?

Second, does the fact that most moments in athletes' careers are something less than great have a bearing on those relatively few moments (in some cases one, in some cases none) legitimately designated as great? Such questions show how an ancient and especially seminal philosophical problem makes itself felt in apparently banal sports slogans. The problem is called the one and the many. Its origin is found in the work of the pre-Socratics, especially Heraclitus and Parmenides. Plato and Aristotle contributed some of their most profound thinking toward its solution. And many of its ramifications are still discussed today, although the form of these discussions is different from the Greek conception of the problem. Most traditional philosophical treatments of the one and the many involve technical epistemological and metaphysical distinctions, for example, the sense in which a general term for a class (e.g., athlete) may be predicated of many different specific individuals (Wilt, Joe, Bobby, etc.). As such, these distinctions need not be introduced here. But the force of the problem is manifest in the "great moments" phrase and I propose to arrange the following discussion around this problem.

What makes a "great moment in sport" great for the athlete who initiates that moment? I shall suggest an answer to this question by exploring the evaluative criteria whereby an athletic experience can be described as great and also some of the factors comprising the temporal properties which underlie the possibility of such greatness. The most apparent condition required for a great athletic moment is that the athlete perform his own particular sport *well*, that he exercise his body so that the purpose and goals of his sport be realized with a high degree of excellence. Two important corollaries should be appended to this principle. First, the excellence which contributes to such greatness is, as a rule, relative to the level at which the performances occur. The excellence of the high school athlete is not the excellence of the college athlete, nor does the college athlete excel to the same extent as the professional. Also, excellence displayed at one level of competition in no way implies excellence at any higher level. Thus, sandlot athletes who excel only when the contest is organized in the rough-and-ready way pick-up games are organized frequently cannot cope with the more rigorous training regimen of high school athletic programs, not to mention the finer calibre of play. The number of athletes who do excel in high school and then fail at the collegiate level is significant. Similarly (although the number is proportionately fewer), the collegiate star is commonly found wanting in the professional ranks. One great moment for an athlete need not breed other great moments at either the same or higher levels of competition. Now although excellence is relative to the level on which competition occurs, the problem remains of explaining how this excellence contributes to the greatness of a great moment. A great moment for a high school athlete will not coincide with the excellence of a great moment for a professional, but for each the relation between his own activity and the greatness of the moment is identical and must be analyzed.

The second corollary is the frequently asymmetrical relation between the athlete (or team) enjoying the great moment and the athlete (or team) against whom the greatness is achieved. Thus, the great moment of athlete A can often be realized only at the expense of a lack of greatness on the part of his opponent athlete B. There are occasions when greatness can be attributed to both sides in a contest, but normally the great moment as such is reserved for the winner rather than for both winner and loser of such struggles. This asymmetry is absent when the contest is not man against man (or team against team) but man against nature, as in track and field. In these cases, the struggle is not just between individuals but also between man and the physical restrictions present in natural laws. It makes little sense to assert that nature "loses" if a sprinter betters the existing mark for the 100-yard dash, whereas it does make sense to say that the other contestants in the race lost and are thereby precluded from having great moments, even if one (or more) of the contestants himself bettered the record. Although many seek the goal of athletic excellence, the fact that normally only one can succeed implies that many will fail, or at least not succeed to the extent required for the success to be designated as a great moment. The presence and pressure of failure is an integral factor in the constitution of a great moment, even for those skilled athletes who achieve more than a few such moments. In baseball, the .400 hitter performs with an awesome degree of excellence —but he still fails to hit safely six times out of ten.

But are displays of athletic skill sufficient in themselves to constitute a great moment in sport? I suggest that the answer is no. The basis for this contention is derived from the apparently accidental fact that the vast majority of great moments are witnessed by spectators, frequently in crowds numbering in the tens of thousands. Now this fact appears to be accidental because the mastery involved in achieving a superlative performance has no intrinsic connection with the crowd witnessing that performance. Although a partisan crowd has an affect on an athlete, occasionally to the point where it can be asserted with some plausibility that the crowd "causes" a superior performance, the athlete may well be able to achieve the same performance without any assistance from the crowd. Indeed, it is possible for a stellar performance to occur when the only "crowd" is the performing athlete (or athletes) in isolation. Surely the sprinter who first runs the 100-yard dash in 8.9 seconds will be party to a great moment in sport, regardless whether he does it in the company of himself and an official timer—and no one else—or in the Los Angeles Coliseum before a full house. In what sense then does the presence of a crowd of witnesses constitute a necessary condition for a great moment in sport?

To prepare the way for an answer, visualize the crowd's reaction when an athlete is on the verge of or actually performing in a superlative manner. The crowd is sometimes calm, sometimes droning with anticipation, sometimes cheering, sometimes roaring so powerfully that the volume of sound becomes a palpable force in the athlete's consciousness. The crowd's immediate relation to the performing athlete is realized in this primarily vocal medium. Occasionally crowds become aroused to the point where they gesticulate, jump around, hurl objects at the participants (players and/or officials) and perhaps even riot. But in these latter extreme cases the crowd ceases to be an assembly of sports fans and becomes a mob. In normal circumstances, however, the crowd restricts itself to the verbal dimension. Now crowds become vocal at many moments during a contest, moments when the play is exceptionally good, exceptionally bad, or exceptionally dull. But a great moment in sport is surely never a dull moment, regardless where an individual fan's sentiments lie. The inference is that regardless whether the crowd is cheering or booing, the type and volume of sound produced is only the external manifestation of the crowd's contributing factor to great moments. The relevant feature of the crowd's presence is found by examining a more significant but less visible bond which unites the crowd's many variegated personalities to the athlete as he participates in the contest and as he performs with excellence.

Let us now shift the imaginative focus from the crowd as such to the relation between athlete and crowd. I take it as axiomatic that the athlete always senses the crowd's presence, regardless of the size of the crowd and re-

gardless of the extent of their vocal activity. But such knowledge is generally a pre-reflective awareness that the crowd is "out there," observing his actions. Occasionally athletes will "grandstand," i.e., indulge in antics solely for the amusement (or irritation) of the fans in the stands. But these antics are not strictly related to the proper performance of his athletic functions as such. Normally the activity of the athlete is controlled and dictated by the demands of the game or sport itself and not by the wishes and taunts of the spectators observing that game or sport. Now picture a crucial situation during an important game. The athlete reacts, performs, and excels. The media announcers search for suitable superlatives. The writers strive to capture and immortalize the proceedings in the vagaries of language. And the crowd roars at the display. But to what does the crowd direct its vocal energies? Simply put, to the fact that someone (their favorite, as a rule) has either performed well or, ultimately, won the day. Here care must be exercised in order to grasp why the crowd so reacts. Although athletic contests are usually decided by performances which justify the pre-game sentiment that the best team won, not all winning performances are superior performances in the sense requisite for a great moment. But the conjunction of athletic excellence (although not necessarily excellence resulting in a winning performance) with the approbation of the crowd provides the clue to the constitution of such great moments. We shall pursue that clue by sketching the general reaction of the athlete while in the process of performing with excellence and in the presence of an approving and usually vocal audience.

When performing with excellence, the athlete is normally in a state of positive awareness, if not explicit knowledge, that he is so performing. Frequently such awareness is mute, i.e., it could be verbalized neither at the very moment of performing (assuming verbalization was practically possible under these circumstances) nor after the fact, regardless how glib or perspicuous the athlete may be. Although such awareness may be largely subliminal, it is in the nature of this awareness to guarantee a certain sense of self-satisfaction with his performance and with himself. Now in this state, the self of the athlete is the self as defined by the performance of bodily excellence. Furthermore, this self-satisfaction is not limited to the singularity, the oneness, of his own individuality. For in a crucial respect the crowd is an extension of this aspect of the athlete's self. In observing the excellence of the one athlete or team, the many members of the crowd participate in the human excellence displayed by that one athlete while he is in the process of performing his bodily feats. And this quest for and participation in excellence for both athlete and audience is the source of the greatness of sport's great moments.

What, more precisely, is the nature of this peculiar interpersonal self-extension? First, some observations on what it is *not*. The extension of self from the one performing athlete to the many in the crowd is independent of the activity of the crowd (verbal and otherwise, as discussed above), the size of the crowd, the range of individual motives prompting one, some, or all of that crowd to attend the event, as well as the motivation of the athlete who is himself performing. The greatness of a great moment does not depend on the size of an attendant crowd. A great moment witnessed by an audience of 100,000 is not ten times greater than a great moment witnessed by an audience of 10,000. In fact, as we shall note later, the actual physical presence of the audience is not the most important aspect of the crowd insofar as the multiplicity of the crowd is a necessary condition for the greatness of the moment. Such greatness is not quantitative in nature, does not result from the sheer proximity of masses of onlookers, but is qualitative, depending on the type of bond uniting performing athlete and witnessing crowd.

This bond must also be distinguished from the variety of motives which impel or entice the fan to expend time and money to witness athletic contests and from the variety of motives which drive a relative handful of individuals to seek athletic "stardom." For the fan, these motives are diverse and numerous: to escape a life of drudgery or dullness, to be entertained, to witness violence for the sake of violence. And for the athlete: notoriety (with its attendant blandishments), self-aggrandizement, or money. But the fact that the average fan and average athlete may be an amalgam of the above does not diminish the importance of establishing the difference between these factors and that special link which binds the crowd to excellent athletic performances. My contention is that a qualitative difference can be specified to isolate this link from motives which induce some individuals to pursue athletic excellence by becoming athletes themselves and entice others to observe this pursuit at a distance.

Although the crowd's ensemble of motives is as varied as their wearing apparel, one should not confuse this ensemble with that common pursuit of excellence which provides one of the principal distinguishing characteristics for a great moment. Similarly, the fact that the presence of the crowd is manifested by the crowd's perceptible behavior should not be mistaken as the vital factor in this characteristic. As noted above, such response is only a sign of this characteristic and is not constitutive of it. Where then is this link to be found? The property in question is based on the fact that the human person is embodied, that such bodies can perform a large number of diverse but controlled actions, and that it is possible for some individuals to perform these actions with a high degree of skill. This possibility is real for all individuals, and just as real is the desire to actualize this possibility. But not all individuals have either the chance or the aptitude to realize it. Hence the concern of many to witness this bodily excellence when opportunities are available. We have already seen that winning performances are not necessarily superior performances. But when a superior performance does take place, the propensity in the individual to achieve physical excellence, whether actually or vicariously, is realized in the witnessing of the public event. In the course of such witnessing, the finite limitations of the self (with respect to bodily performance and function) of this or that athlete are transcended, along with the finite limitations of each and every participating member of the crowd observing the excellence. The result is a great moment in sport, an event of fleeting duration, but an event which realizes the inherent urge to excel through the body. This evanescent unity of athlete and audience is itself both one and many; one in the mutual awareness and enjoyment of human bodily excellence by both athlete and audience, many in the different modes through which each member of this rare community—including the athlete on whom the accolade "great moment" is bestowed—actually experiences this moment within his own particular psychological make-up.

This unity between athlete and crowd is present even when the actual crowd is absent (although obviously the vocal external manifestation of the crowd's approval will be lacking). Individuals who persevere to the point where they attain a self-imposed athletic goal also share in a great moment modified by both their own physical limitations and by their relatively private environments. Although large masses of humanity do not witness this moment, such absence does not detract from the moment's greatness. For the purpose of an athletic action intended for excellence is to actualize a humanly physical possibility as if it were an actual possibility for *all* individuals. The duffer who finally breaks 100 has experienced a personal "great moment in sport," even if he is the lone man in the clubhouse with no one to share in his triumph. Hence the importance of distinguishing between the presence of the many as manifested by their primarily verbal behavior and the many as exemplifying any one man's desire to utilize his body with athletic grace and skill. This communal pursuit of athletic excellence and its realization through the actual event of athletic excellence together constitute the greatness of a great moment in sport.

III

The preceding analysis of the "greatness" aspect is more suggestive than conclusive. Many questions can and should be addressed to the assertions in these analyses. But at least it seems clear that there is a fertile confluence between sports parlance and classical philosophical problems such that attention to their interplay will result in pursuit of the right questions. Let me offer yet another and final example showing the efficacy of the one and the many by considering in more detail some of the temporal characteristics in great moments. In this way, a partial confrontation with both basic elements of "great moments in sport" will be achieved—the evaluational factor ("great") and the metaphysical factor ("moments" as relative to time).

To determine the nature of any segment of experienced time, it is helpful to begin by investigating the relation between objectively measurable time (years, hours, minutes, seconds) and what is actually happening *in* that measured time. We then readily discover that the duration of one great moment in sport may require the passage of many moments of measured time. The great moment might be one play in a game, one game in a season, or the entire season itself. Baseball provides prominent examples of each: Willy Mays' catch (sometimes referred to as The Catch) in the 1954 World Series, Don Larsen's perfect game in the 1956 World Series, and the Mets dramatic closing sweep to the eastern division pennant in 1969. All three are legitimate great moments, but obviously the only example corresponding to an intuitive understanding of moment is the first, the Mays catch. As a consequence, our conception of

Larsen's great moment must be broadened so that that moment includes the complete objective duration of the game itself. For if Larsen had walked Dale Mitchell (the 27th man he faced) instead of striking him out, the perfect game would never have existed, the potential great moment just another "might have been." Similarly with the Mets pennant drive, only in this case the duration includes months, the length of an entire season. For if the Mets had been leading or at least in the running for the pennant all during the season, then the drama of their closing surge would have been impossible and the greatness reduced to a successful but mere workmanlike performance. The many (objective) moments comprising the daily rhythm of winning and losing are all necessary (but not sufficient) conditions for one great moment happening as it did. But it is important to preserve the fact that although the actual duration of sports' great moments frequently contain many moments, there is still only *one* great moment. Its singularity imprints an individuating unity on the event, so that regardless how much time measured according to objective standards the event required, the various experienced aspects of that moment can and must be understood as parts of one whole.

Finally, this extension of the duration of a great moment from a few seconds to a half-year is paradigmatic for a similar extension in the athlete's own experience of such moments. The relative infrequency of great moments, even for the most gifted of athletes, sets them off from the many routine and competent performances which comprise most careers. Indeed, some athletes have only one such moment, even when their careers are lengthy and, on the whole, successful. How should we understand such a telescoping affect—the focussing of an entire career into the space of one or perhaps several great moments? Here is one possibility. The fusion of selves between athlete and audience is reflected in the intensification of the principal temporal dimensions in the athlete's own personal history. In a sense, his past, his present, and his future *qua* athlete all coalesce during the actual event of the great moment. For such an athlete, the past comes into the present as an expectation of his success after expending effort, in most cases considerable effort, so that the possibility of greatness may be more than just a hope. The years of training most successful athletes undergo are permeated by this expectation. When the actual moment of greatness is realized, expectation is fulfilled and bears the totality of this (now past) time into the experience of the present moment. The present moment of greatness collects all the fragmented past moments of training, struggling, and hoping and because of the greatness transforms them from (past) moments of expectation into a unified prelude for the greatness of this (present) moment.

The movement from future to present is the possibility of reliving the moment in memory, when the greatness is taken up again and re-experienced as great. In fact, some great moments cannot be fully appreciated until after they have already been concluded as physical events. When Willy Mays was chasing Vic Wertz' long drive, he did not know the outcome of his quest; doubtless the circumstances, the difficulty of the catch, etc., were such that Mays himself could experience the moment as great only in retrospect. An athlete may, when his career is ended, go on to excel in other fields or he may become a derelict: in either case, the glory of the great moment is not affected by what transpires after that moment. Thus, the presence of one great moment radiates into both past and future and into all possible moments that comprise the consciousness of the successful athlete. Past time, the time of training and preparation, becomes an anticipation of greatness, known as an anticipation of greatness only when the great moment is realized. Future time becomes the time of memory, when whatever happens to the individual will be affected by the recognition, a recognition always available to the athlete, that there was once a moment when he embodied the human desire to perform a sport with excellence.

As mentioned at the outset, my contention is not that sport and sport alone offers these moments of intensity. Other types of human endeavor also afford this peculiar coalescence of past and future. And to elicit the distinguishing characteristics between sport and these other endeavors is an important and difficult conceptual problem. But the preceding descriptive account at least provides an introductory framework to begin such an analysis. And it does so in virtue of the mutually suggestive interplay between an ancient philosophical problem and the contemporary wisdom of the popular language of sport.

Play and Seriousness*

KURT RIEZLER

We say: this is merely play; he is merely playing. We differentiate between play and something that is not merely play but is serious. What does this "merely" mean?

But is not the answer obvious? We say "merely playing" whenever we are not serious. We say we are not merely playing so far as we are serious though playing. Unfortunately, the simple answer does not get us very far. What, for heaven's sake, is serious, and why? The "merely" points to a deficiency, to something that is absent in playing. When we say "not merely play" we indicate that this something is present despite our playing. Thus explaining this something whose absence the "merely" asserts, the "not merely" denies, means explaining our seriousness. The question grows.

That seems to be an inquiry into the usage of a word. But the "merely," asserted or denied, accompanies all playing throughout the countries, ages, and languages. It tends to indicate something in man, the queer being, that is able to play and bound to be serious.

The "merely" or "not merely" resides in the attitude of man, not in things, matters, actions, that we could subsume under play and seriousness. The "merely" differentiates attitudes. Man may decide according to his own will or mood whether he should deal playfully or seriously with a person, a thing, a task, a situation, or a game. Man does not decide which attitude of his is playful and which

* From *Journal of Philosophy*, XXXVIII, (September, 1941), 505-517.

serious. Though man's mood can move things to and fro over the borderline between play and seriousness, he can not move the borderline itself, which demarcates attitudes, not things.

I begin with the most simple case. We play games such as chess or bridge. They have rules the players agree to observe. These rules are not the rules of the "real" world or of "ordinary" life. Chess has its king and queen, knights and pawns, its space, its geometry, its laws of motion, its demands, and its goal. The queen is not a real queen, nor is she a piece of wood or ivory. She is an entity in the game defined by the movements the game allows her. The game is the context within which the queen is what she is. This context is not the context of the real world or of ordinary life. The game is a little cosmos of its own.

We may call this little cosmos a world—the "playworld." The term, however, is misleading. "World" suggests certain features the playworld lacks. "World" means or should mean the totality of a something "in" which we live. We ourselves are part of this something. Though the world is always our world, it is intended to mean a world that is not and never will be ours. It means everyone's world. It embraces all other worlds of all other beings. So it is the real world.

We are free to play or not to play, to enter or to leave the "playworld." Our relation to the real world is of a different kind. We have been thrown into it willy-nilly; we can leave but never re-enter it. As the real world differs from the playworld, so a real queen differs from the queen in chess. In the real world all things are connected with all things, every effect is a cause, every end a means. Not so in the playworld. Here the chains of causes and effects are thought of as having limits. Events within the game are separated from events in the real world. To the player the game is not a part of the real world. The "merely" may have to do with this separation.

In playing chess we can be more or less serious. A bridge player may be chided by his partner for lack of seriousness. She feels he is not paying sufficient attention to the game or that he does not live up to its spirit. Still, mere lack of seriousness should not be called a playful attitude toward the game. Play or playfulness is not a negative term. We could speak of a playful attitude if a player were to play a play within the game itself, whether by pursuing a goal of his own or by superimposing rules of his own on the rules of the game—replacing the spirit of the game by the caprices of his mood, which are at odds with the spirit of the game, although not forbidden by its rules. For example, a bridge-player might try to get as many kings as possible in his tricks. He could be said to play with the play. We say that he merely plays so far as he substitutes demands of his own for the demands of the game. Here playfulness stresses the detachment of a sovereign mood—which in this case is detachment from the spirit of the game. Thus the "merely" seems to indicate a detachment from demands that seriousness commands us to respect.

The story of our playing has still other aspects. Though the playworld may be separated from the real world, the goal of the game can be connected with the real world, our ordinary life, our substantial interests. Money, honor, even life, may depend on our winning or losing. The gambler can raise his stakes to a point at which losing would mean serious harm. He has not much use for the "merely," though we might say that he deals seriously with the play but playfully with his money. It is he himself who links his serious interests with the play. To the football champion the victory of Lions over Tigers may be the only thing that matters. Glory, honor, career may depend on his success, according to the customs and codes of the society in which he lives. Since he has to submit to these codes, his football is not merely a play, perhaps no play at all—at least to him. It is an institution of the real world or ordinary life. The playful attitude, if there is any, is on the side of a society that connects a mere play with the glory, honor, and career of its members.

A fashionable gentleman trifles away his day and gambles at night. His gambling is his only seriousness. Here at least he faces the reality of life: fear and hope, risk, action, passion, need for caution and self-control. It may even be that the very thirst for real concern drives him to the gambling table—away from his day of non-committing trifles. Now play and seriousness exchange places. We may conclude: play can be serious, ordinary life need not be serious at all. The "real world" or "ordinary life" may be used to differentiate things belonging to play from those belonging to seriousness; they can not be used to differentiate a playful from a serious attitude.

There are, however, many games of another sort. In some the emphasis lies not on obeying but on inventing or changing rules. After all, chess and bridge also were invented in a playful mood. We might even dare to say that in the present American form, bridge has taken on the character of work by being fettered to so many elaborate rules and conventions that obedience to them threatens to suffocate the playful mood. We never enjoy a playful attitude more than when making or changing the rules or conventions to which we submit. We do it rarely, because we are lazy or lack inventiveness.

This is clear in the case of children's play. What they enjoy most is their own inventive activity. Long before they play games children play with or without toys. They invent and perform stories, determine the meaning of things, assume for themselves the rôle of a king or a queen. This chair is a mountain, the doll in the blue dress and with pink cheeks is Aunt Geraldine. The child disregards the fact that Aunt Geraldine has neither a blue dress nor pink cheeks. She enjoys her activities in determining the meaning of the doll or in forcing Aunt Geraldine to sit straight in her doll chair.

Grownups, watching the child, say: she plays. In their world the child's play is "merely" play. There may be, however, no "merely" for the child herself—no playful attitude, no "merely" that could hint at a deficiency. The distinction between play and seriousness is still in the making, the real and the imaginary world are not yet separated. For the child, things do not yet have their own definite meaning, which demands to be respected and is put aside when we merely play. Things, as separated from their meanings, are as yet unknown. They are what they mean. To children their little activity in playing seems to share in a seriousness in which, in between anxiety and curiosity, they discover the world and its things, themselves and their relation to the world, their power and its limitations. It is the share they enjoy, since in playing alone are they acting.

The "merely" enters the scene when children begin to be capable of, and granted, a first consistent activity in a consistent reality. Now the things of the real world begin to raise their voices, impose their demands, and be conceived in the horizon of an order in which things are no longer what you choose them to be. Now the doll and Aunt Geraldine, play and seriousness, part company. This process may take considerable time.

A four-year-old boy plays railroad with a series of chairs. He sits on the first chair and is the engine. His father enters the room and kisses him. "Don't kiss me," protests the boy, "the chairs could see it and forget that they are railroad cars." Huyzinga[1] [sic] uses the case to support his thesis that children realize that they merely play. The example, however, is dubious. It shows only how the real and the imaginary world still interpenetrate each other.

A girl, we say, plays around with the boys. Or this man merely plays with that girl. We may pity the girl who takes herself or her love seriously and demands to be not merely played with. The girl or the social group sets a standard of love to which this man should but does not conform. His merely playing means disregarding this standard. In some cases both the male and the female merely play. They play with each other a very old play, each knowing that the other merely plays and both enjoying the charm of the game. "Why not? After all, it is not so serious a matter." We say they merely play though they may pretend or even believe themselves to be serious. We say so if we know that neither would go a few steps out of his way for the other's sake. We set a standard of love to which intimate relations between a boy and girl should conform. The "merely" means that an obligation inherent in the relations between the sexes has been disregarded. In some languages, as older Low German and Dutch, the term for an illegitimate child is "playchild," suggesting that only marriage is serious. But play is not the mere negation of seriousness. A love affair that lacks seriousness need not even be play. The amorous life of societies that succeeded in bestowing some charm on love as a game tells another story. There are winners and losers,

[1] In his *Homo ludens*.

goals and rules. The two players may play with each other; the prize may be to be loved and not love. It may be mere vanity, honor, reputation, in a leisure class engaged in a collective battle against boredom. Or the lovers may play not only with each other but with the danger that at any moment one may commit him- or herself seriously and really fall in love. The game has its rules. These rules—the moral code of illicit love—tend to separate the game from ordinary life, its commitments, its interests, titles, rights, and its knowledge. The rules demand "discretion" in all the shades of the term, which range from separation through freedom to courtesy. It may happen that both players lose and really fall in love. Then they no longer merely play, though they may go on observing some rules of the game and try to isolate their love from ordinary life. Out of mutual respect for their self-defense they may even go on pretending to play, using the ruse of a playful attitude to cloak their seriousness.

In some Catholic countries of an old tradition a few weeks of carnival festivities put the relations between the sexes under the exceptional rules of a play. Visitors from countries without such a tradition usually assume that all they have to do is to rid themselves of an habitual restraint. Though nowadays the actual practice of the natives themselves does not quite live up to the idea, the natives still dislike these visitors because their failure to observe the rules spoils the game. Here a social code demands the playful attitude. You are in disguise, wearing a mask and a costume. You are not yourself. You play a rôle. No one is expected to ask or answer serious questions. The stories you tell, the promises you make, the love you profess need be true but for the moment—in a fictitious world. No consequences should be drawn, no obligations remembered, beyond Mardi Gras. The favors you may consummate give you no titles. They do not count in ordinary life. A really jealous husband who does not merely act the part of a jealous husband violates the rules of the play.

Here a society plays, watching in common agreement over rules meant to separate the game from the real world or ordinary life and its chains of causes and effects, ends and means.

The example of love is ambiguous—the ambivalence of love between play and seriousness being the charm of the game. Other examples are simpler.

A writer's cunning and skill may be remarkable. He forces the language to follow his moods. Yet we blame him for merely playing with the language. What do we mean? He only wants to display his skill, enjoys moving along the boundary of what is still allowed, startles us by his artifices. He is an acrobat, not an artist. He merely plays so far as he disregards, for purposes of his own mood, obligations that the correlation of subject-matter and language silently imposes.

We say that a conductor deals but playfully with a Beethoven symphony. We mean that the desire to show off his craftsmanship overpowers the devotion the work demands.

Statesmen, whose job it is to consider all sides of a situation, often complain of experts who isolate the interests of their fields. Once in a while they may sigh angrily; the generals or the diplomats are merely playing their game. The statesman may be right or wrong; he means that the diplomat, educated in the traditions of the European balance of power, the rules of diplomacy and its craftiness, looks at Europe as the playground of a diplomatic game that is an end in itself, and is unable to realize demands beyond his game or requirements of a situation that can not be mastered by his means, methods, or goals. In an analogous way the general, educated as a staff officer by playing war games on maps or in manoeuvres, regards the surface of the earth as a playground for moving armies and navies. Both separate a playworld from the real world, absolutize their own rules and goals, and disregard every horizon that is beyond the limited horizon of their game. Even in such cases play and its "merely" retain the shadow of their meaning. Such examples can be multiplied; the "merely" continues to accompany the playful attitude.

I venture a preliminary thesis. The diversity of our playing seems to suggest two ways of defining the "merely," the one starting from the player, the other from the play. In a playful attitude the manner of our being concerned has specific features, as has the object with which we are concerned. Since these two sorts of specificity correspond to each other the two ways of defining the "merely" converge; they explain each other.

In a playful attitude we are "not really" concerned. But it is just this "not really" that must be explained. Moreover, "not really" is wider than "merely playfully." We are "not really" concerned in many cases when there is no playfulness in our attitude. We may try to say: in a playful attitude things do not matter so much—we are only partly concerned, not with the whole of our interest. But this again is doubtful.

We are often partly concerned in matters of ordinary life, yet this our partial concern need not be playful. If "partial" is to be used this partialness must be of a peculiar kind. We are partly concerned but without linking this partial concern to other parts or to the whole of our concern. It does not count. In severing the link that connects this part with other parts we treat a "partial" concern as if it were no part of anything. Thus the part, not being conceived of as part, is not a part. In the seriousness of ordinary life all partial concern remains partial because it is connected with some of or all our other concerns. The "merely" in our playing seems to point not to a partial concern, but to a distinction in which our concern in playing is separated from our other concerns.

If we start from the game or from the object with which a playful attitude is concerned, a different aspect tells the same story. An area of playing is isolated by our sovereign whim or by man-made agreement. Things within this area mean what we order them to mean. They are cut off from their meanings in the so-called real world or ordinary life. No chains of causes and effects, means and ends, are supposed to connect the isolated area of play with the real world or ordinary life. If there still are such chains they are disregarded. So far as we do not disregard them our attitude is no longer merely playful. An area that under the aspect of ordinary life would be conceived of as only a part is regarded not as part of a wider area but as a cosmos of its own. Thus the two aspects tell the same story.

In merely playing we forget the "real world," our ends, our dependence on things. We often play only for the sake of diversion. At any rate, we disregard the context of ordinary life, the meaning of things, their demands, our obligations, and put in their place meanings, demands, and obligations of our own making. In playing we enjoy being our own masters.

Playing, if it is merely playing, is never a means. The goal of playing is part of the game. It is not an end to which our playing is the means—it serves only to direct our activity, to measure the skill, to differentiate between winner and loser. Playing, our activity in playing is its own end, though we are capable of linking the goal of the game to means and ends in our life outside the game. If we do, we usually drop the "merely." The chains of causes and effects, means and ends, are meant to be cut at the boundaries of the play. No more than causes from outside are allowed to interfere, lest they spoil the game, should consequences be drawn to the life outside the play.

So it seems that with respect to both the how and the what of our concern the "merely" could be explained as follows: things, in their relation to us, are surrounded by a horizon that depends on our attitude toward them. In different attitudes we see things in different horizons. The horizon makes things what they are to us. In the seriousness of our daily activity we look at things within the horizon of our interests in the various concatenations of causes and effects, means and ends. Here every horizon seems to be partial, pointing beyond itself, intended to mean something in connection with other things and other possible horizons. When in serious life we say that we are only partly concerned, we look at our own concern as but a greater or smaller part of our concernedness—in the horizon of something that is more than this part. In a playful attitude the horizon does not point at anything beyond itself, though it is the horizon of a limited area or of a limited concern that is not yet connected with, and not a part of, a wider area or a broader concern: the horizon of a play that is merely a play.

This thesis, however, is preliminary indeed. It may be of some service to differentiate playfulness from the average seriousness of our daily life. But it has no reason to offer why this kind of ordinary life should be serious at all. Why should or could a man not deal playfully with all the chains of means and ends in this dubious seriousness? The question grows out of the answer.

Ere I proceed, I permit an antithesis to speak and to sweep the thesis away in a burst of rage.

At last, so the argument runs, you seem to discover the shortcomings of a thesis that takes for granted the seriousness of ordinary life. In starting from the "merely" you presuppose a standard of seriousness that may be only the standard of the kind of society that thinks in terms of means and ends, in terms of business. It may be that the "merely" is only a habit of speaking. There need not be an absolute "merely" in playing as such—no deficiency. If there is deficiency it may be a deficiency not in play but in the man who utters the "merely" and thus shows that he can not rid himself of his puny sort of seriousness. Your start from the "merely" distorts the story of play.

There is no "merely"—rather an "even." Play is man's triumph—he, the greatest of all beings, can even play. Only the lowest animals do not play. All higher animals, wild or tame,

play. The reasons for which we call them higher or lower may account for their playing and not playing. We assume that worms do not play, though we can not know what movements, actions, things are to worms in their worm world, if there is such a thing. We think of worms as closely tied up with their actual environment at any given moment. They live in the dark. The demands they put upon and receive from their environment are dumb pressures. They can not detach themselves from their environment, change the meaning of things and their functions, as play implies. Dogs and cats, most higher animals, undoubtedly can. They can fight for the love of fighting and not "mean it seriously." They chase a ball, push it away and capture it again, for the fun of chasing; give it importance for a while and leave it as something that is of no interest. Their playing is detachment from the environment and its demands, a sort of freedom the worm seems to lack. The way from worm to cat is but the first and minor part of the way from slavery to freedom. From dog to man is another, and the history of man's culture is again another part. Man's playing is his greatest victory over his dependence and finiteness, his servitude to things. Not only can he conquer his environment and force conditions to comply with his needs and demands far beyond the power of any other animal. He can also play, i.e., detach himself from things and their demands and replace the world of given conditions with a play-world of his own mood, set himself rules and goals and thus defy the world of blind necessities, meaningless things, and stupid demands. Religious rites, festivities, social codes, language, music, art—even science—all contain at least an element of play. You can almost say that culture is play. In a self-made order of rules man enjoys his activities as the maker and master of his own means and ends. Take art. Man, liberated from what you call the real world or ordinary life, plays with a world of rhythms, sounds, words, colors, lines, enjoying the triumph of his freedom. This is his seriousness. There is no "merely."

The antithesis plays havoc with our preliminary thesis. If the shattered thesis is to survive, it must be reshaped in order to withstand the violent assault.

We must make a new start. The "merely" may be misleading. What about the "not merely"? There are cases in which play, though play, is not merely play; and not only because the result of the play is connected by agreement with means and ends in ordinary life, such as money or honor, but in itself, by its inherent seriousness, which is not the seriousness of the real world or ordinary life. But is there such a thing? Why is it serious?

Art is play, though not merely play. Some put the emphasis on play, others on the "not merely." To the artist, if he is a real artist, it is deadly earnest, as earnest as religion to the religious man. But what is art? If we define art as the class of things called art—by some minimum conditions to which the elements of this class must submit,—we find works of art that are not even play, others that are merely play, and again others that certainly are not merely play. In search of the "not merely" we can not start from a definition of minimum conditions. There is something—whatever it may be, call it quality or value,—by virtue of which a work of art is "real art" or "great" or more or less "good." Toward this something both the artist and the art connoisseur are looking, the one in creating, the other in judging, the work. Though both may be equally unable to say what this mysterious something is, they presuppose that there is some thing. Whoever honestly denies it is not an artist or an art connoisseur. Obviously the "not merely" refers to this mysterious something.

If we apply to art the standards of the preliminary thesis, art is merely play. It separates things from the real world, disregards their demands, puts things in an imaginary context, within which they mean what art orders them to mean. The artist is the center of his own rules and laws, which are not the rules and laws of ordinary life and are conceived of as being severed from its endless chains of means and ends, causes and effects. Thus, he merely plays.

And yet he does not play. There is not and can not be a playful attitude, be it in the artist who creates or in the connoisseur who enjoys and judges a work of art. It seems even that this play can not be played in a playful attitude. There is, in art itself, a demand, an ultimate obligation, with which no artist plays. It is devotion to this demand and detachment from all other demands that makes him an artist. With respect to this detachment you may say that he merely plays; with respect to this devotion, he simply can not help being serious indeed. This obligation is there ere the artist becomes an artist and creates his particular style and his works. It is the supreme lead, taken on in reverence and obeyed in judging, choosing, rejecting. It is not man-made, not the creation of any arbitrary mood, not part of the rules of the play, but prior to

any rules. There is no such thing in playing games. Thus, art is not play. The "not merely" points at an unconditional obligation.

Here, however, we are likely to run into a peculiar difficulty. We use and certainly need the term "playful" to characterize a style, a work, the individuality of an artist. Mozart is more playful than Beethoven. Rafael sometimes seems to be; Michelangelo is never playful. The history of art abounds in examples. The term, used in this way within art, need not have any bearing on "good" or "bad"—there is no "merely" in this playfulness, no differentiation of any kind. We mean only an apparently effortless ease that makes creativity look like the play of a sovereign mood. Both *King Lear* and *Midsummer Night's Dream* are called plays, though the former is certainly less playful than the latter. We are tempted to say that compared with *King Lear Midsummer Night's Dream* is "merely" a play: it is a dream in a playworld that does not claim to represent the real world. But we certainly do not mean that Shakespeare's attitude toward his poetry and its inherent demands is merely playful.

In the *Merchant of Venice* the relation itself between play and seriousness is the core of the work. Hence its difficulties. In most performances the tragedy of Shylock is put to the fore as the center of the work framed by a playworld of love, fun, music, and sweetness. Such performances can hardly be convincing. If the relation is reversed the performance convinces—a world of play and love put to the fore against the background of a world in which Shylocks hate and suffer. The poet, however, does not deal playfully with the tension between play and seriousness or with human life, of which this tension is part, or with his poetry.

Whenever in the history of art artists not only seem to have but really have an attitude toward their art that could be called merely playful, this "merely" indicates decay, second-rate work, or the end of a style. Playfulness in art is "not merely" playful at the beginning and "merely" playful at the end of a stylistic period—not in all but in many cases.

Art, whether playful or not, is never merely play. If the mysterious something we call good or quality or value means an obligation that is unconditionally serious, this seriousness is certainly not the seriousness of ordinary life and its horizons of means and ends. If the lead of the term "horizon" is to be followed the "horizon" in art is of another kind.

Listen to a Beethoven symphony. You are

in a world of sounds—nowhere else. This world embraces you. It is present as a whole. There is nothing beyond. The "real world" or ordinary life with all its endless chains of aspects, causes, means, in which every step is finite and none the last, disappears. Something else appears—which can be grasped with your senses but not put into words. If unfortunately a philosophical context or a question that continues to grow compels you to describe it you search for words in a kind of despair. One of the words you are likely to hit upon is "horizon."

This horizon includes a whole. This whole seems present at whatever point we touch this horizon. It is just this that the term "horizon" suggests or should suggest. We apply the term to the sky: south or north, west or east—only one horizon borders the sky. It is the same horizon all around. Thus the term implies the oneness of a whole. Here "whole" does not mean completeness of several elements. It means a Gestalt, present in every part, and not only by virtue of the presence of all other parts. You look only southward and yet the horizon you see embraces a whole. In art the horizon of the whole can still be visible in a torso or a fragment.[2]

The horizon embracing a whole is an ultimate horizon. It does not limit a part as part. It is not a particular horizon, pointing beyond itself. If there is infinity this infinity is within the horizon—an inward infinity.

While you listen to the symphony you are not partly concerned—the whole of your being is listening, you are moved to the core, open to something the term "ultimate horizon" is intended to indicate. The term does not claim to answer the unanswerable question of the mysterious something by virtue of which a work of art is more or less good. Its only claim is descriptive power. We might say that Leonardo or Michelangelo or Shakespeare in their Mona Lisa or Adam or Caesar succeeded in making visible an ultimate horizon that forces the human cosmos as a whole to become transparent in the portrait of a lady, in the movement of a body, in verses uttered by actors that are not Caesars on the boards of a stage that is not the world.

Reformulating the preliminary thesis I may say: Man acts and is acted upon as a being directed in itself toward a "whither" whatever

[2] I refer to the logical tools of Gestalt psychology which realizes the insufficiency of a logic that starts from a multitude of elements and their relations.

this whither may be or at any given moment seems to be. He lives in a world on which he depends. His life is his relation to his world. The world, however, is not merely the sum total of the things in the world. Nor is our relation to our world the sum total of our relations to the things in the world. Single things are to us what they are in the context of our world as a whole. In all our meddling and wrestling with things we wrestle with and woo the world as a whole in a loud or mute give and take, understanding and misunderstanding, power and devotion. So far as we deal with single things, all our "whithers" are finite, though behind each stands another that again is finite—in an endless finiteness. So far as we relate single things to the whole of our being or to our world as a whole (we can not do the one without the other) an ultimate horizon and in it an ultimate whither become visible, which is not the next step. In fact, it is no step at all, not even the last one, because it is not an element of a sequence.

Art is but an example. Though nowadays registered under entertainment business, it was born as a child of religion and entrusted with making visible its ultimate horizon. Art could outlive any religious faith but never the ultimate horizon. The ultimate horizon is not a monopoly of either religion or art. You love someone. The ultimate horizon is present though your theories about love may prevent you from recognizing its presence. You are confronted with a cause you would fight for, whatever words you choose to use. It is by referring the cause to an ultimate horizon, embracing your world as a whole, that you would fight for it. You "evaluate." You do it in two ways: by relating single things or actions to other things or actions in the endless finiteness of your chains of means and ends; or by referring one thing to the whole of your world, to an ultimate horizon bordering this whole. In the second, you may happen to use the term "value." Again it does not matter which terms you use. Let us assume that a social scientist tries honestly to prove that there are no values, but only wants and desires that bring about valuations. He may even succeed. Yet he can not help either looking at his own honesty in an ultimate horizon or admitting that he is not serious.

An any moment any link in one of the endless chains of our ordinary life can be referred to an ultimate horizon of our world as a whole. Without such reference it need not be serious. None of our games that are merely play, such as bridge or chess, has an ultimate horizon;

nor have the endless chains of causes and effects, means and ends, in the so-called seriousness of our ordinary life, as far as you conceive of life as a linkage of chains in which any horizon is only particular and no end ultimate. Whenever an ultimate horizon grips the whole of our being our playing is no longer "merely" playing, ordinary life is bound to be serious, and our concern with whatever it is is really real concern.

It is the ultimate horizon that lets both our play and ordinary life be serious—as the one thing nobody can play with, unless it disappears.

Thus the preliminary thesis, reshaped, can deal with the antithesis. Play may be a triumph of freedom; culture may contain an element of play. Since, however, the very life of culture is nothing else than an ultimate horizon, made visible, this playing never acknowledges a "merely." But the question goes on growing and the thesis remains preliminary. Heraclitus, watching boys playing in the holy grove of the temple of the Ephesian Diana, said: "Aeon is a boy who plays and moves the pawns to and fro." Though you may think of the world as God's play, you are not God. What is "merely" to such a God is "not merely" to you.

Philosophy on the Bleachers*

GEORGE SANTAYANA

In this early summer there is always an answer ready for the man who asks you, "Why do you go to games, why do you waste your time upon the bleachers?" The balm of the air, the lazy shadows of the afternoon, when it is too warm for a walk and too early for dinner, the return of the slack tide between lectures and examinations—all form a situation in which the path of least resistance often leads to Holmes Field. But although these motives lie ready as an excuse, and we may find them plausible, there remains a truer and less expressible interest behind. Motives are always easy to assign, unless we wish to get at the real one. Those little hypocrisies of daily life by which we elude the evils of self-analysis can blind us to our most respectable feelings. We make ourselves cheap to make ourselves intelligible. How often, for instance, do people excuse themselves, as it were, for going to church; the music is so good, the parson such an old friend, the sermon so nearly a discourse of reason. Yet these evasions leave untouched the ultimate cause why churches exist and why people go to them—a cause not to be assigned without philosophy. And it seems to me that similarly in this phenomenon of athletics there is an underlying force, a power of human nature, that commonly escapes us. We talk of the matter with a smile as of a fad or a frolic, a meaningless pastime to which serious things are in danger of being sacrificed. Towards the vague idea of these "serious

* From *Harvard Monthly*, XVIII (July, 1894), 181-190.

things," which might upon inspection be reduced almost without a remainder to the getting of money, we assume an attitude of earnest concern, and we view the sudden irruption of the sporting spirit with alarm and deprecation, but without understanding. Yet some explanation of the monster might perhaps be given, and as I have here a few pages to fill and nothing of moment to communicate, I allow my pen to wander in the same direction as my feet, for a little ramble in the athletic field.

If it is not mere indolence that brings the spectators to our games, neither is it the mere need of healthy exercise that brings the players. The least acquaintance with them or their spirit is enough to convince one of this truth; and yet both friends and enemies of athletics are sometimes found speaking of them as a means of health, as an exercise to keep the mind clear and the body fit for work. That is a function which belongs rather to gymnastics, although the training for games may incidentally accomplish it. If health was alone or chiefly pursued, why should we not be satisfied with some chest-weights in our bedroom, a walk, or a ride, or a little swimming in summer? What could be gained by organized teams, traditional rivalries, or great contests where much money is spent and some bones possibly broken? It is amusing to hear people who are friendly to athletics by instinct or associations labouring to justify them on this ground. However much one may love buoyancy and generosity, and hate a pinched and sordid mind, one cannot help yielding the victory to the enemy when the battle is waged upon this utilitarian ground. Even arguments like those which the *New York Nation*, a paper often so intelligent, propounded not long ago on the subject of football, might then seem relevant, and if relevant conclusive. We should be led to believe that since athletics outrun the sphere of gymnastics, they have no sphere at all. The question why, then, they have come to exist would then pertinently occur, and might lead to unexpected results; but it is a question which the *Nation* and those of like mind need not answer, since to be silent is an ancient privilege of man of which the wise often avail themselves.

Now athletics have a higher function than gymnastics and a deeper basis than utility. They are a response to a natural impulse and exist only as an end in themselves. That is the reason why they have a kind of nobility which the public is quick to recognize, and why "professionalism" is so fatal to them. Professionalism introduces an alien and mercenary motive; but the valetudinarian motive is no less alien, and only harmless because so limited in scope. When the French, for instance shocked at the feeble health and ugliness of their school-boys, send commissioners to England and America to study athletics and the possibility of introducing them into France, the visitors return horrified at the brutality of Anglo-Saxon youth, and recommend some placid kind of foot-ball or some delightful form of non-competitive rowing, as offering all the advantages of fresh air and exercise, without the dangers and false excitements of the English practices. Any gymnastics, with or without pink tights, the French may easily introduce; they are no whit inferior to other nations in this field, as the professional circus can testify. But to introduce athletics into France there must be more than a change of ministry; there would have to be a change of ancestry. For such things are in the blood, and the taste and capacity for them must be inborn or developed by national experiences.

From a certain point of view we may blame athletic enthusiasm as irrational. The athletic temper is indeed not particularly Athenian, not vivacious, sensitive, or intelligent. It is rather Spartan, active, courageous, capable of serious enthusiasm and more ready to endure discipline than to ask for an ultimate reason for that devotion. But this reproach of irrationality ultimately falls upon every human interest, since all in the last analysis rest upon an instinct and not upon a rational necessity. Among the Greeks, to be sure, games had a certain relation to war; some of the contests were with weapons, and were valued for developing martial qualities of soul and body. The relation of athletics to war is intimate, but it is not one of means to end, but more intrinsic, like that of the drama to life. It was not the utility of athletics for war that supported the Greek games; on the contrary, the games arose from the comparative freedom from war, and the consequent liberation of martial energy from the stimulus of necessity, and the expression of it in beautiful and spectacular forms. A certain analogy to war, a certain semblance of dire struggle, are therefore the essence of athletics. Like war, they demand an organization of activities for the sake of victory. But here the victory is not sought for the sake of any further advantage. There is nothing to conquer or defend except the honour of success. War can thus become a luxury and flower into artistic forms, whenever the circumstances of life no longer drain all the energy native to the character. For this reason athletics flourish only among nations that are comparatively young, free, and safe, like the Greek towns and those American and Australian communities which, in athletics as distinguished from private sport, bid fair to outdo their mother country.

The essential distinction between athletics and gymnastics may help us to understand some other characteristics of our sports. They must, for instance, be confined to a few. Where so much time, skill and endurance are required, as in great athletic contests, the majority is necessarily excluded. If we were dealing with an instrument of health, a safety-valve or balance wheel to an overstrained system, the existence of an athletic aristocracy would be an anomaly. But the case is otherwise. We are dealing with an art in which only the few, the exceptionally gifted, can worthily succeed. Nature must be propitious, circumstances must be favourable, patience and inspiration must not fail. There is an athletic aristocracy for the same reason that there is one of intelligence and one of fashion, because men have different endowments, and only a few can do each thing as well as it is capable of being done. Equality in these respects would mean total absence of excellence. The analogy of moral and practical things would mislead us in this sphere. Comfort or happiness would seem to lose nothing of their value if they were subdivided, and a proportional fraction given to each individual: such an equal distribution of them might even seem a gain, since it would prevent envy, and satisfy a certain sense of mathematical justice. But the opposite happens in the arts. The value of talent, the beauty and dignity of positive achievements, depend on the height reached, and not on the number that reach it. Only the supreme is interesting: the rest has value only as leading to it or reflecting it. Still, although the achievement is rare, the benefit of it is diffused; we all participate through the imagination in the delight and meaning of what lies beyond our power of accomplishment. A few moments of enjoyment and intuition, scattered throughout our lives, are what lift the whole of it from vulgarity. They form a background of comparison, a standard of values, and a magnet for the estimation of tendencies, without which all our thought would be perfunctory and dull. Enthroned in those best moments, art, religion, love, and the other powers of the imagination, govern our character, and silently direct the current of our common thoughts.

Now, in its sphere, athletic sport has a parallel function. A man whose enthusiasm it has stirred in youth, has one more chamber in his memory, one more approach to things, and a manlier standard of pleasures and pains. An interesting task for somebody with adequate knowledge of antiquity would be to trace the influence which athletics had among the Greeks; I fancy it might be shown to permeate their poetry, to dominate their sculpture, and strangely to colour their sentiment. And this influence would come not chiefly from the practice but from the spectacle of games, just as the supposed brutalizing tendency of bull fighting is not conceived to stop with the performers within the ring, but to cross the barrier and infect the nation. Athletic sports are not children's games; they are public spectacles in which young men, carefully trained and disciplined, contend with one another in feats of strength, skill, and courage. Spectators are indispensable, since without them the victory, which should be the only reward, would lose half its power. For as Pindar, who knew, tells us:

Success
Is half the prize, the other half renown.
Who both achieves, he hath the perfect crown.

A circumstance which somewhat perplexes this whole matter is the prevalent notion that athletics have a necessary relation to colleges. They have, indeed, a necessary relation to youth, because the time of greatest physical pliability and alertness is soon over; and as those of our youth who unite leisure with spirit are generally at some university, it happens that universities and colleges have become the centres of athletic interest. But this is an accident; a military or local organization of any sort would be as natural an athletic unit as a college. That athletic teams should bear the name of an institution of learning, and materially influence its reputation and fortune, is at first sight very strange; but the explanation is not far to seek. The English academic tradition, founded upon the clerical life of the middle ages, has always maintained a broad conception of education. All that an aristocratic family might wish to provide for its boys, that the schools and colleges provided. They contained the student's whole life, and they allowed a free and just development to all his faculties. The masters' province did not stop in the schoolroom, nor the professors' in the lecture hall. When possible they shared in the social and athletic life of the boys, and when not possible they at least gave it their heartiest support, making every reasonable concession to it; or, rather, not feeling that such friendliness was a concession at all, since they did not undertake merely the verbal education of their pupils, but had as broad an interest in their pursuits as the pupils themselves, or their parents. I remember a master at Eton, a man of fifty and a clergyman, running along the towpath in a sweater to watch the eight, a thing considered in no way singular or beneath his dignity. On the same principle, and on that principle alone, religious teaching and worship fall within the sphere of a college. To this system is due that beauty, individuality, and wealth of associations which make English colleges so beloved and venerable. They have a value which cannot be compensated or represented by any lists of courses or catalogues of libraries—the value of a rounded and traditional life.

But even in England this state of things is disappearing. If we renounce it in this country, we need not suffer a permanent loss, provided the interests which are dropped by the colleges find some other social embodiment. Such a division of functions might even conduce to the efficiency of each; as is observed in the case of the German universities which, as compared with the English, are more active in investigation and more purely scientific in spirit, precisely because they have a more abstract function and minister to but one side of the mind. The real loss would come if a merely scientific and technical training were to pass for a human one, and a liberal education were conceived to be possible without leisure, or a generous life without any of those fruits of leisure of which athletics are one. Plato, who was beginning to turn his back upon paganism and held the un-Greek doctrine that the body should be cultivated only for the sake of the mind, nevertheless assigns in his scheme of education seven years to the teacher of the arts and seven to the athletic trainer. This equality, I fancy, would seem to us improper only because the study and cultivation of bodily life is yet a new thing among us. Physically we are barbarians, as is proved by our clothes, our furniture, and our appearance. To bathe was not Christian before this century. But the ascetic prejudice which survives in some of our habits no longer governs our deliberate judgments. Whatever functions, then, we may wish our colleges to have we shall not frown long upon athletic practices altogether. The incoherences of our educational policy cannot permanently alter our social conditions or destroy the basis which athletics have in the instincts of the people.

Into physical discipline, however, a great deal can enter that is not athletics. There are many sports that have nothing competitive in them. Some of them, like angling, involve enough of mild excitement and of intercourse with nature to furnish good entertainment to the lovers of them, although not enough to amuse a looker-on. The reason is that angling is too easy; it requires, no doubt, a certain skill, but the effort is not visible and glorious enough, it has no relation to martial or strenuous qualities. The distinction between athletics and private sport is that between an art and an amusement. The possibility of vicarious interest in the one and its impossibility in the other are grounded on the meaning which athletics have, on their appeal to the imagination. There is in them a great and continuous endeavour, a representation of all the primitive virtues and fundamental gifts of man. The conditions alone are artificial, and when well combined are even better than any natural conditions for the enacting of this sort of physical drama, a drama in which all moral and emotional interests are in a manner involved. For in real life the latter are actually superposed upon physical struggles. Intelligence and virtue are weapons in life, powers that make, as our Darwinian philosophy has it, for survival; science is a plan of campaign and poetry a cry of battle, sometimes of one who cheers us on, sometimes of one who is wounded. Therefore, when some well-conceived contest, like our foot-ball, displays the dramatic essence of physical conflict, we watch it with an interest which no gymnastic feat, no vulgar tricks of the circus or of legerdemain, can ever arouse. The whole soul is stirred by a spectacle that represents the basis of its life.

But besides the meaning which athletic games may have as physical dramas, they are capable, like other tragedies, of a great aesthetic development. This development they have not had in modern times, but we have only to conceive a scene at Olympia, or in a Roman amphitheatre, to see what immense possibilities lie in this direction. Our own games, in which no attention is paid to the aesthetic side, are themselves full of unconscious effects, which a practiced eye watches with delight. The public, however, is not sufficiently trained, nor the sports sufficiently developed, for this merit to be conspicuous. Such as it is, however, it contributes to our interest and helps to draw us to the games.

The chief claim which athletics make upon our respect remains yet unmentioned. They unite vitality with disinterestedness. The curse of our time is industrial supremacy, the sacrifice of every spontaneous faculty and liberal art to the demands of an overgrown material civilization. Our labour is servile and our play frivolous. Religion has long tended to change from a consolation into a puzzle, and to substitute unnatural checks for supernatural guidance. Art sometimes becomes an imposition, too; instead of delight and entertainment, it brings us the awful duty of culture. Our Muse, like Donna Inez, makes

Her thoughts a theorem, her words a problem,
As if she deemed that mystery would ennoble
'em.

One cannot read verse without hard thought and a dictionary. This irksome and cumbrous manner in the arts is probably an indirect effect of the too great prevalence of practical interests. We carry over into our play the principles of labour. When the stress of life and the niggardliness of nature relax a little and we find it possible for a moment to live as we will, we find ourselves helpless. We cannot comprehend our opportunity, and like the prisoner of Chillon we regain our freedom with a sigh. The saddest effect of moral servitude is this atrophy of the spontaneous and imaginative will. We grow so accustomed to hard conditions that they seem necessary to us, and their absence inconceivable, so that religion, poetry, and the arts, which are the forms in which the soul asserts its independence, languish inwardly in the midst of the peace and riches that should foster them most. We have regained political and religious liberty, but moral freedom—the faculty and privilege of each man under the laws to live and act according to his inward nature—we scarcely care to have. The result is that while, in Greece, Sparta could exist beside Athens, Socrates besides Alcibiades, and Diogenes beside Alexander, we have in the United States seventy millions of people seized with the desire of absolutely resembling one another in dress, speech, habits, and dignities, and not one great or original man among them, except, perhaps, Mr. Edison.

It may seem a ridiculous thing, and yet I think it true, that our athletic life is the most conspicuous and promising rebellion against this industrial tyranny. We elude Mammon only for a few years, which the Philistines think are wasted. We succumb to him soon after leaving college. We sell our birthright for a mess of pottage, and the ancestral garden of the mind for building lots. That garden too often runs to seed, even if we choose a liberal profession, and is overgrown with the thistles of a trivial and narrow scholarship. But while we are young, and as yet amount to nothing, we retain the privilege of infinite potentiality. The poor actuality has not yet taken its place, and in giving one thing made everything else for ever unattainable. But in youth the intellectual part is too immature to bear much fruit; that would come later if the freedom could be retained. The body alone has reached perfection, and very naturally the physical life is what tends to occupy the interval of leisure

with its exuberances. Such is the origin of our athletics. Their chief value is that they are the first fruits of that spontaneous life, of which the higher manifestations are not suffered to appear. Perhaps it is well that the body should take the lead, since that is the true and safe order of nature. The rest, if it comes, will then rest on a sounder basis.

When I hear, therefore, the cheering at our great games, when I watch, at Springfield or at New London, the frenzy of joy of the thousands upon one side and the grim and pathetic silence of the thousands upon the other, I cannot feel that the passion is excessive. It might seem so if we think only of what occurs at the moment. But would the game or the race as such be capable of arousing that enthusiasm? Is there not some pent-up energy in us, some thirst for enjoyment and for self-expression, some inward rebellion against a sordid environment, which here finds inarticulate expression? Is not the same force ready to bring us into other arenas, in which, as in those of Greece, honour should come not only to strength, swiftness, and beauty, but to every high gift and inspiration? Such a hope is almost justified by my athletic philosophy, which, with little else, perhaps, to recommend it, I herewith submit to the gentle reader. It may help him, if he receives it kindly, to fill up the waits at a game, while the captains wrangle, and to see in fancy greener fields than Holmes's from the bleachers.

Why Men Run*

J. KENNETH DOHERTY

Why do men run? The wisest answer would undoubtedly be given by a child, or by a runner, or by a Zen Master; without saying a word, they each would start running. Men do run. That may be the most penetrating reason of all as to why they run. It tells us, beyond all words and abstractions, they are made *for* running, and have been made as they are *by* running.

Why do men run? A physiologist might answer that they run because they have running bodies: running hearts, running lungs, running muscles, running bones. Without a long racial history of running, these would not be what they are.

Man is a land animal. His use of other land animals for transportation has been limited and part-time. His use of machines is a last-minute innovation. For untold ages he has had to depend upon himself whenever and wherever he wanted to go. Sometimes he wanted to go in a hurry. Thus, he ran, and by running he became a man-that-runs. Had he stuck to walking, he would not be as he is today. The maximum stroke volume of his heart would never have reached the 200 cc of blood, nor its effective number of beats the 180 or so per minute that a trained runner's heart puts forth. His muscles would have contained only a fraction of the current 317 billion blood capillaries.

A historian might explain that men run because running is deep in our social history. We are all familiar with the glorious run of Pheidippides from the battle ground of Marathon to cry, "Victory!" in the market-place of Athens. All peoples have such tales of great running. Students of the ancient Inca civilization have become aware that the very extensive system of roads throughout the widespread Inca territory was entirely for foot travel, and more specifically, for running. They had no horses or other animals for rapid transportation. Messages were sent by relay runners, each of whom ran about a mile in distance, carrying knotted ropes by which to refresh their memories of the details they were to transmit by word of mouth. Much of this running was done at 9000 feet or more over the Andes mountains, so that training must have been a matter of studious concern. Other examples from other lands could be cited.

Why do men run? A sociologist might explain man's running on the basis of the strong awareness of need that modern nations have for running, and therefore of the high recognition they give to those who succeed in it. Running is the foremost activity of all the Olympic Games. It attracts more spectators, more world-wide attention, and more representatives from more nations than any other (8:62). The rising new nations of the world are keenly aware of this showcase and of society's tendency to accept the victory of even one man as proof of the virility of an entire nation (12:47). It has not been by chance that the 1960 Olympic marathon was won by an unknown from Ethiopia, or that most of the recent world-records in running have been made by men from Australia and New Zealand.

* From *Quest*, II (April, 1964), 61-66.

To understand why men run, a sociologist also might well turn to Finland where, between 1912 and 1952, a total of a mere four millions of people produced more Olympic champions in running than any other nation. A great social need and readiness, born out of Finland's struggle for independence from the heavy hand of Russia is in evidence. Our sociologist would find that it was individual achievement which turned this social readiness into widespread participation and dedication. The victories of Kohlemainen and Stenroos over the 1912 Olympic world excited the Finnish people tremendously. They made heroes of their runners. Villages even a hundred miles north of the Arctic circle set up running clubs and excellent running facilities.

Why do men run? Psychologists might answer that to run is satisfying to the individual, that it is a "natural" activity providing a sense of achievement for its own sake. Psychologists might quote Roger Bannister, M.D., who found in running—win or lose—". . . a deep satisfaction that I cannot express in any other way . . . . I sometimes think that running has given me a glimpse of the greatest freedom that a man can ever know, because it results in the simultaneous liberation of both body and mind" (1:229). Or they might quote a great coach of runners, Arthur Lydiard of New Zealand, who said of running, "It is a simply unalloyed joy to tackle yourself on the battlefield of your own physical well-being and come out the victor" (10:46).

Psychologists also may find great resources for study in the small-group dynamics of running. England's former mile champion, Bill Nankerville, has written (11:26) of a closely-knit group of non-school running enthusiasts who nourished each other toward international levels of performance. Such great Irish runners as R. M. N. Tisdall, Ron Delany, and Noel Carroll developed out of small running clubs and the leadership and energy of individuals such as Billy Morton of Dublin. The great Gunder Haegg of Sweden probably never would have run competitively if his own father and his friends had not been interested in running and in turn motivated him (6:14). Herb Elliott also has written of his father's passion for running fitness and of their jogs on the long sea beaches when Herb was but a boy of seven (5:9). Examples could be extended endlessly.

But even more endless would be the research to ferret out the cross-currents of racial inheritances, social customs and mores, institutional incentives, famliy expectations, encouragements of friends, as well as the personal aggressions, impulsions, insecurities, and frustrations that can and do motivate men to run.

One of the most discerning stories of long distance running is by Alan Sillitoe, *The Loneliness of the Long Distance Runner*. When the big race is about two-thirds over, the "hero's" impulsion to prove his worth forced him to pour it on, ". . . so by the haystack I decided to leave it all behind and put on such a spurt, in spite of the nails in my guts, that before long I'd left both Gunthorpe and the birds a good way off" (13:34). Yet his sense of what he called honesty and realness would not let him win; or rather, would not let his dishonest trainer-jailer win through his efforts. In full sight of the finish line and the crowd, he deliberately slowed down, waited for his opponent to break the tape, then finished with his back straight and his eyes looking disdainfully into those of his trainer.

Few readers will suffer or even understand the twisted life that produced such a twisted motivation, but many will run with a similar tangle of likes and dislikes, tenacity and weakness, of which they are quite unaware and certainly could never put into words.

When a boy first starts to run competitively, his motives tend to be of as low an order as are his performances: to win a medal or a varsity letter, to make the team, to be one of the gang, to get one's picture in the school paper or yearbook. At this stage he is likely to understand verbal motives that are only a short step beyond what he has already experienced. The coach who emphasizes only the deeply hidden satisfactions that lie in hard work and self-discipline will find his words wasted. Even such a sensitive person as Roger Bannister admitted that, as a boy, he took up running as an escape from the gibes of his school-mates so that he would be free to do what really interested him: to be active as a student, a musician, and an actor (1:35).

Some obstacle becomes a challenge to these boys, some annoyance becomes a hobby, some inspiration cries out, "Begin!" But inspiration produces only the first few steps. During early stages, the runner may need a sort of baby's walker to hold him erect, and a fatherly voice to give encouragement. Until he was sure Gunder could go it alone, Haegg's father devised endless ways, even falsifying times on one occasion, to develop his son's confidence and belief in his future as a runner.

In the later stages, motivation emerges holistically in ways that remind us of Coghill's concept of individuation (4:19-20, 88). In fact, in a few instances, running becomes almost an inescapable way of life, and certainly the focus of life. In 1957, at the age of 68, Clarence DeMar competed in a 10-mile race, notwithstanding the presence of a surgical colostomy (2:81). In 1963, at the age of 65, Percy Cerutty of Australia offered to run from Los Angeles to New York simply to demonstrate the values of running (14:8).

Of course, some men, by body structure and chemistry, are better made for and by running than others. For these men, distance running is a challenge even when it is a hardship; play even when they slave at it; fun, even when they hate it. Cerutty wrote, "Running at its best is an outpouring, a release from tensions. . . . An hour, two hours of hard training slips away as so many minutes. We become tired, exhaustingly tired, but never unhappy. It is work but it seems only fun. Exhilarating, satisfying fun" (3:17).

We may understand this statement when we realize that such attitudes were developed at Camp Portsea, Australia, where men ran along the beautiful seacoast, up great sand dunes, across open country, sometimes nude, then back, following Cerutty's uninhibited methods, to plunge at last in the cold sea. It may be harder to understand the motivations of the Englishman, W. R. Loader, who has described his early training experiences through the sooty brick and stone deserts of Clyneside, Tyneside, and Merseyside, with their coke ovens, foundries, shipyards, blast furnaces, and machine shops. In one instance he had to run through a certain tough district of his town where the handicaps of terrain were as nothing compared with the derisive jeers of the onlookers, especially of the girls:

"Yah, look at the runner coming! . . . Mary Ann, look, it's a runner! He's got nae claes on!" Faces rose up all around, derisive, jeering, insulting. A scabby mongrel dog snapped at the heels, delighted for once to discover that someone else's life was being made a misery. Urchins sprinted alongside, mocking the runner's strides with their own exaggerated movements. It was a torment of the soul far more bitter than any torture of the body. And through it all one had to run with measured step, eyes fixed ahead as if unaware of the tumult, trying to abolish it by ignoring it. . . . But it is a hard thing for youth to set itself alone against spite and hostility. I did that run a number of times and never faced it without a premonitary chill of the spine. Having stood the jeers to the point where I could persuade myself I wasn't giving up through cowardice, I quietly abandoned the practice. (9:61)

Although Loader's experiences and his way of relating them may seem unusual, the hindrances and distractions of social environment often are deterrents to why men run, or better, why men continue to run. Herb Elliott was only 22 when he retired from running; his best running years potentially were still ahead of him. But following his world-record at Dublin in 1959, he was granted a three-year scholarship at Cambridge University and, along with his regular studies, had to cram a four-year Latin course into nine months. He met and married Ann Dudley and had a son and often found himself thinking of his family debts while listening to Cerutty's exhortations toward greater running efforts.

Percy and I weren't on the same wave-length . . . . It surely wasn't indolence that kept me from training. It was my realization that as a family man . . . training was not as important in my career . . . . Running was a job that had to be fitted in between my other activities. (5:88)

We must accept the fact, therefore, that the demands of vocation and family and everyday fun do limit the kind and amount of running that men do. That amateur running is avocational is an even more essential concept than that it must receive no material reward.

I began this article by saying that men, even modern men, are men-that-run, that their vital organs and systems and chemistry are as they are partly because man ran long before he became homo sapiens. To say that running is socially recognized or personally satisfying cheapens the argument, makes running an artificial action that waits upon cultural whims and gadgets. Running is not so much a tool of the new emerging nations as an inherent part of man-society-nature interactions. Not to run, even to a modern man, is as unthinkable as not to eat, or not to sleep, or not to make love.

But try as I may, I shall never say it as well as did Brutus Hamilton, head coach of the University of California and the 1948 U.S. Olympic track team:

People may wonder why young men like to run distance races. What fun is it? Why all that hard, exhausting work? Where is the good of it? It is one of the strange ironies of this strange life that those who work the hardest, who subject themselves to the strictest discipline, who give up certain pleasurable things in order to achieve a goal, are the happiest of men. When you see 20 or 30 young men line up for a distance race in some meet, don't pity them, don't feel sorry for them. Better envy them instead. You are probably looking at the 20 or 30 best "bon vivants" in the world. They are completely and joyously happy in their simple tastes, their strong and well-conditioned bodies, and with the thrill of wholesome competition before them. These are the days of their youth, when they can run without weariness; these are their buoyant, golden days; and they are running because they love it. Their lives are fuller because of this competition and their memories will be far richer. That's why men love to run. That's why men do run. There is something clean and noble about it. (7:7)

REFERENCES

1. Bannister, Roger. *The Four Minute Mile.* New York: Dodd, Mead & Company, 1955.
2. Bock, Arlie V. "The Circulation of a Marathoner," *The Journal of Sports Medicine and Physical Fitness, III* (June-September, 1963).
3. Cerutty, Percy. "Running with Cerutty," *Track and Field News,* 1959.
4. Coghill, G. E. *Anatomy and the Problem of Behavior.* New York: Cambridge University Press, American Branch, 1929.
5. Elliott, Herb, as told to Alan Trengrove. *The Golden Mile.* London: Cassell & Company, Ltd., 1961.
6. Haegg, Gunder. *Gunder Haegg's Dagbook.* Stockholm: Tidens Forlag, 1952.
7. Hamilton, Brutus. "Why Men Like To Run," *Coaching Newsletter,* II (July, 1957).
8. Jokl, Ernst, et al. *Sports In The Cultural Pattern Of The World.* A paper prepared for the Institute of Occupational Health, Helsinki, 1956.
9. Loader, W. R. *Testament Of A Runner.* London: William Heinemann Ltd., 1960.
10. Lydiard, Arthur and Garth Gilmour. *Run To The Top.* London: Herbert Jenkins, Ltd., 1962.
11. Nankeville, Bill. *The Miracle Of The Mile.* London: Stanley Paul and Co., Ltd., 1956.
12. Natan, Alex. "Sport and Politics," *Sport And Society.* London: Bowes & Bowes, Ltd., 1958.
13. Sillitoe, Alan. *The Loneliness of the Long Distance Runner.* New York: New American Library of World Literature, 1959.
14. *Track and Field News,* September, 1963.

The Symbolic Power of Sport*

ELEANOR METHENY

For some years now I have been trying to enrich my own understanding of the educational potential of sport by talking with people who know much more about sport than I do. I have talked with football players who have told me that playing football is one of the most meaningful experiences of their lives. I have heard one lineman talk about "the explosion of joy" he experiences whenever he brings every ounce of his 240 pounds into play. "It's beautiful," he said; and then he added: "I've never said that word out loud before—but it is the right word, and I want to say it."

I have seen a gymnast's eyes grow bright with tears of genuine emotion as he talked about the feeling of wholeness he finds in doing a giant swing. And I have heard a ping pong player say: "Maybe this sounds silly—but somehow for me its the greatest—the most. I don't know how to say this, but somehow all of me is there when I knock that silly little ball back and forth across the table—and it is important in a way I can't describe."

I asked her if she knew Wallace Stevens' lines about an experience that was "like a flow of meanings with no speech—and of as many meanings as of men." She liked these lines, and she wrote them down, saying: "Yes, that's what ping pong is. Was Wallace Stevens a ping pong player?"

And again and again these men and women

* Presented at the Annual Convention of the Eastern District Association for Health, Physical Education and Recreation, Washington, D.C., April 26, 1968.

—and boys and girls—who have found such important meanings in sport competition said: "I've never said these things out loud before." And most of them said: "Thank you for giving me a chance to talk about these things." And one veteran coach said: "It is good to know that one physical educator understands and cares about sport in this way. How wonderful it would be if they could all stand up and 'tell it like it is' without yakking around about physical fitness and character building."

None of them quoted the poetry of Wallace Stevens to me—but many of them recognized this bit of verse as a statement of their own feelings about sport competition.

> I measure myself
> Against a tall tree.
> I find that I am much taller,
> For I reach right up to the sun
> With my eye. . .
>
> Nevertheless, I dislike
> The way the ants crawl
> In and out of my shadow.

Tonight I want to talk about some of the meanings I have found in my own experiences as a competitor on the symbolic field of sport, as a spectator, and as a physical educator. Much of what I shall say is a composite of what I have learned in many conferences with men and women who love sport as much as you do —and with the same ambivalence—and for the same reasons. So perhaps you may wish to validate some of my generalizations by exploring your own feelings about your own favorite form of sport competition as we go along.

No one knows how long men have been competing with each other on the rule-governed field of sport. No one knows when the first rule-governed sport contest was held. But certainly the custom of holding sport contests at funerals was well established by the time of the Trojan Wars—which were fought during the 12th century B.C. And fortunately for all historians, Homer did describe one of these symbolic contests in the *Iliad*—which was written some four hundred years later. So I shall start with this chapter in the long and always controversial history of sport.

As you probably remember, Patroclus was a nobleman, a warrior, and a hero who died on the bloody plains of Troy. In his brief lifetime, he had done well and gloriously all that the gods might expect of such a man; he had done well and gloriously all that such a man might expect of himself. And so, at his funeral, his companions thought it fitting to remind the gods of "the excellence of Patroclus" by re-enacting some of his glorious deeds on the man-made field of sport.

Thus, his companions threw javelins, hurled stones, drove horse-drawn chariots at full speed, ran as fast as they could run, and wrestled with each other in hand-to-hand combat. But they did not perform these actions in the same way that Patroclus had performed them in the heat of battle.

On the battlefield a warrior is not interested in demonstrating how far he can throw a spear. He is interested in killing his enemies, and in saving his own life. As he throws his spear at other men who may be running toward him with their own spears at the ready, he must adjust his aim and force to the requirements of the moment, and he must keep his own guard up to ward off the spears and arrows of the enemy. As he throws, other warriors may jostle him, his feet may slip in the muck, he may be off balance, or his throw may be hampered or hindered by any one of a dozen other circumstances. Thus, he seldom gets a chance to throw his spear as far as he can possibly throw it by giving it everything he has.

In the funeral competitions, the Greek warriors created this chance for themselves. They ruled out the hindering and hampering requirements of war by defining the act of spear throwing as a voluntary action, which a man might choose to perform for his own reasons. They abstracted the pattern of the spear throwing action from the confusion of warfare

and described it as the inconsequential act of throwing a stick at empty space.

They specified when and where this action was to be performed by announcing a time for the competition and defining the boundaries of the field. They eliminated all need to debate about the motives and intentions of other men by imposing the same standards of conduct on all competitors—and by appointing an official judge who was empowered to enforce these man-made rules. And they answered all questions about how each man's performance might be evaluated by spelling out what "counted" in unequivocal terms.

Thus, as each man stepped up to the starting line on the rule-governed field of sport, he knew precisely what he was going to try to do; he knew how the outcomes of his efforts were to be evaluated—and by whom; and he knew that he had a fair chance to perform that action as well as he could perform it—a fair chance to exert his own utmost effort in the performance of one human action.

Freed of all the hampering effects of war, he was free to go all out, holding nothing back—free to focus all the energies of his being on one supreme attempt to hurl his javelin at the nothingness of empty space.

He was free to throw his stick as far as he could throw it. He was free to run as fast as he could run—to hit as hard as he could hit—to leap, to jump—as high, as far—as he could leap and jump. He was free to match his strength with the strength of other men in open combat. He was free to involve every fiber of his mortal being in the performance of one human action. He was free to focus all the forces of his being on one supreme attempt to impose his own man-made design on the universe of his existence.

The Greek warriors created this moment of freedom for themselves—and for all men—by devising the most restrictive set of rules men have ever made for themselves. They devised the prototype of the man-made rules that now govern all sport competition.

These rules are paradoxical. They restrict in order to free. They impose restrictions on human behavior, and they limit human action; but within those restrictions they offer every man an opportunity to know the feeling of being wholly free to go all out—free to do his utmost—free to use himself fully in the performance of one self-chosen human action.

These paradoxical rules create this man-made moment of freedom by ruling out the conditions and considerations of human reality, and by ruling in the pattern of an idealized world in which every man might be and do whatever he is capable of being and doing—an ideal world in which every man might be free to pursue his own interests—an ideal world in which every man might function at his best—an ideal world in which every man might make full use of all the energies of his mortal being, unhampered and unhindered by the demands imposed by the realities of his existence.

Or we might say, in the words of Wallace Stevens, the rules of sport propose

A new text for the world,
A scribble of fret and fear and fate,
From a bravura of the mind,
A courage of the eye . . .
A text of intelligent men
At the center of the unintelligible . . .

In the funeral competitions, the Greek warriors did not show the gods how well Patroclus had actually performed the actions of his life in the heat of battle. They showed the gods—and other men—how well each competitor actually did perform the empty action of throwing a javelin through space under ideal circumstances which offered each competitor a fair chance to do his utmost as a man among men.

Perhaps we would all like to think that the Greek warriors performed these symbolic actions with great dignity. Perhaps we would like to think that all men exhibit their best behavior on the symbolic field of sport. But Homer's description of the funeral games does not support this exalted theory. And neither do our own experiences.

So let it be said to the glory of the Greek warriors—and to the glory of all competitors from that day to this—that most of them did honor their own restrictive man-made rules. They did give every man who entered into the competitions a fair chance to function at his utmost. But they also argued with the officials and with each other. They boasted; they bragged; they belittled the powers of other men; they devised strategies that gave them advantage over other competitors; and some of them cheated when the officials were not looking. They were aggressive; they displayed their hostilities; and they revealed all their anxious doubts and fears about themselves, their gods, and other men on the symbolic field of sport.

The actions men perform in sport are indeed symbolic actions—but a sport contest is not a ritual. It is not a symbolic pageant. It is not a cool-headed philosophical debate about human motives and values. It is an emotional moment of commitment to the values of human action—and the emotions aroused by that commitment and those actions are powerful emotions.

In that moment of commitment to the values he attaches to his own human actions, no competitor has time to rationalize about his own feelings and his own motivations. In that moment of all-out action he must experience himself as he is, in all the complexity of his own feelings about himself, his gods, and other men who claim the right to share the universe of his existence.

Or, as the competitors in the early Olympic Games put it, on the symbolic field of sport "every man stands naked before his gods" and reveals himself as he is in the fullness of his own human powers. Stripped of all self-justifying excuses by the rules of sport, he must involve himself in the performance of one self-chosen task. Naked of all pretense, he must use himself as he is, and he must demonstrate his ability to use himself fully, under circumstances which permit him to function in the wholeness of his being as a man.

If he is a proud man, he must experience his own pride. If he is a domineering man, he must experience his own need to dominate the lives of other men. So, too, a neurotic man must use sport to satisfy his own neurotic needs; a resentful man must know his own resentments; and an anxious man his anxieties. An idealistic man must recognize his ideals—and the conflicts he experiences as he tries to live up to those ideals; a loving man will reveal his love; and a fearful hating man will experience his own fearful hate.

Yes, a man may learn much about himself—and about all men—on the symbolic field of sport. In those self-revealing moments of commitment to the values of human action he may know himself at his best—but equally he must also know himself at his worst. And he cannot escape the implications of either image because this is what he is, this is how he feels, and this is what he does in a situation that offers him a fair chance to use himself fully in the performance of one self-chosen human action.

Yes . . .   I measure myself
Against a tall tree.
I find that I am much taller,
For I reach right up to the sun
With my eye . . .

Nevertheless, I dislike
The way the ants crawl
In and out of my shadow.

Many of the sport contests invented by the companions of Patroclus have endured for more than three thousand years—and most of them were hotly contested in Mexico City. But human inventiveness in sport was not exhausted by the ingenuity of the Greeks.

During the Middle Ages, the kings and noblemen of feudal Europe found new ways to compete with each other in the colorful tournaments that symbolized their own excellence as warriors. They, too, took some of the practical and effective actions of their lives and redefined them as impractical and futile actions that produced nothing of material value. They, too, devised rules that gave every competitor a fair chance to use himself fully in the performance of one symbolic action.

For example, they converted the useful and necessary actions a nobleman might perform as he rode his horse into the thick of battle into a series of "knightly exercises;" and they competed with each other in the performance of these actions. In Mexico City, men and women still competed with each other in terms of their ability to perform those twisting, turning, hanging, swinging, and vaulting actions—but they did not ride into the arena on the back of a spirited horse. Rather, they performed those symbolic actions on the back of a stationary and leather-covered horse, and on other equally symbolic pieces of apparatus—familiar to all persons who have ever attended a gymnastic meet.

The hard-working peasants who tilled the fields of the feudal lords did not compete in their tournaments. In time of war they did not ride into battle on horseback. They slogged it out on foot, hurling huge rocks at the enemy, and pooled their strength in attempts to push heavy battering rams through the gates of neighboring strongholds.

Perhaps these hard-working peasants recognized the values of cooperative effort. Perhaps they recognized that men who are individually inconsequential can sometimes achieve their purposes by working together as a team. More probably they did not. But in either case, they did devise sport forms that exemplify this principle—for these hard-working peasants invented the prototype of all team sports.

Initially, these team competitions were little more than mass mayhem—because there were few rules and no officials in those days. One group of peasants tried to push a huge boulder in one direction; an opposing group tried to **push it in the opposite direction; and surely**

every peasant worked out many of his frustrations, his aggressions, and his hostilities as he got into the act. But gradually, rules were defined, the boundaries of the field were marked out, and sticks were set up to represent the gates of the enemy's castle—and you may see those symbolic gates today on the goal lines of every soccer, football, and hockey field. Gradually, too, the heavy rock was reduced in size, and took on the shape of a sphere—and eventually this sphere-shaped ball became the object of contest in many different team sports.

Much has been written about the ball as a symbolic representation of our ball-shaped earth. Perhaps the peasants who threw and kicked such balls on the symbolic field of sport noticed this resemblance; more probably they were not consciously aware of it. But in either case it may be noted that the ball did become a familiar object of contest at about the time Columbus proved that the world of man's existence is indeed a sphere.

As feudal Europe was gradually reorganized into the more complex social patterns of the Renaissance, the old feudal lords were transformed into a new class of human beings called gentlemen. These gentlemen did not work with their hands; they did not maintain their social position by displays of muscular power. Rather, they prided themselves on their ability to deal with the world by using their wits—and by employing all manner of strategic devices.

These gentlemen exhibited little interest in the rough team sports of the muscular peasants. Rather, they developed new sport forms which symbolized their own ways of dealing with the forces of mass, space, and time.

In the sports that symbolized the actions of gentlemen—as exemplified by tennis and golf—each man performed alone, or perhaps with one partner, and his opponents were always men of equal social rank. The rules for these sports prohibited any bodily contact between players, and there was little direct contact with the object of contest. Rather, a light ball was manipulated with a device or implement which greatly extended the player's reach and force; and this implement was wielded with skill, dexterity, and strategy, rather than with the greatest possible muscular effort.

Did these gentlemen recognize the resemblance between their sport effort and their conception of themselves as gentlemen who manipulated the things of earth with ease, skill, and light implements? Probably not. But we may conjecture that they found satisfaction in these sports because they were consonant with their own self-image.

Moving now toward our own time, we may note that the invention of new ball games came to an end during the 19th century—with the invention of basketball in 1891 and the invention of volleyball in 1895. And we may note that the new sports of the 20th century exhibit very different patterns of organization.

Today, men have extended their concern for the earthly globe to a vision of the farthest reaches of the universe, and their expectations of exploring that universe are based on their mastery over complex machines and atomic sources of power. Both of these conceptions are reflected in the new sport forms that have been developed in recent years.

In sky diving, for example, the diver utilizes the man-made power of mechanical flight to carry himself to the heights of the sky—from which he descends with great skill, using his parachute only in the final moments of the dive. In scuba diving, the diver uses the discoveries of modern science and technology to equip himself for his descent into the depths of the sea. And in all forms of mechanized racing, men control the power of motorized vehicles on land, on sea, and in the air—even as they may use these vehicles in machine-to-machine combat in such events as the destruction derby.

These new sports symbolize "the excellence of Patroclus" in terms that reflect the hopes, dreams, and accomplishments of men now living in the latter days of the 20th century—and it seems likely that many men and women, boys and girls, are interested in them for that reason. But, equally, many other men and women, boys and girls, are interested in performing the symbolic actions that the Greek warriors performed three thousand years ago. So we must not try to account for the symbolic power of sport by describing it in terms of the work men do.

Perhaps a contestant may find a particular sport particularly meaningful because it does formulate his conception of himself as a man who performs certain kinds of work. Perhaps he may also choose a sport because it formulates the basic patterns of his own personality structure—as some psychologists and psychiatrists have suggested. Perhaps he finds a particular sport particularly interesting because his own physical being is so admirably designed for the performance of that action. Perhaps he chooses it because he was introduced to it at an early age and became involved in the challenge it provided. Or perhaps he chooses it for the same reason a mountain climber may choose to scale Mt. Everest—simply because it is there.

Perhaps he chooses to ski because he likes the feeling of cold air as it stings his face, or because he likes the whiteness of snow and the blueness of the sky. Perhaps he chooses to swim because he likes the sensation of being supported by water—or the feeling of being engulfed by its oceanic depths. Perhaps he likes contact sports because he likes the feeling of slamming his body against the body of another person with all his force—or perhaps he avoids the contact sports for the opposite reason. Perhaps he likes the open air and sunlit greenness he finds on the golf course. Perhaps he likes the smell of sweat—or the feeling of being confined in a closed space. Perhaps, perhaps, perhaps . . . for who can account for all the likes and dislikes of human beings?

I think that all of these factors are relevant to the choices men may make in sport. I think all of them provide some insight into men's reasons for preferring one sport rather than another. But I also think they are secondary to men's interest in the symbolic power of sport, as such.

During the past ten years I have talked with many men and women, and many boys and girls, about the dimensions of their interest in the rule-governed competitions of sport. In those conversations, I have heard many explanations—but always, sooner or later, I have heard the word "freedom." Freedom to go all out, holding nothing back—freedom to focus all the energies of my own mortal being on the voluntary performance of one self-chosen human action—freedom to experience myself at my own utmost as a whole-hearted, fully motivated, fully integrated, and fully functioning human being.

Many of these performers testified that their all-out efforts in sport had improved their physiological functioning and made them more fit for the rigors of their daily lives. Others mentioned permanently damaged ankles, knees, hip joints, shoulder joints, necks and fingers. One was wearing a steel plate in his skull; another was wearing a back brace. But none of them told me that they had entered into competition for the purpose of becoming physically fit. Rather they had become more fit—or less fit—because they had engaged in competition for its own sake. (And in all truth, all of them knew that there are many quicker and easier and more efficient ways to develop muscular strength, flexibility, speed, and cardio-respiratory endurance.)

Yes, of course, the all-out effort of sport competition can improve physiological functioning—and I am interested in improving the physiological functioning of every school child. But this is not why I want to give every child a fair chance to compete on the symbolic field of sport during the school day.

The meanings I have found in my own involvement in sport are important meanings. I value them as I value the meanings I have found in my own involvement in poetry, drama, music, science, philosophy, history, mathematics, sculpture and dance. I value them with the most important meanings I have found in my own commitment to the values of human action. I value them as some of the most important meanings I have found in my own commitment to the values of education.

I think you do too. I think every member of the Eastern District Association for Health, Physical Education and Recreation values the meanings he has found in sport in this way.

And so I am doing my own utmost to persuade my colleagues in education—and particularly my colleagues in health education, physical education, and recreation—that sport is truly "a flow of meanings without speech"—and "of as many meanings as of men." I am telling my colleagues that they have been undervaluing the educational potential of sport for a long, long time. And I am urging them—as I am urging you—to re-examine the meanings they have found in their own glorious moments of all-out effort on the symbolic field of sport. And I am urging you, too, to stand up proudly in the forums of education and "tell it like it is."

Man, Nature and Sport

JAN PROGEN

There is a universal appeal in nature. Whether it be found in the magic of water, the magnetism of mountains, the beckoning of the sky or the power of an unknown world beneath the surface of the earth, the attraction is there and it is very real. The Homeric Greeks' love for the sea shows this interest to be deep-rooted in the history of man. The current ecological movement to save the natural environment from an affluent and over-productive society indicates a modern concern for nature as well as its great appeal expressed by increasing numbers of people seeking sports activities away from the cities and gymnasiums and in natural settings.

I see this trend toward natural sports not so much as an escape *from* daily life as an escape *to* nature: not so much to forget, but rather to remember.(23:9) For the surf, mountains, open sky, etc. have always provided a challenge to man, and the existence of challenge has always stimulated a response from him (13:57)—a desire to do the undone, to see the unseen, to push beyond the previous limitations of his abilities and accomplishments. This drive and need for adventure is unique to man.

To make a definition of sport which would be comprehensive enough to include games, with their highly structured, rule-orientated form and natural sports, with their free form, is not feasible. Therefore, a special definition of natural sport is offered for the purposes of this paper. Natural sports are activities which involve human participation as a response to the challenge offered primarily by the physical, natural world such as hills, air currents and waves. They are bounded by the personally constructed goals of the participant as, for example, to climb the mountain, explore the cave or ski down the hill. This paper explores the relationship of man to natural sports. Through the use of recorded commentary by parachutists, mountaineers, surfers, soarers, skiers, hikers, sailors, canoeists and spelunkers, the meaning of the natural sport experience is revealed and clarified.

The Aesthetic Experience. The primary motive for many who engage in natural sports is the sheer enjoyment of the beauty of nature. One mountaineer found a great pleasure in renewing his senses in the natural beauty of clean air, sparkling snow and brilliant sunsets and sunrises, and found it satisfying just to be surrounded by trees, grass, flowers and bare, honest rock.(12:631) There is an abundant amount of visual beauty in nature, and all that needs to be done is to open oneself up to it.

One aspect of beauty is the great pleasure and special thrill in being the first one to enter a cave.(6:160) One spelunker who found a virgin room in a new cave filled with tall, white stalagmite formations was not primarily impressed by the beauty of it all. "What really excited me was the floor of the room. There wasn't a print in the sand. I was the first human to ever set foot there."(28:54) Skiing more commonly provides this opportunity to touch "untouched" nature—to know it in a new

237

way. By making one's tracks in the snow, "this possibility of touching nature as the first person is provided since the evidence brought down by newly fallen snow precludes any contamination of this evidence of nature by anything else."(18:642) Styles sees this as a contribution to mankind: "He enlarges it [the mountain] by a first ascent, from a remote wedge of upheaved rock and ice into a field for the adventure and pleasure of other men; he adds it to the accessible delights of the human heritage." (25:3)

The sensation of being finite in the cosmos is also part of the aesthetic experience. Challenging the mighty forces of nature, a surfer with only a sliver seems very small (20:130) Jim Whittaker's feelings on the top of Everest were very similar. "Not expansive. Not sublime. I felt like a frail human being."(27:78) In contrast to this, sport in nature has offered man an opportunity to feel alive, full and significant. "Who's afraid of the universe? It's midnight on the desert or the coast or high above the timberline; the Milky Way is close and the stars are singing. I tremble before the cosmos no more than a fish trembles before the tide."(23:109) But there is something beyond this expansive feeling. "The jumper has his brief moment of exhilaration, his fleeting illusion of omnipotence. But there is more. A man can find a sound and abiding satisfaction in jumping—perhaps a new and better sense of what he is."(5:669)

Challenge. But for numerous others, beauty is not the major reason. Overwhelming beauty can be viewed from easily attainable summits. (13:49) For some there must be something more, and this something is often challenge. Challenge is a concept which transcends competition. It is a personal response to one's environment, a willingness to test oneself within various contexts and media. While sometimes it takes the form of rivalry, it often has no element of strife, no need to declare victor or defeated. David Smith "paraswamdoveranbiked" in his own peace pentathlon of nonwar, fun events to satisfy his need for challenge without competing against anyone else, and to make his statement about the absurdity of competition.(16:50-61)

Some spelunkers are driven to discovery, to put up with great physical and psychological ordeals, to brave the hardships and hazards of seemingly unscalable walls, deep abysses and steep and slippery slopes of caves like Schoolhouse in West Virginia and Neff Canyon Cave. The attraction is the many kinds of challenges offered there. (6:173,176) The names of features in Schoolhouse Cave such as "Groan Box," "Sam's Struggle," "Nick of Time," and "Grind Canyon" express the essence of their activities.(6:173)

Houston recognized the constant striving of man to do the ultimate, to reach beyond his grasp, as a response to challenge and the primary motive for mountaineering.(12:633) John Hunt, leader of the first successful climb of the world's highest peak, stated: "There was the challenge, and we would lay aside all else to take it up." (15:231) Mallory spoke of self-knowledge, development and satisfaction in mountaineering and indicated that mountains, as all other natural elements, are not conquered or an enemy to battle against. "Whom have we conquered? None but ourselves. Have we won a kingdom? No—and yes. We have achieved the ultimate satisfaction, filled a destiny. To struggle is to understand, never the last without the other."(13:58) Houston also noted that "men do not conquer mountains any more than mountains conquer men, in the pursuit of what mountains offer, men find more than victory."(13:634)

> Mountaineering is more a quest for self-fulfillment than a victory over others or over nature. . . . The aim is to transcend a previous self. . . . A true mountaineer knows he has not conquered a mountain by standing on its summit for a few fleeting moments. Only when the right men are in the right places at the right time are the big mountains climbed, never are they conquered. (12:57)

Hunt also recognized man's need to respond to other challenges of nature and expressed his faith in the spirit of man to accomplish his goals:

> I also believe that we cannot avoid the challenges of other giants. Mountains scarcely lower than Everest itself are still "there," as Mallory said. They beckon us and we cannot rest until we have met their challenge too. And there are many other opportunities for adventure; whether they be sought among the hills, in the air, upon the sea, in the bowels of the earth, or on the bottom of the ocean bed. . . . There is no height, no depth, that the spirit of man, guided by a higher Spirit, cannot attain. (15:232)

There are many examples of men designing more intense challenges into those already proffered by nature. In mountaineering "to add to stress and its headiness, climbers now make ascents at night or in winter, alone, or deliberately in bad weather."(13:51) Participants of soaring, which is a sport like surfing and sailing in that the thrill is experienced by "harnessing" the energy of nature, find that "power flight isn't fun any more. The challenges are gone."(8:101) The challenge of accomplishing a difficult feat motivated ten men to jump from an airplane one after another and join hands in the form of a star—the first ten-man star ever made—before opening their parachutes. (10:66)

Stress-Risk. Many of the sports occurring in natural, non-competitive settings involve a relatively high degree of stress and risk in the spirit of adventure which provides a sense of thrill in danger, exhilaration, confidence, control and self-satisfaction in the participant. Voluntarily "the stress-seeker struggles under heavy baggage and against severe hardships to 'stretch his capacity' to do what few others can do—his capacity to bear the fear of falling and endure thirst, sunburn, frostbite, blisters, fatigue, and the effects of altitude where 'simple tasks become major struggles'."(13:49) But it must be made clear that these hardships are not the goal, and the mountaineer is not a masochist; rather, he accepts these hardships as part of the game in order that he might know the pleasures of mountaineering.(12:634)

Nor are the activities performed *because* of the risks. Alvarez pointed out that "what looks like absurd risk is usually quite different to the expert: it is justifiable control."(1:10) Comparing the degree of control in daily life to that of a skilled mountaineer, he stated:

In America there are more daily risks and violence than mountain climbers see in a lifetime. I would rather commit myself ten times over to El Capitan than go alone into Harlem or Watts or try to cross Central Park after dark; on a mountain at least you have some control over disaster. (1:12)

Control is the key factor which separates the difficult from the dangerous:

No true mountaineer ever courted danger for its own sake. The whole point of any sport is that it demands the acquisition of a special skill which cancels out the danger. It was the mountaineer's justification that he climb by routes where his skill in mountaincraft, supported by courage and resolution of no mean order, made him competent to ascend and descend safely. (25:129)

Houston distinguished between risk and danger giving a very clear example of the role of control. "Experienced climbers understand,

enjoy, and seek risk because it presents a difficulty to overcome and can be estimated and controlled. He equally abhors danger because it is beyond his control."(13:52) Manageable risks that make a route difficult, such as difficult mountain faces or deep sea waters, attract participants; uncontrollable dangers such as are found in areas with a high incidence of avalanches or shark-infested waters, are not popular with sportsmen.

Speaking especially of the lonely, risky sports, Alvarez showed that "intentional, planned risk demands all the qualities most valuable in life: intelligence, skill, intuition, subtlety, control." (1:12) Robert Kennedy recognized the abilities characterizing the men with whom he climbed Mt. Kennedy as they "possessed qualities of the best mountain men: keen intelligence, an obvious willingness to undergo pain and discomfort for an objective, and a very high degree of courage. Theirs is not blind, inescapable, meaningless courage. It is courage with ability, brains, tenacity of purpose."(17:22)

Dr. Sol Roy Rosenthal introduced the idea that there is a specific reason, perhaps chemical, why people participate in risk-action sports. His thesis suggests that calculated risks as provided by these activities are necessary for daily well-being. He observed that the exhilaration and even euphoria resulting from risk-exercise is absent from the non-risk, gamelike sports such as tennis and golf, and he noted that the degree of exhilaration resulting varied with the competence of the individual and with the degree of difficulty of the sport, the more dangerous sports producing the greatest uplift in spirit.(7:52-53) Further, he stated that "the feeling, characteristic of many of the most demanding, risk-exercises, is so intense that you almost feel hooked. It is like being addicted, you feel you must go back and know it again."(7:53) This is supported by Robert Gannon's comment about soaring: "I'm hooked, and it seems for good. I look out my window and see a cloud hanging, beckoningly, over the distant mountains and I long to spread my wings and get under it to circle with the other hawks."(8:204) The tantalization may be due to the fact that the experience, while usually satisfying, is not totally so. There are so many questions to be answered and aspects of the experience which could be perfected; the development of control is a slow and challenging one.

Another part of the reason for the addictive quality of these sports may be that they call forth "lost traces of strength and courage that daily life does not afford."(12:631) Sylvian Saudan established life-death situations in which he skied down 14,000-foot peaks in the Alps into the unknown, alone and without mountaineering equipment. He claimed that this gave him an opportunity not often found in normal life enabling him to dominate his fears and passions.(4:61,72) Such sports afford an attitude of "complete" living as the purpose is to escape death not life, for death is an accident in sport.(24:204-206) Alvarez stated that essentially all risky sports are "like a close up on your life, in which the essentials are concentrated and defined. You deliberately set up a situation in which, in order to survive, you must respond as fully as you know how to."(1:12)

Natural sports require total involvement and commitment. "It is like playing chess with your body, a sort of physical strength which demands not courage but sheer concentration." (1:10) Leydet showed his complete involvement in the description of his first run down the rapids of the Colorado River. "We were committed—there was no way to turn back or to try a different approach. And oddly enough with that realization my apprehension ceased, giving way to a feeling of aliveness and exhilaration."(19:38)

Freedom-Independence. The absence of organization and rules in such non-competitive sports as skiing and surfing allows for a very high degree of independence which is a great appeal, particularly to young people. "One of the greatest attractions of surfing is that it is an individual sport and you don't have to belong to anything to do it. Kids resent organization. In surfing you just pick up your board and go—no rules, no uniforms, no one you have to compete with."(22:108)

Concomitantly, in natural sports there is a great degree of freedom; "you take complete responsibility for your own life. You choose and are responsible."(1:12) Coutts claimed that "one basic underlying reason why man engages in sport is the sense of freedom which he finds there."(2:68) He pointed out that "non-game sports, such as mountain climbing, skiing, sky diving and scuba diving, allow for a greater feeling of being free in the sense of being dependent on self for survival or success and in providing for more creative expression through choices and action."(2:70) How many ways can a baseball player play right field? Certainly a mountaineer has much more freedom—more alternatives in how he engages in his sport, allowing for greater creativity.(24:189) Perhaps the characteristic simplicity of

mountaineering, surfing and the like as compared to game and team sports enables this greater degree of freedom and creativity. Renny and Terry Russell found that in camping they had an opportunity to act rather than being acted upon:

> The elemental simplicities of the wilderness travel with thrills not only because of their novelty, but because they represent complete freedom to make mistakes. The wilderness gave them their first tastes of the rewards and punishments for wise and foolish acts. . . .

Slusher noted that "the surfer is endlessly free. . . he determines his own destiny. . . . Failure cannot be blamed on a sudden gust of wind or a strong current. This is part of the sport. In fact it is the sport. . . . Each and every encounter is new and fresh. Man stands on his own and faces the unstructured and unique forces of nature."(24:178)

Union with Self, Nature and Other Men. Responding to the question, "What is a National wave?" an Australian surfer gave this answer:

> A series of incidents that add, tie up to a tale, a being. One minute a pressure, then a cruise of ease, euphoria, next a calculus, finally, always, a satisfaction. One pure slice of existence. Being. (3:122)

Slusher established that "there is a certain feeling that comes to the body through involvement in sport that is a sense of being. In the straining and alteration from normal pursuits, man feels his body as he never knew it before."(24:36)

Slusher said that being is "a total expression of the wholeness of man." (24:12) This oneness is often expressed in sports of nature:

> Autonomy of existence can be achieved by the body *knowing* the object in a way that is not known by others or by other objects. Through the process of transcendence he no longer perceives the self as is. The skin diver becomes part of the sea, the skier part of the mountains . . . *In the body* and *by the body* man learns *existenz* as an exciting new way. (24:36)

As Nuuhiwa said, "you must try to blend into the wave, you match the wave's movements, you become part of it."(21:27) The peace pentathloner expressed a similar idea:

> The rhythm of movements. A relaxation of flow of the inner essence—continuity of being, moving through any movement, harmony. I run up the mountain. I flow down the mountain. In time with the moment. In pace with the universe. Watching from inside and out. Unity with all. (16:52)

In sport there is an I-thou relationship in which "man finds himself, man becomes, man is, only in relation to his thou" [possibly some element of nature].(9:90) It is a very personal and loving thing. Julius Kugy said, "I leaned on mountains as upon strong friends. They were so kind to me as to bring me comfort and restoration after grave earthly sorrow. Such is the love and trust with which I turn to them." (12:633) Ricky Grigg felt the same way about the sea. "The sea absorbs me and provides every passion I know. There's intense interest, excitement, love, fear, deep respect. . . the sea is very personal to me."(3:93)

No wonder natural sportsmen become addicted to their sport. It is not strange that they often experience a touch of sadness when their adventure is over, as Hillary did at the end of that Everest expedition.(11:248) Flying in the warmth of a plane over Canada's Back River, whose rapids he had just canoed down, Austin Hoyt stated that already he "had begun to miss the bite of the wind in his face and the fury of the river."(14:41)

Yet during those expeditions both of these men must have felt some anxiety in their freedom—an anxiety which assisted them in their efforts. It's like the surfer in relation to the wave who "while he needs to 'ride it in,'. . . would like nothing better than to relieve himself of his situation."(24:179)

Sometimes man finds a deep union with other men after sharing a sports experience in nature, particularly because man is dependent upon his fellow man and is depended on in a survival, life-death situation. Mountaineering provides a very vivid example. "Each man deliberately places his life in the hands of his companions. . . . After many or arduous climbs together, individuals feel deeply this kinship of the rope."(13:51)

Together two or three or four can do what is impossible for one to accomplish. Slusher noted that in sports like mountaineering there is both a quality of cooperation between the participants and a struggle for survival where man just wants to exist.(24:39) Teamwork is essential to ascents like Everest, and it provided John Hunt with one of the greatest sensations he had ever known. "Comradeship, regardless of race or creed, is forged among high mountains, through the difficulties and dangers to which they expose those who aspire to climb them, the need to combine their efforts to attain their goal, the thrill of a great adventure shared together."(15:231)

Contrast with Ordinary Life. Part of the beauty of sports occurring in natural settings is the marked absence of spectators, who dominate most of the game sports with their artificial standards and scores. Aloneness doesn't have to be the same as sheer loneliness. Sometimes it's good to be alone. Joseph Krutch recognized this when he asked the question: "How many more generations will pass before it will become nearly impossible to be alone even for an hour, to see anywhere nature without man's improvements upon her?"(19:30) Parachuting enables man to be very much alone. In fact, it's a very private thing to do. (26:85) The sportsman is in control of the situation of aloneness. Though he may be anxious, fearful or excited, he knows the reason for these emotions, which is often not the case in daily life where "floating" anxieties plague many. Being alone for the first time in soaring brought this reaction from Gannon: "It's a funny thing, but you just don't know the thrill, the real thrill of soaring—you never become lightheartedly alive with joy—until you're up there alone."(8:100)

Aloneness is only one of the sudden contrasts in natural sport. An exciting and strenuous 160-foot belay into a cave is very different from the utter calm and beauty discovered once inside it.(6:156) The quiet, motionless temperament of water is quite a contrast to the anxious exhilaration of the unknown just around the bend in the river.(14:40) Parachuting provides this contrast as well as a sense of freedom and a desire to make time and the world stand still, if for only an instant:

> The physical sensations of the jump occur as sudden contrasts. From noise, vibration, immobility and confinement, the jump brings rapid motion, and suddenly, as the canopy opens, suspension in what seems for the moment an absolute quiet in endless time and space. The subjective release of tension with a surge of exhilaration. . . . You feel free when you jump. And when that old canopy opens, it's like the hand of God has caught you up. You look down on the world, and you think how nice it would be to stay up there. (5:663)

In man's exhilaration from the release of such earthly holds he recognizes himself as a complete and united being. Life is restored to him and man is important to himself. (24:10, 22)

By accepting and seeking the challenges of nature in the natural sports experience, the participant has the opportunity to know himself and the world in new ways. In an aesthetic sense, man can open himself up to great visual beauty, virgin experiences and the sensation of being finite in the cosmos. There is an opportunity to meet challenges which demand the development of control in risky and stressful situations not often found in ordinary life. Man has a chance to know freedom and to be dependent upon and responsible for himself. Ultimately, he has the unique opportunity to unite with himself, nature and other men in the world of natural sports.

BIBLIOGRAPHY

1. Alvarez, A. "I Like to Risk My Life." *Saturday Evening Post*, 240 (September 9, 1967), 10-12.
2. Coutts, Curtis A. "Freedom in Sport." *Quest*, X (May, 1968), 68-71.
3. Dixon, Peter. *Men Who Ride Mountains*. New York: Bantam Books Inc., 1969.
4. Edwards, Harvey. "Daredevil of the Alps: He Skis the Steepest." *Ski*, 34 (Spring, 1970), 61, 72.
5. Farrell, Dennis. "The Psychology of Parachuting." *Motivations in Play, Games and Sports.* Edited by Ralph Slovenko and James A. Knight. Springfield, Illinois: Charles C Thomas, 1967.
6. Folsome, Franklin. *Exploring American Caves*. New York: Collier Books, 1962.
7. Furlong, William. "Danger as a Way of Life." *Sports Illustrated*, 30 (January 27, 1969), 52-53.
8. Gannon, Robert. "Half-Mile Up Without an Engine." *Popular Science*, 192 (April, 1968), 98-101.
9. Gerber, Ellen W. "Identity, Relation and Sport." *Quest*, VIII (May, 1967), 90-97.
10. "Go and Make a Falling Star." *Esquire*, 70 (July, 1968), 66-67.
11. Hillary, Edmund. *High Adventure*. New York: E. P. Dutton & Company, Inc., 1955.
12. Houston, Charles S. "Mountaineering." *Motivations in Play, Games and Sports.* Edited by Ralph Slovenko and James A. Knight. Springfield, Illinois: Charles C Thomas, 1967, 626-636.
13. ————. "The Last Blue Mountain." *Why Men Take Chances*. Edited by Samuel Z. Klausner. Garden City, New York: Anchor Books, Doubleday & Company, 1968, 49-58.
14. Hoyt, Austin. "Down the Back to the Arctic." *Sports Illustrated*, 19 (August 26, 1963), 34-41.
15. Hunt, John. *The Ascent of Everest*. London: Hodder & Stroughton, 1953.
16. Jones, Robert F. "The World's First Peace Pentathlon." *Sports Illustrated*, 32 (May 11, 1970), 50-60.
17. Kennedy, Robert F. "Our Climb Up Mt. Kennedy." *Life*, 58 (April 9, 1965), 22-27.
18. Knight, James A. "Skiing." *Motivations in Play, Games and Sports.* Edited by Ralph Slovenko and James A. Knight. Springfield, Illinois: Charles C Thomas, 1967, 637-648.
19. Leydet, Francois. *Time and the River Flowing: Grand Canyon.* Edited by David Brower. San Francisco: Sierra Club & Ballantine Books, 1968.
20. Mitchell, Carleton. "The Fad and Fascination of Surfing." *Holiday*, 35 (May, 1964), 122-130.
21. Ottum, Bob. "The Charger Sinks the Dancer." *Sports Illustrated*, 25 (October 10, 1966), 26-29.
22. Rogin, Gilbert. "An Odd Sport and an Unusual Champion." *Sports Illustrated*, 23 (October 18, 1965), 94-110.
23. Russell, Terry and Russell, Renny. *On the Loose*. San Francisco: Sierra Club & Ballantine Books, 1967.
24. Slusher, Howard S. *Man, Sport and Existence*. Philadelphia: Lea & Febiger, 1967.
25. Styles, Stowell. *On Top of the World*. New York: The Macmillan Company, 1967.
26. "The Joys of Falling Through Space." *Saturday Evening Post*, 239 (June 18, 1966), 82-85.
27. Ullman, James Ramsey. "At the Top—and Out of Oxygen." *Life*, 55 (September 20, 1963), 68-92.
28. "Wonders of a Cave Find: A Big Spelunking Jackpot in the Ozarks." *Life*, 57 (December 18, 1964), 49-54.

Play: A Non-Meaningful Act*

JOSEF PIEPER

How can we visualize something that serves nothing else, that by its very nature has meaning only in its own terms?

Almost inevitably there comes to mind a notion that has been much discussed in anthropological literature of recent decades—although it has been the subject of considerable romantic speculation, as well as of sound analysis. I am referring to the concept of *play*. Does not play epitomize that pure purposefulness in itself, we might ask? Is not play activity meaningful in itself, needing no utilitarian justification? And should not festivity therefore be interpreted chiefly as a form of play?

Obviously, these are extremely complex questions which cannot be settled merely in passing. Nevertheless, we would hazard that the term *play* does not adequately define the distinguishing feature of free activity, let alone of festivity. To be sure, Plato closely associates the two ideas when he speaks of "the graciousness of play and festival." And if "seriousness," as Hegel says, "is work in relation to the need," then it does seem logical to equate play with festivity in similar fashion. In fact a real festival can scarcely be conceived unless the

*From *In Tune With The World* by Josef Pieper, copyright © 1963 by Kösel-Verlag KG München; English translation by Richard and Clara Winston. New York: Harcourt, Brace & World, 1965. © by Kösel-Verlag GmbH & Co., München, and reprinted with their permission.

ingredient of play—perhaps also, although here I am not so sure, the ingredient of playfulness —has entered into it. But all this has not answered the crucial question of whether the element of play makes an action meaningful in itself. Human acts derive their meaning primarily from their content, from their object, not from the manner in which they are performed. Play, however, seems to be chiefly a mere *modus* of action, a specific way of performing something, at any rate a purely formal determinant. Thus it is natural enough that people inevitably flounder in phantasms and unrealities when they try to regard all those human activities that are obviously not just work as play and nothing more: the work of the artist, too—of the writer, musician, painter —or even religious worship. For suddenly everything that was "meaningful in itself" slips through their fingers and becomes a game empty of all meaning. Significantly, one good argument against Huizinga's book on *homo ludens*, which represents the religious festivals of primitive peoples purely as play, is that this view is tantamount to saying that all sacred acts are meaningless. Incidentally, this objection has not been made by a theologian; the critic is an ethnologist, protesting against distortion of empirical observation.

The question, then, remains open: By what virtue does an act possess the inner quality of being meaningful in itself?

Seeing "t'United" Play*

J. B. PRIESTLEY

These caps have just left the ground of the Bruddersford United Association Football Club. Thirty-five thousand men and boys have just seen what most of them call "t'United" play Bolton Wanderers. Many of them should never have been there at all. It would not be difficult to prove by statistics and those mournful little budgets (How a Man May Live—or rather, avoid death—on Thirty-five Shillings a Week) that seem to attract some minds, that these fellows could not afford the entrance fee. When some mills are only working half the week and others not at all, a shilling is a respectable sum of money. It would puzzle an economist to discover where all these shillings came from. But if he lived in Bruddersford, though he might still wonder where they came from, he would certainly understand why they were produced. To say that these men paid their shillings to watch twenty-two hirelings kick a ball is merely to say that a violin is wood and catgut, that *Hamlet* is so much paper and ink. For a shilling the Bruddersford United A.F.C. offered you Conflict and Art; it turned you into a critic, happy in your judgment of fine points, ready in a second to estimate the worth of a well-judged pass, a run down the touch line, a lightning shot, a clearance kick by back or goalkeeper; it turned you into a partisan, holding your breath when the ball came sailing into your own goalmouth, ecstatic when your forwards raced away towards the opposite goal, elated, downcast, bitter, triumphant by turns at the fortunes of your side, watching a ball shape Iliads and Odysseys for you; and what is more, it turned you into a member of a new community, all brothers together for an hour and a half, for not only had you escaped from the clanking machinery of this lesser life, from work, wages, rent, doles, sick pay, insurance cards, nagging wives, ailing children, bad bosses, idle workmen, but you had escaped with most of your mates and your neighbours, with half the town, and there you were, cheering together, thumping one another on the shoulders, swopping judgments like lords of the earth, having pushed your way through a turnstile into another and altogether more splendid kind of life, hurtling with Conflict and yet passionate and beautiful in its Art. Moreover, it offered you more than a shilling's worth of material for talk during the rest of the week. A man who had missed the last home match of "t'United" had to enter social life on tiptoe in Bruddersford.

* Excerpt from *The Good Companions*, Vol. I. New York: Harper & Brothers, 1929.

BIBLIOGRAPHY ON SPORT AS A MEANINGFUL EXPERIENCE

Alvarez, A. "I Like to Risk my Life." *Saturday Evening Post*, 240 (September 9, 1967), 10–12.

Amsler, J. Essai pour le sport et le sacre. *Education Physique et Sport*, 483–488 (1958).

Banham, Charles. "Man at Play." *Contemporary Review*, 207 (August, 1965) 61–64.

Bannister, Roger. "What Makes the Athlete Run?" *The Australian Journal of Physical Education*, (March, 1964), 31–36.

———. "The Meaning of Athletic Performance." *International Research in Sport and Physical Education*. Edited by E. Jokl and E. Simon. Springfield, Illinois: Charles C. Thomas, 1964.

Beisser, Arnold R. "Psychodynamic Observations of a Sport." *Psychoanalytic Review*, 48 (Spring, 1961), 69–76.

———. The Madness in Sports. New York: Appleton-Century-Crofts, 1967.

Blumenfield, Walter. "Observations Concerning the Phenomenon and Origin of Play." *Philosophy and Phenomenological Research. I* (June, 1941), 470–478.

Bouet, M. "Basic Principles of an Interpretation of High-Performance Sport." *Sport in the Modern World—Chances and Problems*. Edited by Ommo Grupe, Dietrich Kurz, and Johonnes Teipel. New York: Springer, Verlag, 1973.

———. Signification du Sport. Paris, 1968.

Coomaraswamy, A. K. "Play and Seriousness." *Journal of Philosophy*, XXXIX (September, 1942), 550–552.

Davis, John Eisele. "The Utilization of Play in the Construction of Healthy Mental Attitudes." *Mental Hygiene*, 20 (January, 1936), 49–54.

Desmonde, William H. "The Bull-Fight as a Religious Ritual" *American Imago*, 9 (June, 1952), 173–195.

"The Difficult Art of Losing." *Time*, 92 (November 15, 1968), 47–48.

Doherty, J. Kenneth. "Why Men Run." *Quest*, II (April, 1964), 61–66.

———. "Motivation in Endurance Running" in *Modern Training for Running*. New Jersey: Prentice-Hall, 1964.

Felshin, Jan. "Sport and Modes of Meaning." *Journal of Health, Physical Education, and Recreation*, 40 (May, 1969), 43–44.

Franke, E. "Sporting Action and Its Interpretation." *Sport in the Modern World—Chances and Problems*. Edited by Ommo Grupe, Dietrich Kurz, and Johonnes Teipel. New York: Springer-Verlag, 1973.

Furlong, William. "Danger as a Way of Joy." *Sports Illustrated*, 30 (January 27, 1969), 52–53.

Genasci, James E. and Klissouras, Vasillis. "The Delphic Spirit in Sports." *Journal of Health, Physical Education, and Recreation*, 37 (February, 1966), 43–45.

Gerber, Ellen W. "Identity, Relation and Sport." *Quest*, VIII (May, 1967), 90–97.

Gilbert, Bill. "When Games Were for Fun." *Sports Illustrated*, 31 (November 24, 1969), E7–10.

Gregg, Jerald Rex. "A Philosophical Analysis of the Sports Experience and the Role of Athletics in the Schools." Unpublished Ed.D. dissertation, University of Southern California, 1971.

Harper, William A. "Man Alone." *Quest*, XII (May, 1969), 57–60.

Harris, Dorothy V. Involvement in Sport: A Somatopsychic Rationale for Physical Activity. Philadelphia: Lea & Febiger, 1974.

Hoffman, Shirl J. "The Athletae Dei: Missing the Meaning of Sport." *Journal of the Philosophy of Sport*, III (Sept., 1976), 42–51.

Houston, Charles S. "The Last Blue Mountain." *Why Man Takes Chances*. Edited by Samuel Z. Klausner. New York: Anchor Books Edition, 1968.

Houts, Jo Ann. "Feeling and Perception in the Sport Experience." *Journal of Health, Physical Education, and Recreation*, 41 (October, 1970), 71.

Huizinga, Johan. Homo Ludens. London: Routledge & Kegan Paul, 1950.

Kahn, Roger, "Intellectuals and Ballplayers." *American Scholar*, 26 (Summer, 1957), 342–349.

Kenyon, Gerald S. "Sport Involvement: A Conceptual Go and Some Consequences Thereof." *Aspects of Contemporary Sport Sociology*. Proceedings of C.I.C. Symposium on the Sociology of Sport. Edited by Gerald S. Kenyon. Illinois: The Athletic Institute, 1969.

Klausner, Samuel Z., Ed. Why Man Takes Chances. New York: Anchor Books Edition, 1968.

Kleinman, Seymour. "The Significance of Human Movement: A Phenomenological Approach." National Association for Physical Education of College Women Report of the Ruby Anniversary Workshop. Interlochen, Michigan, 1964.

———. "Sport as Experience." Unpublished paper presented at the Annual Convention of the American Association for Health, Physical Education, and Recreation, Seattle, Washington. April, 1970.

———. "Is Sport Experience?" (Part IV of "Sport: Whose Bag?") *Quest*, XIX (January, 1973), 93–96.

Kretchmar, R. Scott and Harper, William A. "Why Does Man Play?" *Journal of Health, Physical Education, and Recreation*, 40 (March, 1969), 57–58.

Kretchmar, R. Scott. "From Test to Contest: An Analysis of Two Kinds of Counterpoint in Sport." *Journal of the Philosophy of Sport*, II (September, 1974), 23–30.

———. "In Defense of Indefensible Sports and Sportspersons." Proceedings of the National College Physical Education Association for Men, Hot Springs, Arkansas, 1976.

Lawton, Philip. "Sports and the American Spirit: Michael Novak's Theology of Culture." *Philosophy Today*, XX (Fall, 1976), 196–208.

Lorenz, Konrad. "Avowal of Optimism" in *On Aggression*. New York: Harcourt, Brace & World, 1966.

Mackay, Afred F. "Interpersonal Comparisons." *Journal of Philosophy,* 2 (October, 1975), 535–549.

McMurty, John. "Philosophy of a Corner Linebacker." *The Nation,* 212 (January 18, 1971), 83–84.

———. "The Illusions of a Football Fan: a Reply to Michalos." *Journal of the Philosophy of Sport,* IV (Fall, 1977), 11–14.

Mitchell, Robert. "Sport as Experience." *Quest,* XXIV (Summer, 1975), 19–27.

Metheny, Eleanor. *Connotations of Movement in Sport and Dance.* Iowa: Wm. C. Brown, 1965.

———. "The Symbolic Power of Sport." Unpublished paper presented at the annual convention of the Eastern District Association for Health, Physical Education, and Recreation, Washington, D.C., April 26, 1968.

———. *Movement and Meaning.* New York: McGraw-Hill, 1968.

Miller, David L. *Gods and Games: Toward a Theology of Play.* New York: World Publishing Company, 1970.

Morford, W. R. "Is Sport the Struggle or the Triumph?" (Part I of "Sport: Whose Bag?") *Quest,* XIX (January, 1973), 83–87.

Norbeck Edward. "Human Play and its Cultural Expression." *Humanitas,* V (Spring, 1969), 43–55.

Ortega y Gasset, José. "Uber des Lebers Sportloch-festlichen Sinn." In DSB (ed.): Jahrbuch des Sports, 9–20, Frankfurt, 1955/56.

Park, Roberta J. "Raising the Consciousness of Sport." *Quest,* XIX (January, 1973), 78–82.

Parker, Franklin. "Sport, Play and Physical Education in Cultural Perspective." *Journal of Health, Physical Education, and Recreation,* 36 (January, 1965) 29–30.

Pavlich, Mary. "The Power of Sport." *Arizona Journal of Health, Physical Education, and Recreation,* 10 (Fall, 1966) 9–10.

Phillips, Patricia A. "The Sport Experience in Education." *Quest,* XXIII (January, 1975), 94–97.

Pieper, Josef. *In Tune With the World: A Theory of Festivity.* Translated by Richard and Clara Winston. New York: Harcourt, Brace & World, 1965.

Priestley, J. B. "Seeing 't'United' Play" in *The Good Companions,* Vol. 1. New York: Harper & Brothers, 1929.

Rahner, Hugo, S. J. *Man at Play.* New York Herder and Herder, 1967.

Riezler, Kurt. "Play and Seriousness." *Journal of Philosophy,* XXXVIII (September, 1941), 505–517.

Rupp, Adolph. "Defeat and Failure to Me are

Enemies." *Sports Illustrated,* 9 (December 8, 1958), 100–106.

Sadler, William A. Jr. "Alienated Youth and Creative Sports' Experience." *The Journal of the Philosophy of Sport,* IV (Fall, 1977), 83–95.

Santayana, George. "Philosophy on the Bleachers." *Harvard Monthly,* VIII (July, 1894), 181–190.

Schwartz, Thomas. "On the Utility of Mackay's Comparisons." *Journal of Philosophy,* 2 (October, 1974), 549–551.

Slovenko, Ralph and Knight, James A., Eds., *Motivations in Play, Games and Sports.* Springfield, Illinois: Charles C Thomas, 1967.

Slusher, Howard S. *Man, Sport and Existence.* Philadelphia: Lea & Febiger, 1967.

———. "To Test the Waves is to Test Life." *Journal of Health, Physical Education, and Recreation,* 40 (May, 1969), 32–33.

Sarani, Roberts. "The Flash of Spirit." *Quest,* XXIII (January, 1975), 78–82.

Stevenson, Christopher L. "The Meaning of Movement." *Quest,* XXIII (January, 1975), 2–9.

Stewart, Mary Lou. "Why Do Men Play?" *Journal of Health, Physical Education, and Recreation,* 41 (November-December, 1970), 14.

Stone, Roselyn E. "Human Movement Forms as Meaning—Structures: Prolegomenon." *Quest,* XXIII (January, 1975), 10–19.

———. "Meanings Found in the Acts of Surfing and Skiing." Unpublished Ph.D. dissertation, University of Southern California, 1970.

Studer, Ginny L. "The Language of Movement is in the Doing." *Quest,* XXIII (January, 1975), 98–100.

Thomas, Carolyn. "Personal Equations of Sport Involvement." Proceedings of the NCPEAM/NAPECW National Conference, Orlando, Florida, January 6–9, 1978.

Tiger, Lionel. "A Note on Sport" in *Men in Groups.* New York: Random House, 1969.

Toohey, Margaret S. "Is the Movement Experience a Profound Encounter of One's Being?" Proceedings of the NCPEAM/NAPECW National Conference, Orlando, Florida, January 6–9, 1978.

Vernes, Jean Rene. "The Element of Time in Competitive Games." Translated by Victor A. Velen. *Diogenes,* 50 (September, 1965), 25–42.

Weiss, Paul. *Sport: A Philosophic Inquiry.* Carbondale: Southern Illinois University Press, 1969.

Wenkart, Simon. "The Meaning of Sports for Contemporary Man." *Journal of Existential Psychiatry,* 3 (Spring, 1963), 397–404.

———. "Sports and Contemporary Man." *Motivations in Play, Games and Sports.* Edited by Ralph Slovenko and James A. Knight. Springfield, Illinois: Charles C Thomas, 1967.

White, David A. " 'Great Moments in Sport:' The One and Many." *Journal of the Philosophy of Sport,* II (September, 1975), 124–132.

SECTION V

Sport and Value—Oriented Concerns

Many philosophical questions are somewhat abstract and seem not actually to touch upon the life of an individual. However, the subject of values is relevant to every thinker. Since each person has his or her own idea of what is good, discussion about the value of any subject such as sport often is nothing more than a series of statements of beliefs and attitudes. This, in fact, has been the approach used by many philosophers. They have conceived of their role as the setting forth of a recommended system of values, i.e., a coherent set of beliefs and attitudes which suggest attendant behaviors. Moral and socio-political philosophy (which together with aesthetics—allotted separate treatment in this volume—exhaust the sub-discipline of axiology) have been, to some, the most important branches of the discipline in that they deal with recognizable and practical issues.

This modus operandi is not as didactic as might first appear. Philosophers base their value systems on their views of reality and truth; this enables them to answer the most immediate and consequential question: "What is the ultimate source of human values?" Depending upon one's philosophical view, the answer might be God, the physical or natural world, society, eternal or classical truths, or the individual. For instance, those who believe that the world of material objects is the real world tend to think that value derives from natural law. Thus, Herbert Spencer, a scientist and philosopher who tried to extend the theory of evolution to other spheres, chose to justify amusements by the famous "'surplus energy' theory." In "The Ethics of Pleasure" it is easy to see the justification of sports based upon ethical principles stemming from Spencer's interpretation of the importance of the physical world.

Josiah Royce, on the other hand, was the leading American idealist of his time. He was most definite in stating that "the rational solution of moral problems rests on the principle: Be loyal." In his article he values physical training, i.e., sports, because he believes it tends to train people to be loyal. Richard McCormick's article, in turn, is a classical treatment of applying "an immutable moral principle" to a current question.

In a somewhat different vein, Keating argues that sportsmanship is not the all encompassing moral category that it is commonly taken to be. Indeed, according to Keating its moral applicability is limited to the realm of sport (where it functions by cultivating the festive spirit of sport) thereby removing athletics (where it functions exclusively as a legal device to constrain the competitive temper of athletics) from its proper moral jurisdiction. Pearson's work presents an interesting analysis of the ethical status of deception in sport. Based on her distinction between "strategic deception" (which she defines as the attempt to build up in one's opponent the expectation that a certain act will occur when, in fact, another act that disappoints the expectation is intended) and "definitional deception" (which she defines as the illicit overturning of the game contract), Pearson concludes that only the latter form of deception is morally unsound in that it vitiates the purpose of sport which is to test one's skill. Delattre develops an ethical account of sport in terms of the notion respect for the game which he identifies as a necessary condition of competitive success in sport. On this account, the violation(s) of the rules constitutes a moral impropriety because it reduces competition to an excessive egoistic order in which one's opponents are treated as "means" ignoring their moral status as "ends."

Osterhoudt's essay suggests the terms in which Kant's and Hegel's respective moral systems provide a suitable normative guide for the conduct of sport. Considering first the merits of Kant's moral philosophy, Osterhoudt argues that a commitment to Kant's categorical imperative as a moral guide for sport enjoins us to regard the laws of sport (its rules and regulations) for their own sake, as self-legislated laws which derive their moral sustenance from the athlete's free decision to abide by them. From this initial line of argument, Osterhoudt next takes up a consideration of Hegel's *Sittlichkeit* which is shown to reform the abstract character of the Kantian imperative by suffusing the latter with content. The content supplied in this case is the historical content of socio-cultural institutions referred to by Hegel's notion of *Sittlichkeit*. Given the historical thrust of the *Sittlichkeit*, its implementation as a moral principle in sport leads, as Osterhoudt so elegantly shows, to a philosophy of sport history in which the evolution of sport itself, of its ownmost possibilities, is revealed.

More contemporary philosophical viewpoints have strayed away from formal value systems of the sort proposed previously. For example, the existentialists, particularly those of the Sartrean school of thought, reject the notion that the individual should act in accordance with some preset system of values. They maintain that each individual chooses what he or she values in accordance with his or her being. Ironically, this has led to the development of existentialist values, in that authenticity, being oneself, doing one's own thing, etc. have become "universal" existential values. In "Morality as an Intimate of Sport," Howard S. Slusher points to the ways in which sport and values juncture in an existentialist mode.

Analytical philosophers refuse to deal with values in the usual normative manner. They assert that the role of the philosopher is to analyze propositions to determine their necessary implications (although G. E. Moore, whose work *Principia Ethica* inaugurated the analytic movement in ethics, considered the linguistic analysis of moral terms to be a preliminary to the question, "What things are good?").

Unlike a moral principle, which is true only in accord with a previously accepted value system, an analytical proposition is inherently true. That which is inherent, is necessary; that which is contingent, is a choice. For example, the statement that "basketball is a team game" is an inherently true proposition, while the statement that "basketball should be a cooperative endeavor" is an ethical principle. The article by John Rawls is illustrative of this type of axiological reasoning. Rawls' rules of practice are constitutive rules that constitute and regulate forms of activity, such as sport, the existence of which is logically dependent on the rules. Therefore, to agree to play the game is to agree to abide by the rules because they are an inherent part of the game. Rawls concludes, on the above grounds, that it is immoral to disobey the rules. In an interesting challenge to Rawls' central thesis, Anthony Ralls argues that such a premise implies acceptance of the morality of keeping a promise (to play the game). He puts forth his own proposition relating to rules-keeping. The article by B. J. Diggs is an attempt to clarify the moral position of sport rules by focusing on the necessary relation of game rules to utilitarian game goals.

The selection by Lenk, "Toward a Social Philosophy of Achievement and Athletics," is the only essay included herein that deals exclusively with the socio-political value of sport. In this regard, Lenk proffers a critical response to the Neo-Marxist claim that sport merely instantiates the so-termed "performance principle" operative in achievement-oriented societies. Such an extreme view, argues Lenk, overlooks the potential for individual development and self-confirmation in sport, a potential nurtured on the athlete's free decision to express himself or herself through the medium of sport. This potential for self-development in sport exhibits none of the repressive features associated with achievement-motivated behavior by the Marxists, and their failure to account for this quite different form of human performance behavior seriously damages, according to Lenk, the credibility of their attack on achievement performance in general and sportive achievement performance in particular.

One of the contradictions which arises in any discussion on morality and socio-political philosophy is the apparent difference between conceived and operant values, the difference, for example, in believing in neighborly love and in practicing it. Does the coach who conceives of the use of sport to teach obedience to social rules (conceived value), contradict herself when she orders her players to "foul for profit" (operant value)? Or, is this merely a good example of the hierarchical nature of values? In other words, the value of winning may be higher on the coach's hierarchy than the value of teaching ethical principles. Since most modes of behaving involve a choice between various action possibilities, inevitably choices are made in accordance with values held to be most important.

In assessing the moral and socio-political status of sport, it is useful to consider the two categories of value traditionally used in axiology (theory of value): extrinsic and intrinsic value. Extrinsic valuation ascribes value to a person or thing based upon its function in a class or system. Hence, to value something extrinsically is to value that "thing" as a means to an end(s). In contrast, intrinsic valuation ascribes value to things as ends-in-themselves. To value something intrinsically, then, is to invest that "thing," whatever it might be, with primary value in lieu of any reference to its possible instrumental use. Using these two categories of value as a frame of reference, numerous questions can be asked regarding the moral and socio-political standing of sport. The most obvious question that comes to mind is what category of value is most appropriate to the sportive realm. Those who espouse an extrinsic value framework determine the value of sport in terms of its capacity to secure ends external to it. The history of sport is, of course, replete with instances of such valuation (a cursory perusal of sport's historical record reveals that it has been variously employed as a biological, psychological, social, political, military and economic instrument). Others, however, have argued that the good-making properties of sport reside within, and are peculiar to sport itself, and not in any extrinsic capacity it might possess. According to this value reference, sport is best treated as an intrinsic good, as something of value in and of itself. In fact, those of the latter value persuasion argue that an extrinsic regard for sport, taking note that such a regard places primary emphasis not on sport itself but its instrumental effects, is itself an exploitative value stance in that it lays sport open to, and makes possible, the sort of political and economic corruption that beset it today.

Other questions relating to sport and value-oriented concerns come easily to mind: Is sport good for people? Is it good to have to learn various sports? Is that good more important than the good accruing to freedom of choice? Is each or any of the practices associated with sport, good? Which ones and according to what source of values? Is it better to play well or to win? Are there right and wrong ways to play sports?

There has been much interest of late in the topic of morality and sport. Morgan's essay (1976) exemplifies much of the work in this area in its attempt to locate a suitable moral guide (in this instance Sartre's "Ethic of Ambiguity" is recommended) for the practice of sport. Osterhoudt's article (1973) incorporates the same analytic approach in arguing for the implementation of Kant's categorical imperative as a principle of moral conduct in sport. In a similar vein, Roberts and Galasso (1973) build on Cunningham's thesis that all conscious, intentional acts are inescapably moral by arguing that all sporting acts, given the latter's general nature, are necessarily moral. Zeigler (1973) develops the ethical implications of pragmatism for education, sport, and physical education. Suits (1973) presents a provocative account of the moral status of game-playing in which he argues that the play state is the ideal all human beings "ought" to aspire to. Sadler (1973) and Broekhoff (1973) argue that the moral character of sport can be assessed only in terms of its cultural situation. Keating (1973) rehearses some of the arguments he previously levelled against the use of sportsmanship as an all-encompassing moral principle and concludes that it only properly applies, in its fully moral sense, to the play domain. Osterhoudt (1973) unfolds a different view of the moral scope of sportsmanship by considering the implications of Keating's position for the "common good," a perspective which leads him to suggest that the moral virtues of magnanimity and generosity generated by sportsmanship apply for that matter to all other spheres of human life insofar as such virtues best fulfill the "common good."

The socio-political value dimension of sport is a subject that to date has not managed to attract serious philosophic attention. Most of the substantive work that has been done in this area has focused on the question whether sport reflects the political and ethical ideology of modern industrial society or whether sport in some sense subverts this ideology and therefore provides an expressive alternative to it. Those who argue for the former view include: Rigauer (1969), Oelschlägel (1968), Gehlen (1965), Krockow (1962), Habermas (1958), Plessner (1956), Ellul (1954), and Peters (1927). Those who argue for the latter view comprise: Suenens (1973), Lenk (1973), and Magnane (1964).

There remains much study to be done about sport and ethical and socio-political situations. First of all, the relationship between sport and ethical and social value is badly in need of clarification. The assumption that these subjects are inherently linked together must be examined. The values from sport need definition, particularly with reference to specific kinds and levels of sport. The kinds of ethical and socio-political principles taught through sport, again with reference to various types of sport experiences, need delineation. In this case, the conclusions derived from philosophical analysis can and should be subjected to empirical testing.

Ethics and socio-political philosophy, as aspects of philosophy and sport, have been allowed to remain a jumbled bag of assertions which have not been subjected to either philosophical or empirical analysis. It is a subject worthy of the attention of those who love sport, and also of those who are its critics.

The Ethics of Pleasure*

HERBERT SPENCER

To the great majority, who have imbibed more or less of that asceticism which, though appropriate to times of chronic militancy and also useful as a curb to ungoverned sensualism, has swayed too much men's theory of life, it will seem an absurd supposition that amusements are ethically warranted. Yet unless, in common with the Quakers and some extreme evangelicals, they hold them to be positively wrong, they must either say that amusements are neither right nor wrong, or, they must say that they are positively right—are to be morally approved.

That they are sanctioned by hedonistic ethics goes without saying. They are pleasure-giving activities; and that is their sufficient justification, so long as they do not unduly interfere with activities which are obligatory. Though most of our pleasures are to be accepted as concomitants of those various expenditures of energy conducive to self-sustentation and sustentation of family; yet the pursuit of pleasure for pleasure's sake is to be sanctioned, and even enjoined, when primary duties have been fulfilled.

So, too, are they to be approved from the physiological point of view. Not only do the emotional satisfactions which accompany normal life-sustaining labours exalt the vital functions, but the vital functions are exalted by those satisfactions which accompany the superfluous expenditures of energy implied by amusements: much more exalted in fact. Such satisfactions serve to raise the tide of life, and taken in due proportion conduce to every kind of efficiency.

Yet once more there is the evolutionary justification. In § 534 of *The Principles of Psychology*, it was shown that whereas, in the lowest creatures, the small energies which exist are wholly used up in those actions which serve to maintain the individual and propagate the species; in creatures of successively higher grades, there arises an increasing amount of unused energy: every improvement of organization achieving some economy, and so augmenting the surplus power. This surplus expends itself in the activities we call play. Among the superior *vertebrata* the tendency to these superfluous activities becomes conspicuous; and it is especially conspicuous in Man, when so conditioned that stress of competition does not make the sustentation of self and family too laborious. The implication is that in a fully developed form of human life, a considerable space will be filled by the pleasurable exercise of faculties which have not been exhausted by daily activities.

. . . .

Throughout the foregoing class of pleasures, resulting from the superfluous excitements of faculties, the individual is mainly passive. We turn now to the class in which he is mainly active; which again is subdivisible into two classes—sports and games. With sports, ethics has little concern beyond graduating its degrees of reprobation. Such of them as involve the direct infliction of pain, especially on fellow-

* From *The Principles of Ethics*, Vol. I. New York: D. Appleton and Company, 1910.

beings, are nothing but means to the gratification of feelings inherited from savages of the baser sort. That after these thousands of years of social discipline, there should still be so many who like to see the encounters of the prize-ring or witness the goring of horses and riders in the arena, shows how slowly the instincts of the barbarian are being subdued. No condemnation can be too strong for these sanguinary amusements which keep alive in men the worst parts of their natures and thus profoundly vitiate social life. Of course in a measure, though in a smaller measure, condemnation must be passed on field-sports—in smaller measure because the obtainment of food affords a partial motive, because the infliction of pain is less conspicuous, and because the chief pleasure is that derived from successful exercise of skill. But it cannot be denied that all activities with which there is joined the consciousness that other sentient beings, far inferior though they may be, are made to suffer, are to some extent demoralizing. The sympathies do, indeed, admit of being so far specialized that the same person who is unsympathetic towards wild animals may be in large measure sympathetic towards fellow-men; but a full amount of sympathy cannot well be present in the one relation and absent in the other. It may be added that the specializing of the sympathies has the effect that they become smaller as the remoteness from human nature becomes greater; and that hence the killing of a deer sins against them more than does the killing of a fish.

Those expenditures of energy which take the form of games, yield pleasures from which there are but small, if any, drawbacks in the entailed pains. Certain of them, indeed, as football, are as much to be reprobated as sports, than some of which they are more brutalizing; and there cannot be much ethical approbation of those games, so-called, such as boat-races, in which a painful and often injurious overtax of the system is gone through to achieve a victory, pleasurable to one side and entailing pain on the other. But there is ethical sanction for those games in which, with a moderate amount of muscular effort, there is joined the excitement of a competition not too intense, kept alive from moment to moment by the changing incidents of the contest. Under these conditions the muscular actions are beneficial, the culture of the perceptions is useful, while the emotional pleasure has but small drawbacks. And here I am prompted to denounce the practice, now so general, of substituting gymnastics for games—violent muscular actions joined with small concomitant pleasures, for moderate muscular actions joined with great pleasures. This usurpation is a sequence of that pestilent asceticism which thinks that pleasure is of no consequence, and that if the same amount of exercise be taken, the same benefit is gained: the truth being that to the exaltation of the vital functions which the pleasure produces, half the benefit is due.

Of indoor games which chiefly demand quickness of perception, quickness of reasoning, and quickness of judgment, general approval may be expressed with qualifications of no great importance. For young people they are especially desirable as giving to various of the intellectual faculties a valuable training, not to be given by other means. Under the stress of competition, the abilities to observe rapidly, perceive accurately, and infer rightly, are increased; and in addition to the immediate pleasures gained, there are gained powers of dealing more effectually with many of the incidents of life. It should be added that such drawbacks as there are, from the emotions accompanying victory and defeat, are but small in games which involve chance as a considerable factor, but are very noticeable where there is no chance. Chess, for example, which pits together two intelligences in such a way as to show unmistakably the superiority of one to the other in respect of certain powers, produces, much more than whist, a feeling of humiliation in the defeated, and if the sympathies are keen this gives some annoyance to the victor as well as to the vanquished.

Of course, such ethical sanction as is given to games, cannot be given where gambling or betting is an accompaniment. Involving, as both do, in a very definite way, and often to an extreme degree, the obtainment of pleasure at the cost of another's pain, they are to be condemned both for this immediate effect and for their remote effect—the repression of fellow-feeling.

Before passing to the altruistic aspect of amusements, there should be noted a less familiar egotistic aspect. Unless they have kept up during life an interest in pastimes, those who have broken down from overwork (perhaps an overwork entailed on them by imperative duties) usually find themselves incapable of relaxing in any satisfactory way: they are no longer amusable. Capacities for all other pleasures are atrophied, and the only pleasure is that which business gives. In such cases recovery is, if not prevented, greatly retarded by the lack of exhilarating occupations. Frequently dependents suffer.

This last consideration shows that these, like other classes of actions which primarily concern the individual, concern, to some extent, other individuals. But they concern other individuals in more direct and constant ways also. On each person there is imposed not only the peremptory obligation so to carry on his life as to avoid inequitably interfering with the carrying on of others' lives, and not only the less peremptory obligation to aid under various circumstances the carrying on of their lives, but there is imposed some obligation to increase the pleasures of their lives by sociality, and by the cultivation of those powers which conduce to sociality. A man may be a good economical unit of society, while remaining otherwise an almost worthless unit. If he has no knowledge of the arts, no aesthetic feelings, no interest in fiction, the drama, poetry, or music—if he cannot join in any of those amusements which daily and at longer intervals fill leisure spaces in life—if he is thus one to whom others cannot readily give pleasure, at the same time that he can give no pleasure to others, he becomes in great measure a dead unit, and unless he has some special value might better be out of the way.

Thus, that he may add his share to the general happiness, each should cultivate in due measure those superfluous activities which primarily yield self-happiness.

Physical Training and Moral Education*

JOSIAH ROYCE

The rational solution of moral problems rests on the principle: *Be loyal.* This principle, properly understood, involves two consequences. The first is this: Have a cause, choose a cause, give yourself over to that cause actively, devotedly, whole-heartedly, practically. Let this cause be something social, serviceable, requiring loyal devotion. Let this cause, or system of causes, constitute a life-work. Let the cause possess your senses, your attention, your muscles,—all your powers, so long as you are indeed active and awake at all. See that you do not rest in any mere sentiment of devotion to the cause. Act out your loyalty. Loyalty exists in the form of deeds done by the willing and devoted instrument of his chosen cause. This is the first consequence of the commandment: *Be loyal.* The second consequence is like unto the first. It is this: *Be loyal to loyalty.* That is, regard your neighbor's loyalty as something sacred. Do nothing to make him less loyal. Never despise him for his loyalty, however little you care for the cause that he chooses. If your cause and his cause come into some inevitable conflict, so that you indeed have to contend with him, fight, if your loyalty requires you to do so; but in your bitterest warfare fight only against what the opponent does. Thwart his acts where he justly should be thwarted; but do all this in the very cause of loyalty itself, and never do anything to make

*Excerpted from *Some Relations of Physical Training to the Present Problems of Moral Education in America.* Boston: The Boston Normal School of Gymnastics, *ca.* 1908.

your neighbor disloyal. Never do anything to encourage him in any form of disloyalty. In other words, never war against his loyalty. From these consequences of my central principle follow, as I maintain, all those propositions about the special duties of life which can be reasonably defined and defended. Justice, kindliness, chivalry, charity,— these are all of them forms of loyalty to loyalty.

Even while I have set forth this sketch of a general ethical doctrine, I have intentionally illustrated my views by some references to your professional work. But at this point I next have briefly to emphasize the positive relations which physical education may have and should have to the training of the loyal spirit. Here I shall simply repeat what others, more expert than I am, have long since, in various speech, set forth.

The first way in which systematic physical training of all grades and at all ages may be of positive service in a moral education is this: Loyalty, as we have seen, means a willing and thoroughgoing devotion of the whole active self to a chosen cause or to a chosen system of causes. But such devotion, as we have also seen, is a motor process. One must be in control of one's powers, or one has no self to give to one's cause. One must get a personality in order to be able to surrender this personality to anything. And since physical training actually has that relation to the culture of the will which your leaders so generally emphasize, while some physical expression of one's personality is an essential accompaniment of the existence of every human personality,—for both of these reasons, I say, the training of physical strength and skill is one important preparation for a moral life. There is indeed a great deal else in moral training besides what physical training supplies; but the physical training can be a powerful auxiliary. Here I come upon ground that is familiar to all of you, and that I need not attempt to cover anew with suggestions of my own. The positive relation of good physical training to the formation of a sound will is known to all of you. The only relatively new aspect of this familiar region that may have been brought to light by the foregoing considerations is this: Loyalty, as you see, on its highest levels involves the same general mental features which are present whenever a physical activity, at once strenuous and skilful, is going on. As a skilful and difficult physical exercise demands that one should keep his head in the midst of efforts that, by reason of the strain, or of the excitement,—by reason of the very magnitude and fascination of the task, would confuse the untrained man, and make him lose a sense of what he was trying to do, even so the work of the effectively loyal person is always one which requires that he should stand in presence of undertakings large enough to threaten to cloud his judgment and to crush his self-control, while his loyalty still demands that he also should keep his head despite the strain, and should retain steady control of his personality, even in order to devote it to the cause. Loyalty means hard work in the presence of serious responsibilities. The danger of such work is closely similar to the danger of losing one's head in a difficult physical activity. One is devoting the self to the cause. The cause must be vast. For its very vastness is part of what gives it worth. I cannot be loyal to what requires of me no effort. But the consciousness of the vastness and difficulty of one's cause tends to crush the self of the person who is trying to be loyal. And a self crushed into a loss of self-possession, a self no longer aware of its powers, a self that has lost sight of its true contrast with the objects about it, has no longer left the powers which it can devote to any cause. Mere good will is no substitute for trained self-possession either in physical or in moral activities. And self-possession is a necessary condition for self-devotion. When the apostle compared the moral work of the saints to the running of a race, his metaphors were therefore chosen because of this perfectly definite analogy between the devotion of the trained organism to its physical task and the devotion of the moral self to its

cause. In both classes of cases, in loyal devotion and in skilful and strenuous physical exercise, similar mental problems have to be solved. One has to keep the self in sight in order to surrender it anew, through each deed, to the task in hand. Meanwhile, since the task is centred upon something outside of the self, and is a serious and an imposing task, it involves a tendency to strain, to excitement, to a loss of a due self-possession, to disturbance of the equilibrium of consciousness. The result is likely to be, unless one is in a state of physical or of moral training, just a primary confusion of self-consciousness, accompanied by fear or by a sense of helplessness. Against such a mood the mere sentiment of devotion is no safeguard. To hold on to one's self at the moment of the greatest strain, to retain clearness, even when confronted by tasks too large to be carried out as one wishes, to persist doggedly despite defeats, to give up all mere self-will and yet to retain full self-control,—these are requirements which, as I suppose, appear to the consciousness of the athlete and to the consciousness of the moral hero in decidedly analogous ways. And in both cases the processes involved are psycho-physical as well as psychical, and are subject to the general laws of physiology and of psychology.

. . . .

The second way in which physical training may serve the purposes of moral training is a more direct way. It is the one which Dr. Luther Gulick had in mind when he lately asserted in a paper in the *School Review* that "athletics are primarily social and moral in their nature." Dr. Gulick is well known to you as one of the protagonists in the cause of the moral importance of physical education; and you know his main argument. Social training, in boys about twelve years of age, naturally takes the form of the training which gangs of boys give to their members. A gang of boys with nothing significant to do may become more or less of a menace to the general social order. A gang of boys duly organized into athletic teams, in the service of schools, and of other expressions of wholesome community activity, will become centres for training in certain types of loyalty. And this training may extend its influence to large bodies of boys who, as spectators of games or as schoolmates, are more or less influenced by the athletic spirit. *Mutatis mutandis*, the same considerations apply to the socially organizing forces that belong to college athletics. The plans of those who are engaged in physical education may therefore well be guided, from the first, by a disposition to prepare young people to appreciate and to take part in such group activities as these. Thus both the physiological and the intellectual aspects of physical training would appear to be subordinate, after all, to the social, and in this way to the moral, aspects of the profession. In speaking of these moral aspects, one would not even emphasize, as much as many do, the central significance of the self-denial, of the personal restraints and sacrifices, of the morally advantageous physical habits, which attend athletic training. One would rather more centrally emphasize the view that athletic work is not merely a preparation for loyalty, but that in case of the life of the organized athletic teams, and in case of any physical training class of pupils who work together, the athletic work *is* loyalty itself,—loyalty in simple forms, but in forms which appeal to the natural enthusiasm of youth, which are adapted to the boyish and later to the adolescent phases of evolution, and which are a positive training for the very tasks which adult loyalty exemplifies; namely, the tasks that imply the devotion of a man's whole power to an office that takes him out of his private self and into the great world of real social life. The social forms of physical training in classes or in teams require, and so tend to train, loyalty.

.   .   .   .

The third positive relation of physical training to moral training is suggested by what I have said about the need of an enlightened form of loyalty. Merely blind loyalty may do mischief; but it does so, we have said, not because it is loyalty, but because it is blind. It turns into enlightened loyalty in so far as it reaches the stage of loyalty to loyalty,—the stage where one certainly does not tend merely to take over into one's own life and directly to adopt the special cause that one's neighbor has happened to choose as his own, but where one regards the spirit of loyalty, the willingness to devote the self to some cause, as a precious common moral good of mankind,—a good that we can indeed foster in our neighbors even when their individual causes are not, or are even, by accident, opposed to our own. I can respect, can honor, I can help, my neighbor's family loyalty without in the least wishing to become a member of his family. And just so I can be loyal to any aspect of my neighbor's loyalty without accepting his special cause as my own. He may be devoted to what I cannot and will not view as my individual cause; and

still, in dealing with him, I can be loyal to his loyalty.

Now I have already pointed out that the spirit of loyalty to loyalty is finely exemplified by the spirit of fair play in games. For true fair play does not merely mean conformity to a set of rules which chance this season to govern a certain game. Fair play depends upon essentially respecting one's opponent just because of his loyalty to his own side. It means a tendency to enjoy, to admire, to applaud, to love, to further that loyalty of his at the very moment when I keenly want and clearly intend to thwart his individual deeds, and to win this game, if I can. Now in the complications of real life it is hard to keep the spirit of loyalty to loyalty always alive. If my passions are aroused and if I hate a man, it is far too easy to think that even his faithful dog must be a mean cur, in order to be able to be so devoted to his master as he is. And real life often thus confuses our judgment through stirring our passions. But it is a very precious thing when you can keep your head so clearly as to be able to oppose even to the very death, if needs must be, your enemy's cause, even while you are able to love his loyalty to that cause, and to honor his followers for their devotion to their leader and his friends for their fidelity to him.

Now it is just such loyalty to loyalty that can be trained in true sport very much more readily than in real life, because, in sport, the social situation is simple. And because the spirit of fair play, in an athletic sport, can constantly express itself by definite physical deeds, and because the passions aroused by wholesome athletic contests ought never to be as blind, as violent, or as enduring, as those which real life unhappily so often fosters, the training in fair play ought to be much easier in the world of athletic sports than the training of loyalty to loyalty is in our daily life,—much easier, much simpler, and much more definite. Hence, if games were in all cases rightly conducted, if confusing passions were properly kept from unnecessary interference with the joyous devotion of the players to their respective sides, if the general physical training of all those who are to engage in school and in college sports were conducted from the first by teachers who had a serious interest in the moral welfare of their classes,—well, if these conditions were realized, physical education ought to contribute its important share to what we have now seen to be the very crown of human virtue; namely, to the spirit of loyalty to loyalty,—to the spirit that honors and respects one's very enemies for their devotion to the very causes that one assails. The result should be the spiritual power to appreciate that common good for which even those who are mutually most hostile are contending. We human beings cannot agree as to the choice of our individual causes. We can learn to honor one another's loyalty.

.   .   .   .

And with these words I am indeed brought to the central problem amongst all those with which this discussion is concerned. I have set forth the three sorts of positively helpful relations that a sound physical training can develop in its bearing upon the work of moral training. First, because skilful and serious physical exercise involves true devotion, a sound physical training can help to prepare the organism and the personality for loyal types of activity. Secondly, physical training, in so far as it is a part of the life of a social group, can more directly aid the individual to learn to be loyal to his group. Thirdly, physical training, in so far as it can be used to give expression to the spirit of fair play, may be an aid towards the highest types of morality; namely, to those which embody that spirit of loyalty to loyalty which is destined, we hope, some day to bring to pass the spiritual union of all mankind. I have pointed out that all these three forms are simply possible forms in which the moral usefulness of physical training may appear. There is nothing that fatally secures the attainment of any of these three results. All depends upon the spirit, the skill, and the opportunities of the teacher, and upon the awakening of the right spirit in the learners. Instead of these good results, a failure to reach any of these three sorts of good results, in any tangible form, is in case of any given pupil or class of pupils perfectly possible. And, as we have just seen, the failure of certain forms of athletic sports to further, in certain well-known cases, the high cause of loyalty to loyalty has of late been far too conspicuous.

Is Professional Boxing Immoral?*

RICHARD A. McCORMICK, S.J.

Professional boxing is a part of us. Yet every now and then a tragedy (such as the death of Benny Paret) shocks us into enquiry. It revives and reveals the morality of professional boxing as a legitimate question. This is in some ways unfortunate. The outbursts surrounding tragedy tend to obscure the real issue by focusing exclusively on fatalities. They also provoke us to continue to think with our hearts rather than our heads. Rarely has morality been clarified in such an atmosphere.

Boxing can be and has been defined as a giving and parrying of light blows with no intention of striking the opponent severely. If no one has ever questioned the morality of this type of thing, neither has anyone ever thought it a realistic definition of modern professional boxing. Recent moral theologians who have reflected on the matter wisely restrict their considerations to "professional boxing as it is today." When the theologian says *as it is today,* he is trying to highlight an existing situation, perhaps not an inevitable one. Some, possibly many, elements of professional boxing could be radically altered, in which case it is quite conceivable that a different moral evaluation of the sport would have to be made.

By using the phrase *professional boxing as it is today* the theologian does not mean to concentrate on the fight-for-pay element which distinguishes amateur from professional; his intention is to emphasize the characteristics of professional boxing once the distinction has

* Reprinted by permission from *Sports Illustrated,* 17 (November 5, 1962), 70-82. © 1962 Time Inc.

been made. He is trying to paint a picture in a single phrase. Among these characteristics there is the element of a career involving a whole series of fights with cumulative effects. There is the admitted effort of most professionals to win by a KO—or at least a TKO—rather than by decision. There is the medical report of injury, particularly to the brain. There is the synthetic notion of courage wherein confession of injury followed by retirement from a fight invites derision by a crowd that enjoys a beating, clamors for the kill and lustily boos evasive tactics. There are the undeniable benefits that boxing has brought to the lives of many individuals. There are television contracts which create severe scheduling demands; there are boxing commissions and control groups. Finally, there is a specific set of rules. Professional boxing involves more and longer rounds, lighter gloves and sometimes different scoring criteria. These are the things the moralist attempts to evoke with the phrase *professional boxing as it is today.* It is not an individual fight that is his immediate concern. Individual fights may not contain the elements widely present in the sport as a whole. Nor is his concern boxing at the level of the Golden Gloves, the CYO and the private club. Still less is it a judgment of the individual fighter and his motives. It is a whole institution as it touches human conduct.

The defenders of professional boxing regard boxing as a science demanding skill, strength and discipline. In boxing there is splendid opportunity for physical development, alertness, poise, confidence, sportsmanship, initiative and character-building in general. Statistically professional boxing is, they point out, far less dangerous than auto racing, college football and several other sports. Furthermore, the game has given underprivileged youngsters a chance to better themselves. In summary, the advantages outweigh the disadvantages.

With an eye to these claims, some earlier moral evaluations of professional boxing were at times relatively tolerant. In fairness to these earlier views, it must be pointed out that they were formulated before widespread publication of pertinent medical findings. In fairness to professional boxing, however, it should be said that even those who now regard the sport as immoral concede the above advantages. Their objections are elsewhere.

The application of an immutable moral principle will vary with the variation of concrete fact or its understanding. Thus in the past 20 years or so there has been a growing consensus among theologians that the sport will not survive moral scrutiny. The three most recent American studies (Hillman, Bernard, Laforet) conclude that the current version of professional boxing is immoral. Most moral theologians would endorse and defend this position, not as the official position of the Catholic Church (the Church has never spoken officially on the matter) but as their own conviction after thoughtful application of their principles to the facts as they see them. If they have been less than enthusiastic about publicizing their conviction it is not because of reluctance to take publicly an unpopular stand. That would be cowardice. Rather it is because the conviction has matured slowly and painfully and because even now some uncertainties still cling to it. But as the subject receives intensified study, it is increasingly difficult to find defenders of the sport among theologians.

Professional boxing is unique among the sports. It is admittedly the only sport whose primary objective toward victory is to batter and damage an opponent into helplessness and the incapacity to continue. In a sport where the infliction of damage is rewarded, one would expect a wide variety of injuries.

Ophthalmic injury is far from unknown, even to the extent of actual blindness. Maxillofacial and aural trauma, including damage to the jaw, teeth, nose and hearing apparatus, are more common. Boxer's nose and cauliflower ear are commonplaces. There is also the possibility of renal damage. Studies (*Journal of Urology*, 1954) have concluded that acute kidney trauma occurs in 65% to 89% of boxers during a fight and is manifested by postbout hematuria. A more recent study (*The Journal of the American Medical Association*, 1958), however, shows these symptoms to be innocent, transitory and painless. The long-term effects in terms of kidney scar and permanent impairment do not seem to exist.

While these and other types of injury do occur, it is craniocerebral injury that recently has engrossed the attention of the medical world. Because of the premium placed on the KO and the TKO, the head has always been the prime target in professional boxing. Blows directed to the head or face comprise about 85% of all blows delivered in the ordinary bout. Body blows are principally diversionary tactics to lay open this prime target. The injuries caused by head blows have provided excellent opportunity for medical investigation because, as noted in *The Lancet* (1937), "unlike accidents these injuries are caused by traumas almost always of the same kind and acting with almost laboratory exactness."

Scientists indicate that the human brain weighs about three pounds. It is fluid-packed but not secured within the skull. A blow to the head causes it to wobble, slide and bounce back and forth inside its cranial container. If a moderate blow can bang the brain against its sidewall, a more severe blow can bring it into contact with the bony sphenoidal ridge to produce selective damage to the frontal lobes, either bleeding or bruising. Where there is destruction of nerve cells the damage is permanent and, when repeated, cumulative.

Medical scientists also call attention to another injury not infrequently suffered by boxers: the punctate (small) hemorrhages in the pons and medulla, probably caused by the jamming of cerebrospinal fluid. Again, where such hemorrhages destroy nerve tissue the damage is permanent, though this need not imply that malfunction of the brain ensues. Such a symptom would be a matter of extent and degree. The possibilities for brain damage appear to be as multiple as the organ is delicate.

What are the noticeable results of brain injury? The most sensational, if not the most tragic, is death, generally associated with hemorrhage. Depending on how one reads statistics, will one conclude with Dr. Arthur H. Steinhaus, former chief of the Division of Physical Education and Health Activities of the U.S. Office of Education, that "professional boxing is 83 times more deadly than high school football and 50 times more deadly than college football"? Or with T. A. Gonzales that "32 years of boxing competitions . . . have produced fewer deaths in proportion to the number of participants than occur in baseball or football"? The point is not clear.

But if death is a relative rarity, the same does not seem to be true of brain damage. In 1928 H. S. Maitland concluded his discussion of the punch-drunk syndrome with the statement that 50% of fighters will develop the condition in mild or severe form if they stay in the game long enough, and that this "seems to be good evidence that some special brain injury due to their occupation exists." Dr. Edward J. Carroll Jr., who came to know fighters intimately through professional and nonprofessional contacts, estimated that after five years of boxing 60% of the boxers will develop mental and emotional changes which are obvious to people who know them. He stated (*American Journal of The Medical Sciences,* 1936) that "no head blow is taken with impunity and . . . each knockout causes definite and irreparable damage. If such trauma is repeated for a long enough period, it is inevitable that nerve cell insufficiency will develop ultimately . . . ." The recent work of La Cava in Italy and Pampus in Bonn tends to substantiate these claims. Findings such as these received fresh emphasis by sparring partner Ben Skelton's report (SI, Sept. 24) that Liston's left jab is so hard "that for a week after being hit with it I was taking pills to kill the pain."

Dr. Steinhaus has been so impressed with the medical evidence concerning brain damage in boxing that he feels a second foul line must be created at the shoulder. He cites a noted brain surgeon with wide experience with boxers as contending that every head-pommeling is likely to leave some small portion of the brain tissue permanently damaged, even though this may not be noticed for some time. The treacherous aspect of such injury is that it apparently does not manifest itself clinically until rather late in the degenerative process. Furthermore, there are obvious reasons why professional fighters would be reluctant to report symptoms of brain damage.

When one reads these statements—and there are many more of the same—one has an indefinable sense of uneasiness, of inconclusiveness. There is almost the sense of being in the presence of a crusader. Is it really this bad? Could it be that the admirable tendency of the doctor to regard *any* disease or injury as *too much* has expanded these statements? H. A. Kaplan (*The Journal of the American Medical Association,* 1959) contends that "a blow from a human being with a padded gloved fist probably is not forceful enough to produce any direct damage to the brain." In an area such as this, the theologian admits to hopeless incompetence. To complete his understanding of professional boxing he must rely completely on medical specialists. With this in mind I submitted the following statement, attributed to a prominent brain specialist, to 10 of the top neurosurgeons in the U.S. and Canada: "The brain is so constructed that it cannot suffer a series of head blows over the years in boxing without certainly or at least very probably incurring thereby some permanent injury." These experts agreed that the statement could be endorsed as a general statement. One was at pains to indicate that the statement, while it is probably correct, is poorly written. He could not accept the inference in it that malfunction of the brain follows brain damage. Such a symptom would be a matter of degree.

If these specialists are incorrect in their estimate about brain damage, then the moral theologian would desire to reexamine certain aspects or emphases of his argumentation, as we shall see. But it is this type of evidence that makes one take a long second look at the words of Abe Simon, former heavyweight contender: ". . . jarring of the brain. That's what causes the trouble—my headaches and those of every fighter who has taken punishment. It's not a single punch; it's the constant jarring. . . . [The fighter] is always soothed by the falsehood that he will be just as good as new after a short rest. He never is, and no fighter living today who has had 50 or more reasonably hard fights can honestly make the claim."

Such a medical review was necessary preparation for a moral estimate. Since everyone familiar with the sport concedes its advantages, the moral discussion boils down to this: Are the arguments against professional boxing conclusive? Of the many moral objections one hears, the most serious are reducible to three.

1) *The knockout.* It is simply unrealistic to deny that most professional fighters aim for a knockout. This is regarded as the most decisive and impressive way to win a fight. It is what the fighter wants and very often what the fans want. The long climb to contender status or the comeback often hinges on it. As Nat Fleischer wrote in *The Heavyweight Championship* of Louis' comeback tour after his 1936 loss to Max Schmeling: "There was only one way to do that—to roll up victory after victory over the knockout route."

Not a few moral theologians find it difficult to admit that the knockout is justifiable. They frequently formulate this as follows: directly and violently to deprive oneself or another of the use of reason is morally reprehensible except for a sufficient cause. It is the rational faculties, intellect and free will that distinguish man from the brute. Directly to deprive man of these faculties without a sufficient reason is to dehumanize. These theologians are reluctant to admit that sport, money, fame qualify as sufficient reason. If such violent deprivation of higher controls is reprehensible, then the intent to do so is equally reprehensible. Hence a sport in which this intent plays such an integral role must be condemned.

Is the argument convincing? I do not believe it is. First of all, the knockout is understood in the rather limited sense of "rendering unconscious." This is not a necessary sense of the word. A knockout is, more realistically, beating a fighter to the point where he is physically incapable of continuing. This is what the ordinary professional desires. Deprivation of the use of reason is not essential to this. Hence, practically, it is hard to show how the knockout in this limited sense is an essential aim of most fighters. Second, even if it were the fighter's aim, it would be difficult to show how the knockout of itself (independent of injury) is sufficient to condemn the sport. It can be argued that, generally, deprivation of the use of reason lasts only a few seconds at most (8 to 10 usually) and that this is so little as to be negligible. If this were the only thing at stake, it is highly doubtful that there would be as much objection to boxing as there seems to be.

2) *The intent of injury.* If the argument concerning the knockout is not satisfying, the objection from injury is much more arresting. Professional boxing is the only sport where the immediate objective is to damage the opponent. A puffed or cut eye, a lacerated cheek, a bleeding nose—these are signals for an intensified attack on the vulnerable area. When Jimmy Doyle died after being knocked out by Sugar Ray Robinson, Robinson was asked if he noticed that Doyle was in trouble. He is widely quoted as answering: "Getting him into trouble is my business." In all other sports the immediate objective is to cross a goal line, tip in a basket, throw a strike. Injury and incapacity to continue are incidental. A knee to the groin, a fist to the face in football, bean balls and deliberate spiking in baseball are penalized and would unhesitatingly be branded as immoral by the theologian. Patterson was simply describing the unique character of professional boxing when he wrote (*Victory over Myself*), after the first Johansson knockout, of his desire

never to be vicious again. "At the same time I know that I must be, because I am in a business of violence." If direct damage to the opponent is immoral in all other sports, why not in this business of violence?

It is here that the medical evidence assumes some importance. Were the injury passing and negligible, theologians might perhaps mitigate their judgment. But if the specialists are right in their claims about injury, particularly brain injury, this must give us pause. The sport as now practiced tends directly to inflict this damage. When injury to the cranium and its contents occurs, it is, as Blonstein and Clarke note (*British Medical Journal*, 1954), "a direct product of boxing and not an accident as in all other sports." Since this is true, then these effects are also the direct object of the fighter's intention. This is not to say that the fighter explicitly desires to maim or cause lasting damage. Few would be that inhuman. As a rule, the fighter's only explicit desire is to win as decisively as possible. But the means he chooses are means that are damaging. Hence he implicitly intends this damage as a means. How could he disown it? The point might seem a bit fine, but can one choose to pound and sink a nail and yet disown the hole in the wood?

At this point professional boxing encounters the disapproving frown of many a moralist. Man, they argue, does not possess the right directly to inflict damage on himself or another in this way. He is not the absolute master of his person with the power to destroy or mutilate as he wishes. Absolute dominion over man's integrity is possessed by God alone. As a creature, man is an administrator charged with the duty and privilege of reasonable administration. His ability directly to mutilate himself is severely limited.

This is a cardinal principle of sound moral thought. If there is indecisiveness here, there will inevitably be ambiguity or error in the evaluation of many aspects of modern living. Once the limit on man's ability to mutilate himself is obscured, the condemnation of suicide, euthanasia, reckless medical experiment, useless surgery and so on tends to lose rational defense. The novelist knows that the first chapters profoundly affect the outcome of the final chapters of his book. Similarly, moral theology is jealous of her basic principles because they contain the germ of practical conclusions.

Applying these principles, theologians believe that when a man pounds another into helplessness, scars his face, smashes his nose, jars his brain and exposes it to lasting damage, or when he enters a contest where this could happen to him, he has surpassed the bounds of reasonable stewardship of the human person. Surely there are equally—or more—effective ways for men to learn the art of self-defense.

Does the fact that this is done for money affect the moral analysis? Certain medical experiments on the human body, even if done for money, would remain objectionable. In fact, is there not a legitimate sense in which it is true to say that the greater the spoils, the more objectionable the whole business? For as the cash at stake increases, so does the danger of viewing the integrity of the human person as salable at a price. Money can be overvalued. When it is, something else is undervalued. If this something else happens to be the integrity of the human person, have we not made a wrong turn somewhere?

3) *Fostering of brutish instincts.* Man is a delicate combination, midway between animal and angel, with a bit of both in him. His characteristic balance is achieved when he harmonizes these elements. When he fosters one to the neglect of the other, he tends to become either a disengaged dreamer or a savage. Thomas Aquinas knew nothing of professional boxing; but with an unerring knowledge of human nature he pointed out that to take pleasure in the unnecessary sufferings of another man is brutish.

Anyone who has watched professional fights will know what Aquinas was talking about. The crowd too often has come for blood and the knockout. The knockout is the touchdown pass, the home run of boxing. The nearer it is, the more frenzied the howling of the crowd. As Nat Fleischer said simply of the first Patterson-Johansson fight: "The crowd, sensing the kill, went wild." We occasionally hear the referee urge the boys to mix it up, give the fans their money's worth. When a boy is being mauled around the ring, the arena comes alive and emotions run high. The fighter is goaded by the crowd; his own fury further stimulates them. The brutish instinct is in command. At this pitch the finest moves in boxing are missed or—worse—greeted by a chorus of hissing and booing. Tunney was so disgusted with this type of thing in one of his fights that he created the phrase, "the bloodthirsty yap of the mob." The modern prizefight is increasingly the canonization of brute force—and that at a time when we are struggling with all our might to understand the meaning of force in the world.

Is not man too weak a creature to unleash and give free play to these forces with impunity? Does he not tend to grow in the image of that which he cheers? If this is true, how long can he cheer these exhibitions without acting at variance with the demands dictated by his own rational nature? To many, this is the strongest indictment of professional boxing, an objection sufficient in itself as a stricture of the game.

These arguments are not frivolous. Any discussion of professional boxing which ignores them is playing the ostrich. They are drawn from natural law; whatever validity they have would surely be intensified by the Christian revelation through which man becomes conscious of an even more startling personal dignity. It was probably arguments such as these that led the Vatican Radio to announce its conviction that professional boxing is objectively immoral. *L'Osservatore della Domenica* insinuated the same thing. Informed Catholics, however, are rightly distressed at the implications in the assertion that these views are "semiofficial" ecclesiastical positions.

The Catholic Church has not condemned professional boxing. Many have wondered why not. The eager expectation of ecclesiastical intervention could easily contain a distorted notion of the function of the Church. While she jealously guards the purity of morals, it does not follow that condemnations do or should issue from her at the slightest provocation—if for no other reason than that this discourages intellectual effort in the ranks by seeming to render it unnecessary. We stand to learn a great deal from this controversy.

Many reasons suggest themselves in explanation of the Church's official silence on the matter. First of all, and most important perhaps, the matter simply is not clear to her. While the Church speaks frequently on changeless moral principles, she is generally quite content to leave the application of these to her theologians. But theological opinion has been, possibly still is, somewhat divided, or at least hesitant. Most of the serious writing has been unfavorable to boxing, but there are many voices yet to be heard.

Second, professional boxing is largely, but not exclusively, a local American problem. The U.S. champion is the world champion, the big gate is here and the big fights are generally here. If public statements are called for, it is reasonable to think that this would be left to local bishops.

Finally, even should the Church desire to take a strong stand, there is the difficulty of formulating a statement which will avoid the impression that all boxing is being censured. It is foolish to lump the pillow fights of the sixth grader with the hard smashes of the professional. And even at the professional level the differences between individual fighters are tremendous. There are those in superb condition who fight once or twice a year to defend a title—and these are the champions who are hit the least. Then there are those who all but drag themselves into the ring to have their brains rattled on a month-to-month basis. To group these together in a single sweeping rejection would be unrealistic and hazardous.

Not only is the central moral issue challenging; there are also many fringe problems no less tantalizing. One that is increasingly aired: Is the victorious fighter guilty when his opponent dies as a result of blows received in the ring? Though boxing is different from other sports in its direct aim (the infliction of damage), death is such a departure from the average that its occurrence should be regarded as an undesired byproduct of the sport. Morally it is an accident.

Problematic too are the possibilities involved in allowing a man with a past record to contend for the crown (SI, Feb. 12). The issue is scarcely one of Christian forgiveness or rehabilitation. Surely we can hope that we are both humble enough and large enough for this. The problem is rather the defenselessness of our children against their own hero-worshiping simplicity. On the other hand, a clear break with an unfortunate past might actually provide a very helpful example to youngsters. What ever the answer may be, there is a moral dimension even here.

The question of professional boxing is a vexing one. The issues seem clear. Defenders of the sport insist that the advantages outweigh the disadvantages. Those who censure it, while admitting the advantages, believe that the moral discussion must begin with the sport itself, not only its circumstances. They see the sport as directly injurious and as one which tends unduly to foster the instinct of brutality in all concerned. Perhaps this is not *necessarily* true; there are many laudable attempts being made to supervise the sport more thoroughly (SI, April 23). Nor is it *factually* true of all professional fights; but it is too *generally* true of the sport today. Thus the majority vote among those who have written on the moral question is unfavorable.

Unless the arguments leveled at professional boxing as it is today can be answered, I believe the sport would have to be labeled immoral. I realize that other theologians may take a different point of view. It could be that not all the facts are in. Perhaps, too, we have a great deal to learn about our own principles. Premature conviction slams the door to enlightenment as effectively as refusal to face the moral issue.

If there remain some uncertainties to haunt us, the general implications of our sincere and honest interest are clear. For, regardless of what answer we come up with, it is both a sign and guarantee of our abiding spiritual health to face issues at their moral root. It is never easy to question the moral character of our own pleasure and entertainment. Since, however, moral issues are not defined by the convenient and inconvenient, the pleasant and the annoying, but reach to the division between good and evil, they are too important to receive less than an earnest, but calm and dispassionate, treatment. Failure to do this would be a collective shrug-of-the-shoulder at moral values and, as such, a threat to the spiritual goods upon which we have built our dignity and freedom.

Sportsmanship as a Moral Category*

JAMES W. KEATING

Sportsmanship, long and inexplicably ignored by philosophers and theologians, has always pretended to a certain moral relevancy, although its precise place among the moral virtues has been uncertain. In spite of this confusion, distinguished advocates have made some remarkable claims for sportsmanship as a moral category. Albert Camus, Nobel prize winner for literature in 1957, said that it was from sports that he learned all that he knew about ethics.[1] Former President Hoover is quoted as saying: "Next to religion, the single greatest factor for good in the United States in recent years has been sport."[2] Dr. Robert C. Clothier, past president of Rutgers University, paraphrased the words of Andrew Fletcher and commented: "I care not who makes the laws or even writes the songs if the code of sportsmanship is sound, for it is that which controls conduct and governs the relationships between men."[3] Henry Steele Commager, professor of history at Columbia University, has argued that it was on the playing fields that Americans learned the lessons of courage and honor which distinguished them in time of war. Commager sums up: "In one way or another, this code of sportsmanship has deeply influenced our national destiny."[4] For Lyman Bryson, of Columbia University, sportsmanship was of extraordinary value:

> The doctrine of love is much too hard a doctrine to live by. But this is not to say that we

have not made progress. It could be established, I think, that the next best thing to the rule of love is the rule of sportsmanship. . . . Some perspicacious historian will some day write a study of the age-old correlation between freedom and sportsmanship. We may then see the importance of sportsmanship as a form of enlightenment. This virtue, without which democracy is impossible and freedom uncertain, has not yet been taken seriously enough in education.[5]

Pope Pius XII, speaking of fair play which is widely regarded as an essential ingredient of sportsmanship, if not synonymous with it, has said:

> From the birthplace of sport came also the proverbial phrase "fair play"; that knightly and courteous emulation which raises the spirit above meanness and deceit and dark subterfuges of vanity and vindictiveness and preserves it from the excesses of a closed and intransigent nationalism. Sport is the school of loyalty, of courage, of fortitude, of resolution and universal brotherhood.[6]

Charles W. Kennedy was a professor of English at Princeton University and chairman of its Board of Athletic Control. His small volume, *Sport and Sportsmanship*, remains to this day probably the most serious study of sportsmanship conducted in America. Kennedy's commitment to sportsmanship was not merely theoretical and scholarly. As chairman of Princeton's Board of Athletic Control, he severed athletic relations with Harvard when unsportsmanlike conduct marred the relationship.[7] For

Kennedy it was not sufficient that sportsmanship characterize man's activities on the athletic field; it must permeate all of life.

> When you pass out from the playing fields to the tasks of life, you will have the same responsibility resting upon you, in greater degree, of fighting in the same spirit for the cause you represent. You will meet bitter and sometimes unfair opposition. . . . You will meet defeat [but] you must not forget that the great victory of which you can never be robbed will be the ability to say, when the race is over and the struggle ended, that the flag you fought under was the shining flag of sportsmanship, never furled or hauled down and that, in victory or defeat, you never lost that contempt for a breach of sportsmanship which will prevent your stooping to it anywhere, anyhow, anytime.[8]

Similar eulogies by other distinguished men with no professional or financial interest in sport or athletics could be multiplied without difficulty, but perhaps the point has already been made. The claims for sportsmanship as a moral category deserves some investigation. It is surprising that the experts in moral theory, the philosopher and the theologian, have seen fit to ignore so substantial an area of human conduct as that occupied by sport and athletics.

Three interrelated problems will be considered in this study: (1) the source of the confusion which invariably accompanies a discussion of sportsmanship and the normal consequences resulting from this confusion; (2) the essence of genuine sportsmanship, or the conduct and attitude proper to sport, with special consideration being given to the dominant or pivotal virtues involved; (3) sportsmanship as applied to athletics—a derivative or analogous use of the term. Once again special attention will be directed to the basic or core virtues which characterize the conduct and attitude of the well-behaved athlete.

THE SOURCE OF CONFUSION AND ITS CONSEQUENCES

What is sportsmanship? William R. Reed, commissioner for the Big Ten Intercollegiate Conference, is most encouraging: "It [sportsmanship] is a word of exact and uncorrupted meaning in the English language, carrying with it an understandable and basic ethical norm. Henry C. Link in his book 'Rediscovery of Morals' says, 'Sportsmanship is probably the clearest and most popular expression of morals.' "[9] Would that this were the case. Reed, however, does not define sportsmanship or enumerate the provisions of its code, and the briefest investigation reveals that he is badly mistaken as to the clarity of the concept. The efforts of no less a champion of sportsmanship than Amos Alonzo Stagg presage the obscurities which lie ahead. In addition to a brilliant athletic career at Yale and forty years as head football coach at the University of Chicago, Stagg did a year of graduate work in Yale's Divinity School and would thus seem to have the ideal background of scholarly training in moral theory and vast practical experience to discuss the problem. Yet his treatment leaves much to be desired. He defined sportsmanship as "a delightful fragrance that people will carry with them in their relations with their fellow men."[10] In addition, he drew up separate codes of sportsmanship, or Ten Commandments of sport, for the coach and for the football player and held that both decalogues were applicable to the business world as well. The second, and by far the most unusual, commandment contained proscriptions seldom found in codes of sportsmanship. "Make your conduct a worthy example. Don't drink intoxicants; don't gamble; don't smoke; don't use smutty language; don't tell dirty stories; don't associate with loose or silly women."[11] Stagg's position is undoubtedly an extreme one, but it calls attention to a tendency all too common among the champions of sportsmanship—the temptation to broaden the concept of sportsmanship until it becomes an all-embracing moral category, a unique road to moral salvation. As always, there is an opposite extreme. Sportsmanship, when not viewed as the pinnacle of moral perfection, can also be viewed as a moral minimum—one step this side of criminal behavior. "A four point program to improve sportsmanship at athletic events has been adopted by the Missouri State High School Activities Association."[12] The first and third provisions of by-law No. 9 detail penalties for assaults or threats upon officials by players or fans. Such legislative action may be necessary and even admirable, but it is a serious error to confuse the curtailment of criminal activities of this sort with a positive promotion of sportsmanship.

What, then, is sportsmanship? Another approach is by way of the dictionary, everyday experience, and common-sense deductions. Sportsmanship is conduct becoming a sportsman. And who is a sportsman? One who is interested in or takes part in sport. And what is sport? Sport, Webster tells us, is "that which diverts and makes mirth"; it is an "amusement, recreation, pastime." Our problem, then, is to determine the conduct and attitude proper to this type of activity, and this can be done only after a more careful consideration of the nature of sport. Pleasant diversion? Recreation? Amusement? Pastime? Is this how one would describe the World Series, the Masters, the Davis Cup, the Rose Bowl, the Olympic Games, or a high-school basketball tournament? Do the "sport" pages of our newspapers detail the pleasant diversions and amusements of the citizenry, or are they preoccupied with national and international contests which capture the imaginations, the emotions, and the pocketbooks of millions of fans (i.e., fanatics)? It is precisely at this point that we come face to face with the basic problem which has distorted or vitiated most discussions of sportsmanship. Because the term "sport" has been loosely applied to radically different types of human behavior, because it is naïvely regarded as an apt description of (1) activity which seeks only pleasant diversion and, on the other hand, (2) of the agonistic struggle to demonstrate personal or group excellence, the determination of the conduct proper to a participant in "sport" becomes a sticky business indeed. Before proceeding with an analysis of sportsmanship as such, it is necessary to consider briefly an all-important distinction between sport and athletics.

Our dictionary definition of sport leans upon its root or etymological meaning. "Sport," we are told, is an abbreviation of the Middle English *desport* or *disport,* themselves derivatives of the Old French *desporter,* which literally meant to carry away from work. Following this lead, Webster and other lexicographers indicate that "diversion," "recreation," and "pastime" are essential to sport. It is "that which diverts and makes mirth; a pastime." While the dictionaries reflect some of the confusion and fuzziness with which contemporary thought shrouds the concept of athletics, they invariably stress an element which, while only accidentally associated with sport, is essential to athletics. This element is the prize, the *raison d'être* of athletics. Etymologically, the various English forms of the word "athlete" are derived from the Greek verb *athlein,* "to contend for a prize," or the noun *athlos,* "contest," or *athlon,* a prize awarded for the successful completion of the contest. An oblique insight into the nature of athletics is obtained when we realize that the word "agony" comes from the Greek *agonia*—a contest or a struggle for victory in the games. Thus we see that, historically and etymologically, sport and athletics have characterized radically different types of human activity, different not insofar as the game itself or the mechanics or rules

are concerned, but different with regard to the attitude, preparation, and purpose of the participants. Man has probably always desired some release or diversion from the sad and serious side of life. This, of course, is a luxury, and it is only when a hostile environment is brought under close rein and economic factors provide a modicum of leisure that such desires can be gratified. In essence, sport is a kind of diversion which has for its direct and immediate end fun, pleasure, and delight and which is dominated by a spirit of moderation and generosity. Athletics, on the other hand, is essentially a competitive activity, which has for its end victory in the contest and which is characterized by a spirit of dedication, sacrifice, and intensity.

When this essential distinction between sport and athletics is ignored, as it invariably is, the temptation to make sportsmanship an all-embracing moral category becomes irresistible for most of its champions. In 1926 a national Sportsmanship Brotherhood was organized for the purpose of spreading the gospel of sportsmanship throughout all aspects of life, from childhood games to international events.[13] Its code consisted of eight rules:

1. Keep the rule.
2. Keep faith with your comrades.
3. Keep yourself fit.
4. Keep your temper.
5. Keep your play free from brutality.
6. Keep pride under in victory.
7. Keep stout heart in defeat.
8. Keep a sound soul and a clean mind in a healthy body.

The slogan adopted by the Brotherhood to accompany its code was "Not that you won or lost—but how you played the game." In giving vigorous editorial support to the Sportsmanship Brotherhood, the *New York Times* said:

> Take the sweet and the bitter as the sweet and bitter come and always "play the game." That is the legend of the true sportsmanship, whether on the ball field, the tennis court, the golf course, or at the desk or machine or throttle. "Play the game." That means truthfulness, courage, spartan endurance, self-control, self-respect, scorn of luxury, consideration one for another's opinions and rights, courtesy, and above all fairness. These are the fruits of the spirit of sportsmanship and in them . . . lies the best hope of social well-being.[14]

Dictionaries that have suggested the distinction between sport and athletics without explicitly emphasizing it have remained relatively free from this type of romantic incrustation and moral exaggeration in their treatment of sportsmanship. Beginning with nominal definitions of sportsmanship as the conduct becoming a sportsman and of the sportsman as one who participates in sport, they proceed, much more meaningfully, to characterize the sportsman by the kind of conduct expected of him. A sportsman is "a person who can take loss or defeat without complaint or victory without gloating and who treats his opponents with fairness, generosity and courtesy." In spite of the limitations of such a description, it at least avoids the inveterate temptation to make sportsmanship a moral catch-all.

THE ESSENCE OF GENUINE SPORTSMANSHIP

Sportsmanship is not merely an aggregate of moral qualities comprising a code of specialized behavior; it is also an attitude, a posture, a manner of interpreting what would otherwise be only a legal code. Yet the moral qualities believed to comprise the code have almost monopolized consideration and have proliferated to the point of depriving sportsmanship of any distinctiveness. Truthfulness, courage, spartan endurance, self-control, self-respect, scorn of luxury, consideration one for another's opinions and rights, courtesy, fairness, magnanimity, a high sense of honor, co-operation, generosity. The list seems interminable. While the conduct and attitude which are properly designated as sportsmanlike may reflect many of the above-mentioned qualities, they are not all equally basic or fundamental. A man may be law-abiding, a team player, well conditioned, courageous, humane, and the possessor of *sang-froid* without qualifying as a sportsman. On the other hand, he may certainly be categorized as a sportsman without possessing spartan endurance or a scorn of luxury. Our concern is not with those virtues which *might* be found in the sportsman. Nor is it with those virtues which *often* accompany the sportsman. Our concern is rather with those moral habits or qualities which are essential, which characterize the participant as a sportsman. Examination reveals that there are some that are pivotal and absolutely essential; others peripheral. On what grounds is such a conclusion reached? Through the employment of the principle that the nature of the activity determines the conduct and attitudes proper to it. Thus, to the extent that the conduct and attitudes of the participants contribute to the attainment of the goal of sport, to that extent

they can be properly characterized as sportsmanlike. The primary purpose of sport is not to win the match, to catch the fish or kill the animal, but to derive pleasure from the attempt to do so and to afford pleasure to one's fellow participants in the process. Now it is clear that the combined presence of such laudable moral qualities as courage, self-control, co-operation, and a spirit of honor do not, in themselves, produce a supporting atmosphere. They may be found in both parties to a duel or in a civil war. But generosity and magnanimity are essential ingredients in the conduct and attitude properly described as sportsmanlike. They establish and maintain the unique social bond; they guarantee that the purpose of sport—the immediate pleasure of the participants—will not be sacrificed to other more selfish ends. All the prescriptions which make up the code of sportsmanship are derived from this single, basic, practical maxim: Always conduct yourself in such a manner that you will increase rather than detract from the pleasure to be found in the activity, both your own and that of your fellow participants. If there is disagreement as to what constitutes sportsmanlike behavior, then this disagreement stems from the application of the maxim rather than from the maxim itself. It is to be expected that there will be differences of opinion as to how the pleasurable nature of the activity can best be maximized.

The code governing pure sport is substantially different from a legalistic code in which lawyers and law courts are seen as a natural and healthy complement of the system. In fact, it is in direct comparison with such a system that the essence of sportsmanship can best be understood. In itself, sportsmanship is a spirit, an attitude, a manner or mode of interpreting an otherwise purely legal code. Its purpose is to protect and cultivate the festive mood proper to an activity whose primary purpose is pleasant diversion, amusement, joy. The sportsman adopts a cavalier attitude toward his personal rights under the code; he prefers to be magnanimous and self-sacrificing if, by such conduct, he contributes to the enjoyment of the game. The sportsman is not in search of legal justice; he prefers to be generous whenever generosity will contribute to the fun of the occasion. Never in search of ways to evade the rules, the sportsman acts only from unquestionable moral right.

Our insistence that sport seeks diversion, recreation, amusement does not imply that the sportsman is by nature a listless competitor. It is common practice for him, once the game is under way, to make a determined effort to win. Spirited competitor that he often is, however, his goal is joy in the activity itself and anything—any word, action, or attitude—which makes the game itself less enjoyable should be eliminated. He "fights" gallantly to win because experience has taught him that a determined effort to overcome the obstacles which his particular sport has constructed, adds immeasurably to the enjoyment of the game. He would be cheating himself and robbing the other participants of intense pleasure if his efforts were only halfhearted. Yet there is an important sense in which sporting activity is not competitive but rather co-operative. Competition denotes the struggle of two parties for the same valued object or objective and implies that, to the extent that one of the parties is successful in the struggle, he gains exclusive or predominant possession of that object at the expense of his competitor. But the goal of sporting activity, being the mutual enjoyment of the participants, cannot even be understood in terms of exclusive possession by one of the parties. Its simulated competitive atmosphere camouflages what is at bottom a highly co-operative venture. Sport, then, is a co-operative endeavor to maximize pleasure or joy, the immediate pleasure or joy to be found in the activity itself. To so characterize sport is not to indulge in romantic exaggeration. It is indisputable that the spirit of selfishness is at a very low ebb in genuine sport. Gabriel Marcel's observation concerning the relationship of generosity to joy may even have a limited applicability here. "If generosity enjoys its own self it degenerates into complacent self-satisfaction. This enjoyment of self is not joy, for joy is not a satisfaction but an exaltation. It is only in so far as it is introverted that joy becomes enjoyment."[15] In comparison with sport, athletics emphasize self-satisfaction and enjoyment; sport is better understood in terms of generosity, exaltation, and joy.

Although there is no acknowledgment of the fact, the concern which has been shown for sportsmanship by most of its advocates has been almost exclusively directed to its derivative meaning—a code of conduct for athletes. To the extent that the Sportsmanship Brotherhood was concerned with athletics (and their code of conduct would indicate that was their main concern), their choice of a slogan seems singularly inappropriate. "Not that you won or lost—but how you played the game." Such a slogan can be accommodated in the world of sport, but even there the word "enjoyed"

should be substituted for the word "played." Application of this slogan to athletics, on the other hand, would render such activity unintelligible, if not irrational.

"SPORTSMANSHIP" IN ATHLETICS

Careful analysis has revealed that sport, while speaking the language of competition and constantly appearing in its livery, is fundamentally a co-operative venture. The code of the sportsman, sportsmanship, is directed fundamentally to facilitating the co-operative effort and removing all possible barriers to its development. Mutual generosity is a most fertile soil for co-operative activity. When we move from sport to athletics, however, a drastic change takes place. Co-operation is no longer the goal. The objective of the athlete demands exclusive possession. Two cannot share in the same victory unless they are team mates, and, as a result, the problems of competition are immediately in evidence. "Sportsmanship," insofar as it connotes the behavior proper to the athlete, seeks to place certain basic limitations on the rigors of competition, just as continual efforts are being made to soften the impact of the competitive struggle in economics, politics, international relations, etc. But we must not lose sight of an important distinction. Competition in these real-life areas is condoned or encouraged to the extent that it is thought to contribute to the common good. It is not regarded as an end in itself but as the only or most practicable means to socially desirable ends. Friedrich A. Hayek, renowned economist and champion of competition in economics, supports this position:

> The liberal argument is in favor of making the best possible use of the forces of competition as a means of co-ordinating human efforts, not an argument for leaving things just as they are. It is based on the conviction that, where effective competition can be created, it is a better way of guiding individual efforts than any other. It does not deny, but even emphasizes, that, in order that competition should work beneficially, a carefully thought-out legal framework is required and that neither the existing nor the past legal rules are free from grave defects. Nor does it deny that, where it is impossible to create the conditions necessary to make competition effective, we must resort to other methods of guiding economic activity.[16]

A code which seeks to mitigate the full force of the competitive conflict can also be desirable in athletics. While an athlete is in essence a prizefighter, he seeks to demonstrate his excellence in a contest governed by rules which acknowledge human worth and dignity. He mistakes his purpose and insults his opponent if he views the contest as an occasion to display generosity and magnanimity. To the extent that sportsmanship in athletics is virtuous, its essence consists in the practice of fairness under most difficult conditions. Since the sportsman's primary objective is the joy of the moment, it is obvious from that very fact that he places no great emphasis on the importance of winning. It is easy for him to be modest in victory or gracious in defeat and to play fair at all times, these virtues being demonstrated under optimum conditions for their easy exercise. The strange paradox of sportsmanship as applied to athletics is that it asks the athlete, locked in a deadly serious and emotionally charged situation, to act outwardly as if he were engaged in some pleasant diversion. After an athlete has trained and sacrificed for weeks, after he has dreamed of victory and its fruits and literally exhausted himself physically and emotionally in its pursuit—after all this—to ask him to act with fairness in the contest, with modesty in victory, and an admirable composure in defeat is to demand a great deal, and, yet, this is the substance of the demand that "sportsmanship" makes upon the athlete.

For the athlete, being a good loser is demonstrating self-control in the face of adversity. A festive attitude is not called for; it is, in fact, often viewed as in bad taste. The purists or rigorists are of the opinion that a brief period of seclusion and mourning may be more appropriate. They know that, for the real competitor, defeat in an important contest seems heartbreaking and nerve-shattering. The athlete who can control himself in such circumstances demonstrates remarkable equanimity. To ask that he enter into the festive mood of the victory celebration is to request a Pagliacci-like performance. There is no need for phony or effusive displays of congratulations. A simple handshake demonstrates that no personal ill-will is involved. No alibis or complaints are offered. No childish excuses about the judgment of officials or the natural conditions. No temper tantrums. To be a good loser under his code, the athlete need not be exactly gracious in defeat, but he must at least "be a man" about it. This burden, metaphorically characterized as sportsmanship, bears heavily upon all athletes—amateur or professional. But there are added complications for the professional. Victories, superior performances, and high ratings are essential to financial success in professional athletics. Too frequent defeat will result in forced unemployment. It is easy,

therefore, for a professional athlete to view his competitors with a jaundiced eye; to see them as men who seek to deprive him of his livelihood. Under these circumstances, to work daily and often intimately with one's competitors and to compete in circumstances which are highly charged with excitement and emotion, while still showing fairness and consideration, is evidence of an admirable degree of self-mastery.

Attempts have been made to identify sportsmanship with certain games which, it is contended, were the private preserve of the gentleman and, as a result, reflect his high code of honor.

> Bullying, cheating, "crabbing" were all too common in every form of sport. The present movement away from muckerism probably should be attributed in large measure to the growing popularity of golf and tennis. Baseball, boxing, and many of our common sports trace their origin to the common people who possessed no code of honor. On the other hand, golf and tennis, historically gentlemen's games, have come down to us so interwoven with a high code of honor that we have been forced to accept the code along with the game. . . . The effect of the golf code upon the attitude of the millions who play the game is reflected in all our sports.[17]

It is true that in England the terms "gentleman," "sportsman," and "amateur" were regarded as intimately interrelated. The contention that the common people, and consequently the games that were peculiarly theirs, had no comparable code of honor may be correct, but it awaits the careful documentation of some future social historian. One thing is certain, however, and that is that there is nothing in the nature of any game, considered in itself, that necessarily implies adherence to a moral code. Some games like golf and tennis in which the participants do their own officiating provide greater opportunity for the practice of honesty, but if a high code of honor surrounds the "gentleman's games," it is due principally to the general attitude of the gentleman toward life rather than to anything intrinsic to the game itself. The English gentleman was firmly committed to sport in the proper sense of that term and eschewed the specialization, the rigors of precontest preparation, the secret strategy sessions, and professional coaching which have come to be regarded as indispensable for the athlete. "The fact that a man is born into the society of gentlemen imposes upon him the duties and, to some extent, the ideas of his class. He is expected to have a broad education, catholic tastes, and a multiplicity of pursuits. He must not do anything for pecuniary gain; and it will be easily seen that he must not specialize. It is essentially the mark of the bourgeois' mind to specialize."[18] Moreover, "too much preparation is contrary to all English ethics, and secrecy in training is especially abhorrent. Remember that sport is a prerogative of gentlemen. And one of the ear-marks of a gentleman is that he resort to no trickery and that he plays every game with his cards on the table—the game of life as well as the game of football."[19]

It is the contestant's objective and not the game itself which becomes the chief determinant of the conduct and attitudes of the players. If we take tennis as an example and contrast the code of conduct employed by the sportsman with that of the athlete in the matter of officiating, the difference is obvious. The sportsman invariably gives his opponent the benefit of the doubt. Whenever he is not sure, he plays his opponent's shot as good even though he may suspect that it was out. The athlete, however, takes a different approach. Every bit as opposed to cheating as the sportsman, the athlete demands no compelling proof of error. If a shot seems to be out, even though he is not certain, the athlete calls it that way. He is satisfied that his opponent will do the same. He asks no quarter and gives none. As a result of this attitude and by comparison with the sportsman, the athlete will tend toward a legal interpretation of the rules.

The athletic contest is designed to serve a specific purpose—the objective and accurate determination of superior performance and, ultimately, of excellence. If this objective is to be accomplished, then the rules governing the contest must impose the same burdens upon each side. Both contestants must be equal before the law if the test is to have any validity, if the victory is to have any meaning. To the extent that one party to the contest gains a special advantage, unavailable to his opponent, through an unusual interpretation, application, or circumvention of the rules, then that advantage is unfair. The well-known phrase "sense of fair play" suggests much more than an adherence to the letter of the law. It implies that the spirit too must be observed. In the athletic contest there is a mutual recognition that the rules of the game are drawn up for the explicit purpose of aiding in the determination of an honorable victory. Any attempt to disregard or circumvent these rules must be viewed as a deliberate attempt to

deprive the contest of its meaning. Fairness, then, is rooted in a type of equality before the law, which is absolutely necessary if victory in the contest is to have validity and meaning. Once, however, the necessary steps have been taken to make the contest a true test of respective abilities, the athlete's sole objective is to demonstrate marked superiority. Any suggestion that fair play obliges him to maintain equality in the contest ignores the very nature of athletics. "If our analysis of fair play has been correct, coaches who strive to produce superior teams violate a fundamental principle of sportsmanship by teaching their pupils, through example, that superiority is more greatly to be desired than is equality in sport. . . . But who today would expect a coach to give up clear superiority—a game won —by putting in enough substitutes to provide fair playing conditions for an opposing team?"[20] Thus understood, sportsmanship would ask the leopard to change its spots. It rules out, as illegitimate, the very objective of the athlete. Nothing shows more clearly the need for recognition of the distinction between sport and athletics.

CONCLUSION

In conclusion, we would like to summarize our answers to the three problems set down at the outset.

1. The source of the confusion which vitiates most discussion of sportsmanship is the unwarranted assumption that sport and athletics are so similar in nature that a single code of conduct and similar participant attitudes are applicable to both. Failing to take cognizance of the basic differences between sport and athletics, a futile attempt is made to outline a single code of behavior equally applicable to radically diverse activities. Not only is such an attempt, in the nature of things, doomed to failure but a consequence of this abortive effort is the proliferation of various moral virtues under the flag of sportsmanship, which, thus, loses all its distinctiveness. It is variously viewed as a straight road to moral perfection or an antidote to moral corruption.

2. The goal of genuine sport must be the principal determinant of the conduct and attitudes proper to sporting activity. Since its goal is pleasant diversion—the immediate joy to be derived in the activity itself—the pivotal or essential virtue in sportsmanship is generosity. All the other moral qualities that may also be in evidence are colored by this spirit of generosity. As a result of this spirit, a determined effort is made to avoid all unpleasantness and

conflict and to cultivate, in their stead, an unselfish and co-operative effort to maximize the joy of the moment.

3. The essence of sportsmanship as applied to athletics can be determined by the application of the same principle. Honorable victory is the goal of the athlete and, as a result, the code of the athlete demands that nothing be done before, during, or after the contest to cheapen or otherwise detract from such a victory. Fairness or fair play, the pivotal virtue in athletics, emphasizes the need for an impartial and equal application of the rules if the victory is to signify, as it should, athletic excellence. Modesty in victory and a quiet composure in defeat testify to an admirable and extraordinary self-control and, in general, dignify and enhance the goal of the athlete.

NOTES

1. *Resistance, Rebellion and Death* (New York: Alfred A. Knopf, Inc., 1961), p. 242.
2. In Frank Leahy, *Defensive Football* (New York: Prentice-Hall, Inc., 1951), p. 198.
3. "Sportsmanship in Its Relation to American Intercollegiate Athletics," *School and Society,* XLV (April 10, 1937), 506.
4. Henry Steele Commager, in *Scholastic,* XLIV (May 8-13, 1944), 7.
5. Lyman Bryson, *Science and Freedom* (New York: Columbia University Press, 1947), p. 130.
6. Pope Pius XII, *The Human Body* (Boston: Daughters of St. Paul, 1960).
7. "Athletic Relations between Harvard and Princeton," *School and Society,* XXIV (November 20, 1926), 631.
8. Charles W. Kennedy, *Sport and Sportsmanship* (Princeton, N.J.: Princeton University Press, 1931), pp. 58-59.
9. William R. Reed, "Big Time Athletics' Commitment to Education," *Journal of Health, Physical Education, and Recreation,* XXXIV (September, 1963), 30.
10. Quoted in J. B. Griswold, "You Don't Have To Be Born with It," *American Magazine,* CXII (November, 1931), 60.
11. *Ibid.,* p. 133.
12. "Sportsmanship," *School Activities,* XXXII (October, 1960), 38.
13. "A Sportsmanship Brotherhood," *Literary Digest,* LXXXVIII (March 27, 1926), 60.
14. *Ibid.,* pp. 60-61.
15. Gabriel Marcel, *The Mystery of Being,* Vol. II: *Faith and Reality* (Chicago: Henry Regnery Co., 1960), pp. 133-34.
16. Friedrich A. Hayek, *The Road to Serfdom* (Chicago: University of Chicago Press, 1944), p. 36.
17. J. F. Williams and W. W. Nixon, *The Athlete in the Making* (Philadelphia: W. B. Saunders, 1932), p. 153.
18. H. J. Whigham, "American Sport from an English Point of View," *Outlook,* XCIII (November, 1909), 740.
19. *Ibid.*
20. Frederick R. Rogers, *The Amateur Spirit in Scholastic Games and Sports* (Albany, N.Y.: C. F. Williams & Son, 1929), p. 78.

Deception, Sportsmanship, and Ethics*

KATHLEEN M. PEARSON

At the heart of every athletic activity is the attempt to successfully deceive one's opponent. The thesis presented here is that deception in athletics is not a simple, unitary event. Deception can be analyzed into at least two types: (a) Strategic Deception and (b) Definitional Deception. Finally, a rule of thumb can be established for deciding on the ethics of acts of deception which fall into those two categories.

STRATEGIC DECEPTION

Strategic deception occurs when an athlete deceives his opponent into thinking he will move to the right when he actually intends to move left—that he will bunt the baseball when he intends to hit a line drive—that he will drive the tennis ball when he actually intends to lob it. Examples of this sort of deception are replete in athletic events and need not be elaborated here. The important question is whether these acts of strategic deception are ethical or unethical.

In order to deal with this question, we need a rule of thumb for deciding on the ethics of an act. A standard for deciding if an act of deception is unethical is as follows: If an act is designed by a willing participant in an activity to deliberately interfere with the purpose of that activity, then that act can properly be labeled unethical.

What is the purpose of athletic activities? Why even have such things as basketball games, football games, tennis games? I suggest that the purpose of these games, in an

*From *Quest*, XIX (January, 1973), 115–118.

athletic setting, is to test the skill of one individual, or group of individuals, against the skill of another individual, or group of individuals, in order to determine who is more skillful in a particular, well-defined activity.

How is any particular game defined? A particular game is no more (in terms of its careful definition) than its rules. The rules of one game distinguish it as being different from all other games. Some games may have quite similar rules; however, there must be at least one difference between the rules of one game and those of all other games in order for that game to be distinguished from all other games. If we were to find another game with exactly the same rules between the covers of its rulebook, we would naturally conclude that it was the same game. Thus, problems of identity and diversity of games are decided by the rules for each game. Identical games have identical rules and diverse games have differing rules. A game is identified, or defined, as being just that game by the rules which govern it.

If the purpose of athletics is to determine who is more skillful in a particular game, and if an unethical act is one which is designed to deliberately interfere with that purpose, it is difficult to see how acts of strategic deception could be called unethical. In fact, this sort of deception is at the heart of the skill factor in athletic events. It is the sort of activity which separates the highly skilled athlete from the less skilled athlete, and therefore, is the sort of activity that makes a significant contribution to the purpose of the athletic event. Strategic deception is in no way designed to deliberately interfere with the purpose of athletics.

DEFINITIONAL DECEPTION

Definitional deception occurs when one has contracted to participate in one sort of activity, and then deliberately engages in another sort of activity. An example of this sort of deception might occur if one were to sign a contract to teach political science, be assigned to a political science class, and then proceed to campaign for a particular political candidate.

How does this parallel an act which might be committed in an athletic setting? The paradigm used here suggests that: (a) Under certain circumstances, the commission of a foul in a game falls into the category of definitional deception; (b) Under certain circumstances, the act of fouling can be labeled as unsportsmanlike; and, (c) Certain kinds of fouls can be linked to acts which can be properly labeled as unethical.

It was established earlier that a game is identified, or defined, as being just that game by the rules which govern it. Furthermore, we are all familiar with the fact that it is in compliance with the rules of a particular game that we commit certain acts, while it is against the rules to commit other acts. When one commits an act that is not in compliance with the rules, he is said to have committed a foul, and a prescribed penalty is meted out in punishment for that act. The ways in which fouls are committed in athletic contests can be separated into two categories. The first category consists of those fouls which are committed accidentally, and the second is composed of those fouls which are committed deliberately.

Let us first consider the case of accidental fouls. According to our rule of thumb, an act must be designed to deliberately interfere with the purpose of the activity in order for that act to be labeled unethical. Since the criterion of intentionality is missing from the accidental foul, that act has no ethical significance. We would ordinarily expect a person to accept the penalty for that foul, but we would not place moral blame on him.

Next, let us turn to the person who deliberately commits a foul while participating in an athletic contest. If the purpose of the contest is to determine who is more skillful in that game we can say that a player has entered into a contract with his opponent for the mutual purpose of making that determination. In other words, he has contracted with his opponent and the audience (if there is one) to play football, for instance, in order to determine who is more skillful in a game of football.

I have argued earlier that a particular game is defined by its rules—that the rules of a game are the definition of that game. If this is the case, a player who deliberately breaks the rules of that game is deliberately no longer playing that game. He may be playing "smutball," for instance, but he is not playing football. This is a case of deliberate definitional deception. These kinds of acts are designed to interfere with the purpose of the game in which they occur. How can it be determined which of two players (or teams) is more skillful in a game if one of the players (or teams) is not even playing that particular game? If the arguments presented here are correct thus far, we can conclude that the intentional commission of a foul in athletics is an unethical act. Ordinarily, when we refer to unethical acts on the part of athletes, we call these acts unsportsmanlike.

Someone might argue, at this point, that the penalties for fouling also are contained within the rulebook for a particular game, and therefore, fouls are not outside the rules for the game. The obvious rebuttal to this position is that penalties for breaking the law are contained within the law books, but no sensible person concludes, therefore, that all acts are within the law. If this were the case, there would be no sense in having laws at all. Similarly, if this were the case with games, there would be no sense in having rules for games. However, since the definition of a game is its rules, if there were no rules for that game there would be no game. Therefore, even though the penalties for fouling are contained within the rulebook for a game, the act of deliberate fouling is, indeed, outside the rules for that game.

A variety of elegant arguments can be produced to indict the deliberate foul. It violates the ludic spirit, it treats the process of playing as mere instrument in the pursuit of the win, and it reflects a view of one's competitor as both enemy and object rather than colleague in noble contest. All of these pleas, however, fall short of the ultimate and most damaging testimony; deliberate betrayal of the rules destroys the vital frame of agreement which makes sport possible. The activity even may go on in the face of such fatal deception, but neither the logic of analysis, nor the intuition of experience permit us to call whatever is left a game—for that is shattered.

Some Reflections on Success and Failure in Competitive Athletics*

EDWIN J. DELATTRE

The initial objects of my reflections are the great and transporting moments of participation in competitive athletics. Reflection on these moments draws our attention to the conditions under which they are possible and to the kinds of people who are capable of achieving them. Reflection on these, in turn, enables us to see at once the touchstone relationship of competitors, and the moral and logical incompatibility of competing and cheating. Most of all we are reminded throughout these reflections that success in competitive athletics is not reducible to winning, nor failure to losing.

Richard Harding Davis was sensitive to the great and transporting moments of participation in competitive athletics. In the late fall of 1895, he wrote a gripping account of the recently contested Yale-Princeton football game. He captured both the involvement of the spectators and the struggle of the participants in revealing ways.

With the score at 16–10 in favor of Yale, but amidst a Princeton comeback, the description proceeds:

> It was obviously easy after that to argue that if the Tigers had scored twice in ten minutes they could score at least once more . . . or even snatch a victory out of defeat. And at the thought of this the yells redoubled, and the air shook, and every play, good, bad, or indiffer-

*From *Journal of the Philosophy of Sport,* II (Sept., 1976), 133–139.

ent, was greeted with shouts of encouragement that fell like blows of a whip on one side and that tasted like wine to the other. People forgot for a few precious minutes to think about themselves, they enjoyed the rare sensation of being carried completely away by something outside of themselves, and the love of a fight, or a struggle, or combat, or whatever else you choose to call it, rose in everyone's breast and choked him until he had either to yell and get rid of it or suffocate. (2:p. 9)

Forgetting "for a few precious moments to think about" oneself, being "carried completely away," can be among the high points of human existence. Yet being so transported in the wrong way, or in the wrong context, becomes fanaticism, irresponsible loss of self-control, even madness. Here we will not concern ourselves with the problematic dimensions of being "carried completely away," since they are not relevant to our reflections.

As the objects of eros are many, we can become passionately involved in diverse pursuits and activities, concerns, persons, even places. Inquiry can be transporting, the quest to discover—was anyone ever more obviously carried completely away than the Leakeys at Olduvai George? The love of another, a symphony, dance; the range of our passionate concerns is virtually endless. In this list, of course, is the game: competitive athletics. Because of its special place on this list, which will emerge in our discussion, competitive athletics merit our attention and reflection.

Let us return then to Davis' description, for it becomes even more revealing about the transporting moments in competitive athletics:

> The clamor ceased once absolutely, and the silence was even more impressive than the tumult that had preceded it. It came toward the end of the second half, when the light had begun to fail and the mist was rising from the ground. The Yale men had forced the ball to within two yards of Princeton's goal, and they had still one more chance left them to rush it across the line. While they were lining up for that effort the cheering died away, yells, both measured and inarticulate, stopped, and the place was so still that for the first time during the day you could hear the telegraph instruments chirping like crickets from the side line. (2:p. 9)

What is crucial in this passage is not the silence of the crowd, but the occasion for it. The silence is occasioned by the resolution of the game into this moment, this spellbinding moment when the competition is most intense. Think of the moment not as a spectator, but as a competitor. Think of the overwhelming silence of the moments when the game is most of all a test, the moments of significance in the game, the turning points, which all the practice and diligence and preparation point to and anticipate.

Such moments are what make the game worth the candle. Whether amidst the soft lights and the sparkling balls against the baize of a billiard table, on the rolling terrain of a lush fairway or in the violent and crashing pit where linemen struggle, it is the moments when no let-up is possible, when there is virtually no tolerance for error, which make the game. The best and most satisfying contests maximize these moments and minimize respite from pressure. When competition achieves this intensity it frequently renders the outcome of the contest anti-climactic, and it inevitably reduces victory celebrations to pallor by contrast.

We see here the basic condition of success in competitive athletics. We must be able mutually to discover worthy opponents, opponents who are capable of generating with us the intensity of competition. Exclusive emphasis on winning has particularly tended to obscure the importance of the quality of the opposition and of the thrill of the competition itself. It is of the utmost importance for competitors to discover opponents whose preparation and skill are comparable to their own and who respect the game utterly.

We are recalled to this insight by the applicability to competitive athletics of the phrase "testing one's mettle." The etymological roots of "mettle" are the same as those of metal; indeed these were originally variant spellings of the same word. Just as the quality of a metal ore was determined long ago by the intensity of the color streak produced by rubbing it against a mica-like material called a touchstone, so in competition, one's opponent is his touchstone. In rubbing against a worthy opponent, against his skill, dedication and preparation, the quality of a competitor's mettle is tested.

As all philosophers know, Socrates employed the metaphor of the touchstone in the dialogues. Fellow participants in dialogue are the touchstones by which one tests the epistemic quality of his beliefs. That I have used the same metaphor must not be allowed to obscure the point that inquiry, dialogue, is, without qualification, not competitive. To view inquiry as competition, argument as something won or lost, is to misunderstand both. Dialectical inquiry is the shared and cooperative pursuit of the best approximation of the truth. In successful dialogues, false and confused beliefs are exposed as such, and those who held them benefit by the disclosure of their inadequacy. The testing of one's mettle in competitive athletics is quite another thing. The distinction is vital because when inquiry is treated as competition it is destroyed as inquiry.

Competition, contesting, if you will, thus requires commensurate opponents. The testing of one's mettle in competitive athletics is a form of self-discovery, just as the preparation to compete is a form of self-creation. The claim of competitive athletics to importance rests squarely on their providing for us opportunities for self-discovery which might otherwise have been missed. They are not unique in this by any means—the entire fabric of moral life is woven of such opportunities—but there is no need for them to claim uniqueness. They provide opportunities for self-discovery, for concentration and intensity of involvement, for being carried away by the demands of the contest and thereby in part for being able to meet them, with a frequency seldom matched elsewhere. It is in the face of these demands and with respect to them that an athlete succeeds or fails. This is why it is a far greater success in competitive athletics to have played well under the pressure of a truly worthy opponent and lost than to have defeated a less worthy or unworthy one where no demands were made.

We may appreciate this last point through a final look at Davis' chronicle:

> And then, just as the Yale men were growing fearful that the game would end in a tie, and while the Princeton men were shrieking their lungs out that it might, Captain Thorne made his run, and settled the question forever.
>
> It is not possible to describe that run. It would be as easy to explain how a snake disappears through the grass, or an eel slips from your fingers, or to say how a flash of linked lightning wriggles across the sky. (2:p. 9)

We cannot separate the significance of the Yale victory and the Princeton defeat from the fact that there was involved a player capable of such a run. For Princeton to have played well against a team with such a back, to have held a back of such quality to a single long run, to have required magnificence of Thorne for him to score, is a great success in itself.

How different this is from the occasion for Jack London's concluding lament in his coverage of the Jack Johnson-Jim Jeffries fight:

> Johnson is a wonder. No one understands him, this man who smiles. Well, the story of the fight is the story of a smile. If ever man won by nothing more fatiguing than a smile, Johnson won today.
>
> And where now is the champion who will make Johnson extend himself . . . (4:p. 513)

Jeffries was game in that fight, and he took a terrible beating. But the fight was no real competition because the opponents were not commensurate. Worse, Jeffries was ill-prepared, he was not the opponent he might have been. Accordingly, the extent of success possible for Johnson was extremely limited by the time the fight began.

As we noted previously, more is required for successful competition than commensurate opponents. Opponents, to be worthy, must utterly respect the game. Let us return now to explore that claim, for it involves not only important moral considerations but also rather more subtle logical or conceptual ones. An example will help us to expose and deal with both.

It is well known that during his career as a golfer, Bobby Jones several times called penalty strokes on himself. By 1926, he had won the American and British Opens and the American amateur title. In that year he granted an interview on golf style to O. B. Keeler, who asked Jones about those self-imposed penalties:

> 'One thing more, Bobby. There is a lot of interest in those penalty strokes you have called on yourself. At St. Louis and Brookline and at Worcester—they say that one cost you the championship—and the one at Scioto, in that awful round of 79 when the ball moved on the green—' Bobby held up a warning hand. 'That is absolutely nothing to talk about,' he said, 'and you are not to write about it. There is only one way to play this game.' (3:p. 222)

From the point of view of morality, competitors must consider it unworthy of themselves to break deliberately the rules of the game. When a person violates the rules which govern competition, he treats his opponents as means merely to his end of victory. The symbols of victory have status or meaningfulness only because they stand for triumph in competition; without the opposition, they are worthless. Attainment of these symbols by cheating is therefore the exploitation of those who competed in good faith. Competitors are equally reduced to means merely in cases where the end of the cheater is prize money or gambling profit. Without the competition there can be neither prize nor wager, and the cheater simply uses the bona fide competitors solely for his own gain. Cheating is thus a paradigm case of failure to act with respect for the moral status of persons as ends.

From the point of view of logic, the need for the players' utter respect for the game is equally crucial. Competing, winning and losing in athletics are intelligible only within the framework of rules which define a specific competitive sport. A person may cheat at a game or compete at it, but it is logically impossible for him to do both. To cheat is to cease to compete. It is for this reason that cheaters are the greatest failures of all in competitive athletics, not because of any considerations of winning or failing to do so, but because they fail even to compete.

In the case of golf, as in the Bob Jones example, failure to impose a penalty on oneself where it is required by the rules is to cease to compete at golf. For one can compete with others only in accordance with the rules which govern and define the competition.

Or consider the case of pocket billiards. In all pocket billiard games it is a rule violation to touch any object ball or the cue ball with one's hands or clothing, etc. during play. It is also a violation for the cue to touch any object ball in the execution of a shot; any player who violates these rules has committed a foul. The penalty for a foul in all cases is termination of one's inning or turn. Now suppose that during a game of straight pool in the execution of a shot where the cue ball must be struck at a steep angle because of an object ball immediately behind it, a player knowingly touches that object ball with his finger, undetected by his opponent or a referee. If he continues to shoot, if he does not terminate his inning voluntarily, he has ceased to compete at straight pool. And because he is no longer competing, he cannot win at straight pool. He may appear to do so, he may pocket the prize money or collect on the wager or carry off the trophy, but since he is not competing any longer, he cannot win. The cheater is logically prohibited from competing and therefore from winning. He can lose by disqualification.[1]

We may wish here to recall Bernard Suits' discussion of rules in "The Elements of Sport." Suits distinguishes the constitutive rules of a game, those which proscribe certain means of achieving the end of the game, from rules of skill which apply to how to play the game well or effectively. He points out that to ". . . break a constitutive rule is to fail to play the game at all." (5:p. 52) He mentions also a third kind of rule, namely the kind of rule which if violated requires the imposition of a specific penalty, the sort of rule we have been discussing. He urges rightly that violating such a rule is neither to fail to play the game nor to fail to play it well, since the penalized action may be nonetheless advantageous to the competitor. But he also notes that such rules are extensions of the constitutive rules. This is the emphasis of my argument. In particular, to commit an act which merits a penalty, to do so knowingly and *not* to incur the penalty is to cease to play the game. To ground a club in golf or to commit a foul in pool is not to cease to play the game. But to ignore the penalty imposed by the rules surely is, and it is in this sense that we understand rules with penalties as extensions of constitutive rules.

Both morally and logically, then, there is indeed only one way to play a game. Grantland Rice makes clear his appreciation of this insight in his autobiography, *The Tumult and the Shouting*. For emphasis, he employs the example of a rookie professional offensive lineman. The athlete responds to Rice's praise for his play during his rookie year by observing that he will be better when he becomes more adept at holding illegally without being caught. Of course, to Rice this confused vision of successful competition is heartbreaking.

We have seen now that success in competitive athletics requires being and discovering worthy opponents, and that worthy opponents must be relative equals with utter respect for the game and their fellow competitors. We have related success to competing well, performing well, under pressure. No one can be a success in competitive athletics if he fails to compete, either by avoiding worthy opposition or by cheating.[2]

Of course, our treatment of competitive athletics is rather narrow; it does not deal with the variety of reasons and purposes people have for engaging in competitive athletics. Our reflections do not really pertain to people who play at competitive games merely for fun or relaxation or exercise, who use, as it were, the format of competitive games for purposes largely indifferent to competing and to winning. We are talking only about people who seek to compete with those whose investment in a game, whose seriousness of purpose and talent, are comparable to their own and who therefore play to win.

Now people vary greatly in talent and available time for preparation, opportunity, training and so on. This means that success in competitive athletics cannot be tied unconditionally to absolute quality of performance. Whether a competitive athlete is a success hinges on numerous relevant factual considerations. We acknowledge this point as part of our sense of fairness through handicapping, establishment of weight divisions in boxing and wrestling, age divisions in junior and senior competition, and division of amateur and professional, to mention only a few.

What then of the athlete as competitor, the athlete who competes with equals, who, in the very act of competing, sets victory among his goals? Is winning everything in such competition, the only thing, the sole criterion of success?

We have been told so often enough, and we have seen the young encouraged to believe that winning and success are inseparable, that those who win are "winners" and those who lose, "losers." This view, however, must be tempered by our previous insights; we must not become preoccupied with individual victories to the exclusion of recognition of the importance of patterns of outstanding performance. As Thackeray saw, "The prize be sometimes to the fool. The race not always to the swift." (6:p. 57)

Sometimes performance in victory is mediocre, in defeat awesome. Many super bowls are testimonial to the former. There are countless other examples of mediocrity in victory, from little league games to professional contests. So too of excellence in defeat. To cite only one:

> Anyone who saw Wohlhuter's heroic performance in Munich won't soon forget it. In the first qualifying heat, he tripped, and his pipe-stem body scraped along the track. Scrambling to his feet, he chased after the field—but was shut out by a stride.
>
> 'I was startled,' he recalls. 'To this day, I don't even know why or how I went down. When there're 80,000 people watching you, you want to have a good day. I had a choice —walk off the track or give it a try. I chose to be competitive.' (1:p. 48)

To stress victory to the point of overlooking quality of performance is to impoverish our sense of success in competitive athletics.

It matters whether we win or lose. It also matters whether we play the game well or badly, given our own potential and preparation. It matters whom we play against and whether they are worthy of us, whether they can press us to call up our final resources. Satisfaction in victory is warranted only when we have played well against a worthy opponent. Otherwise victory is no achievement, and pride in it is false.

NOTES

1. We might ask whether other members of a team are competing if one member is cheating. We would ask immediately whether they knew of it, and deny that they were competing if they knew and did nothing. We would be more perplexed if they did not know. But we would still deny, I think, that the team as a unit was competing. Notice that a team can

be disqualified for the violations of one member. The same considerations apply to cheating in the form, say, of recruiting violations.

2. Obviously there is no failure involved in the decision not to participate in athletic or nonathletic competition. Some people are constitutionally unsuited for athletics, some for competition, while others find the demands of games artificial or fabricated and therefore unsatisfying. That there is failure in cheating or in constantly playing unworthy opponents neither suggests nor entails that there is anything wrong with unwillingness to enter at all into competition.

BIBLIOGRAPHY

1. Bonventre, Peter. "The Streaker," *Newsweek* (February 17, 1975).
2. Davis, Richard Harding. "Thorne's Famous Run," *The Omnibus of Sport*. Grantland Rice and Harford Powel (eds.). New York: Harper and Brothers, 1932. Reprinted from: "How the Great Game Was Played," *The Journal* (November 24, 1895).
3. Keeler, O. B. "Bobby Jones on Golf Style," *The Omnibus of Sport*. Grantland Rice and Harford Powel (eds.). New York: Harper and Brothers, 1932.
4. London, Jack. "The Story of a Smile," *The Omnibus of Sport*. Grantland Rice and Harford Powel (eds.). New York: Harper and Brothers, 1932.
5. Suits, Bernard. "The Elements of Sport," *The Philosophy of Sport: A Collection of Original Essays*. Robert G. Osterhoudt (ed.). Springfield, Illinois: Charles C Thomas Publisher, 1973.
6. Thackeray, William M. "Sportsmanship," *The Omnibus of Sport*. Grantland Rice and Harford Powel (eds.). New York: Harper and Brothers, 1932.

In Praise of Harmony:
The Kantian Imperative and Hegelian Sittlichkeit
As the Principle and Substance of Moral
Conduct in Sport*

ROBERT G. OSTERHOUDT

The purpose of this essay is to examine the terms in which Kant's categorical imperative provides a principle by which moral conduct in sport is properly guided; and to study as well Hegel's *Sittlichkeit* as giving this principle concrete life, or substance, and so providing its use as a moral principle for practical action in sport with content. Hegel criticized the imperative as vacuous, or lacking content, and thought himself to have provided the content of morality with his *Sittlichkeit*. He was in any case much indebted to Kant, whose thought in general provides the modern springboard for Hegel's celebrated system. Among his foremost debts to Kant is what he owes to Kant's ethics, and to the view of humanity that it contains. The general outline of Kant's ethics and its significance for sport is considered in the second section of the essay. The terms in which Hegel takes up, modifies, and extends the Kantian imperative is the subject of the third section. The fourth section introduces Hegel's *Sittlichkeit* as a natural outgrowth of his response to the imperative. In section five the historical development of human reason, morality, and freedom generally and their development in sport more particularly are dis-

*From *Journal of the Philosophy of Sport*, III (Sept., 1976), 65–81.

cussed. And the final section is reserved for a brief summary of earlier discussions, and the drawing of conclusions with respect to these discussions.

In order to provide adequate foundation for the final leaps, the sweep of issue discussed here is unavoidably wide—from Kant's imperative in general and the notions which underlie it (most importantly, his view of humanity, reason, and freedom), as well as the significance of this principle for sporting activity; to Hegel's *Sittlichkeit* and his view of humanity, reason, freedom, the state, and history, views which conclude in an argument for the harmony of humanity generally, and of humanity in sport more particularly. At its end—when the entire line of its argument is apparent—the essay comes to a philosophy of sport history, which, under the influence of its Hegelian roots, is tantamount to a philosophy of sport at the formal completion of its development. This is to say that the essay comes to a synoptic account, not merely of human possibilities in sport, but of the historical development of these possibilities as well. And this after all is only to call attention to the latter's necessarily providing the primitive data for the former—it is only by these data that such possibilities become visible. What is intended at bottom is a demonstration of the terms in which sport has been and ought to be an expression of man's fundamental nature, and an articulation of a moral posture which secures an authentically human condition in sport.

II

Kant had held, with Aristotle, that reason provides human existence with its distinctive, or originative ground. According to this view man's reason constitutes his fundamental nature, and sets him apart from mere sensuous existence. By this account, reason is the determining basis, or power of human life—it governs the current of our distinctly human actions. Among the most prominent of these actions are moral judgments, wherein man acts out of a concept of law, and not out of a thoughtless obedience to natural law (of which an acting out of mere impulse or caprice are disguised instances). The concrete fact of such judgments presupposes human freedom in Kant's view. That is, Kant finds in our unrelenting consciousness of moral duty (our inclination to act so as to deserve happiness) an indication, or practical proof of our freedom. Moral duty itself requires as a necessary prior condition the freedom to act in accord with what are taken as one's moral obligations or contrary to them.

This freedom, then, furnishes a distinction for Kant between a world of sense and a world of understanding. The form of the former is variant among persons and is determined by the natural law, while the form of the latter is invariant among persons and is free both from the natural law and for itself. Thus, Kant has connected reason and freedom (and morality as well)—a connection that Hegel will want to preserve, though in a somewhat different form. As a rational being, or subject, consequently, man is free, as a sensuous being, he is a mere object of empirical determinations. In accord with Aristotle's general principle of axiology, that a species ought to cultivate most fully (primarily) that which is distinctive of it, Kant further argues that: man must regard himself from the side of reason and freedom, for this is the side which is characteristic of, or essential to him, and the side which makes morality possible.

Since reason is therefore the determining ground of man's authentic action, we may say that the moral laws spun out by it (and so consonant with the fundamental character of reason, and so themselves in this sense rational) are self-determined in a way in which

laws which are the expression of sensuous impulse are not. Which is to say, that what stands at the center of human nature (namely, reason) is one and the same with what determines moral laws. The determining principle of these laws is therefore inherent to oneself (in fact, the ground of oneself), as distinct from residing in an external agency. In the latter case these laws could not be said to be self-determined in any authentic sense. They would instead need to be thought of as presenting largely external, or alien applications to oneself, and so not free, nor then moral determinations at all. The laws to which man is therefore morally obligated are his own—they are self-legislated. He is also subject to empirical law of course, though in this there is nothing of positive moral significance according to Kant. The moral significance of this relationship, insofar as it has such significance, is instead negative. More precisely, the significance of this relationship resides in its sketching out the limits (and so in negative part the nature) of moral action, and so in its stipulating that to which moral action and freedom are constrained (that over and against which they become what they are—that to which they are opposed).

Kant conceives of man, then, as a unified consciousness at once a participant in the world of sense by which he is determined and in the world of reason by which he is free. He has both a sensuous (natural) and rational aspect. By the former he is drawn from freedom, and so from moral duty and his fundamental self, and by the latter he is turned to them. By the former he is compelled to the particularity of idiosyncratic inclination, caprice, and desire, and by the latter he is impelled to the universality of moral obligation. Kant argues, in the form of his celebrated imperative, that the moral law, characteristically unlike the natural law, commands unconditionally, or categorically, to "act only according to that maxim by which you can at the same time will that it should become a universal law." (16: p. 39) Put more accessibly, "act so that you treat humanity, whether in your own person or in that of another, always as an end and never as a means only." (16: p. 47) The imperative commands that we universalize our respect for each person as a free moral agent, and so withhold regarding him as a mere object externally bound to, and thereby exploited by our sensuous or egoistic inclinations. This notion entails extending to others what we, as free, self-determining, rational beings, would have extended to ourselves. Kant therefore proposes a union of all rational beings in a realm of common law (a "realm of ends") in which the general ends of all become the ends of all others. In this the individual and common goods coalesce. Accordingly, it follows that a willful violation of this principle is humanistically self-destructive in a general fashion, let alone in a fashion particular to sport.

The use of the imperative in sport secures an internal relationship with the laws (rules and regulations) which define and govern it, and with those other persons who also freely participate in it. A regard for these laws as self-legislated, and an intrinsic respect for those others is nonetheless presupposed by a free entry into sporting activity. In fact, this is what is meant by such an entry; that is, the taking of the laws of sport as one's own, and the cultivation of a divining sympathy for all others who have also made such a choice. The categorical imperative commands that we abide by these laws for their own sake (for they are expressions of our most fundamental nature), and that we consequently treat others with a regard that we ourselves would prefer —that is, treat others as ends-in-themselves. Only insofar as persons make such a treatment do they stand in a positive and viable relation to reason, and so to one another.

Since we have willed, by the terms of the imperative, that our lawful acts are proper for all who locate themselves in circumstances of a given determination, to act other than lawfully is to violate and so to destroy the activity into which we have freely entered, to violate the laws we ourselves have legislated, to overturn our unique participation in the world of understanding (in this case with respect to sport), to act contrary to our own nature and so to act inauthentically and to be inauthentic or alienated from ourselves—succinctly, to be other than we fundamentally are. Such conduct is, then, destructive of the humanistic spirit necessary to sport authentically undertaken, necessary to the genuinely humanistic dispositions of sportspersons. The relations among sportspersons thereby fall into antagonism, intemperance, inequality—into an impoverished and despotic war of the one against the many. We could not, according to our interpretation of Kant's moral imperative, opt for the disregard or, even the instrumental treatment of law in sport, or for the antipathetic treatment of others in sport so as to exploit them in effect. For to do this is to will that such conduct become universally legislated, in which case sport, and man himself for that matter, become sterile instruments of

something external to them. Their essential ground in such a circumstance is veiled by an untoward attention to, and acclaim for external ends—they work actively toward their own demise.

III

Hegel's response to Kant on these matters issues both from his interest in taking on Kant's anthropology and from his interest in "reforming" the imperative, which, as we have seen, was a product of that anthropology.[1] With Kant, Hegel was of the view that reason[2] provides the constitutive ground of human existence, and is as such self-contained (that is, having its being within itself, as distinct from the extrinsic character of sensuous existence), or having the faculty of grasping and so realizing its own fundamental nature as such. Also with Kant, he held that freedom is the acting in accord with one's determining principle (i.e., with reason). That is to say, genuinely free acts are self-determined, which goes on this count as being rationally determined. They are therefore distinct from those acts which are the product of external, sensuous laws. As Schacht observes with regard to the Kantian and Hegelian notions of freedom:

Human freedom, therefore, is to be conceived not simply in terms of the self-determination of one's action in accordance with one's will,[3] but rather in terms of their rational self-determination, or determination, in accordance with a will the principle of which is a law of thought rather than a law of mere nature. (29: p. 298)

Freedom is therefore not merely a negative and empty flight from empirical determination, but is as well the rich positivity of a self-conscious discovery of one's rational nature and an acting in accord with that nature. For Hegel, then, as for Kant, moral actions are essentially and fundamentally of this vintage; i.e., free, self-conscious, and rational.

It was with Hegel's rejection of what he took to be the dualistic-tending cleavages in Kant's thought generally (as well as in his anthropology and ethics more particularly) that the Hegelian philosophy turns away from its Kantian foundations. Hegel argues with respect to Kant's moral philosophy that the worlds of sense and understanding, as obtained by Kant, dissect man into a "unity" of antithetic aspects, which is no unity at all but a mere collection of disparate parts.[4] For Hegel, the dispute with Kant, as it persists at this level (recognizing that its status at this level is itself the product of yet more general disagreements), is the consequence of Kant's view that only the form of moral law derives from reason and that its content comes to us from our natural inclinations and faculties. Hegel holds instead that only a law which derives wholly from reason (both in its form and in its content) can be rightly said to be rational, self-determined, free, and so moral. From this Hegel concludes that virtually any moral commandment (principle, law, or maxim) having nature as its source can be universalized and that the Kantian imperative, which claims in itself to command without reference to contingent circumstance, and to command to all persons, has nothing *categorical* to so *command,* for it "commands" virtually all actions governed by the laws of nature, which are, by Kant's view, unendowed with the finely differentiated choices of reason. The imperative is in this sense empty, or without content.

In order to have erected a principle of moral obligation at all, however, Kant had to have stipulated "in what moral duty consists —that is, . . . [to have stated] what is the concept of duty simply as regards its form." (5: p. 214) And, Kant achieved the construction of his imperative, not by failing to consult the world of practical moral action, as commonly supposed, but *through* such a consultation. The formal concept of moral duty was therefore discovered by abstracting from its matter. In this, Hegel can have no objection, for it is not unlike the method used in preparing his own position—that is, erecting general principles from particular cases and allowing the principle and its instances to mutually and dialectically refine one another. Neither, as has been showed, is Hegel's objection to the imperative an objection to Kant's conception of man as primarily rational, nor is it to Kant's notion of freedom as self-conscious, self-determining reason, nor to Kant's view of morality as presupposing and being founded on freedom; for in these Hegel is in agreement with Kant. The dispute is instead more general; that is, of a metaphysical and anthropologic order. More precisely, it is over the constitution of that matter from which the principle is drawn; namely, a "nature" which has, in Hegel's view, no organic connection to reason and is resultantly alien to it and so foreign to freedom, self-determination, and moral obligation. In sum, Hegel's objection to the Kantian imperative is an objection for one, to the principles which undergird it as dividing man and as promoting an unsympathetic regard for nature; and for another yet unmentioned reason, to its failure to show the *development* of its own content.

Hegel's "reform" of the imperative is therefore at bottom a metaphysical reform. His "nature" is not that over and against which reason is qualitatively distinguished and so fundamentally different, but is itself a stage, albeit a primitive stage, in the development of reason and so is itself basically rational. The imperative, then, as it is freed from the fetters of Kant's tacit dualism, and as its development is made explicit, stands. A case can even apparently be made for the view that the rational content of moral life as conceived by Hegel yields the imperative as its principle; and consequently, that it is the imperative which is the formal ordering principle of this content. The imperative is, by this account, reason knowing itself as moral obligation. The moral life of Hegel is the life of rational self-conscious self-determination, and so freedom. It is founded on an unrestrained, a universal respect for all persons—on a treatment of humanity always as an end and never as a means only—as exhorting a realm in which all persons treat one another as ends-in-themselves and never as means only, which goes in turn as seeking oneself and treating others equally as seekers of a commonly held fundamental nature, as being self-conscious, self-determining, rational, and so free beings. This is what is meant by an intrinsic regard for "something"; that is, the making of "its" fundamental nature the primary object of our respect for "it." The system of reason, consequently, as it is dialectically actualized, searches out and embodies the rational, self-determinations which constitute the imperative.

IV

For Hegel, then, both the form and content of moral law must derive from reason. He "finds a basis for the determination of action other than a configuration of 'the modes which nature gives,' yet one that accords with the individual's own essential self, in the objective and determinate system of 'ethical life' (*Sittlichkeit*)[5]—and only in it." (29: p. 316) Hegel's reference to *Sittlichkeit* is a reference to the living systems of socio-cultural law and institution (to the nation-states)[6] which have punctuated the historical development of humanity. Insofar as these living systems have been endowed with reason they have aspired, as have individuals authentically in themselves, to self-conscious self-determination, freedom, and a moral posture and this is that toward which all culture, and individuals, authentically disposed move. As in Kant, the opposition of the individual and the public interests dissolves in this notion, and an organic conception of the state emerges. Unlike the Kantian formulation of this organicism, however, its Hegelian form is promulgated so as to overcome the dualistic tendencies in Kant, and to show the historical development of freedom in the nation-states which have contributed significantly to its maturation. In effect, Hegel's *Sittlichkeit* is an argument for the harmony of humanity and a demonstration of the historical development of this harmony. We will first take up the argument for harmony, then show the intimately related general form, and finally the particular content of its development.

The argument for harmony is essentially a discussion of human life as liberated from the abstractly absolutized and so artificial half-truths and discords of excess, deficiency, and division. It is an affirmation of the unity and tolerance of man as over and against his fragmentation and intolerance. This affirmation is consonant with the general Hegelian longing for harmony—for the living unification of separated opposites. The fragmentation of humanity to which the Kantian program implicitly holds gives way in Hegel to a monistic notion of humanity as a harmonious whole in which ostensibly antagonistic aspects yield to living, forthflowing form—to the balanced and unified development of ethical personality. And with this the *Sittlichkeit*, or cultural and dynamic individualism of the Greeks and "romantic" German poets, displaces the *Moralitat*, or isolated and static individualism, of Kant and Christianity.[7] This view is much reminiscent of Aristotle's *Golden Mean*[8] which Hegel interpreted as a dynamic, a dialectical quest for balance and harmony, by which emphasized extremes produce discord, unhappiness, injustice, a pervasive and self-destructive impoverishment. In fact, for Hegel, "life, whether political, historical or personal is the dialectical struggle to achieve balance and harmony [a lost wholeness, or completeness] without disrupting and negative extremes." (22: pp. 101-102)

As earlier implied, the general form of this harmony and tolerance takes the shape of a developmental dialectic, by process of which separated opposites, contradictions, or antithetical tendencies are unified (though their opposition is in some sense also preserved) by means of contending with one another for domination of the whole. Humanity develops

in this way by placing its faculties in opposition to each other. The very character of our experience, which is constituted by the movement of thinking, presupposes such opposites as well as their dialectical search for unity.[9] The fundamental nature of this search is therefore demonstrated by the terms of our historical development according to Hegel. Owing to this, "the essence of morality can be understood only if morality is taken as a branch of the historical development of the essence of man." (20: p. 84) Morality can be understood only in the concretely unfolding development of human history.

History is conceived by Hegel as the concretion of the fundamental principle and form of reality. It shows the particular terms of one's self (and one's cultural fabric; indeed, reality itself) creatively becoming what one (and "it") essentially is; namely, self-consciously self-determining, rational, and so free agent. History observes the particular events of this development, and in the end reveals the continuity and form of these events, or the rational course of these results—provides their general form with dynamic substance, or content. This form and this substance appear in a hierarchy (actually a circle) of succeeding stages, from primitive forms of consciousness in which all things appear differentiated to absolute forms of consciousness in which all things are apprehended as a unity. Each of these stages, save the final one, contains certain inherent inadequacies which become more apparent as the stage develops, and which in the end manifest themselves as the negation of the stage itself and its sliding away to the positive consequence of a higher stage, as Hartmann observes:

The People is a concretion of Spirit[10] or, logically speaking, an instance of it. Inasmuch as it develops its principles, it grows into its universality. When it forgets and neglects them, it falls away from it. In these principles the People finds its own consciousness of itself. At the height of its development, by the very dialectic of the process— for otherwise the development would not be at its height—it ceases to strive onward. It leans backward and, as it were, enjoys what it has achieved. Thus it turns culmination into decline. At that point reflection flourishes, arts and philosophy arise, but the will—the temporal actualization of the divine will in this form and fashion— slackens. Gradually the People dies off. In this very act, however, the national and thus particular spirit returns to its universality, enriched by the latest experience. It thus elevates itself over the actual phase reached, and prepares itself for the next phase, in another people. Thus history, through national cultures, is the process of the Spirit progressing to its own self, its own cumulative concept of itself, from nation to nation. (13: p. xxix)

In this way, then, each stage is understood to be presupposed by all prior stages and to be the necessary consequence of those stages.[11] Each of these stages is therefore necessarily dependent on the previous one, and each succeeding stage develops progressively toward pure rationality— reason knowing itself as such, or freedom. This is the sense in which the world is not blind or mindless, not abandoned to mere accident, but understood as seeking a qualitative end—an end very much like that envisioned by Kant's "realm of ends."

History, then, takes the form of a gradual awakening of reason to itself—of a gradual actualization of freedom, from the ancient Orient in which only one, the ruler, was free, to classical antiquity where some, the citizens, were free, to the modern world in which "all" men are free (man as man is free). As earlier implied, this awakening works itself out as a dialectical unity of world-historical opposites. With his *Sittlichkeit*, Hegel demonstrates that this unification, this harmony, and freedom gain objective existence through a rational, self-determined system of customs, laws, and institutions—through the nation-state. The independent criterion of right for these customs comes in large measure to an absolutization of the cultural life of the Greeks as refined by Christianity and the modern European states— to a restoration of the substantial content of life in classical antiquity. *Sittlichkeit* is here interpreted, then, as showing the development of the imperative and as filling it with the rich material in which all cultural (and individual) life of merit appears. It demonstrates the unification of opposites, the integration of seemingly disparate insights into a larger, unified vision of the world, the unity of men's differentiated determinations, and so effects a comprehensive synthesis which restores man to his totality. It stands in praise of harmony. Most instructively for this examination of sport, it attempts to show the enduring unity of man's impulse to physical vigor and his inclination to contemplation and wisdom.

V

What remains here is to stipulate the content of these historical developments generally, as well as with respect to sport more particularly—to traverse these developments in detail—to show the general form and content of the reconciled antithesis, not as an empty generality, but as something general that is essentially particular and determinate. The principal intent here is to reveal sport as an activity properly guided by the principle and the substance of moral reflection and action which direct humankind at its best, in its noblest activities and aspirations, in its authentic life generally. It is to unveil sport as an activity in which humankind fulfills itself individually and as a community; and so, to deliver it from the excessive influence of partisanship and negation by which it maintains no viable relation with the fabric of genuine human life and culture. It is to promote a spirit of universal tolerance and harmony in sport— to demonstrate the full continuity of sport with the whole of life, and so the rightful place that sport takes beside the other integral forms of human activity.

In the ancient (as well as in the modern) primitive cultures the human circumstance is elevated but a little above animality. The level to which humanity has risen in these cultures is barely human in that, like animal inclination, it is necessarily and almost entirely taken up with securing the basic conditions of bio-psychological survival. Only the germ of religious, artistic, scientific, and philosophic insight is to be found here, and then only as fragmented attenuations of the most basic aspects of life generally. The full richness of the higher faculties is caught only glimpse of and then not as potential forms of human fulfillment—not as man realizing himself as such. Sport too in these cultures is largely an instrument of survival, either in the form of providing a medium of preparation for it, or in the form of expressing an extension of it. The fullness of its humanity is not yet seen, let alone accomplished. It is from this relatively barren foundation, full as it nevertheless is with human possibilities, that humanity generally, its sporting activity in particular, upbuilds itself.

The first genuinely historical contributions to this development were the products of the ancient Semitic (principally, the Egyptian, Mesopotamian, Hebrew, and Phoenician) and Oriental (principally, the Chinese, Indian, and Persian) cultures. In these, the potentialities of human existence are first recognized, though the positive unity of these potentialities is not yet noticed. In fact, "the harshest antitheses are apparent in these developments—the conception of the purely abstract unity of God, and of the purely sensual Powers of Nature." (11: p. 113) With the possible and partial exceptions of the Hebrews and Persians (who moved culture nearer its rational groundings, and so provided the transition to Western life), the various aspects of the human are thereby conceived as over and against one another, as alien to one another, as in external relationship to one another. And as such the antitheses remain unreconciled— the terms of their harmonization has not yet been developed—they remain contending elements. The recognition of such antitheses is nonetheless the first, necessary stage in bringing about their conciliation—in bringing about the conciliation of nature and reason, substance and subject, individuality and sociality, the finite and the infinite. The mere shadow of freedom is therefore apparent here. Sport in these cultures serves as an isolated and vacuous instrument of political, commercial, social, religious, or military significance. It has not yet become conscious of itself as such—it remains here in the service of the external, and so is itself external, even to itself—the point of its own existence is obscured to it. Hegel summarizes these developments and their passing over into the Greek consciousness:

This undeveloped reconciliation exhibits the struggle of the most contradictory principles which are not yet capable of harmonizing themselves, but, setting up the birth of this harmony as the problem to be solved, make themselves a riddle for themselves and for others, the solution of which is only to be found in the *Greek* world. (11: p. 115)

It was the great genius of the Greeks (principally, the Athenians) to have summoned humanity in general to self-knowledge, and so to freedom. The Greeks, unique among the ancients, conceived of the various aspects of reality—most notably and generally, the natural and the rational; and more particularly, the biological, psychological, social, scientific, artistic, religious, and philosophic—not as fragmented bits and pieces of knowledge having nothing but an external, and so largely alien relation to one another, but as participants in an organic union, which explains each, not merely in isolation by itself alone, but in internal relation with all other things as well. By this view, the various aspects of reality are understood as progressively developing interpenetrations which deliver individuality and culture alike to themselves—to an awareness of their fundamental natures, and to emancipation. In this, reason shows the

unity among natural differentiations, and individual excellence is understood as an enduring harmony of one's physical vigor and action and one's intellectuality. The two sides of man's constitution are no longer conceived as antipathetic constituents, but as the natural seen through the gaze, and providing the stuff of reason; that is, as *separated opposites giving way to a synthetic harmony.*

Importantly numbered among the integral aspects of human life for the Greeks is the impulse to physicality, which expresses itself in its most refined terms in sport (and dance). Sport, consequently, is conceived as one among the various aspects of reality that participates in the organic union of events earlier talked about—a union which can now be known as human life properly so-termed. As such, it is not in its basic disposition an instrument to be employed in the service of external ends, but a self-sustaining aspect of the lot of activities by which humankind expresses and fulfills itself as such.

Sport presents the higher seriousness; for in it Nature is wrought into Spirit, and although in these contests the subject has not advanced to the highest grade of serious thought, yet in this exercise of his physical powers, man shows his Freedom. (11: p. 243)

Sport is neither then a diversion from, nor an aside to, nor is it therefore outside of the mainstream of authentic individual and cultural life and in extrinsic relation to such life; rather, it occupies a central place in, and has an intrinsic "relation" to this life.

The decline of Greek greatness was in some measure accelerated by its own attentions to the movement, or to the dynamic of dialectic, which is taken as the procedural form of life and thought itself. This cultivation of the moving and developing by its nature propels individuals and cultures out of certain inclinations and into others, and so does not make the preservation of these certain inclinations as such their chief aim (as in most of the ancient Semitic and Oriental cultures). In the case of the Greeks, these other inclinations took on a progressively more excessive and extreme character. Most significantly, the substantial individuality of ancient Greece's most enlightened period gave way to the excess of idiosyncratic subjectivity by which self-interest is held little to at all in relation to public interest, but as externally and negatively contrasted to it. The intellectual severs its full living relationship with the physical, the instrumentality of the commercial and the military comes to dominate and cover over the internal richness of the intrinsic, and education and sport become themselves tools of the commercial, political, military and exhibitionary.

In Sparta (and in similar measure in Thebes and Macedonia as well) and in Rome the fragmentation characteristic of the late Greek pre-eminence continues, though in a moderately different fashion. Here a comparatively fixed and lifeless preservation of the prevailing order dominates. This order is not resultantly constructed in the full and harmonious image of human nature, but in significant contrast to it. Persons were either indifferent to life or devoted to a capricious indulgence of it. In this circumstance, the cultural and the individual—let alone the physical and the intellectual—oppose one another, and so strain at obtaining a viable articulation. There are everywhere divisions and separations and nowhere the harmony nor freedom of the synthetic. Sport in these cultures again takes on an instrumental and so incidental disposition. It is used largely for military, political, and entertainment purposes, and is thereby alienated from itself (and genuine human life) as such, and so without redeeming individual or cultural value.

With the negativity, the degeneration of the life of reason in the Roman world, the way had been prepared for a new positivity—the turning of life back to its self-conscious ground. The domination of the medieval period by the Christian and Islamic religions again brought the focus of human life to its rational underpinnings. But this focus is more so Hebrew and to a lesser extent Persian than Greek, in that, by it, the natural is again trammeled under a virtually exclusive emphasis on religiosity. The sensuous or mindless excesses of the Roman experience now pass over into an excess of a different order, but an excess nonetheless. The Middle Ages not only failed to make institutional provision, let alone suggest the terms of unity, for many forms of fundamental human impulse—most prominently for the impulses to physicality, aestheticality, sociality, even intellectuality, at least as these are free from the fetters of religion to openly explore, not to mention realize the scope of their own natures—but actively suppressed these as drawing one away from religious fulfillment. The effect of this was to divide man utterly, to divide him from himself and from others. The bodily aspect was conceived through much of this period as the principle of evil itself; and sport, foremost

among those activities engaging this aspect, was much condemned. Sport was again, as it had been throughout its history, but for its Greek practice, in external relation to itself, outside itself, in violation of itself, an activity at odds with itself. Again, man found himself alienated from much that he is, and so yet found himself much in search of himself.

This search bore its first fruit of promise in the humanism of the early Renaissance. Here the transcendent abstractions and religious exclusivity of medievalism are gradually replaced[12] by a thisworldly attention to the human circumstance; that is, to the human becoming aware of, and actualizing itself as such—as self-conscious, self-determining, rational, and so free being. The general sweep of modern history is constructed of the general form of this awareness and actualization. An exuberance for the whole organic of human life, an exuberance significantly reminiscent of the Greek[13] emerged, and learning properly so-termed (as an odyssey in and for itself, which goes for Hegel as a dialectic journey after reason knowing itself as such—after freedom) was revived. Sport was again seen in more sympathetic relief, as an integral participant in the authentic life of humanity, though it never again actually achieved the status it had been given by the Greeks.

The treatment of sport in the past century in particular has turned notably away from Greek possibilities. It has fashioned, or has had fashioned for it, an ardent imbalance of human faculty, and has been vigorously *employed in the service of an* ominous number of external ends.[14] The perilous consequences of these developments are now increasingly evident. If we are to preserve ourselves, let alone "preserve" sport as an authentic expression of ourselves, the reconciliation of the alienations discussed here must be achieved, painful as such restorations inevitably are.

VI

The intent of this essay has been to show the terms in which Kant's categorical imperative provides a principle by which moral conduct in sport is properly guided, and to demonstrate as well the manner by which Hegel's *Sittlichkeit* gives the imperative concrete content. The merits of the position obtained here can be summarized as: 1) human moral action and freedom generally (as well as their expression in sport more particularly) finding its originative source in itself (in the fundamental nature of human existence), and not in an external agent, in the latter case of which moral principle and action are separated and their articulation occurs in the form of an alien application of the former to the latter— a mindless determination of the latter by the former; 2) the resultant coalescence of the individual and the public interests, by which a humanistic or intrinsic respect among all persons and their self-legislated laws and institutions generally, as well as in sport more particularly (as distinct from a mutual antagonism among persons and their state characteristic of extrinsic conceptions), is secured; 3) the provision of a singular, universal principle by which our moral conduct in general (as well as in sport more particularly) may be governed, as distinct from the multiplicity and relativity of conventionalism which has no independent ethical principle, and so can have no such guide, and so can neither satisfactorily distinguish the 'ought' from the caprice of the 'is'; 4) the working out of the creative flow and record, the continuity of this principle throughout history generally, as well as sport history more particularly—the demonstration of its concrete development, as distinct from its stipulation as an empty and lifeless exhortation; 5) the recognition that this creative flow is itself a display of the reconciled antitheses of once separated human aspects—most notably, the harmonization of the physical and the intellectual aspects, which is, by Hegel's view, the supreme need of the human spirit—and so a restoration of man to his unified totality; and, 6) the location of sport in the full context of genuine human event, by which its necessarily intrinsic and humanistic character is unveiled—a type of account which provides the only basis by which sport and the human can even so much as tolerate, let alone fulfill one another.

If the philosophy of sport can be said to have adduced a singularly and an immensely significant conclusion, it is surely this latter. For it has understood well that only by such an insight may sport be sufficiently well understood and appreciated to command the sort of respect that can preserve it in its authenticity. That this sort of treatment is so infrequently extended to sport (to say nothing of culture generally) is at once a testimony to its perilous status, and a call to its reform. The present effort represents an attempt to provide the right root of moral conduct in sport (to provide the right root of this reform) that it seems the active conspiracy of our age to eliminate.

Notes

1. The line of argument referred to here extends even deeper into the roots of Kant's philosophy than to his anthropology; namely, to his accounting of the problem of knowledge which is the cornerstone of his thought.

2. By 'reason' (*vernunft*) Hegel means strictly that synthetic faculty of mind which unites separated opposites or disparate facts by interpretation, as distinct from 'understanding' (*verstand*) which separates by analysis and which provides the stuff of interpretation. Both reason and understanding together comprise the human faculty of apprehending ideas by means of other ideas. The term is used here to refer to consciousness generally, as being that and only that capable in the end of turning itself back onto itself, thus revealing and fulfilling itself.

3. The will is conceived throughout, not as an intellectual faculty distinct from reason though nonetheless attached to reason in some circumstances, but reason itself insofar as it is concerned with action. Reason and action do not therefore exclude one another, but the latter is rather an instance of the former, as that by which the former expresses itself, or "receives" the intention of actualization.

4. This is a view which Hegel importantly shared with the great poets and dramatists of the German Enlightenment (most notably, Lessing, Goethe, Schiller, and Holderlin), all of whom exercised a major influence over his work.

5. From the German 'Sitte' meaning 'custom' referring to the historical life of human culture, as distinct from what Hegel took as the isolated and static individualism of the imperative, the *Moralitat*.

6. The reference here is to the cultures, or states, which have organized freedom, both with respect to its form and its content, and have advanced it (or contributed to its concrete actualization) in some significant way.

7. The position that Hegel actually takes in the end mediates the Kantian view (from which many basic distinctions are preserved) and that of the extreme romantics (not the German "romantics," Lessing, Goethe, Schiller, and Holderlin, earlier referred to as greatly influencing Hegel in a positive fashion) of the late eighteenth and early nineteenth centuries (who generally saw only an undifferentiated harmony of qualities).

8. Which stipulates that: moral virtue or excellence is a characteristic involving choice, and that it consists in observing the mean relative to us, a mean which is defined by a rational principle, such as a man of practical wisdom would use to determine it. It is the mean by reference to two vices: the one of excess and the other of deficiency. (1: p. 43; 1106b-1107) . . . the nature of moral qualities is such that they are destroyed by defect and by excess. (1: pp. 35-36; 1104a)

9. As Hegel avers: An organic life requires in the first place One Soul, and in the second place, a divergence into differences, which became or-

ganic members, and in their several offices develop themselves to a complete system; in such a way, however, that their activity reconstitutes that one soul. (11: p. 144)

10. By 'Spirit' Hegel means the system of reason concretely manifest.

11. By necessary consequence it is not meant that the same events could not have occurred otherwise, nor that subsequent stages are in every detail the "necessary" products of prior ones (for there is abundant irrationality, or arbitrariness in the world), but that the actual development of the world can be generally explained only by such a connection of events as history has recorded.

12. This replacement can be traced through the moralistic humanism of the Reformations, the realistic humanism of the seventeenth century, and the naturalistic humanism of the Enlightenment. The moralistic interlude aside, this development represents in general a gradual liberalization of the early Renaissance humanism, and so a gradual turning away from the constraints of the medieval.

13. It is nonetheless the case that the egalitarian spirit of the modern period exceeded that of the Greek, and that the political, economic, and educational franchise was gradually broadened in greater measure than in the Greek circumstance, largely under the mediating influence of Christianity.

14. It has been employed most notably as a chauvinistic, cultural, economic, military, scientific, pedagogical, political, psychological, and social instrument.

Bibliography

1. Aristotle. *Nicomachean Ethics.* Translated by Martin Ostwald. Indianapolis: The Bobbs-Merrill Co., 1962.
2. Bannister, Roger. *The Four Minute Mile.* New York: Dodd, Mead, and Co., 1958.
3. Copleston, Frederick. *A History of Philosophy: Modern Philosophy: Fichte to Hegel.* Garden City, N.Y.: Doubleday and Co., 1965.
4. Duruy, Victor. *A History of the World.* Cleveland: The World Syndicate Pub. Co., 1937.
5. Ebbinghaus, Julius. "Interpretation and Misinterpretation of the Categorical Imperative," *Kant: A Collection of Critical Essays.* Edited by Robert P. Wolff. Garden City, N.Y.: Doubleday and Co., 1967.
6. Findlay, J. N. *Hegel: A Re-Examination.* New York: Humanities Press, 1964.
7. Friedrich, Carl J., ed. *The Philosophy of Hegel.* Second edition. New York: Random House, 1954.
8. Friedrich, Carl J., ed. *The Philosophy of Kant: Immanuel Kant's Moral and Political Writings.* New York: Random House, 1949.
9. Hegel, G. W. F. *Encyclopedia of Philosophy.* Translated by Gustav E. Mueller, New York: Philosophical Library, 1959.
10. Hegel, G. W. F. *The Phenomenology of Mind.* Translated by J. B. Baillie. New York: Harper and Row, Publishers, 1967.
11. Hegel, G. W. F. *The Philosophy of History.* Translated by J. Sibree. New York: Dover Publications, 1956.
12. Hegel, G. W. F. *The Philosophy of Right.* Translated by T. M. Knox. London: Oxford University Press, 1967.
13. Hegel, G. W. F. *Reason in History.* Translated by Robert S. Hartmann. Indianapolis: The Bobbs-Merrill Pub. Co., 1953.
14. Hegel, G. W. F. *Science of Logic.* Translated by A. V. Miller. London: George Allen and Unwin, 1969.
15. Kant, Immanuel. *Critique of Pure Reason.* Translated by Norman K. Smith. New York: St. Martin's Press, 1965.
16. Kant, Immanuel. *Foundations of the Metaphysics of Morals.* Translated by Lewis W. Beck. Indianapolis: The Bobbs-Merrill Co., 1959.
17. Kaufmann, Walter. *Hegel: A Reinterpretation.* Garden City, N. Y.: Doubleday and Co., 1965.
18. Kaufmann, Walter, ed. *Hegel: Texts and Commentary.* Garden City, N.Y.: Doubleday and Co., 1966.
19. Lessing, Gottfried E. *Nathan the Wise.* Translated by Bayard Q. Morgan. New York: Frederick Ungar Pub. Co., 1955.
20. Maier, Joseph. *On Hegel's Critique of Kant.* New York: Columbia University Press, 1939.
21. Metheny, Eleanor. *Connotations of Movement in Sport and Dance.* Dubuque, Iowa: William C. Brown Co., Publishers, 1965.
22. Mueller, Gustav E. *Hegel: The Man, His Vision and Work.* New York: Pageant Press, 1968.
23. Mure, G. R. G. *An Introduction to Hegel.* London: Oxford University Press, 1940.
24. Osterhoudt, Robert G. "An Hegelian Interpretation of Art, Sport, and Athletics," *The Philosophy of Sport: A Collection of Original Essays.* Edited by Robert G. Osterhoudt. Springfield, Ill.: Charles C Thomas, Publisher, 1973.
25. Osterhoudt, Robert G. "The Kantian Ethic as a Principle of Moral Conduct in Sport," *Quest,* No. 19 (January, 1973), 118-123.
26. Paton, H. J. *The Categorical Imperative: A Study in Kant's Moral Philosophy.* Sixth edition. London: Hutchinson and Co., 1967.
27. Santayana, George. "Philosophy on the Bleachers." *Howard Monthly,* 18 (July, 1894), 181-190.
28. Schacht, Richard L. *Alienation.* Garden City, N.Y.: Doubleday and Co., 1970.
29. Schacht, Richard L. "Hegel on Freedom," *Hegel: A Collection of Critical Essays.* Edited by Alasdair MacIntyre, Garden City, N.Y.: Doubleday and Co., 1972.
30. Schiller, Friedrich. *On the Aesthetic Education of Man.* Translated by Reginald Snell. New York: Frederick Ungar Pub. Co., 1965.

31. Singer, Marcus G. *Generalization in Ethics*. New York: Alfred A. Knopf, 1961.
32. Smith, William, trans. *The Popular Works of Johann Gottlieb Fichte*. Fourth edition. London: Trubner and Co., 1889.
33. Stace, W. J. *The Philosophy of Hegel: A Systematic Exposition*. New York: Dover Publications, 1955.
34. Thilly, Frank and Wood, Ledger. *A History of Philosophy*. Third edition. New York: Holt, Rinehart and Winston, 1957.
35. Van Dalen, Deobold B. and Bennett, Bruce L. *A World History of Physical Education: Cultural, Philosophical, and Comparative*. Second edition. Englewood Cliffs, N.J.: Prentice-Hall, 1971.
36. Watson, John. *Schelling's Transcendental Idealism: A Critical Exposition*. Chicago: S. C. Griggs and Co., 1882.
37. Williams, T. C. *The Concept of the Categorical Imperative*. London: Oxford University Press, 1968.

Morality as an Intimate of Sport[*]

HOWARD S. SLUSHER

Working within the structure of *personal concern* the morality decisions that face man in sport are most personal. They provide the *intimate* fiber of communication between man and the activity. In order to actualize the ethic man must ask where he *is* within the totality of the sport experience. For all of life begins and ends with what he experiences in existence. If one espouses the thesis that you "treat your opponent as you would desire to be treated," then the *meaning of the truth* of that statement is a dependent variable. Its validity is determined by the *intimateness* of man to the experience.

The word "intimate" is being used to connote that which is beyond human thought. The value is not achieved, *really*, if man just *thinks* that is the way to act. Or even if he says that is the way I would like to be treated. This quality of the "intimate" goes into the depths of existence and certainly extends itself beyond modern Christian Ethic. The implication is that man *cares*, not merely intellectually, but with an involvement that extends to the very root of his personhood. If man is not treated in this manner, one is not *just* disappointed, he becomes *nauseated*. He *suffers* because his involvement was more than what was stated—it was *all* of life. Sport is, generally, an act of initial volition. Man participates with *all* of his complexities. This completeness leads to a seriousness of involvement. Only too often the "intermediate" goal of victory blinds man from

seeing the eventuation of his participation. To become intimate is to initiate morality. Real morality cannot be achieved until man is willing to *risk* his self in the sport experience.

In achieving this morality man cannot treat man according to usual role expectancy. One does not treat one as an umpire, bowler, boxer, jockey, skier, or basketball player. One is treated *intimately*, as an *individual*. Too often, in our complicated and mass culture of mechanization, we forget that man is not a collective noun. He is a person with a unique identity. Sport must be wary that, in its zest for *ends* and results that are indicated on the scoreboard, man is not relegated to a *mean*. Again, I trust this thought is in keeping with Buber's moral imperative:

> One cannot treat either an individual or a social organism as a means to an end absolutely, without robbing it of its life substance. . . . One cannot in the nature of things expect a little tree that has been turned into a club to put forth leaves.[1]

The *intimate* relationships of sport provide the raw material for the most "humane" of all ethical structures. However, one must wonder if the potential is being realized or prostituted. The question is not one of the normal means/ends dichotomy. No matter how good or bad is either the means or ends, man is *immoral* if he attempts to structure any form of dualism

[*] From *Man, Sport and Existence*. Philadelphia: Lea & Febiger, 1967.

[1] Martin Buber. *I and Thou*. Translated by Ronald Gregor Smith. (Edinburgh: T. & T. Clark, 1953), p. 17.

which segments, and thereby injures, the authentic existence of man. Our experiences and our goals need be one. Our dreams and our realities need be fused. To say they *are* not is to admit *reality*. To say they *cannot* is to admit *defeat*. We might make choices that are less than what we would hope them to be. But we must not close our eyes and our hearts to those that are *not* chosen. An ethic of *existence* is personal; it is intimate. In sport man can free himself *in* the closeness of another: in his relations with man, in his empathy for skill development, in his appreciation of dedication. All these qualities *bring* him closer to the door of being. Whether he *enters* into life or stays behind a closed partition is a matter of *choice*. A choice of none less than life or death, for man and sport.

In making the choice we cannot run away from the obvious question. Is the authentic life both "good" and "right"? When man is trying to find *real* self in the world of sport, does the *sport* itself encourage man in a world of good and right? In talking about modern sports, The Rev. Edward Hildner, who at ninety-three years of age is the sole surviver of the first basketball game, said, "There are too many whistles, too many interruptions because some silly little rule is broken. The same is true about baseball—all that baloney that makes the game too long."[2] Well the game may now be "right." But is it "good"? Is this what James would call a difference that makes no difference and therefore it makes no difference? I think not. Man does not find any sure and clear roads to follow in journeying toward the *real* life. The subtle differentiation between "right" and "good" affords insights into the sport situation as an arena for the development of *being*. Choices are difficult to make when the scope of the question is clear. But in the complexity of the sport world we are talking of another issue. It is easy to see how man could "settle" for a world of absolutes. When life becomes intimate, man needs to deal with the "gray areas." Black and white will not do. The importance of *relatives* becomes both obvious and terrifying. But now the decisions cannot be avoided. They are close. They are intimate. How do you regulate between the good of the team and the rightness of man? It might be right for man to hunt (the deer will be injured due to overpopulation is the usual reason that is given); but few would say it is good to kill a defenseless animal. Hopefully the reader is not expecting any type of ethical

[2] "Scorecard." *Sports Illustrated,* 25 (1966), p. 22.

panacea. The only answer I know is that man must do what *he* feels is good. Values and ethics, as moral derivatives, need be unclouded so that man can act with a decisiveness that indicates position and reflection. But this is only the start. For the more immediate and intimate man becomes to sport, the greater will be the effort to reach the zenith.

Physical Fitness as a Moral Quality. To talk of *physical* fitness as an aspect of sport is to be obviously and almost hopelessly out of date. Obviously man needs some form of physical tonus to engage in all activities of life. But in sport it is all the more imperative. Yet to talk of *physical* fitness is to relate to an "old" concept. Now the vogue is *total* fitness. But really one can't help but hear the intonations of a guilty dualistic culture giving mouth service to those elements that *also* compose man.

Fitness is basically a survival technique. It is necessary for day-to-day living and receives special attention during a period of increased stress. War and sport have been special modes of human life that have stressed the demands of fitness. To talk of the importance of fitness to any individual concerned with survival is much like "bringing coals to Newcastle." But to see fitness receive extensive stress is to recognize the moral structure of survival.

Since fitness is necessary for survival, we can understand that fitness is a desired *means* for the achievement of a specific end. Accordingly, it becomes a *relative* dimension of morality. How fit should one be for football? How fit should one be for squash? Is the same type of fitness required for sailing as mountain climbing? Obviously, the answer to the dimensions of fitness are dependent upon the *ends*. What is your aim? Obviously the end is not mere participation. Nor is it victory. Somewhere, someplace we come to recognize there is *more* to life than the obvious. We have not forgotten fulfillment, righteousness and self-realization. All this indicates that when we conceive of fitness for the purposes of a sport we are saying it is a *means for a means*. The question that needs to be asked deals with the end to which fitness is an appropriate mean. Is fitness a moral quality, serving as a handmaiden, of sport?

Darwinism has established the principle of survival of the fittest. But the "fit" in sport are not those with qualities of concern, love, empathy, care, passion and respect for personhood. To survive in the world of sport man better *not* have these qualities. To be hard, to be tough, to be strong and to be rough—these are the qualities that pay dividends. Again, the accent is in different kinds of strength or relative values. The truth of the matter is that the Bible would not have a chance against the likes of Darwin in a war or in sport.

Now the preceding conversation begins to haunt us. It might be "right" to develop a level of fitness that enables man to conquer; but is it good? Is it good for *mankind?*

Much is often said of the *social values* of sport. Certainly such moral structures facilitate our social life. About this there can be no complaint. Love, warmth and kindness assist man in his attempt to be human. Yet the qualities of fitness lead man to anything but a social life. They serve as a means, not to the ends of actualization, but rather toward achieving a conquering soul. I think few would deny the apparent necessity for fitness in sport. In so demanding we must readily see that the original choice commits us to further choice. We select sport. We must choose fitness. When we select fitness, we commit ourselves to a "war-like" environment. From this choice little in the way of "tender loving care" can emerge. Morality assists us toward social awareness and compatibility. Fitness facilitates our preparation for war. Since social harmony and war are opposites, it follows that morality and fitness are also at polar extremes. I cannot go quite as far as some who insist fitness is *immoral* (since it is nonsocial). But, from the immediate discussion, it is obvious that I can *almost* go that far.

The morality of man is a consequence of the *existing* social order. Alter the order and you possibly alter the morality. This does not necessitate that the morality be recognized by the social order at the time it existed. To be there is to demonstrate its existence. If it is "right" and "good," it will activate the society toward the appropriate end. But it never will be right for all.

The preceding has demonstrated the social dimension of morality; however, basically, morality is a personal and individual matter. In this regard sport gives man the choice of participating in "individual" activities such as golf, riding, swimming, bowling and skiing. If man desires the social setting, he turns his attention to team sports such as baseball, basketball, football, volley ball, hockey and soccer. It is interesting to note that no matter whether man participates in individual or team activities the social code continues to dictate. Officials, umpires, referees are employed to make certain the "just" receive their due. They are a symbol of the rules. In essence they represent what is *right*. Although they have little direct con-

cern with the *good,* at times they temper their decisions *with what ought to be.* It is quite frequent for an official to "miss" a foul (not right) when it does not affect the direct play of the game (the good). When this action becomes repeated, it soon becomes an expected tradition or custom of the game. Thus, as the social order changes, sport, and the concept of right and good, makes similar modifications. While morality is not completely a servant to changing times, one could hardly deny the rightful effect of the environment upon the morality of any given time.

Allowing for the Existing Morality

Morality is directly related to its environment. However, this does not mean the social matrix always affords assent to the expressed value. Since the realm of sport is atypical from many other endeavors of life—one would expect a varied ethic. That is to say, it is hard to believe that one would even dream that the sport participant would exhibit the same value structure on the gridiron as he does when visiting friends. Each situation calls for its own judgments. This is not to say that this system of relatives is right or wrong. But it does say that it is internally consistent with prior analysis. We might not like ourselves for making certain value decisions. Nevertheless, man makes the choice. Yet, it has been my impression that educators, laymen, sportswriters, and sometimes even coaches act surprised and even shocked when a value is demonstrated that is contrary to the Judea-Christian Ethic. All of this in spite of the accepted thesis of situational ethics.

This expressed horror is not naiveté. In fact, it is more probably a reflection of associated guilt which is manifested in another. Any individual who has been around football for any period of time knows that "elbows fly" on the first play from scrimmage. This is when each man tells his opponent "who is boss." Yet let a player get "caught" for punching and everyone exhibits great shock. "How could such a nice boy do a thing like that? Why he goes to church every Sunday." Yes. But this is Saturday. And on Saturday the name of the game is *kill*. Do we really expect him to practice the Ten Commandments in front of 60,000 people? I think not. We might *like* him to. But we don't *expect* him to. Yet overtly we give the impression that the morality of sport is identical to the morality of the choir. It seems it is high time we either change the nature of sport (which is highly unlikely), or stop the hypocrisy and *admit* to ourselves the existing ethic. To condone, covertly, and punish, overtly, is not my idea of authenticity.

Our expressed purpose and preference in sport is clear. It is not comradeship, self-discovery or aesthetics. I don't care what the "level" of participation is—be it six-year-olds or sixty-year-olds—man plays to succeed. And success is measured by pushing the other guy down, just a little, so that you, as you harness the forces of nature, climb a little higher. Each time we climb a little higher. Each child learns that some day if he works hard and is lucky (but he also learns he has to *make* his own "breaks"), he might grow up to be the champion.

The athlete *knows* the acceptable moral code; however, within this frame he might make many varied value decisions. While he might select to play professional baseball as opposed to seeking a college education, it is not an unethical decision. It is simply an expressed preference. This is what he *likes*. Values are *not* moral imperatives. Since man is *not*, in any sense, forced into action, it would seem wise that we make room for the values we locate in sport. Again, no one is saying this is what we *want*. All that is being said is this is what *is*. Let us not make the mistake of so many who preceded us. Let us recognize *situations* in sport as they exist; and let us stop in the game of self-deception. No life could be more immoral than where one refuses to be aware of his own existence.

The Practice Conception of Rules*

JOHN RAWLS

The other conception of rules I will call the practice conception. On this view rules are pictured as defining a practice. Practices are set up for various reasons, but one of them is that in many areas of conduct each person's deciding what to do on utilitarian grounds case by case leads to confusion, and that the attempt to coordinate behavior by trying to foresee how others will act is bound to fail. As an alternative one realizes that what is required is the establishment of a practice, the specification of a new form of activity; and from this one sees that a practice necessarily involves the abdication of full liberty to act on utilitarian and prudential grounds. It is the mark of a practice that being taught how to engage in it involves being instructed in the rules which define it, and that appeal is made to those rules to correct the behavior of those engaged in it. Those engaged in a practice recognize the rules as defining it. The rules cannot be taken as simply describing how those engaged in the practice in fact behave: it is not simply that they act as if they were obeying the rules. Thus it is essential to the notion of a practice that the rules are publicly known and understood as definitive; and it is essential also that the rules of a practice can be taught and can be acted upon to yield a coherent practice. On this conception, then, rules are not generalizations from the decisions of individuals applying the utilitarian principle directly and independently to recurrent par-

ticular cases. On the contrary, rules define a practice and are themselves the subject of the utilitarian principle.

To show the important differences between this way of fitting rules into the utilitarian theory and the previous way, I shall consider the differences between the two conceptions on the points previously discussed.

1. In contrast with the summary view, the rules of practices are logically prior to particular cases. This is so because there cannot be a particular case of an action falling under a rule of a practice unless there is the practice. This can be made clearer as follows: in a practice there are rules setting up offices, specifying certain forms of action appropriate to various offices, establishing penalties for the breach of rules, and so on. We may think of the rules of a practice as defining offices, moves, and offenses. Now what is meant by saying that the practice is logically prior to particular cases is this: given any rule which specifies a form of action (a move), a particular action which would be taken as falling under this rule given that there is the practice would not be *described as* that sort of action unless there was the practice. In the case of actions specified by practices it is logically impossible to perform them outside the stage-setting provided by those practices, for unless there is the practice, and unless the requisite proprieties are fulfilled, whatever one does, whatever movements one makes, will fail to count as a form of action which the practice specifies. What one does will be described in some *other* way.

* Excerpted from "Two Concepts of Rules." *The Philosophical Review*, 64 (January, 1955), 3-32.

One may illustrate this point from the game of baseball. Many of the actions one performs in a game of baseball one can do by oneself or with others whether there is the game or not. For example, one can throw a ball, run, or swing a peculiarly shaped piece of wood. But one cannot steal base, or strike out, or draw a walk, or make an error, or balk; although one can do certain things which appear to resemble these actions such as sliding into a bag, missing a grounder and so on. Striking out, stealing a base, balking, etc., are all actions which can only happen in a game. No matter what a person did, what he did would not be described as stealing a base or striking out or drawing a walk unless he could also be described as playing baseball, and for him to be doing this presupposes the rule-like practice which constitutes the game. The practice is logically prior to particular cases: unless there is the practice the terms referring to actions specified by it lack a sense.[1]

2. The practice view leads to an entirely different conception of the authority which each person has to decide on the propriety of following a rule in particular cases. To engage in a practice, to perform those actions specified by a practice, means to follow the appropriate rules. If one wants to do an action which a certain practice specifies then there is no way to do it except to follow the rules which define it. Therefore, it doesn't make sense for a person to raise the question whether or not a rule of a practice correctly applies to *his* case where the action he contemplates is a form of action defined by a practice. If someone were to raise such a question, he would simply show that he didn't understand the situation in which he was acting. If one wants to perform an action specified by a practice, the only legitimate question concerns the nature of the

practice itself ("How do I go about making a will?").

This point is illustrated by the behavior expected of a player in games. If one wants to play a game, one doesn't treat the rules of the game as guides as to what is best in particular cases. In a game of baseball if a batter were to ask "Can I have four strikes?" it would be assumed that he was asking what the rule was; and if, when told what the rule was, he were to say that he meant that on this occasion he thought it would be best on the whole for him to have four strikes rather than three, this would be most kindly taken as a joke. One might contend that baseball would be a better game if four strikes were allowed instead of three; but one cannot picture the rules as guides to what is best on the whole in particular cases, and question their applicability to particular cases as particular cases.

3 and 4. To complete the four points of comparison with the summary conception, it is clear from what has been said that rules of practices are not guides to help one decide particular cases correctly as judged by some higher ethical principle. And neither the quasi-statistical notion of generality, nor the notion of a particular exception, can apply to the rules of practices. A more or less general rule of a practice must be a rule which according to the structure of the practice applies to more or fewer of the kinds of cases arising under it; or it must be a rule which is more or less basic to the understanding of the practice. Again, a particular case cannot be an exception to a rule of a practice. An exception is rather a qualification or a further specification of the rule.

It follows from what we have said about the practice conception of rules that if a person is engaged in a practice, and if he is asked why *he* does what *he* does, or if he is asked to defend what he does, then his explanation, or defense, lies in referring the questioner to the practice. He cannot say of *his* action, if it is an action specified by a practice, that he does it rather than some other because he thinks it is best on the whole.[2] When a man engaged in a practice is queried about his action he must assume that the questioner either doesn't know that he is engaged in it ("Why are you in a hurry to pay him?" "I promised to pay him today") or doesn't know what the practice is. One doesn't so much justify one's particular

---

[1] One might feel that it is a mistake to say that a practice is logically prior to the forms of action it specifies on the grounds that if there were never any instances of actions falling under a practice then we should be strongly inclined to say that there wasn't the practice either. Blue-prints for a practice do not make a practice. That there is a practice entails that there are instances of people having been engaged and now being engaged in it (with suitable qualifications). This is correct, but it doesn't hurt the claim that any given particular instance of a form of action specified by a practice presupposes the practice. This isn't so on the summary picture, as each instance must be "there" prior to the rules, so to speak, as something from which one gets the rule by applying the utilitarian principle to it directly.

[2] A philosophical joke (in the mouth of Jeremy Bentham): "When I run to the other wicket after my partner has struck a good ball I do so because it is best on the whole."

action as explain, or show, that it is in accordance with the practice. The reason for this is that it is only against the stage-setting of the practice that one's particular action is described as it is. Only by reference to the practice can one *say* what one is doing. To explain or to defend one's own action, as a particular action, one fits it into the practice which defines it. If this is not accepted it's a sign that a different question is being raised as to whether one is justified in accepting the practice, or in tolerating it. When the challenge is to the practice, citing the rules (saying what the practice is) is naturally to no avail. But when the challenge is to the particular action defined by the practice, there is nothing one can do but refer to the rules. Concerning particular actions there is only a question for one who isn't clear as to what the practice is, or who doesn't know that it is being engaged in. This is to be contrasted with the case of a maxim which may be taken as pointing to the correct decision on the case as decided on *other* grounds, and so giving a challenge on the case a sense by having it question whether these other grounds really support the decision on this case.

If one compares the two conceptions of rules I have discussed, one can see how the summary conception misses the significance of the distinction between justifying a practice and justifying actions falling under it. On this view rules are regarded as guides whose purpose it is to indicate the ideally rational decision on the given particular case which the flawless application of the utilitarian principle would yield. One has, in principle, full option to use the guides or to discard them as the situation warrants without one's moral office being altered in any way: whether one discards the rules or not, one always holds the office of a rational person seeking case by case to realize the best on the whole. But on the practice conception, if one holds an office defined by a practice then questions regarding one's actions in this office are settled by reference to the rules which define the practice. If one seeks to question these rules, then one's office undergoes a fundamental change: one then assumes the office of one empowered to change and criticize the rules, or the office of a reformer, and so on. The summary conception does away with the distinction of offices and the various forms of argument appropriate to each. On that conception there is one office and so no offices at all. It therefore obscures the fact that the utilitarian principle must, in the case of

actions and offices defined by a practice, apply to the practice, so that general utilitarian arguments are not available to those who act in offices so defined.[3]

Some qualifications are necessary in what I have said. First, I may have talked of the summary and the practice conceptions of rules as if only one of them could be true of rules, and if true of any rules, then necessarily true of *all* rules. I do not, of course, mean this. (It is the critics of utilitarianism who make this mistake insofar as their arguments against utilitarianism presuppose a summary conception of the rules of practices.) Some rules will fit one conception, some rules the other; and so there are rules of practices (rules in the strict sense), and maxims and "rules of thumb."

Secondly, there are further distinctions that can be made in classifying rules, distinctions which should be made if one were considering other questions. The distinctions which I have drawn are those most relevant for the rather special matter I have discussed, and are not intended to be exhaustive.

Finally, there will be many border-line cases about which it will be difficult, if not impossible, to decide which conception of rules is applicable. One expects border-line cases with any concept, and they are especially likely in connection with such involved concepts as those of a practice, institution, game, rule, and so on. Wittgenstein has shown how fluid these notions are.[4] What I have done is to emphasize and sharpen two conceptions for the limited purpose of this paper.

[3] How do these remarks apply to the case of the promise known only to father and son? Well, at first sight the son certainly holds the office of promisor, and so he isn't allowed by the practice to weigh the particular case on general utilitarian grounds. Suppose instead that he wishes to consider himself in the office of one empowered to criticize and change the practice, leaving aside the question as to his right to move from his previously assumed office to another. Then he may consider utilitarian arguments as applied to the practice; but once he does this he will see that there are such arguments for not allowing a general utilitarian defense in the practice for this sort of case. For to do so would make it impossible to ask for and to give a kind of promise which one often wants to be able to ask for and to give. Therefore he will not want to change the practice, and so as a promisor he has no option but to keep his promise.

[4] *Philosophical Investigations* (Oxford, 1953), I, pars. 65-71, for example.

The Game of Life*

ANTHONY RALLS

1. ON PLAYING THE GAME

I wish to continue the discussion of the question *Ought I to be moral and if so why?*, and to do so by referring to a metaphor, analogy or example that has been used occasionally in the contemporary literature, that of *playing a game*. The point of the metaphor, analogy or example is roughly this: if you are playing a certain game (usually it's baseball, although a recent article makes a similar point about chess) you *can't* break the rules. Analogously, if you are playing the moral game, the Game of Life, then you've got to stick to the rules. Now it is obvious that the compulsion to adhere to the rules of a game is not, or not normally, physical; but it is alleged that there is some kind of compulsion or necessitation involved, and that this, rightly understood, will illumine the nature of morality and moral discourse.[1] In addition to its occurrence in the literature, it is clearly an analogy that is, or has been, entrenched in English moral language, as in the Lifeboy motto To Play The Game, the expression "It's not cricket," and the significantly famous verses of Rudyard Kipling about the Great Scorer.

* Excerpted from "The Game of Life." *The Philosophical Quarterly*, 16 (January, 1966), 23-34.
[1] See, e.g., John Rawls: "Two Concepts of Rules," *Philosophical Review*, 1955, esp. pp. 25 ff; John Searle: "How to Derive 'Ought' from 'Is'", *Philosophical Review*, 1964, esp. p. 56; Max Black: "The Gap between 'Is' and 'Should'", *Philosophical Review*, 1964, pp. 165-181 *passim*.

In this paper I want to raise doubts about the premises that this form of argument requires, namely *that so-and-so is playing the game*, and *that playing the game necessitates keeping the rules*. I consider what justifications these premises themselves require, and in this context I discuss the suggestion made in several quarters recently, that by virtue of the performative nature of moral utterances, all persons, or all members of society, or all language-users, are committed to a moral point of view, or to some moral position in particular. I try to turn the force of this argument against its supporters, and finally consider again some reasons why one might hold that everyone ought to be moral, and just how one could avoid this conclusion. The upshot is that talking of morality as a kind of super-game does not serve the purpose intended, for it does not show us why we *should* play *that* game.

2. ON GETTING OUT OF THE GAME

Consider an argument of the form:
> If you are playing a game, you must keep the rules of that game;
> So-and-so is playing a game;
> THEREFORE so-and-so must keep the rules of that game.

Such an argument is plainly valid provided that the modal 'must' is properly kept within the consequent of the major premiss, and that we can avoid a *Quaternio Terminorum*. But if we are to accept the conclusion, we must first be convinced of the truth of the premises.

Now in the case of the games of cricket, baseball and the like, it is normally a voluntary matter whether one decides to play or not. And if I agree to play cricket, it would not *be* cricket for me to give up playing half way through, or to break the rules and refuse to accept the consequences as specified in the Laws of Cricket. But you can avoid having to keep the rules, by the simple expedient of not playing; and *this* expedient is supposed not to be available when the question at issue is, Ought I to keep the rules of the Game of Life, that is, to be moral?

Why can I not avoid playing the Game of Life?

One answer need be mentioned only to be dismissed. I mean the claim that I ought to keep the rules, i.e. to be moral, because all men, including me, are proper subjects for making moral judgments *about*. This claim is either question-begging or irrelevant. It is question-begging in that, in making the claim, there is presupposed what is at stake, namely that moral rules are rules to which all men, including me, ought to subscribe. It is irrelevant in that, no matter how many people judge me morally, *I* am not thereby committed to judging myself.

More pertinent might be the contention that everyone plays *some* game, since everyone has some guiding principles or other. But unless it could be shown that to have some guiding principles or other is, *eo ipso*, to be moral, this would not show that everyone is playing the moral game; and even if they were, how would this show that they ought to be doing so, and therefore must keep the rules? I return to this point later.

For the present I observe that the clear inadequacy of these moves seems to be what drives some philosophers into producing allegedly empirical grounds for saying that everyone is actually playing the Game of Life. These moves represent it as a plain *fact*, or a consequence of a plain fact, that everyone plays that game. It would follow that refusing to obey the rules would be inconsistent with the acceptance of some obviously true statement which it would be absurd not to accept; and thus that the refusal to obey the rules would itself be absurd. There are at least three such obviously true statements:

(*a*) Everyone speaks some language;
(*b*) Everyone is a member of some community;
(*c*) Everyone is a human being.

Schematically, I would argue concerning any such general statement, first, that it carries no weight unless regarded *ascriptively*;[2] that is, unless we *already* accept some moral viewpoint which gives moral weight to that feature of the human condition. Secondly, that either such a statement is not universal or not necessarily universal, and so does not or need not bind everyone, or that it *is* necessary, in which case it does not *morally* bind anyone, since a necessarily true statement can have no prescriptive force of itself.

These retorts are expressed in terms too general to carry conviction, and the arguments are better dealt with in particular. I propose to deal at some length with an argument of Searle's which will illustrate these points; but shall first examine the major premiss of the Games argument, in order to narrow down the point at issue.

3. ON KEEPING THE RULES

The major premiss needed to substantiate the conclusion *that everyone must keep the rules* would be the major premiss of the argument in (2), namely *that if you are playing a game, you must keep its rules*. I think this is always intended to be analytically true (it certainly is by Searle); it is worth noticing that it serves no purpose if it is not analytic. Treating it as a synthetic statement it presumably amounts to one of two possible claims. The first might be:

> If you are playing a game, then it'll be a bad thing, a poor show, not cricket, if you don't keep the rules.

But this is itself a piece of explicitly moral reasoning, which of course substantiates a moral conclusion, but not in the manner desired. If we question the conclusion, of course we'll question this premiss too.

The alternative reading of this premiss might be:

> If you are playing a game, then it'll be the worse for you, you'll catch it, if you don't keep the rules.

The first comment on this claim must be, that if it is genuinely factual it is hard to see how it could be substantiated. The second, hardly less obvious, comment is, that this alleged fact is strictly irrelevant to establish-

[2] I have tried to say something about *ascriptive judgments* in "The Ascription of Personal Responsibility and Identity," *Australian Journal of Philosophy*, 1963, esp. pp. 347-8, developing a feature of ascription which is implicit in Hart's account (H. L. A. Hart, "The Ascription of Responsibility and Rights," in *Logic and Language* (1st series), ed. Antony Flew, Oxford, 1951).

ing the moral conclusion desiderated. **For no matter how** certainly it is demonstrated that acting thus will be in my interests, will achieve what I really want to have or avoid what I really want not to have, the question necessarily remains to be asked: Should I act thus? Should I consider my own interests here? Indeed it is hard to see what is left to 'should' if we exclude the possibility cf setting 'I want' over against 'I should.' So that while it may be the case that in fact what I want to do is always what I should do, or even that what everybody wants to do is always what everybody should do, this has to be shown; hence this version of the major premiss won't support by itself the conclusion that one should or that one must obey the rules, but stands in need of support.

I think we are left with the analytic reading of the major premiss as the only one possible, but the consequences of this are almost equally disastrous. It might go somewhat as follows:

> If you are playing a game, then you cannot without self-stultification, or self-contradiction, not keep its rules.

But this, which still seems to be saying something interesting, in fact only amounts to this:

> If you are to be said to be playing a game, then you must (among other things) be keeping its rules.

This makes keeping the rules a necessary condition of playing the game, with the inevitable consequence that the fact that you are playing the game cannot be adduced as *a reason why* you must keep the rules. It immediately follows that the alleged argument, from the consideration of which this paper got going, is quite insubstantial. If the analytic account of the major premiss is correct, persuading people to play the game is the same thing as, and therefore not logically prior to, persuading them to keep the rules. If 'everyone is playing the game' is to be true, it *must* be true that everyone must keep the rules.

Rules and Utilitarianism *

B. J. DIGGS

I

The first kind of rule which I shall describe belongs to a large class of rules which I call "instrumental." All rules in this large class are adopted or followed as a means to an end, in order to "accomplish a purpose" or "get a job done." The simplest of these rules is the "practical maxim" which one ordinarily follows at his own pleasure, such as "Be sure the surface to be painted is thoroughly dry" or "Do not plant tomatoes until after the last frost."[1]

The instrumental rule to which I call attention is more complex. On many occasions when one wants a job done, either he is not in a position or not able or not willing to do the job himself. If he is in a position of power or authority, or if he has money, he may simply order or hire others to "do the job" and leave it to them. In numerous cases, however, he himself lays down rules of procedure, and establishes "jobs" or "roles" in the institutional sense. A "job" in this latter sense is not a job to be "done," but a job to be "offered to" or "given" to a person. If a person "takes" or is "assigned" "the job" then we often think of him as under an obligation to "do his job," and this partly consists in his following rules. Instrumental rules of this

* Excerpted from "Rules and Utilitarianism." *American Philosophical Quarterly*, I (January, 1964), 32-44.
[1] Cf. Max Black, "Notes on the Meaning of 'Rule'," *Theoria*, vol. 24 (1958), pp. 121-122; reprinted in his *Models and Metaphors* (Ithaca, N.Y., 1962), pp. 95-139.

kind, unlike practical maxims, have a social dimension: It *makes sense* to ask whether a job-holder (or role-taker) is *obligated* to follow a particular rule, or whether this is one of his *duties*, and the penalty attaching to a breach of the rules does not consist simply in his not "getting the job done."

Rules of this kind are found in very different institutions. Some are rules of a "job" in the ordinary sense. Others apply to anyone who voluntarily assumes a "role," such as "automobile driver." Others characterize a position which one is obliged to take by law, for example, that of private in the army. The goals which the rules are designed to serve may be ordinary products of labor, such as houses, steel beams, etc.; or fairly specific social goals such as "getting vehicles to their destinations safely and expeditiously"; or goals as general as "the national defense." In some cases the rules, differing from job to job, mark a division of labor, as the rules which say what factory workers, or the members of a platoon, are to do. In other cases, the same rules apply more or less equally to all as in the case of (at least some) rules regulating traffic.

Notwithstanding their variety, these rules can be classified together because they share two fundamental characteristics: (1) The rules prescribe action which is thought to contribute to the attainment of a goal. This is the "design" of such rules, at least in the sense that if the prescribed action does not effectively contribute to the attainment of the goal, for the most part, then the rule itself is subject to criticism. (2) The rules are "laid down" or "legislated" or "made the rule" by a party which has power or authority of some kind; one cannot learn "what the rules are" simply by determining what general procedures most effectively promote the goal. This latter characteristic sharply differentiates these rules from what I have called practical maxims, although both share the first characteristic and are "instrumental."[2]

. . . .

III

Rules of common competitive games, such as baseball, chess, and the like, say how a game is to be played. They state the "object of the game," "the moves," "how the counting should go," etc. Often they are stated in "rule books," and sometimes they are enforced by referees appointed by an acknowledged authority. These formalities, however, are not at all necessary. The rules must be "laid down" or "adopted" in some sense, but all that is required (in the case of those games being discussed) is that a group of players "agree" on a

[2] Practical maxims should not be dismissed, however, as "mere rules of thumb" on the one hand, or as "simply stating relations between means and ends" on the other. When one follows a maxim the rule *directs* action and is a *criterion* of certain kinds of rightness and wrongness in acting.

In passing note that Rawls's "summary conception," as a whole, does not properly apply to practical maxims, although several features of this conception do apply. Rawls's analysis, admirable as it is, is very apt to mislead. For the "summary view," as he calls it, is a blend of two quite distinct conceptions: In part it is a confused conception or a misconception of a rule, as a summary or report. In other respects it is an accurate conception of what I have called a practical maxim. This may account for an ambivalence in Rawls's article: Cf. ". . . it is doubtful that anything to which the summary conception did apply would be called a *rule.*" [(p. 23) "Two Concepts . . ."] with "Some rules will fit one conception, some rules the other; and so there are rules of practice (rules in the strict sense), and maxims and 'rules of thumb'." (p. 29). The point is that maxims are rules in a *different* sense from other kinds of rules, whereas no rule, *qua rule*, is a summary or report.

The importance of this point is that there are two possible confusions here, not one: A person may conceive moral rules as summaries or reports, or he may conceive moral rules on the model of maxims. The texts of Austin and Mill, which Rawls cites, together with Rawls's discussion, suggest that the latter, more than the former, was their mistake.

set of rules. This agreement may consist simply in their following and enforcing rules which they all have learned: Think, for example, of a group of small boys playing baseball, and think of the difference between one's knowing the rules and playing the game. In such cases there is no formally agreed-upon authority; each player—in principle—is both rule-follower and rule-enforcer. No player has the authority to modify the rules at will, but the players together can change them in any way they see fit. As one should expect, there are many variations.

In the latter respects game rules of this kind are quite like the rules in (I). These game rules, however, noticeably lack the first major characteristic of those rules: They are not designed to yield a product. More precisely, they are not adopted to promote the attainment of a goal which, in the senses indicated earlier, is "over and beyond" the rules.[3] They do not serve a goal which is "logically independent" of the game which they define.

3.1.1 Of course people who play games do so with various motives, and some of the goals which motivate them are logically independent of the game; for example, exercise, recreation, the opportunity to talk to friends or make a conquest. Undoubtedly games are popular because they serve so many ends. Nevertheless, motives and goals of this kind are not essential. Many players participate (so far as can be determined without psychoanalyzing them) "just because they want to" or simply "from love of the game." Actually this kind of motive, even if it is not typical, is that which is most distinctive of players: One who "loves a game" commonly regards another, who lacks the motive, as poorly appreciating "the quality of the game." This is apt to be missed just because games have been turned into instruments, for exercise, diversion, etc., to such a great degree. The point is, they *need* not be.

Moreover, games *qua* games do not seem to have a design or goal *different* from the motives of the rule-followers, in the way rules of jobs commonly do. What is this goal? One who most appreciates a game speaks about it rather as if it were an aesthetic object, worth playing on its own account and apart from any product or result; and if he is asked to justify his claim that it is good, he seems to have a problem analogous to that of justifying an aesthetic

[3] Some games have become instruments to such a considerable degree, and some instrumental activities have become so much like games, that no description will prevent the intrusion of dubious and borderline cases.

judgment.[4] Sometimes, to be sure, the rules of games are changed, and in particular instances violated, in order to change the consequences. Many official rules, for example, have been changed in order to lessen player injuries; and particular persons may find a game played by the official rules too strenuous, or pursuit of the ball after a bad drive too troublesome. These facts, however, do not imply that the rules are designed to produce consequences, such as the right amount of exercise or exertion, or the good health of the players. Changes of the kind mentioned simply indicate that the rules of a game, like the rules of a job, are adopted in a context by persons who have many desires and many obligations other than "to play the game" and "follow its rules." Games are often altered to make them harmonize better with such contextual features. It is true, of course, that persons who have turned games into instruments change or violate the rules more readily. As we say, these people do not take the game as seriously.

Some philosophers are inclined to say that even when one plays a game "just because he wants to" or "for love of the game," the game is still an instrument—to "his enjoyment" or "pleasure." This stand depends for its cogency on our being able to describe this pleasure or enjoyment without referring to the game, which should be possible if the pleasure or enjoyment really were something separate from playing the game. However, although it is clearly possible to play a game and not enjoy it, the converse does not appear plausible. To be sure, one sometimes says that he gets about the same enjoyment from one game as another, especially when the two are similar. But this is apt to mean that he has no strong preference for one game over another, that he likes one as well as the other, not that there is a kind of pleasurable feeling which in fact results from both, more or less equally, and which *conceivably* could be had from very different activities or even from being acted *on* in some way. (Similarly, when one says that he "likes to talk to one person about as much as another," this clearly does not mean that talking to the two persons produces the same kind of pleasure in him.) Moreover, when we speak of getting about the same enjoyment from two

games, sometimes the "enjoyment" does not appear to be, strictly speaking, the enjoyment "of playing the game," but rather the enjoyment of exercising, talking to friends, etc. I do not deny, however, that games can become instruments. I want to argue that they need not be, often are not, and that in calling them games we do not imply that they are instruments.

The kind of goal the pursuit of which to some degree *is* essential to the playing of the game is the "object of the game," as defined by the rules, and the various sub-goals which promote this object according to the rules. Such goals as these, for example, "to score the most runs," "to get the batter out at second base," obviously are not logically independent of the rules of the game—if there were no rules it would be logically impossible to try to do these things. It is just nonsense to speak of changing the rules so that one can better attain the object of the game.

3.1.2 Since the action within a game is designed to attain goals defined by the rules, the action as well as the goal logically depends on the rules: In important respects a move in the game has the consequences it has because the rules say it has; *in these respects* the rules define the consequences and determine the character of the action.[5] Since the character of instrumental action is fixed at least partly by the goal which the action is designed to serve, the action can be described in this essential respect, as a "trying to get the goal," without refering to or presupposing rules. In the case of play in a game, unless the game has become an instrument, this is not possible; if one describes the action in a game apart from the rules, as a "trying to catch a ball," he leaves out the design. On account of this difference one may feel inclined to say that whereas rules of the kind described in (I) *may* be used to describe an action, game rules by defining new kinds of action just constitute "forms of life."[6]

3.2 However, this is but one side of the story, and if it were the only one it is not likely that the two kinds of rules would be confused. To see the other side, which is equally important, one should attend to the fact that the play in a game is not wholly defined by the rules of the game. "The kind of game he plays" ordinarily does not refer to the game as defined by the rules; "to play a game" ordinarily means more than following

---

[4] This reminds one of the ancient distinctions between "doing" and "making," and between (what the medievals called) "immanent" and "transitive" activity. I do not mean to deny that some jobs are worth doing "on their own account," but even when "one enjoys a job," there is a discernible purpose which it is designed to promote.

[5] This is the point which Rawls emphasized.
[6] Cf. A. I. Melden, "Action," *Philosophical Review*, vol. 65 (1956), pp. 523-541.

the rules. The point is that although the object of the game is defined by the rules, since the action in a game normally consists in "trying to attain that object," and since the game rules do not determine success in this respect, the action in *this* respect is instrumental. Players often develop tactics and strategies and skills in playing. Sometimes they follow what I have called practical maxims, and at other times they follow team rules agreed on among themselves or laid down by the "manager." The latter are, of course, examples of the rules described in (I). Obviously they should not be confused with rules of games, as I have described them. For one can be said to play a game without his following any particular set of instrumental rules.

The point of greatest importance here is that although game rules are not themselves instruments, they support, as it were, a considerable amount of instrumental activity, much of which logically could not be carried on without them. To play a game is typically to follow the rules of the game *and* engage in this instrumental activity; a "good player" does more than just follow the rules. Even one who "loves the game for its own sake" derives his satisfaction from the kind of *instrumental* activity which the rules of the game make possible. Games make new goals, new pursuits, and new skills available to men.

In this situation it is not surprising that some should regard games themselves as instruments. To regard them in this way, however, would be to confuse their function.

Toward a Social Philosophy of Achievement and Athletics*

HANS LENK

To date, no comprehensive philosophy of achievement behavior has been developed. Nevertheless, the new critical generation and the so-called establishment agree about one thing: both believe that we live in an "achieving society" guided by the "performance principle" (or "the principle of achievement"). Social ranks and opportunities, advancement, remuneration, and influence have been assessed and allotted solely on the basis of personal professional performance. A society that assigns roles and ranks to its members on this principle is called an "achieving society" (McClelland).

On the above points both sides are in agreement. However, on other issues there is a parting of minds: While the new protest generation considers all workers to be yoked under the inhuman and also unnecessary pressure or even "terror" of performance and the compulsion of productivity which ought to be eliminated as quickly as possible, the members of the Establishment resolutely plead for the preservation of the "performance principle" which, as they claim, has brought us prosperity and economic security. Anyone who preaches defeatism regarding production, performance, and achievement, is, they say, plainly asocial and irresponsible in view of the need to raise productivity for the future welfare of mankind.

*From *Man and World: An International Philosophical Review*, 9 (July, 1976), 45–59.

There is something "human, all too human" about these all-or-nothing dichotomies which are highly convenient for dividing people into supporters and opponents, into members of ingroups and outgroups: hedonists and hippies versus ascetic puritans. Performance or pleasure? The hedonists plead: "Then we prefer to choose pleasure"; the puritans reply: "We don't want any socioeconomic catastrophe—therefore we are for performance."

Apparently, however, performance, as it is claimed by the critics, always also involves the pressure of productiveness and "pressure for achievement." Pleasure or the compulsion of achievement, this alternative seems to be the only one: puristic thinking in terms of alternatives on both sides—whether from the Left or the Right. Yet thinking in terms of totality is, in fact, always wrong. Reality is not that simple. This line of thought leads too easily to totalitarianism.

This kind of thinking in clichés is typical of that argument which is used ideologically for the apparently theoretical justification of one's own values as well as for the rejection of those of others

"Performance" is strongly imbued with emotions depending upon interests and social values of the person pronouncing upon it: to some people it is a concept of quality, a price tag, which even advertising uses suggestively: in the year of the last Olympic Games some service stations used the slogan "Performance decides" for advertising purposes. By advocating competition and by talking about performance the advertisement created, or attempted to create, the illusion of achievement. The other connotations of this word of many meanings, "Leistung," i.e. performance (achievement), were also—implicitly at least—suggested in one way or another. On the other hand, the social critics, who saw through this trick, rejected all ideas of competition, all merits in training to improve performance, as ideological perfidy on the part of holders of power or the ruling class to maintain their established privileges and positions. They even regarded the reference to successful achievement as conservative ideology.

The criticism of the performance principle and the model of the "achieving society" is transferred ready-made to athletics. Particularly in the so-called late capitalist system athletics are regarded by the critics as a "national and international demonstration of the performance potential and the ideology of achievement of the political and economic system." Athletics would, they say, serve "to restore and preserve physical fitness . . . which, in turn, is exploited in the process of work." This criticism claims that the popular sports find their function in "canalizing aggressions (which mainly arise in the process of work) into harmless channels"; that is to say they have a "bread-and-circus function." Even school sports ("as the acknowledged reservoir for the training of new sports champions," who would also be used by other people as tools of the capitalist system) are alleged to contribute "decisively to the stabilization and consolidation of this capitalist system." These assertions come from a resolution put forward by the Young Socialists of West Germany at their party conference some years ago. This socialist criticism can be summarized as follows: "A society which has made a point of converting the concept of achievement through the performance principle into an ideology cannot avoid applying it in sports, too. This ideologically irrational performance principle is reflected in sport in just the same way as it is in the processes of industrial work and production. The top sportsmen, as muscle-machines and symbolic reflections of the political and economic system that they represent, become mechanical medal-producers." Two years earlier a document of the Socialist German Students' Association (SDS) had already regarded "the performance in sports as an indirect encroachment of social repression" itself. All that the Young Socialists did was to repeat this sweeping judgment in more intelligible language.

Yet even such an otherwise deliberate author as Günter Grass recently expressed the opinion that the "dictatorship of the performance principle" was becoming increasingly reflected in competitive sports. A substitute 'arms race' was taking place in all the nations that go in for sports and especially for the Olympics. The sportsmen were not motivated solely by "personal ambition": "It is the collective performance principle that drives them." "Athletics do not provide a release from pressures. They are the result of the pressures to which competitive societies submit themselves. They have trained crack sportsmen by means of blind compliance in order to be represented by them." Yet, "where achievement does not help to solve social problems it creates additional social problems. Achievement on principle makes excessive demands on those from whom it is extorted, devours and dissipates their strength, their health and their time, senselessly produces a surplus, mixes poison in the air and the water and creates slag piles which not even weeds can make turn green." "Misapplied social ambition" would call for excessive output also in sport. It was not only the professionally employed who were subjected to "professional coercion" and "the terror of performance," but also the crack sportsmen who "make their bodies available for the interests of others."

Are athletics to be regarded as the most conducive instantiating model of the performance principle, as the clear reflection of the "achieving society," as the open embodiment of systematic coercion to compete, with all the manifestations of socio-pathological and psycho-neurotic compulsion? What the performance principle" means, in this alleged interpretation, is compulsion to perform. The total cliché permits no differentiation. Competitive sports are competitive terrorism. Pleasure in performance—that is unknown. One author, Rigauer, had already described the methods of training for sports as "repressive . . . systems of operational instructions": "To practise competitive sports means that one must perform in order to fulfil society's expectations of (one's) performance" (p. 18).

But does performance in sports actually and totally come under the "performance principle" in the sense used by the social critics? Can criticism be transferred from the business sphere to competitive sports so simply without further distinction? As always, analysis is more difficult than general pro-and-contra clichés.

In the first place the talk about *"the* performance principle" is by no means unambiguous. Marcuse uses it in his book *Eros and Civilization* (p. 115) in at least three different meanings. In one place he says: "The definition of the standard of living in terms of automobiles, television sets, airplanes and tractors is that of the performance principle itself." In this first meaning he equates "performance principle" with the principle of economic competition and with the contention that the society is stratified in accordance with the economic criteria of profit and success. In the second meaning Marcuse denotes only the "extra," or surplus, repression exerted above and beyond that required for ensuring an appropriate standard of living, i.e., the enforced, "alienated" labour, as coming under the "performance principle." Finally, in the third case Marcuse also interprets the "performance principle" for our society and for our culture as a principle of the identity of the personality, as a principle of self-presentation and self confirmation, even self-constitution. He does not subordinate artistic achievements to the performance principle but to the "criticism of the performance principle."

What, then, is the Marcusean position which makes sense regarding achievement in sports? The relationship of sports to the "performance principle" naturally differs according to each of the three interpretations. According to the first interpretation the amateur's achievement in sports does not, in fact, belong to the performance principle, apart from few highly earning athletes or professionals who determine and enhance their status on the "performance market" partly through the sale of their mercenary "goods" called "performance." And in the second version, too, achievement in sports does not come under the performance principle if one disregards coercive measures by the directors of associations or sanctions in the form of threats that a sports scholarship would be withdrawn if an athlete does not turn up at a training course or a meet, etc. According to this interpretation normal achievement in sports is even a part of a "libidinally" hued, or tinged, activity in Marcuse's sense: the athlete does, in fact, personally aspire to this particularly strongly and attaches intense emotional value and feelings of delight to it, even if it is to some extent a question of an abstract "delight" at success in the future and a "delight" at the performance achieved. In this interpretation, achievement in sports

would have to be classed, according to Marcuse's definition, precisely with what he calls "criticism of the performance principle"—an obvious absurdity as compared with the normal usage of the language. In competitive sports one would actually have a "libidinally" hued and constituted activity in a culture subordinated to the play impulse, which is what Marcuse calls for in place of the listless monotony of the assembly-line work of factories of today.

It is completely wrong to suppose that every achievement in sport is the result of pressure to perform, that every performance in sport is extorted from the athlete. Hardly anyone makes more demands upon himself than the sportsman himself. This assessment and this experience of the athlete should not be ignored —not even if it is contended that this attitude towards performance was manipulated in his early childhood. The differences between the fact that the athlete aspires to high achievements in sports and strives for success on the one hand and the attitude toward compulsory labour or toward the maintenance of production norms at the assembly-line on the other simply cannot be ignored. Purely sociological criticism all too often fails to take into account this crucial difference. Evaluated attitudes are, however, constitutive for these differences. Mark Twain was puzzled long ago as to why to gum up paper-bags was work, yet the climbing of Montblanc was sport.

In the third interpretation of the performance principle given by Marcuse, in which it is explained as a criterion of self-assertion, achievement in sports is most certainly included in the "performance principle." Everything said about "libidinally" hued and constituted activity would also be applicable here.

Before this explanation can be gone into more fully, however, it is necessary first to discuss, in view of the general criticism of social critics of the "performance principle" in the professional field, how far this criticism applies to performance in sports. This criticism might be briefly summarized: The social-philosophical criticism of the professional "performance principle" is directed, firstly, against the compulsory character of the routine work which is extorted unilaterally from the worker contrary to his interests and abilities; secondly, against the non-attributability of the result of complex production processes, of a "performance," of an accomplished work to the person producing it; thirdly, against the lacking, but falsely claimed equality, of opportunities in education and employment; and, fourthly, against the inhumanity of a hypostasized perfect implementation of the "performance principle."

On the transferability of point 1 of this criticism what may be said is this: Achievement in sports is not as a rule (apart from extreme exceptions) extorted from the individuals under pressure; it corresponds to the maximum extent to the interests and abilities of the athlete.

On point 2: As a result, success or performance as well as achievement in sports is still to be attributed exclusively to the individual as his own work—in contrast to the "performance on the assembly-line." Only the individual athlete can accomplish the achievement, the performance is unmistakably effected by a personal feat—it cannot be accomplished by surreptition and trickery. National help in fostering and funding can facilitate it, but cannot be a substitute for it. Even if the rate of success of the performance decreases in comparison with that of better assisted competitors—the individual accountability for the performance is thereby not diminished nor is its emotional content. Every attraction for the athlete himself, the effort to succeed, the pleasure in performance, and the pride in achievement and the importance of all these for proving and confirming oneself cannot be simply argued away. They are psychic realities.

On point 3: The equality of opportunities in competitive sports is, indeed, also impeded by national and social promotional measures, but it is still more nearly achieved than in the professional "start in life." This certainly applies primarily to the participants from countries somewhat on an equal footing of fostering athletic improvement. However, this also applies to the already motivated and experienced sportsmen themselves, and not to all who could potentially take part in a competition. The points of criticism that were directed against the applicability of the performance principle in the professional sphere can, therefore, hardly be transferred to sports and achievement in sports—and, by the way, also not to professional work in general but only to some specific forms, admittedly still deplorable ones—e.g. assembly-line work. (But there are initiatives under way to improve human conditions of factory work—and they should be supported intensively.) Not only emotional preoccupation but also personal accountability and attributability are completely guaranteed in athletic achievement. Equality of opportunity is, within limits, relatively easier to achieve here than in any other social sphere.

The fourth point of the criticism, which was directed against the all-too-perfect implementation of the performance principle and against a total "achieving society," can likewise not be utilized as an argument against competitive sports as a social phenomenon. For the latter by no means requires a total "achieving society," even if, as a social segment, it is organized in restricted aspects in accordance with the criteria of achievement. Sport by no means requires that all other social spheres should be regulated and evaluated according to the criteria of performance nor that every single person has to be regarded only as an object of productiveness of achievements, even if an evaluation of the individual in his performance role prevails within the very disciplines relating to competitive sports.

Perhaps one could advance some more detailed arguments against the gross conception of athletics as the ideal model of the "achieving society" in general such as was advocated by Adam and v. Krockow.

Adam describes "the attitude towards achievement in sports as a model . . . for . . . the attitude to proficiency in general": Advancement on the social scale as a result of an objective and impartial comparison of performance reconciles the initially seemingly antagonistic principles of equality and of differentiated assignment of ranks. In an ideal "achieving society," according to Adam, "all orders of precedence would be based on comparative performance." Absolute objectivity of comparison (especially of different kinds of performance) is impossible. But this objectivity can most nearly be achieved in a model manner in competitive sports (through measurement, contriving a decisive situation or counting successful attempts—less or hardly at all objectively through assessment of points and scores on the basis of subjective decisions). "The mechanism of self-affirmation" through one's own performance stabilizes, according to Adam, the "feeling of one's own value"—particularly in the overcoming of intentionally induced feelings of listlessness and obstacles in training for sports. In athletics, moreover, the attitude toward achievement is trained in an exemplary manner and, in Adam's opinion, that is essential for the preservation of the species and for the balance of fortune of mankind in view of the problems of the growing population.

Whilst Adam analyses the model of competitive sports more from a sociopedagogic perspective, v. Krockow (1962, p. 58 ff., 52 ff.) goes in more for a sociological and socio-

philosophical interpretation: "Athletics—a product of the industrial society"; v. Krockow expands this almost trivial sociological proposition to the philosophical one "that competitive
sports . . . are the symbolically concentrated
representation of the society's basic principles."
It is in sport that "exactitude," "ideality," "objectivity," equality of opportunities, measura-
bility and comparability, spectacularness and
general intelligibility represent symbolically
more clearly than anywhere else the principles
of differentiation in performance (i.e. attribution of a social rank on the grounds of individual achievements); the same is true, according to v. Krockow, of the principle of
competition and yet also of the equality of
opportunities for success. "Performance, competition and equality. What makes modern
sport so pregnant with symbolism and so fascinating is not at least the exactness, not to
mention the ideality, with which it realizes
these basic principles of the industrial society"
(1972, p. 94). V. Krockow (*ibid.* p. 96) even
asserts: "Sport gives expression to the principles of the industrial society far better than
the latter itself does": the objectivity and also
the transparency of the comparison of performances, which are nearly perfectly realized in
sport, are not exhibited by anything like so
completely and visibly in any of the other
fields of the complex, almost unsurveyable industrial society. The achievements of the re-
search-worker can only be assessed by experts,
the celebrities of our publicity-conscious society create the illusion of achievements, often
through acts of self-advertisement. Yet here—
in sport—"the record jump is transmitted op-
tically into every house, intelligible to everyone and measured three times over" (*ibid.* p.
95).

Thus, we apparently have sport as the ideal-
typical (purely idealized, trenchantly demonstrated) model of the so-called "achieving
society." This model thesis seems attractive:
it not only explains the fascination of sport
and its stormy development parallel with the
industrial society itself. It also enables one to
understand the protest of the new social criticism, which criticizes the so-called performance principle and competitive sports jointly
in a like manner. Moreover, this model thesis
is compatible with the relative separation or
"extra-worldly demarcation" (v. Krockow) of
the sphere of sport from the so-called vicissitudes of life, from the sphere of work. Model
character and relative own-worldliness can
very well go together.

On the other hand, this model thesis also
encounters certain difficulties: What is too
easily overlooked is the fact that the so-called
"achieving society" is intrinsically a "success
society," sometimes of sham achievements sold
by means of publicity and of careers, all the
more so because professional and social
achievement can scarcely be attributed any
longer to the individual alone: team, boom
and system constitute the determinants of general social achievements. Somewhat exagger-
atedly one might say: We no longer live in
the idealized, publicly proclaimed "achieving
society" but in a "success society": the really
personally accomplished achievement counts
less in the acquiring of status than do the
social effect of achievements, the success or
even the semblance of achievement or of talent, or in certain cases the publicity given to
alleged achievements (e.g. election successes).
Publicity as a substitute for achievement? Is
social success already proof of achievement?
Certainly, this overall equating of publicity,
success and achievement applies, if at all, primarily to representatives of the upper middle
classes, to employees laden with responsibilities and to promotion-seeking "performance
men." For the lower classes the requirements
of production are increasingly converted into
standardized and routinized functions of super-
vision of standards which do not allow the individual to stand out from the rest and to
distinguish himself through his own efforts, for
their main requirement seems to be, rather,
the avoidance of acts of disruption and the
adherence to average norms as far as possible
without any loss due to friction. Whereas
social climbers are more inclined to regard
the attitude to performance from the point of
view of ability to achieve social success, for
members of the lower classes the required
"performance orientation" seems to consist exclusively in the postulate of allocation and subordination to complex organizational processes
with as little disruption as possible.

Ichheiser as early as 1930, in his book *Kritik
des Erfolges (Criticism of Success)*, made a
clear distinction between ability to perform
and ability to succeed. He also drew attention
to the mechanism of deception whereby the
Machiavellian exploitation of the ability to
succeed and the concomitant, but mostly concealed, violations of norms imperceptibly favour those who are already able to succeed or
who are privileged, and he pointed out that
this is not regarded as, let us say, a sign of
plain good fortune but is considered by others
(and by those concerned themselves) to be a
personal achievement.

The sociological requirements of the socio-psychological factors of all these variations of the "performance principle" have not yet been sufficiently examined. It is only in the most recent period that the psychological theory of attribution (Weiner and others) has been going more closely into these questions, in that it is examining the cognitive conditions under which particular types of personality attribute success to themselves as personal achievements or are more inclined to believe that they owe it to fortunate circumstances.

Are the above-mentioned deviations from the idealized "performance principle" the reason for the special fascination of athletics? Does achievement in sports still represent relatively purely, as it were, something which is no longer to be found in the assessment of professional and public achievement: the individual accountability and attributability, the "joyful" experience and "pleasure" in success, the fact that the possibility of deception and corruption does not exist as a rule or else is subjected to strict controls, and the absence of real dependence in the sense of submission to power?

The new criticism of sport mostly relates the outlined character of sport (as a model for the ideal principles of an achieving society) exclusively or predominantly to the so-called capitalist or late capitalist societies. This is undoubtedly a biased restriction as socialist industrial societies or, to put it better, state capitalist systems of society are even more dedicated to the raising of production norms and are inclined to make even more severe demands on the individual for the fulfilment of such norms. Naturally, that also applies to athletics in the socialist countries.

The social criticism of sport is not directed against every demand for achievement but only against the ideology of the achieving society which subordinates all other requirements to the raising of production and achievement and which is oriented to the assurance and creation of privileges of a class-conditioned kind: In particular, a striving for achievement that is motivated by the class struggle is expressly approved by the critics.

Admittedly, a total achieving society would be terrible: the competition of all against all in all activities—man preying upon man (homo homini lupus)—would make Hobbes' primordial vision come true. The "achieving society" is only a Utopian model which cannot be truly brought into existence, although in some areas, as in sport, it is one ideal orientational symbol among others and is additional to other models for guidance. It can certainly only be applied to limited social spheres and also only in a restricted degree that would be ideally typical (in the sociological meaning of the word after Max Weber); in fact it applies exclusively to social spheres that are distinguished by their comparative competitiveness. It is certainly not desirable to judge a person as a whole solely by his performances in limited social spheres, whether the latter relate to his profession or, say, to sport. Nor should all the members of a society be subjected to the necessity of achievement even in limited spheres. The "achieving society," which serves as a model in a good many respects, must not become the "compulsorily productive and achieving society" in every respect. A model like this one can only give limited guidelines for limited applicability conditions. Yet, it is true that even our society still cannot dispense with certain constrictions on achievement for quite a long time. That, however, is another matter.

But science, art, and sport could be spheres of performance for individually differentiated possibilities of distinction, and they could be opportunities for enjoyable, libidinally motivated and hued (Marcuse) activities, which could be conducive to self-confirmation, social self-assertion and, in this way, to the stabilizing development of the personality. The pedagogical applications obviously are at hand. The younger Marx's anthropology of the creative, freely evolving human being, as displayed in the ideal image of the scientist and the engineer, is in every way also comparable with the ideal image of the role of the competitive athlete, whose free "self-chosen activity" and whose opportunity to fashion his performance freely and in a certain sense to reflect and unfold his personality therein, ought not to be replaced by a thesis of compulsion for a perfect and excessive performance in competitive sport. That is by no means to deny that in a good many kinds of sports and disciplines, which are especially subjected to public interest and public pressure, one may discern tendencies of a quasi-moral public pressure on performance or the authoritarianism of a corporate dirigistic power and corresponding influences on athletes.

There is no doubt that the new criticism of sport is right in one respect: the concept of the "achieving society" as well as that of the so-called "performance principle" have hitherto been simply taken for granted and have not been more closely examined from the socio-philosophical point of view. This also leads to the partly grotesquely unworldly and excessively incisive black-and-white analysis of athletics. A hitherto nonexistent philosophy of achievement would still have a lot of work to do here in respect to more precise distinctions, necessary differentiations and balanced judgments.

What becomes clear after this analysis is this: one cannot simplify the matter as the German writer Günter Grass does and just assert that the "collective performance principle" impels or compels the athletes as forcefully as it does people in the professional field and that "performance terror" and "compulsion by the object in question" ("Sachzwang") would prevent them from making their own decisions and determining their own actions. Apart from extreme cases which are not to be denied, the athlete identifies himself to a very great extent with his athletic achievements—especially those in training, which scarcely attract public attention. He finds pleasure in the fulfilment of tasks which demand of him all his energy subject to a calculated risk. He identifies himself completely with this subjectively and freely chosen attitude of his.

The thesis of compulsion can, therefore, only fall back on a thesis of manipulation: to the effect that the competitive sportsmen were, in fact, drilled through educational influences in early childhood into adopting the competitive attitude, which our culture positively prizes, and into internalizing the "achieving principle." Certainly, athletes are not more manipulated here than anyone else who has grown up in the Western industrial society. Surely almost all education, then, had to be regarded as manipulation—and nobody could then be called free, for everybody would be "manipulated" in every respect. Viewed empirically, manipulation could hardly be separated from education. In fact, merely relative freedom is identifiable by the fact that the person who is already competent to judge responsibly subscribes to a decision, adopts it as his own, and even defends it. From the point of view of moral philosophy this must be accepted as his opinion, even if the decision to be defended should in some cases prove to be a pleasant illusion.

Obviously, acute problems arise in the case of young adolescents who are not yet able to perceive and assess the problems of an excessive training for performance. Nowadays there are a good many disciplines, ranging from swimming to gymnastics, in which such an intensive regimen of training is required, even at the youthful age of 10 to 12 years, that manifestations of narrow-mindedness, regimentation and dependence on the authoritarian decisions of the parents or coach cannot be precluded in all cases. Nevertheless, the guiding aim in every case should be to avoid forcing even the child to act against his own will, but as often as possible to discuss critically with him (albeit in a preparatory manner) the intelligible problems of the training and gradually to develop his powers of discernment so that the child will later on be able to form his own, relatively independent opinions and to make his own decisions. A coach, too, must be prepared to point out the problems to an athlete and, in some cases, to advise him rather to choose another way of self-development if sports seem to be too onerous to that boy or girl.

Quite apart from that, the achievement of the highest performance is scarcely possible if one does not completely identify oneself with the training and with the significance of this activity.

Self-determined motivation of performance (so far as it is relatively possible) is always preferable in every respect to extraneously determined pressure to perform. Thus, the "democratic" style of coaching founded on the ideal of participatory decisions is by no means a Utopian fiction: It was already introduced and further developed in a good many kinds of team sports quite a long time ago, especially with respect to the Olympic Gold Medal crews of the successful rowing coach, Karl Adam, although it ought to have been more difficult to guide a team towards this objective than, say, an athlete concerned with a single discipline. The possibility of practicing exemplarily "democratic" behavior in a small group of sportsmen shall not be gone into further here.

At any rate, it is clear that the mere system-stabilizing compensatory function of sport and its alleged function to serve only as a vehicle for the regeneration of the labour force, as well as the diverting, manipulating and "depoliticizing" effect of athletics, cannot properly represent *all* the aspects of this complex social and psycho-social phenomenon, as the critics claim.

It is true that the star athletes are also regarded as representatives of the nation, but this function is primarily projected onto them by public opinion. This does not, however, mean that they become just "mechanical medal-producers," "efficient muscle-machines," pampered beasts of top level performance and "reproduced symbols of the political and economic system" and nothing else. Not only are their psychic experiences and the significance of sport for the development and stabilization of their personalities to be looked at in another light, but sport also acquires another meaning in its cultural-philosophical aspect: as a modern Herculean-Promethean myth of daring, energetic action, it embodies the dynamic character of the archetypal roles of the contest and of competitiveness in a symbolical manner resembling the way in which life was reflected for the ancient Greeks in some of their great classical dramas of fate. Yet this interpretation of competitive sport has still only been mentioned. It cannot be presented in detail here; an attempt has been made elsewhere (by the author in 1972) to indicate its main outlines.

The socio-philosophical discussion of sport and of the attitude towards achievement has only just begun. To extricate it from the mere polarization of thinking in black and white, of "pro and contra," is the task of a detailed analysis and criticism in the future. What is particularly noteworthy is the fact that society, which regards itself as an "achieving society," does not possess any kind of elaborated, let alone well-founded, philosophy of the types of attitudes towards achievement. A wide field of activity remains open here for bold philosophical theses and critical considerations.

Bibliography

Adam, K.: Nichtakademische Betrachtungen zur einer Philosophie der Leistung. In *Leistungssport* II (1972) No. 1, pp. 62-68.

Bohme, J.-O., Gadow, J., Güldenpfennig, S., Jensen, J., Pfister, R.: *Sport im Spätkapitalismus*. Frankfurt, 1971.

Gebauer, G.: "Leistung" als Aktion und Prasentation. In *Sportwissenschaft* 1972, pp. 182-203.

Grass, G.: Sport ohne Stoppuhr. In DSB (ed.): *Deutscher Sport* 2, München 1971, p. 18 ff.

Hack, L.: Was heisst schon Leistungsgesellschaft? In *Neue Kritik* 7, No. 3 (1966) pp. 23-32.

Ichheiser, G.: *Kritik des Erfolges*. Leipzig, 1930.

Jungsozialisten: Stellungnahme zum Sport in der Resolution zum Parteitag Bremen 1971. In Jungsozialisten: *Bremer Parteibeschlüsse*. Bonn, 1971, pp. 20-24.

Krockow, C. von: Der Wetteifer in der industriellen Gesellschaft und im Sport. In Ausschuss deutscher Leibesetzieher (ed.): *Der Wetteifer,* Frankfurt/Wien 1962, pp. 48-63 (Limpert).

Krockow, C. von: *Sport und Industriegesellschaft*. München, 1972 (Piper).

Lenk, H.: *Leistungsmotivation und Mannschaftsdynamik*. Schorndorf/Stuttgart, 1970 (Hofmann).

Lenk, H.: *Philosophie im technologischen Zeitalter*. Stuttgart, Berlin, Köln, Mainz, 1971 (2nd ed.) (Kohlhammer).

Lenk, H.: *Werte, Ziele, Wirklichkeit der modernen Olympischen Spiele*. Schorndorf/Stuttgart, 1964, 1972 (2nd ed.) (Hofmann).

Lenk, H.: *Leistungssport: Ideologie oder Mythos?* Stuttgart, Berlin, Köln, Mainz, 1972 (Kohlhammer).

Lenk, H.: Achievement Motivation and Performance Sport. *Journal of World History* XIV 1972 a), pp. 239-249.

Lenk, H.: Sport, Achievement, and the New Left Criticism. In *Man and World* (1972 b), pp. 179-192.

Lenk, H.: Trees, Tournaments, and Sociometric Graphs. *International Review of Sport Sociology* VI (1971), pp. 175-204.

Lenk, H.: Alienation, Manipulation, and the Athlete's Self. In Grupe, O. (ed.): *Sport in our World—Chances and Problems*. (Scientific Conference in the Connection with the Olympic Games in Munich 1972) Berlin, Heidelberg, New York (Springer 1973), pp. 8-18.

Lenk, H. (ed): *Technokratie als Ideologie*. Stuttgart, Berlin, Köln, Mainz, 1973 (Kohlhammer).

Lenk, H., Gebauer, G., Franke, E.: Perspectives of the Philosophy of Sport. In Grupe, O., Kurz, D., Teipel, J. M.: *The Scientific View of Sport*. Berlin, Heidelberg, New York (Springer 1972), p. 29-58.

Lenk, H., Moser, S., Beyer, E. (eds.): *Philosophie des Sport*. Schorndorf/Stuttgart, 1973 (Hofmann).

Lenk, H.: *Social Philosophy of Athletics*. Champaign, Illinois, 1979 (Stipes Publishing Co.).

Marcuse, H.: *Eros and Civilization*. Boston 1955; reprinted: London (Sphere Books).

McClelland, D. C.: *The Achieving Society*. Princeton 1961 (van Nostrand).

Offe, C.: *Leistungsprinzip und industrielle Arbeit*. Frankfurt 1970 (Europäische Verlagsanstalt).

Rigauer, B.: *Sport und Arbeit*. Frankfurt, 1969 (Suhrkamp).

Slusher, H. S.: *Man, Sport, and Existence*. Philadelphia, 1967 (Lea & Febiger).

Vanderzwaag, H. J.: *Toward a Philosophy of Sport*. Reading/Mass. 1972 (Addison & Wesley).

Weiss, P.: *Sport—a Philosophic Inquiry*. Carbondale-Edwardsville, London-Amsterdam, 1969 (Southern Illinois University Press).

BIBLIOGRAPHY ON SPORTS AND VALUE-ORIENTED CONCERNS

American Association for Health, Physical Education, and Recreation, Division for Girls and Women's Sports and Division of Men's Athletics. *Report of a National Conference on Values in Sports,* Interlochen, Michigan, June 17-22, 1962.

Asinof, Eliot. "1919: The Fix Is In." In *The Realm of Sport.* Edited by Herbert Warren Wind. New York: Simon and Schuster, 1966.

"Athletics and Morals." *Atlantic Monthly,* CXIII (February, 1914), 145-148.

Banham, Charles. "Man at Play." *Contemporary Review,* 207 (August, 1965), 61-64.

Beisser, Arnold R. *The Madness in Sports.* New York: Appleton-Century-Crofts, 1967.

Bend, Emil. "Some Functions of Competitive Team Sports in American Society." Unpublished Ph.D. dissertation, University of Pittsburgh, 1970.

Bovyer, George. "Children's Concepts of Sportsmanship in the Fourth, Fifth, and Sixth Grades." 34, (October, 1963), 282-287.

Bowen, Wilbur P. "The Evolution of Athletic Evils." *American Physical Education Review,* XIV (March, 1909), 151-156.

Broekhoff, Jan. "Sport and Ethics in the Context of Culture." *The Philosophy of Sport: A Collection of Original Essays.* Edited by Robert G. Osterhoudt. Illinois: Charles C Thomas, 1973.

Calisch, Richard. "The Sportsmanship Myth." *Physical Educator,* X (March, 1953), 9-11.

Chryssafis, Jean E. "Aristotle on Physical Education." *Journal of Health and Physical Education,* 1 (January; February; September, 1930), 3-8, 50; 14-17, 46-47; 14-17, 54-56.

Clifton, Marguerite. "Values Through Sports." Unpublished paper presented at the annual convention of the Eastern District Association for Health, Physical Education, and Recreation, Philadelphia, Pennsylvania, March 18, 1963.

Comer, G. "Relationships Between Sport and Mental Health." *Physical Education,* 60 (November, 1968), 83-86.

Coon, Roger. "Sportsmanship, A Worthy Objective." *Physical Educator,* 21 (March, 1964), 16.

Deatherage, Dorothy. "Factors Related to Concepts of Sportsmanship." Unpublished Ed.D. dissertation, University of Southern California, 1964.

Delattre, Edwin J. "Some Reflections on Success and Failure in Competitive Athletics." *Journal of the Philosophy of Sport,* II (September, 1975), 133-138.

Diggs, B. J. "Rules and Utilitarianism." *American Philosophical Quarterly, I* (January, 1964), 32-44.

Edwards, Harry. "An Assessment of the Sports Creed" in *Sociology of Sport.* Homewood, Illinois: Dorsey Press, 1973.

Ellul, J.: La technique oul'enjeu du siecle Paris, 1954.

Gehlen, A.: Sport und Gesellschaft. In: Schultz,

U. (ed.): Das grosse Spiel, p. 22-33. Frankfurt. 1965.

Graves, H. "A Philosophy of Sport." *Contemporary Review,* 78 (December, 1900), 877-893.

Habermas, J.: Siziologische Notizen zum Verhaltnis von Arbeit Und Freizeit. In: Funke, G. Ced.: Konkret Vernunft. (Festschr Rothacker). Bonn 1958, 227 sgg.

Hartman, Betty Grant. "An Exploratory Method for Determining Ethical Standards in Sports." Unpublished Ph.D. dissertation, The Ohio State University, 1958.

Hearn, Francis. "Toward a Critical Theory of Play." *Telos,* 30 (Winter, 1976-77), 145-160.

Hoben, Allan. "The Ethical Value of Organized Play." *Biblical World,* XXXIX (March, 1912), 175-187.

Hogan, William R. "Sin and Sports." *Motivations in Play, Games and Sports.* Edited by Ralph Slovenko and James A. Knight. Illinois: Charles C Thomas, 1967.

Hosmer, Millicent. "The Development of Morality through Physical Education." *Mind and Body,* 21 (June, 1914), 156-163.

Johnson, George E. "Play and Character." *American Physical Education Review,* XXXI (October, 1926), 981-988.

Keating, James W. "Sportsmanship as a Moral Category." *Ethics,* LXXV (October, 1964), 25-35.

————. "The Heart of the Problem of Amateur Athletics." *Journal of General Education,* 16 (January, 1965), 261-272.

————. "Athletics and the Pursuit of Excellence." *Education,* 85 (March, 1965), 428-431.

————. "The Ethics of Competition and its Relation to Some Moral Problems in Athletics." *The Philosophy of Sport: A Collection of Original Essays.* Edited by Robert G. Osterhoudt. Illinois: Charles C Thomas, 1973.

Keenan, Francis. "Justice and Sport." *Journal of the Philosophy of Sport,* II (September, 1975), 111-123.

Kehr, Geneva Belle. "An Analysis of Sportsmanship Responses of Groups of Boys Classified as Participants and Non-Participants in Organized Baseball." Unpublished Ed.D. dissertation, New York University, 1959.

Kellor, Frances A. "Ethical Value of Sports for Women." *American Physical Education Review,* XI (September, 1906), 160-171.

Kennedy, Charles W. "The Effect of Athletic Competition on Character Building." *American Physical Education Review,* XXXI (October, 1926), 988-991.

————. *Sport and Sportsmanship.* New Jersey: Princeton University Press, 1931.

Krockow, C. V.: Der Wetteiferin der industriellen Gesellschaft und im Sport. In: Ausschu B Deutscher Leibeserzieher (ed): Dev Wetteifer, 48-63, Frankfurt-Wien, 1962.

Laughter, Robert James. "Socio-Psychological Aspects of the Development of Athletic Practices and Sports Ethics." Unpublished Ph.D. dissertation, The Ohio State University, 1963.

Lee, Joseph. *Plan in Education*. New York: Macmillan, 1920.

Lenk, H. "Alienation, Manipulation and the Self of the Athlete. *Sport in the Modern World—Chances and Problems*. Edited by Ommo Grupe, Dietrich Kurz and Johannes Teipel. New York: Springer-Verlag, 1973.

Lenk, Hans. "Toward a Social Philosophy of Achievement and Athletics." *Man and World: An International Philosophical Review*, 9 (July, 1976), 45-59.

Magnane, G. Sociologie du Sport. Paris, 1964.

McAfee, Robert A. "Sportsmanship Attitudes of Sixth, Seventh, and Eighth Grade Boys." *Research Quarterly*, 26 (March, 1955), 120.

McBride, P. *The Philosophy of Sport*. London: Health Cranton, 1932.

McCormick, Richard A., S. J. "Is Professional Boxing Immoral?" *Sports Illustrated*, 17 (November 5, 1962), 70-82.

McMurty, John. "Philosophy of a Corner Linebacker." *The Nation*, 212 (January 18, 1971), 83-84.

Massengale, John Denny. "The Effect of Sportsmanship Instruction on Junior High School Boys." Unpublished Ed.D. dissertation, The University of New Mexico, 1969.

Montague, Ashley. "Play or Murder" in *The Humanization of Man*. New York: World Publishing, 1962.

Morgan, William J. "An Analysis of the Sartrean Ethic of Ambiguity as the Moral Ground for the Conduct of Sport." *Journal of the Philosophy of Sport*, III (September, 1976), 82-96.

Muhammad, Elijah. "On Sport and Play" in *Message to the Blackman in America*. Illinois: Muhammad Mosque of Islam No. 2, 1965.

Nash, Jay B. "The Aristocracy of Virtue." *Journal of Health, Physical Education, and Recreation*, 20 (March, 1949), 157, 216-217.

"Now Ike's Golf is Legal." *Sports Illustrated*, 12 (January 18, 1960), 24.

Oberteuffer, Delbert. "On Learning Values Through Sport." *Quest*, I (December, 1963), 23-29.

Oberteuffer, Delbert, Michielli, Donald and Carlson, Joseph. "Sportsmanship—Whose Responsibility?" *Anthology of Contemporary Readings*. Edited by Howard S. Slusher and Aileene S. Lockhard, Iowa: Wm C. Brown, 1966.

Oelschlägel, G.: Karl Marx und die Korperkultur. Theorie und Proxis der Korperkultur 17, 394-401, 587-594 (1968).

Osterhoudt, Robert G. "In Praise of Harmony: The Kantian Imperative and Hegelian *Sittlichkeit* as The Principle and Substance of Moral Conduct in Sport." *Journal of the Philosophy of Sport*, III (September, 1976), 65-81.

——. "The Kantian Ethic as a Principle of Moral Conduct in Sport." *Quest*, XIX (January, 1973), 118-123.

——. "On Keating on the Competitive Motif in Athletics and Playful Activity." *The Philoso-*

phy of Sport: A Collection of Original Essays. Edited by Robert G. Osterhoudt. Illinois: Charles C Thomas, 1973.

——. "The Kantian Ethic as a Principle of Moral Conduct in Sport and Athletics." *The Philosophy of Sport: A Collection of Original Essays*. Edited by Robert G. Osterhoudt. Illinois: Charles C Thomas, 1973.

Pearson, Kathleen M. "Deception, Sportsmanship, and Ethics." *Quest*, XIX (January, 1973), 115-118.

Peters, A. Psychologie des Sports. Seine Konfrontation mit Spiel und Kampf. Leipzig, 1927.

Plessner, H.: Die Funktion des Sports in der indistriellen Gesellschaft. Wissenschaft und Weltbild 262 sgg. (1956).

Potter, Stephen. The Theory and Practice of Gamesmanship. New York: Bantam Books, 1965. (First published New York: Holt, Rinehart and Winston, 1948).

Powell, John T. "Culture, Countries and Sport." Unpublished paper presented at the annual convention of the American Association for Health, Physical Education, and Recreation, Detroit, Michigan, April 3, 1971.

Proost, Jan. "The Concept of Fair Play in Homer's Greece." Unpublished Master's thesis, University of Toledo, 1972.

Ralls, Anthony. "The Game of Life." *Philosophical Quarterly*, 16 (January, 1966), 23-24.

Rawls, John. "Two Concepts of Rules." *Philosophical Review*, 64 (January, 1955), 3-32.

Reader, Mark, Wolf, Donald. "On Being Human." *Political Theory*, 1 (May, 1973), 186-202.

"Requiem for a Friend [Pope Pius XII on sport]." *Sports Illustrated*, 9 (October 20, 1958), 27.

Richardson, Deane E. "Ethical Conduct in Sport Situations." *Proceedings of the Sixty-Fifth Annual Meeting of the National College Physical Education Association*. San Francisco, California, 1962.

Rigauer, B.: Sport und Arbeit, Frankfurt 1969.

Roberts, Terry, Galasso, P. J. "The Fiction of Morally Indifferent Acts in Sport." *The Philosophy of Sport: A Collection of Original Essays*. Edited by Robert G. Osterhoudt. Illinois: Charles C Thomas, 1973.

Rogers, Frederick Rand. *The Amateur Spirit in Scholastic Games and Sports*. Albany, New York: C. F. Williams & Sons, 1929.

Royce, Josiah. *Some Relations of Physical Training to the Present Problems of Moral Education in America*. Boston: The Boston Normal School of Gymnastics, ca. 1908.

Rupp, Adolph. "Defeat and Failure to Me Are Enemies." *Sports Illustrated*, 9 (December 8, 1958), 100-106.

Sadler, William A. "A Contextual Approach to an Understanding of Competition. A Response to Keating's Philosophy of Athletics." *The Philosophy of Sport: A Collection of Original Essays*. Edited by Robert G. Osterhoudt. Illinois: Charles C Thomas, 1973.

Scott, Jack. *The Athletic Revolution*. New York: Free Press, 1971.

————. "Ethics in Sport: The Revolutionary Ethic." Unpublished paper presented at the annual convention of the American Association for Health, Physical Education, and Recreation, Houston, Texas, March 28, 1972.

————. "Sport and the Radical Ethic." *Quest* XIX (January, 1973), 71-77.

Shaw, John H., "The Operation of a Value System in the Selection of Activities and Methods of Instruction in Physical Education." *Proceedings of the Fifty-Ninth Annual Meeting of the College Physical Education Association,* Daytona Beach, Florida, 1956.

Shriver, Sargent. "The Moral Force of Sport." *Sports Illustrated,* 18 (June 3, 1963), 30-31, 62-63.

Slusher, Howard S. *Man, Sport and Existence.* Philadelphia: Lea & Febiger, 1967.

————. "Ethics in Sport: The American Ethic." Unpublished paper presented at the annual convention of the American Association for Health, Physical Education and Recreation, Houston, Texas, March 28, 1972.

Spencer, Herbert. "Amusements" in *The Principles of Ethics,* Vol. 1. New York: D. Appleton and Company, 1910.

Stearns, Alfred E. "Athletics and the School." *Atlantic Monthly,* CXIII (February, 1914), 148-152.

Stewart, C. A. "Athletics and the College." *Atlantic Monthly,* CXIII (February, 1914), 153-160.

Suenens, L. "The Alienation and Identity of Man." *Sport in the Modern World—Chances and Problems.* Edited by Ommo Grupe, Dietrich Kurz and Johannes Teipel. New York: Springer—Verlag, 1973.

Suits, Bernard. "Is Life a Game We Are Playing?" *Ethics,* 77 (April, 1967), 209-213.

————. "The Grasshopper: A Thesis Concerning the Moral Idea of Man." *The Philosophy of Sport: A Collection of Original Essays.* Edited by Robert G. Osterhoudt. Illinois: Charles C Thomas, 1973.

"Symposium on Sportsmanship." *Physical Educator,* VI (October, 1949), 1-15.

Thomas, Carolyn E. "Do You 'Wanna' Bet: An Examination of Player Betting and the Integrity of the Sporting Event." *The Philosophy of Sport: A Collection of Original Essays.* Edited by Robert G. Osterhoudt. Illinois: Charles C Thomas, 1973.

Tiede, Tom and Berkow, Ira. "Our Changing Morality," Part 3. *The Springfield Union,* February 24, 1970, p. 17.

Tunis, John R. "The Great Sports Myths" in *Sports: Heroics and Hysterics.* New York: John Day, 1928.

Turbeville, Gus. "On Being Good Sports in Sports." *Vital Speeches,* 31 (June 15, 1965), 542-544.

Ulrich, Celeste. "Ethics in Sport: The Christian Ethic." Unpublished paper presented at the annual convention of the American Association for Health, Physical Education, and Recreation, Houston, Texas, March 28, 1972.

Underwood, John. "The True Crisis [Is Sport Crooked?]." *Sports Illustrated,* 18 (May 20, 1963), 16-19, 83.

UNESCO. *Sport, Work, Culture. Report of the International Conference of The Contribution of Sports to the Improvement of Professional Abilities and to Cultural Development.* Helsinki, Finland, August 10-15, 1959.

Weiss, Paul. *Sport: A Philosophic Inquiry.* Carbondale: Southern Illinois University Press, 1969.

Wilton, W. M. "An Early Consensus on Sportsmanship." *Physical Educator,* 20 (October, 1963), 113-114.

Woods, Sherwyn M. "The Violent World of the Athlete." *Quest,* XVI (June, 1971), 55-60.

Zeegers, Machiel. "The Swindler as Player." *Motivations in Play, Games and Sports.* Edited by Ralph Slovenko and James A. Knight. Illinois: Charles C Thomas, 1967.

Zeigler, Earle F. "The Pragmatic (Experimentalistic) Ethic as it Relates to Sport and Physical Education." *The Philosophy of Sport: A Collection of Original Essays.* Edited by Robert G. Osterhoudt. Illinois: Charles C Thomas, 1973.

SECTION VI
Sport and Aesthetics

Aesthetics as a branch of philosophy coexists with ethics and sociopolitical philosophy in the general category of axiology. Whereas ethics deals with the question of what is good, and sociopolitical philosophy with the question what is the common good, aesthetics is concerned with what is beautiful. Questions concerning beauty, taste, and the nature of the aesthetic experience are among the most complex of philosophical issues.

Much of aesthetic inquiry centers around the appreciation and evaluation of artificial art—that is, objects deliberately created to be beautiful, to catalyze an aesthetic experience. Nevertheless, most people have had the pleasure of experiencing beauty in a natural setting, with no artist intervening. In fact many artists have devoted their work to attempting to recreate or capture scenes of natural beauty. Somewhere between the natural and the created art object is the structure created for utilitarian purposes, such as a building, which also happens to be beautiful and evokes an aesthetic experience.

Sport may be an example of the latter category, or it may be considered a phenomenon of natural beauty. In either case, however, most sporting endeavors have failed to attract artistic attention. The exceptions, of course, are the "form" sports: diving, gymnastics, figure skating, aquatic art, and riding. However, these activities are transitory, they exist as objets d'art only momentarily and are therefore a unique form of art, akin more to the temporal arts of music, theatre, cinema, opera and dance than the spatial arts of architecture, literature, painting and sculpture.

The question of what is art hinges upon the more fundamental problem of what is beauty. As with all other philosophical issues, there are various points of view roughly corresponding to the major philosophical schools of thought. Opinions include the beliefs that beauty is the idealized representation of nature (a concept held by the classical Greeks, for example), and the often-quoted statement that "beauty is in the eye of the beholder." In either case, certain criteria are applied, either those which correspond to the dictates of nature, or those which the individual chooses to apply. The admission of the latter possibility has led aestheticians to question the validity of assuming that art is a subtopic of the theory of beauty. While a person may have an aesthetic response to beauty, a similar reaction may occur when confronted with the ugly or violent or even, if pop artists are to be taken seriously, with the merely ordinary.

Still another complex question is the problem of aesthetic quality. Much of traditional art criticism has been based upon the assumption that certain principles of aesthetics have been established, either classically or in a given time and society. The evaluation of a work of art is then made in conformity to these accepted principles. A competing viewpoint is the notion that basic to quality in art is the object's ability to evoke an emotional response, a reaction, an "experience," a moment of communication between the viewer and the artist via the art object. Although stated in much more sophisticated terms today, the root of this is in the pleasure theories exposited by men like Herbert Spencer in the late nineteenth century. Then the aesthetic response was described in terms of the viewer's enjoyment, a primarily emotional response. However, with the development of aesthetic theories which regard art as deliberately symbolic, as nonverbal language, cognitive responses are also considered to be a part of the aesthetic experience. Meaning, relevance, communication, insight are all terms used in connection with the aesthetic experience. As with the word beauty, the connotations of the term pleasure have been much expanded.

Sport has long been considered a worthy subject for artists. In other words, its potential as an object of beauty to be represented in some created art form has been recognized. Sporting art has been shown to be meaningful, capable of evoking an aesthetic experience. Some of the best examples come from the ancient Greeks who gave particular representation to sport and sportsmen in art.

Perhaps more important than the representation of sport in art is the belief that sport itself is an art form. As a form of cultural expression, it fits the criteria applied to other art forms such as painting and sculpture. The origin of this idea is generally credited to the German romantic philosopher Friedrich von Schiller. He contended that the ideal of beauty is represented in the play-instinct; play, which is the expression of the self at its most complete, can be the highest form of aesthetic culture. Karl Groos, in his classic work *The Play of Man*, expresses a similar point of view.

Schiller and Groos established the relationship between play and aesthetics on the basis of similarities between them. For example, they are both nonproductive and, in a biological sense, removed from the acts of humans necessary for survival. More recent speculations have gone further in attempting to demonstrate that the sport experience is inherently an aesthetic experience. The article by Eugene Kaelin analyzes the aesthetic qualities of sporting events from the point of view of the spectator.

Terry Roberts' essay, "Languages of Sport: Representation," presents an interesting and quite unique approach (one derived from Nelson Goodman's *Languages of Art*) to the general study of sport as well as the more particular study of its aesthetic properties: namely, exploring sport through the medium of established symbol systems such as language and art. In this essay, he restricts his attention to one form of symbolism found in sport, that of representation. Wulk's article, "A Meta-critical Aesthetic of Sport," develops the implications of Monroe Beardsley's critical aesthetic theory for sport.

The final two selections, David Best's "The Aesthetic in Sport," and Joseph Kupfer's "Purpose and Beauty in Sport," consider the aesthetic potential of sport in terms of its purposive structure. In the first essay, Best lays the groundwork for this assessment by distinguishing between the related concepts of the "aesthetic" and the "artistic." The difference between these two concepts, according to Best, lies not in their logical properties, for both are characterized by a fusion of means and ends, but rather in the different ways in which these logical properties are considered. That is, the aesthetic is essentially a spectator concept, and thus broader in scope in that virtually anything can be viewed in the fused manner indicated above; whereas the artistic is principally a participant concept, and thus narrower in scope in that it presupposes that an artifact was made with a definite expressive intent in mind. With respect to the aesthetic concept, Best argues that although any sporting activity can, strictly speaking, be viewed from an aesthetic perspective, only some sport forms claim the aesthetic as a central element of the game (e.g., gymnastics and diving). Indeed, in most sporting activities, as Best points out, the aesthetic element is incidental to the ongoing activity of the game (e.g., competitive sports such as football and basketball). Kupfer's essay, however, argues the opposite view: namely, that competitive sports not only contain an essential aesthetic element, but further, that such sports enhance the aesthetic dimension (through the dramatic contesting of wills) in a fashion that noncompetitive sports cannot. With respect to the artistic concept, Best flatly denies any artistic recognition for sport on the grounds that it lacks, even in those sports that emphasize the aesthetic, the requisite expressive feature. Kupfer, although he doesn't directly address this issue, at least leaves open the possibility of regarding competitive sport (though not necessarily non-competitive sport) as an art form in light of his characterization of its purposive structure and its opposition and scoring features.

One can accept the assumption that sport is an art form, that participating in the sport experience as either player or spectator is potentially an aesthetic experience. But the overriding question in art is when does a phenomenon have the quality to be considered a work of art? In other words, what is the difference between a child's drawing and a Picasso painting? What is the qualitative difference between the action of a Willie Mays and that of a young sandlot player? Is every sport experience an aesthetic experience?

The early literature on sport and art has been concerned principally with attempting to demonstrate the existence of a relationship between sport and art. A number of writers have exposited Schiller's original theories, modifying or expanding them in accord with some philosophical justifications. The articles by Seward (1944) and Hein (1968) are examples of this type of analysis. Two excellent selections which discuss sport as art in cultural terms are those by Maheu (1963) and Jokl (1964). Metzl (1962) analyzes a number of art pieces which take sport as their subject.

More recent efforts, however, have taken on the larger question concerning the aesthetic merits of sport itself. Reid's (1970) incisive work laid the critical foundation for this effort. Osterhoudt's (1973) anthology included a section on aesthetics which considered this question in different theoretical veins: from Aristotle's theory of tragedy to Hegel's philosophy of fine art. Whiting's and Masterson's (1974) anthology also included many pieces that critically examined the aesthetic possibili-

ties of sport. In a major systematic work, Roberts (1976) provided a general vehicle for the examination of the aesthetic properties of sport by reference to established symbol systems such as art and language.

With such a sparse treatment of the subject, there is much room for further research. Most needed are standards for evaluating the quality of movement. Those standards already established in sports such as diving might be reexamined in terms of their faithfulness to artistic principles. Similarly, artistic criteria for games might be developed. A comparison of the art form sport with other art forms might be undertaken with a view to delineating sport's special place within the realm of art. Empirical evidence might be gathered in support of the contention that the sport experience is, in fact, an aesthetic experience according to accepted criteria.

Such analyses may be subjected to the criticism that they are an attempt to exalt sport beyond its simple importance as a source of pleasure and meaning to its millions of participants and spectators. But it is part of human desire to appreciate the value of people's works, and that leads to the discipline of aesthetic criticism.

Play and Beauty[*]

FRIEDRICH VON SCHILLER

I approach continually nearer to the end to which I lead you, by a path offering few attractions. Be pleased to follow me a few steps further, and a large horizon will open up to you, and a delightful prospect will reward you for the labor of the way.

The object of the sensuous instinct, expressed in a universal conception, is named Life in the widest acceptation; a conception that expresses all material existence and all that is immediately present in the senses. The object of the formal instinct, expressed in a universal conception, is called shape or form, as well in an exact as in an inexact acceptation; a conception that embraces all formal qualities of things and all relations of the same to the thinking powers. The object of the play instinct, represented in a general statement, may therefore bear the name of *living form;* a term that serves to describe all aesthetic qualities of phenomena, and what people style, in the widest sense, *beauty.*

Beauty is neither extended to the whole field of all living things nor merely enclosed in this field. A marble block, though it is and remains lifeless, can nevertheless become a living form by the architect and sculptor; a man, though he lives and has a form, is far from being a living form on that account. For this to be the case, it is necessary that his form should be life, and that his life should

* "Letter XV" from *Essays and Letters.* Vol. VIII. Trans. by A. Lodge, E. B. Eastwick and A. J. W. Morrison. London: Anthological Society, 1882.

be a form. As long as we only think of his form, it is lifeless, a mere abstraction; as long as we only feel his life, it is without form, a mere impression. It is only when his form lives in our feeling, and his life in our understanding, he is the living form, and this will everywhere be the case where we judge him to be beautiful.

But the genesis of beauty is by no means declared because we know how to point out the component parts, which in their combination produce beauty. For to this end it would be necessary to comprehend that *combination itself,* which continues to defy our exploration, as well as all mutual operation between the finite and the infinite. The reason, on transcendental grounds, makes the following demand: There shall be a communion between the formal impulse and the material impulse—that is, there shall be a play instinct—because it is only the unity of reality with the form, of the accidental with the necessary, of the passive state with freedom, that the conception of humanity is completed. Reason is obliged to make this demand because her nature impels her to completeness and to the removal of all bounds; while every exclusive activity of one or the other impulse leaves human nature incomplete and places a limit in it. Accordingly, as soon as reason issues the mandate, "a humanity shall exist," it proclaims at the same time the law, "there shall be a beauty." Experience can answer us if there is a beauty, and we shall know it as soon as she has taught us if a humanity can exist. But neither reason nor experience can tell us how beauty can be and how a humanity is possible.

We know that man is neither exclusively matter nor exclusively spirit. Accordingly, beauty as the consummation of humanity can neither be exclusively mere life, as has been asserted by sharp-sighted observers, who kept too close to the testimony of experience, and to which the taste of the time would gladly degrade it; nor can beauty be merely form, as has been judged by speculative sophists, who departed too far from experience, and by philosophic artists, who were led too much by the necessity of art in explaining beauty; it is rather the common object of both impulses, that is of the play instinct. The use of language completely justifies this name, as it is wont to qualify with the word play what is neither subjectively nor objectively accidental, and yet does not impose necessity either externally or internally. As the mind in the intuition of the beautiful finds itself in a happy medium between law and necessity, it is, because it divides itself between both, emancipated from the pressure of both. The formal impulse and the material impulse are equally earnest in their demands, because one relates in its cognition to things in their reality and the other to their necessity; because in action the first is directed to the preservation of life, the second to the preservation of dignity, and therefore both to truth and perfection. But life becomes more indifferent when dignity is mixed up with it, and duty no longer coerces when inclination attracts. In like manner the mind takes in the reality of things, material truth, more freely and tranquilly as soon as it encounters formal truth, the law of necessity; nor does the mind find itself strung by abstraction as soon as immediate intuition can accompany it. In one word, when the mind comes into communion with ideas, all reality loses its serious value because it becomes *small*; and as it comes in contact with feeling, necessity parts also with its serious value because it is *easy*.

But perhaps the objection has for some time occurred to you. Is not the beautiful degraded by this, that it is made a mere play? and is it not reduced to the level of frivolous objects which have for ages passed under that name? Does it not contradict the conception of the reason and the dignity of beauty, which is nevertheless regarded as an instrument of culture, to confine it to the work of being a mere play? and does it not contradict the empirical conception of play, which can coexist with the exclusion of all taste, to confine it merely to beauty?

But what is meant by a *mere play*, when we know that in all conditions of humanity that very thing is play, and *only* that is play which makes man complete and develops simultaneously his twofold nature? What you style *limitation*, according to your representation of the matter, according to my views, which I have justified by proofs, I name *enlargement*. Consequently I should have said exactly the reverse: man is serious *only* with the agreeable, with the good, and with the perfect, but he *plays* with beauty. In saying this we must not indeed think of the plays that are in vogue in real life, and which commonly refer only to his material state. But in real life we should also seek in vain for the beauty of which we are here speaking. The actually present beauty is worthy of the really, of the actually present play-impulse; but by the ideal of beauty, which is set up by the reason, an ideal of the play-instinct is also presented, which man ought to have before his eyes in all his plays.

Therefore, no error will ever be incurred if we seek the ideal of beauty on the same road on which we satisfy our play-impulse. We can immediately understand why the ideal form of a Venus, of a Juno, and of an Apollo is to be sought not at Rome, but in Greece, if we contrast the Greek population, delighting in the bloodless athletic contests of boxing, racing, and intellectual rivalry at Olympia, with the Roman people gloating over the agony of a gladiator. Now the reason pronounces that the beautiful must not only be life and form, but a living form, that is, beauty, inasmuch as it dictates to man the twofold law of absolute formality and absolute reality. Reason also utters the decision that man shall only *play* with beauty, and he *shall only play* with *beauty*.

For, to speak out once for all, man only plays when in the full meaning of the word he is a man, and *he is only completely a man when he plays*. This proposition, which at this moment perhaps appears paradoxical, will receive a great and deep meaning if we have advanced far enough to apply it to the twofold seriousness of duty and of destiny. I promise you that the whole edifice of aesthetic art and the still more difficult art of life will be supported by this principle. But this proposition is only unexpected in science; long ago it lived and worked in art and in the feeling of the Greeks, her most accomplished masters;

only they removed to Olympus what ought to have been preserved on earth. Influenced by the truth of this principle, they effaced from the brow of their gods the earnestness and labor which furrow the cheeks of mortals, and also the hollow lust that smoothes the empty face. They set free the ever serene from the chains of every purpose, of every duty, of every care, and they made *indolence* and *indifference* the envied condition of the godlike race; merely human appellations for the freest and highest mind. As well the material pressure of natural laws as the spiritual pressure of moral laws lost itself in its higher idea of necessity, which embraced at the same time both worlds, and out of the union of these two necessities issued true freedom. Inspired by this spirit the Greeks also effaced from the features of their ideal, together with *desire or inclination*, all traces of *volition*, or, better still, they made both unrecognizable, be-

cause they knew how to wed them both in the closest alliance. It is neither charm, nor is it dignity, which speaks from the glorious face of Juno Ludovici; it is neither of these, for it is both at once. While the female god challenges our veneration, the godlike woman at the same time kindles our love. But while in ecstasy we give ourselves up to the heavenly beauty, the heavenly self-repose awes us back. The whole form rests and dwells in itself—a fully complete creation in itself—and as if she were out of space, without advance or resistance; it shows no force contending with force, no opening through which time could break in. Irresistibly carried away and attracted by her womanly charm, kept off at a distance by her godly dignity, we also find ourselves at length in the state of the greatest repose, and the result is a wonderful impression for which the understanding has no idea and language no name.

Play From the Aesthetic Standpoint*

KARL GROOS

While it is true that undue emphasis of the overflow of energy reduces play to self-indulgence, at the same time it is unfair to art to make too prominent its kinship with play. This is just the position of Guyau in his aesthetic writings; yet he is far from denying the kinship, and I think that he would have concurred to a great extent in Schiller's view if he could have convinced himself of the biological and sociological importance of play by adequate investigation of its phenomena. I at least have been confirmed in my conviction of the close connection between play and aesthetics by the perusal of his book, and there, too, my view stated in the very outset—namely, that this connection obtains in a higher degree than does that between play and artistic production —is also supported by his more thoroughgoing investigation of the facts.

The following points present themselves as the most general results of our observation of aesthetic enjoyment. We have found that all sense organs display numerous impulses to activity, and consequently enjoyment of the response to stimuli is a universal basis of play, varying as to conditions and the quality of the stimuli. Now, since every aesthetic pleasure (except the appreciation of poetry) is connected with sense-perception, we find in it a genuine source of enjoyment, depending on the origin and quality of such perception. Observation merely for its own sake is the lowest

* From *The Play of Man*. New York: D. Appleton and Company, 1901.

form of aesthetic enjoyment, and is so far identical with sensuous play.

On this foundation arises enjoyment of special stimuli. Confining ourselves to sensory play, we can distinguish two groups—namely, sensuously agreeable stimuli and intensive ones. The former, provided higher aesthetic observation does its work of personification, finds its sole object in beauty. Pleasure in intense stimuli is strong enough to subdue the pain which is commonly associated with it, and forms an introduction to enjoyment of what is grotesque, striking, and tragic. It is especially prominent in the trancelike state so common in movement-play as well as in aesthetic enjoyment.

Before going further we must pause to consider the idea so often advanced that such enjoyment is peculiarly the prerogative of the higher senses. Is the pleasure which I feel when I inhale a perfume as much aesthetic as is the perception of beautiful colour? I think the case is like that of the common idea of play. From a psychological standpoint we recognise as such any act that is practised purely for its pleasurable effect, and sham occupation in the higher forms of play may be subjective. Therefore we can affirm that pleasure in perception as such, and not necessarily in agreeable perception, grounds it, and to this extent no one can demur if the beautiful colour is classed with the pleasant odour. For the utmost aesthetic satisfaction, however, more than this is requisite—first, definite form, and second, richer spiritual effect—and since these

321

are perceptible only to the higher senses, it becomes their exclusive prerogative to take in the utmost effects of artistic effort.

To resume our review, we observe that aesthetic enjoyment is not merely a playful sensor experience, but manifests as well the higher psychic grounds of perception. What we said of the pleasure of recognition, the stimulus of novelty, and the shock of surprise need not here be repeated. Illusion remains the most certain mark of higher aesthetic enjoyment, and the important psychological problem connected with it which was referred to in the preceding section has its application here as in other illusion play. The first thing to notice about it here is that it consists partly in the transference of thought from the copy to an original,[1] and that sympathy and the borrowing of qualities which are connected with imitation have also their parts to play. Bearing all this in mind, we are in a position to put the question next in order, What is the principal content of illusion?

Thus we arrive at a point similar to that reached in our study of sensory plays. As the pleasure in stimulus as such surpasses the pleasure in any particular form of stimulus, so here the subjective activity of inner imitation as such is a source of pleasure quite apart from the qualities inherent in the thing copied. Lipps says, in his notice of my *Einleitung in die Aesthetik*, that for me the aesthetic value of the object under observation and personification is not that it is personified, but that it is I who personify it. Part III of the book proves the injustice of this to my general view, yet I do maintain that inner imitation is as such accompanied by pleasurable feelings,[2] and consequently that aesthetic satisfaction possibly finds its first limit when any painfulness connected with the subject outweighs the enjoyment derived from inner imitation.

If, then, the act of inner imitation is in itself pleasurable, it strikes me as self-evident that the degree of satisfaction attained must be proportional to the value of its object. This is clearly illustrated by the highest character of aesthetic intuition, the impression of vital and mental completeness; and inner imitation

shows this, for it delights to act in response to the functions of movement, force, life, and animation. Therefore Lotze is right when he says, after approving the limitations which we have pointed out, "No form is too chaste for the entrance and possession of our imagination." On the other hand, it is evident that the value of this indwelling depends essentially on the peculiarities of the subject. If, for instance, I transform myself into a shellfish and enter into its sole method of enjoyment, opening and shutting its shell, I experience a far narrower sort of aesthetic satisfaction than when I feel with a mother who is caressing her child. It is just because inner imitation is involved that the value of the aesthetic effect is determined by the qualities of the object. But what are the qualities, it may be asked, which augment or detract from this effect? An exhaustive and satisfactory answer to this question is impossible here; such is the extraordinary variety of the contributory factors. It properly belongs, too, to specialized aesthetics. In general, however, it is safe to say that we enjoy imitating what produces agreeable and intense feelings, and we thus find again on higher ground the same conditions which we encountered in sensory play. This distinction is clearly brought out by Lipps in his article on the impression made by a Doric column: "The mechanical effects which are 'easily' attained remind us of such acts of our own as are accomplished without effort or impediment, and likewise the powerful expenditure of active mechanical energy recalls a similar output of our will power. In the first case a cheerful feeling of lightness and freedom results; in the other no less agreeable sensations of our own vigour."[3] In other spheres the value of such indwelling seems to me to be chiefly in the two directions which Schiller has indicated in his comparison of "grace" and "dignity." I would refer again in this connection to what has been said about the importance of poetic enjoyment; if we are right in assigning love and conflict as its chief motives, then here too enjoyment of agreeable and intense stimuli is prominent.

If we ask, finally, how aesthetic enjoyment extends its sway beyond the entire sphere of play, we encroach on the ethical bearings of art. With the introduction of an element of moral elevation and profound insight into life, aesthetic satisfaction ceases to be "mere" play and transcends our present subject. But we must be careful to maintain that it is trans-

---

[1] Lange has treated of the contrary case where Nature is regarded as a work of art. I do not think, however, that it has the significance that belongs to the conversion of appearance into reality.

[2] "À la vue d'un objet expressif," says Jouffroy, "qui me jette dans un état sympathique de soi-même désagréable, il y a en moi un plaisir qui résulte de ce que je suis dans cet état."—*Op. cit.*, 270.

[3] Raumästhetik, p. 6.

cendence and not exclusion, for even when (as is possible to a Shakespeare and a Schiller) the intent toward moral elevation and profound insight is prominent, our enjoyment remains aesthetic only so long as these effects are developed and set forth in connection with playful sympathy.

Our second leading question is that of the relation between play and artistic production. Let us set out by announcing at once that the latter, especially in highly developed art, is further removed from play than is aesthetic enjoyment. This is implied in the fact that, for the genuine artist, practical application of his aptitude is, as a rule, his life's calling; not necessarily his only means of support, of course, but sufficiently absorbing to force the man of creative ability to devote most of his life to an end which to the mass of mankind seems unworthy of serious effort. In such a case art ceases to be playful. But this transformation is not unique. That absorption in an apparently useless form of activity which is so incomprehensible to the average man, but which easily lures its votaries to rapt enthusiasm for their art, is displayed in many forms less exalted than the striving for an ideal. Plays not connected with art hold despotic sway over their victims. Many devote their life's best effort to some forms of sport, and others to mental contests, such as those of chess, whist, etc. E. Isolani says that when Zuckertort was a medical student in Berlin he accidentally became a witness of a match game between two fine chess players, and, although unfamiliar with the rules, he detected a false play. This interested him in the game, and he became a pupil of Anderson. Soon chess instead of medicine became his chief business in life; he thought of nothing but how to improve his play. It kept him awake at night, or, if fatigue overcame him, its problems pursued him in dreams. At twenty-four he was a worn-out man. The demoniac power with which art drives a man so predisposed resides in other games as well; and in this both activities cease to be pure play.

Another basis for our subject is found in the fact that art presupposes a useful field of application for technical skill whose acquirement and improvement are no longer ends in themselves. The acquisition is often a long and painful process, with little that is playful about it. But this is common enough in other play as well when the technical side of any sport is made the subject of serious study and effort.

Our third ground is to be sought in a very real aim, which is ever beckoning to the artist.

It may be designated in a general way as the sympathetic interest of others, manifested in admiring recognition and appreciation of the powers displayed, or in subscribing to the convictions, views, and ideals of the artist. Insofar as this is an effective motive, art is no play. Strictly artistic temperaments are especially liable to its influence at the beginning of their career. Indifference, when sincere, is usually a later development, the product of experience.

Having thus fortified our position against misconstruction, we are prepared to proclaim the proper relationship between artistic production and play. It seems to me to be more and more conspicuous as we approach the springs of art. The primitive festival, combining as it did music and poetry with dancing, had indeed a tremendous effect on its witnessers, and its manifestations were essentially playful. Skill acquired in childhood through playful practice was playfully exhibited with original variations. The epic art, too, was playfully employed by the primitive recounter, with no indication of toilsome preparation or serious treatment, and the case is not widely different with what we know of the beginnings of pictorial art. So long as primitive sculpture served no religious purpose, simple delight in its use was much more prominent, since all inherited the capacity, and none was opposed to the mass as the exponent of a specialty. We meet the same conditions in studying the child's artistic efforts; his poetic and musical efforts as well as those in drawing are essentially playful. The idea of making an impression on others does appear, but it is still very much in the background; enjoyment of his own productive activity predominates in the infantile consciousness. Although highly developed art does so transcend the sphere of play, it too is rooted in playful experimentation and imitation, and we can detect their later growth of joy in being a cause in the work of full-fledged artists of our own day. Indeed, it is present in all creative activity, gilding earnest work with a sportive glitter. In artistic production, however, it has the special office of differentiating it from ordinary toil and making appreciation of the thing created go hand in hand with its production. Each new-found harmony of tone or colour or outline appealing to criticism of its creator causes him intense enjoyment all through the progress of its production, and the indifference sometimes felt toward the finished work results from frequent repetition which has dulled the edge of appetite.

The Well-Played Game: Notes Toward an Aesthetics of Sport*

E. F. KAELIN

When, under the chancellorship of Robert Maynard Hutchins, the University of Chicago "de-emphasized" its commitment to intercollegiate football, reactions to the defection of the Maroons were various. Some critics, recalling the legendary remark of the youthful chancellor—no iron man this—that whenever the desire for physical activity manifested itself, he immediately lay down until it passed off, uttered a resigned "What can you expect?" Others, more rationalistic if less philosophical, pointed out the poor showing of Chicago's gladiators in recent Big-10 competition as sufficient reason for the radical step: better to save face by quitting than to continue bringing up the rear. Both views tended to ignore the corresponding re-emphasis on intramural sport activities intended to keep those egg-heads screwed on to functioning bodies, and not all of them could know of the Manhattan Project developing under the abandoned bleachers of Alonzo Stagg Field. You win some and you lose some; and as all cynics know only too well, if you are the coach and you lose too many, you chance to lose your job as well. Rather than looking for another coach and another site for experimenting on atomic fission, the Chicagoans ended their embarrassment by copping out. The chancellor's tirades against the growing professionalism of the college game were never really heard.

No one was surprised, and only the avid

fans of big-time football mourned the passing of an American institution. The case was different when, about ten years later, the University of Notre Dame made a similar decision. Here was a bigger institution yet. The Fighting Irish with the Polish names were one of the principal reasons for the very existence of South Bend, Indiana. Who were these religious men who decided that a university could be run without the attendant big business of football? Were their souls so hardened that they could no longer respond to the demand of winning one for the Gipper? What else is there to do in the Midwest on a fall Saturday afternoon? No one was naive enough to believe that the lack of distracting spectacles—cultural or otherwise—that is our Mid-western civilization would induce our football-deprived students to pass their time with the books. Thus, not succeeding in their idealism—not even that could make the alumni accept an 8-2 season for the Fighting Irish, where the "8" refers to the number of losses in one season—ND's administration decided to face up to reality: they needed a new coach, someone like Rockne and Layden and Leahy, someone who knew how to win; but they also needed an increased budget to float the necessary football scholarships. The rest of the story is known: they found both, only to have their recent siege on the national championship fended off by the appearance of another national power. Oh, the horror of it: Michigan State University, which

* From *Quest*, X (May, 1968), 16-28.

fills in the beef on its line with the culturally disadvantaged youth of the Southland and which hires its professors to foment counter-revolution in such places as Viet Nam, forced the Irish to play for a tie. They should have done as well in South Vietnam. Who was to console the despondent spirit of the Gipper now? Not Parseghian. He played this one out for his boys who played too hard for too long to accept second place in what turned out to be the only truly national championship competition in college football during recent times. Evidently we build character in our student athletes only by teaching them to win—or at least not to lose—with grace.

Who is to fault such a decision? Shall we repeat it? "It matters not . . . , it's how you play the game. And no one plays for a tie." The desire to win is a necessary part of all competitive sport, as, unfortunately, are the economics and consequently the politics of American universities—always on the make—engaged in big-time football. The question is: does such a mass of interlocking institutions possess a component which is distinctively sporting and distinctively aesthetic? Some of us, spectators and lovers of competitive sports we cannot engage in and participators in those suited to our physical characteristics, claim there is. What we need is a method of inquiry to make clear what we find happening in sport.

I propose to begin my inquiry with some observations on the nature of spectator sports in our American culture. In an affluent society the question of bread is for the most part guaranteed; and where it is not, bread can always be procured if only one is strong enough, agile or skilled enough to perform in the community circus. And there are many circuses in which to perform. Baseball, which lays the oldest and perhaps most fraudulent claim to being America's national pastime, was never played before as great a collective audience as basketball, once it was discovered that an outsized ball could be thrown through a peach basket placed at a suitable height from the floor. Every town in the country has its high school team; every junior college, college, and university that is too small to compete with bigger institutions for the honors of semi-professional football can and does produce basketball teams of acceptable caliber; and some of them rank with the best teams playing anywhere.

But if this were not enough to challenge baseball's claim to supremacy, along came television, which propelled collegiate and professional football into the national consciousness

as never before. Where audiences in the stadia, gymnasia, and field houses across the nation were limited to the hundreds of thousands, the new audience for a single performance is currently being measured in the millions. And if the greedy moguls of professional football do not kill the goose that lays this golden egg by overexposing her, the growing trend of football fanship will make it quite plain even to the most rabid of baseball's fans that football is indeed the currently reigning national sport. Are sport appreciators fickle in their affections? Or is there a deeper reason for the rising disaffection with the game played with a bat?

Yes, Virginia, there is. But it is not the greater violence of football, that, appealing to some dark neurotic drive of the spectators, makes it more popular than nine innings of baseball played in the sun or under the lights. Violence it may be which makes the term "gladiator" more applicable to the participant in the contact sport; after all, the original gladiators fought to the death to appease the neuroses of the Roman citizens. But if the greater popularity of football were attributed to this sort of appeal, then ice hockey or lacrosse or boxing should be more popular than football. Violence, even the vicarious experience of violence on the part of the sports fan, is not what makes it a moral equivalent of war, as were the jousts and tournaments of bored knights. The value of violence in sport to both participant and spectator is not in its expression per se, but in its control toward the achievement of a contested end. Where violence may be sufficient to generate interest in an activity, its control is necessary to sustain our continued interest in its expression.

One of the factors which has worked to reduce interest in the game of baseball, moreover, has been precisely the introduction of more violence. When it was discovered that fans were willing to pay to see home runs instead of closely fought ball games, the era of the king of swat was very swiftly changed to that of the rabbit ball, band box ball parks, and the .260 hitter. Violence in this game was thus found to be one of the factors working toward its undoing as an aesthetic phenomenon and hence as a satisfying spectator sport. Pitchers were converted in this unnatural process into throwers, and their opponents in the struggle for survival into bottle bat bombers whose very cheapness has killed interest in an otherwise intriguing game. Perhaps the game was meant for the Latin Americans and the Japanese after all.

If not the violence of the action, then perhaps the continuity of action, or the lack of it, is the secret of baseball's apparent demise. Consider the experience of introducing a European to the delights of night baseball. Brought up on soccer, in which team, coach, and spectator are all satisfied to win the game by a single goal, 1-0 or 2-1 after a continuous hour's struggle—heaven help the goalie that allows three scores in a single game—our bemused European visitor finds nine innings of walks, hit basemen, home runs, and lengthy rhubarbs an interminable bore. True, it takes some time for him to perceive that the main tension of the game pits the pitcher's power and skill against those of each succeeding batter and that these may be slightly modified by the tension created between the speed of a runner and the "arm" of a defensive fielder; but even when brought to a recognition of these niceties, he can hardly be led to perceive the qualitative character of the game itself. And character discrimination is the essence of aesthetic perception.

In all but a very few instances baseball fails to generate any kind of dramatic unity. Occasionally the loyal fan may wait for the proverbial last inning stand in which the home team overcomes a lead ineptly allowed the visitors in earlier frames, but even this drama is experienced more for itself than as the culmination of many meaningful events leading up to this singular climax of controlled violence. The lack of continuity between the preparation and the climax is all too apparent, and it becomes even more so as viewed on television. Contrast it with a goal line stand in the final seconds of a football game. Who will forget that quarterback sneak of Bart Starr in the last NFL championship game, played on a frozen field, after two prior attempts had failed? Kramer found footing and blocked his man, allowing Starr to penetrate by the distance of half a yard. Twenty-two men were involved in the single action that capped the previous fifty-nine minutes of continuous struggle. The game would have been as beautiful had Dallas's line held; only the irrational support of one team over the other could have changed the character of that game, but then the heroes and the goats would have changed names.

If my observations, though limited, are sufficient to point out one of the differences in appeal between baseball and football (that the action of the one game is diffuse, badly articulated, and rarely climaxing as opposed to the continuous, tightly structured, and usually climaxing action of the other), some ground would have been gained for understanding the greater spectator appeal in the more dramatic game. I propose in what follows to treat my subject from another point of view. I should like to examine the conditions under which the game itself is a vehicle of creative physical activity, akin to that expended in the production and experience of any bona fide work of art.

Such terms as the "superior dramatic action" of the football game over the baseball game may lead one to suspect that the aesthetic properties of athletic contests are to be explained by metaphor or, what amounts to the same thing, by application of a model taken from another context—here, dramatic literature—where the use of the terms is more clearly understood. Such was not my intent. I have referred to the "dramatic action" of competitive sport only to assert for those who have not yet perceived it that the action of organized sports is capable of highly dramatic action. True fans, who are aware of the dramatic content of their sporting events, need no such explanation. What they may lack is a clear understanding of the manner in which those memorable games have achieved the aesthetic character which made them memorable. It is to those fans I now address my efforts.

If I were to use a model of a completely developed aesthetic activity which is understood on its own terms, my choice would not be of a totally dissimilar medium, such as dramatic literature, which works its wonders by the articulation of words and by their meanings, but by the similar medium of dance: human effort expended in kinaesthetic response to the growing needs of a physical situation. In dance, of course, the situation and the responses are mutually determinant and self-contained. My argument will be that competitive sport is capable of the same kind of development, that the sporting event, at its best, is the one which achieves the same sort of mutual determinancy and self-containedness as the most abstract of dance. The "drama" of the sport may indeed produce a more effectively expressive vehicle than what is usually achieved in dance.

The effect of dance, like that of any other art form, is the effect of abstraction. This means only that to make a work of art one needs a medium. Music became an art when sounds were controlled to produce meaningful sequences; painting, when line was used to delineate a form and colored pigments were used to create space tensions. The artwork appears when someone perceives the effects of moving such physical things as sounds, marks, and color pigments out of one context, where they are aesthetically insignificant, into another where they achieve a new interest to perception in a freely created, purely aesthetic context. That the dance itself is rather poorly understood as an art medium is easily grasped, because of the difficulty in our perceiving the abstraction. The dancer moves his body, but so do streetwalkers and ball players; he uses the gestures and movements of his physiological and kinesiological substructure which are already implicit in the acts of walking or swimming or running. If the balletic gesture does nothing more than incorporate our basic bodily movements without an added significance to its occurrence in the aesthetic context, the choreographer or the performing dancer has failed in his task of successful abstraction. For the moment it is sufficient to understand that the medium of the dance and the medium of the sporting event are the same. That is the reason for their comparison.

In another place[1] I have attempted to show the continuous abstraction of human movement from its everyday context, such as walking, stretching, and the like, into the "pure" movements of a creative dance. The abstractive hierarchy runs as follows: at the base is our bodily presence in the natural environment, in which we always move from here to there. The "here" is defined as the center of our own bodily schemata; the "there" may be anything: an object to be grasped or avoided. Under the impulse of our own needs and desires we may wish to kick it, caress it, or merely move it out of the way. Given the necessary sensory-motor coordination we can ordinarily do any of these things. But even at this rather mundane level of human locomotor experience, we may effectuate an abstraction. Having learned to walk to achieve our ends of living, we may begin to play with our motor responses. Here, rather than achieving an end, the activity itself may be changed from means to end. I may walk because I enjoy walking, or I may walk in such a way as to develop a distinctive style of walking.

Whereas walking for the pleasure of walking may develop my muscles or keep them in tone, walking for a distinctive style may develop what traditional aestheticians have always called "grace." It is the abortion of this ideal in the provocative woman's walk which makes her rolling bottom appear obscene, not its invitation to carnal knowledge, which cannot be obscene. When grace is reduced to provocation, the movement is no longer a successful abstraction, being a call to the achievement of another kind of concrete goal. As long as we merely

contemplate the move without entering into its enticement, it may retain the discriminable aesthetic quality I have already named; it is merely provocative. But even they who are incapable of the necessary "aesthetic distance" and accept the proffered gambit to engage in the act of love may yet achieve successful aesthetic abstraction. It suffices to separate the act from its normal consequences, an immediate pleasure or pain and the procreation of the race, to find oneself in possession of a "new" artistic medium, the gentle art of coupling, than which no medium is more powerful in the creation and release of psychic tension, climaxing into a moment of peace. It matters little whether we refer to the medium as the art of making love or as the dance of life; the beauty of it is already apparent in the courting gyrations of birds.

The rhythms of sexual gymnastics would be an odd place to look for a model of sporting aesthetics. Not even the bad joke of referring to lovemaking as America's most popular indoor sport could make the comparison profitable. More to the point, however, is the manner in which the creation and release of psychic tension becomes qualitatively one; or, to put the matter in another way, how man's need for violent activity is expressed in a context in which the partner is not destroyed, but edified in and through the experience. The conventionality or the artificiality added to the natural context allows this expression and develops what is distinctively human. I have already referred to the controlled expression of violence as "the moral equivalent of war," and we are constantly being reminded of this fact by all those protest buttons proclaiming that one ought to "Make LOVE not WAR." The slogan makes sense, but how can you get the generals to see that it does? Or the country parsons, for that matter?

Starting with basic human movements engaged in to achieve a natural goal or end, we may come to understand that the order of significance achievable in this way is "natural"; it grows out of the coordination of our bodies to the achievement of natural ends. Developing grace and learning to experience the aesthetics of love are merely two low-order abstractions on this kind of movement, and man possesses this ability in common with all other natural life forms.

A higher order of significance is reached when physical coordination is related to artificially set goals. Here the significance is "conventional." Man has developed a real taste for playing with his motor responses—for distraction, for the maintenance of physical well-being, or for the moral and aesthetic experiences which play, in its most successful forms, affords. We all know the story: terrains are laid out, rules adopted, equipment standardized. The aim is to perform a physical act with the highest possible degree of efficiency. Significance is attained relative to the attainment of the goal.

Unfortunately for many of our aesthetic interests, this significance is often measured in quantitative terms, and thus in terms of winning or losing. So many points conventionally assigned to the prescribed ways of scoring have often led to ignoring the qualitative aspects of the experience itself. But win or lose, the players must perform their allotted tasks in a specific manner; and all the niceties of movement over and above the strict necessity of scoring—and thus of winning or losing—have come to be called "form." Consider the judging of divers or figure skaters; consider also the graceful movements of a powerful batter—Ted Williams was one—who always looks good with a bat in his hands, even while striking out. This same sort of grace can become the object of the physical performance, as it does in synchronized swimming and team calisthenics. In addition to providing the controlled release of violence, such sports as the latter are capable of producing elaborate visual and spatial configurations of no mean attraction.

Dance is merely the last of the hierarchic series of abstractive human movements. The context created is still artificial, yet not conventional (except for the ballet, which never really achieved its independence from music). I prefer to call the meaning of the dance "auto-significance," intending that expression to refer to the fact that any movement of the dance which achieves any kind of significance at all does so by virtue of the relationship it bears to other movements in the context, considered as both means and end of the kinaesthetic expression. All the significance of the dance is internal to the dance. It may englobe many gestures imitative of everyday human locomotive patterns and even subhuman as well; but the significance of such representational elements is seriously modified for their incorporation into the balletic context. It is not sufficient, for example, for a choreographer to tell his performers to go out and make like a bird or to imitate the actions of a child playing hopscotch; it is the total dance which determines the significance of each of the parts.

Can this model of the self-contained, auto-significant balletic context be applied to our previous understanding of the aesthetic effect of athletic contests? Two considerations are necessary in order to grasp my contention that it can. First, the winning or the losing of the game is irrelevant to its aesthetic evaluation. An honest tie—one which results from an attempt on the part of opposing teams to win—is not therefore an absolute indicator of the failure to achieve aesthetic quality in the performance. Coaches like Parseghian, formerly of Notre Dame, and Peterson, formerly of Florida State, had something else in mind when they decided to play for a tie instead of for victory. Fans with an aesthetic interest can only be disappointed by the calculated decision to accept the tie; even though there is some doubt about the kicker's ability to make the field goal, the decision to go for it instead of for the touchdown which would win the game (as Florida State did against Penn State in the Gator Bowl) is always an anticlimax.

Even when the kicker succeeds, the game itself merely peters out into insignificance. With that decision, the "drama" of the game was lost even if the game itself was not. Thus, although the winning or losing of the game is aesthetically irrelevant, the desire to win is never aesthetically irrelevant.

Besides, the game is made an aesthetic event by the opposition of strength in the wills to win. But desire itself is not sufficient for the highly dramatic sporting event. In any game defined by the opposition of power, skill, and determination in its players, the power and skill cannot be lacking. Expansion teams of professional football and baseball are not aesthetically effective because they can offer no successful competition to the older, more established teams in their respective leagues. They may, of course, succeed in compensating for a lack of power and skill by a superabundance of determination and still participate effectively in the production of an aesthetically meaningful contest of purpose. Worth is still measured in terms of "how you play the game." Playing for a tie is cheating the public.

The second consideration necessary for the understanding of aesthetic quality in sporting events is a point taken from general aesthetic theory. It concerns media and their use to establish significant contexts we call works of art. Someone may have assumed that the previous discussion of abstraction would imply that there are no successful representational art works. This would be a misunderstanding of the process of creation. Some works, and very good ones at that, are highly representational.

But no matter how imitative certain of the discriminable elements within the aesthetic context happen to be, the worth of that work is not measurable in terms of the accuracy of representation. If this were the case, the best painting would be the one which most effectively pictured the events of nature and hardly any so-called "serious" music could be considered beautiful at all.

The truth of the matter is that all works of art are abstract in the sense indicated above—that their significance is perceivable only in the context in which they appear, in spite of the fact that the artist must artificially construct this context out of what he already knows and feels about the things he must work with as a medium and, if he chooses to represent objects of nature, about them as well. All his knowledge and skill, all the materials and technological means of expression at his disposal constitute the initial context from which he is to abstract his significance by manipulating the materials of his craft. Whence the term "transformation"[2] to describe the activity of the artist; he creates by transforming existing materials into something uniquely significant.

Dances too may be non-objective, producing no recognizable natural movement or object; or they may be interpretative and include them. We call the first "surface" expressions; the second "depth" expressions. The term "surface" refers to the organized sensuous features of the experience; and "depth" to recognizable images, ideas, or objects represented in the organization of the surface patterns. Since the value of the depth expressions is not to be found in the accuracy of representation, it can be found only in the tense relationship between expressing surface and expressed depth. Call that "tension" or "total expressiveness" of the artwork in question.

Making aesthetic judgments on works of art, then, proceeds from our attempts to perceive the qualitative relatedness of surface or of surface and depth "counters" (anything discriminable within the context). When we feel the expressiveness of the related counters, we are experiencing the expressive quality of the piece in question. Such judgments are made daily on creative dances. Can the same be done for our perception of the qualitative uniqueness of games?

The answer is obvious: yes, if we can isolate the relevant counters of the experience. And this is a matter of perceiving the tensions where they occur. In baseball it is the continuing struggle between pitcher and successive batters which mounts with runners on the bases and

is qualified by the intermittent tensions between runners and throwers. But, as pointed out before, these tensions fund into qualitative uniqueness slowly, discontinuously, and hardly ever in a meaningful climax. The game of baseball is at best a summation of innings in which the change of offensive and defensive strategies tends to break the continuity of the action. This is possible in football too. But the rules of the game have been set up to maintain aesthetic quality—and hence spectator interest. A change from defensive to offensive strategy in football is allowed by the interception of passes, in which the defensive player himself assumes the offensive; in the recovery of fumbles; and in effective punting, which may put a whole offensive squad on the defensive if the ball may be downed within the five-yard line. The tempo and rhythm of the game are defined in terms of the building up and the release of dynamic tensions, created ultimately by the opposition of equally capable teams.

Controlled violence in which the opponent is not destroyed, but only defeated, and yet somehow morally edified—such is the essence of competitive sport. It reaches its aesthetic heights when the victor narrowly surpasses a worthy opponent. The game itself considered as an aesthetic object is perceived as a tense experience in which pressure is built up from moment to moment, sustained through continuous opposition, until the climax of victory or defeat. The closer this climax occurs to the end of the game, the stronger is our feeling of its qualitative uniqueness. Sudden death playoffs—and perhaps extra-inning games—are as close as a sport may come to achieving this aesthetic ideal.

We are now in a position to evaluate the possibilities of sport to produce aesthetic experiences. To make the point we may summarize the way in which "significance" is achieved within the levels of abstraction discernible in distinctively human locomotive contexts.

At the most basic level, significance is achieved merely by ordering our bodily existence in accordance with the ends imposed upon it by the natural environment and dominated by biological necessity. We have all learned to walk, run, or swim to increase our control of the conditions of our existence, which is often eked out against a hostile environment. Thus, sometimes with the help of the physical environment and sometimes against its tendency to thwart our growth, we learn to fulfill our vital needs. At this level of experience the possibilities of aesthetic perception are already multiple: we may abstract from the necessity to achieve a particular goal and focus on the movement pattern employed in its achievement, thereby developing "natural" grace. This is recognized as much for its maximum efficiency—the greatest amount of result for the least effort—as for the "beauty" of its execution. The feeling of being at one with nature, using it to fulfill our own aims with consummate ease, is a direct aesthetic response of the mover to his motion.

But there is another mode of abstraction possible even at this level of human experience. I have used the provocative walk to illustrate the point. He who gives in to the provocation is once again acting to fulfill a basic human and biological need. We may once more abstract from the naturally imposed end—the propagation of our species or the experience of pleasure as the outcome of the act—and concentrate upon the pattern of significance which develops between the dynamic tensions in the sexual drama, which would remain totally devoid of meaning without the building up and release of psychic tension through mutually determinant masculine and feminine movement sequences. Any pleasure which is not just attendant upon the act must be the consciousness of the many kinaesthetic gestures funding to make up the act. Each act of love is qualitatively unique and aesthetically recognizable for the manner in which it creates tensions, releases them, and terminates in ultimate peace. In their intimate dance of life, the partners to the act create a new human entity: the couple, which is still the basis for the continued existence of our species.

Dissatisfaction with their respective roles in the creation of this entity—due in part to inadequate physical and mental preparation, but in part as well to the failure to perceive its aesthetic aspects—has led many a married person to seek its artificial dissolution in divorce. Because of the religious and moral prejudices placed upon the significance of the act of love, we may never as educators be allowed to participate in any form of physical instruction devised to maximize the attainment of this sort of aesthetic value. Older, more primitive societies do, and their members are quite obviously better adapted to the sexual conditions of life.

My aim, in the pursuit of this example, was not to shock or even to astound, but rather, to point out that even at this level of abstraction the process of humanly-directed, conscious bodily movements is capable of a high degree of aesthetic perfection in which the performers and the performance cannot be differentiated.

The same, of course, is true of the dance, which is not less dramatic for being less sexual in explicit expression. Competitive sporting events are somewhat like the dance and somewhat like an act of love. Like the dance, the athletic competition is defined in terms of the artificiality of its goals; like an act of love, the athletic competition represents an expression of human violence undergone under conditions of control in which the partner or opponent is not destroyed, but morally or humanly edified. Unlike the dance, however, the athletic medium is not "pure." The game does not create its own goals as kinaesthetic responses unfold; rather, these are imposed upon the participants by the rules of the game. To be an aesthetic event, therefore, the athletic contests must within the limits of the rules set down for the game become a unique context of dramatically significant tensional wholes. This it does by building up tension, sustaining and complicating it, and ultimately releasing the percipient into the state of peace. Well-played, i.e., successfully played, games and they alone succeed in this aesthetic ideal.

To abstract from the conventional goal of the game—to win—means only that the manner of playing the game is aesthetically predominant; and skill, power, and desire to win are the factors determining the manner in which the game is played. Thus it has been truthfully said (at least from the aesthetic point of view) that "It matters not whether you win or lose; it's how you play the game."

Unlike the dance, however, the medium of the sporting event cannot be totally abstracted from a pre-existent aim. The dancer or choreographer creates his end in making the dance, within which the performers (their activities) and the performance are one. The form of the game is always more concrete in that, although winning or losing may be irrelevant to its aesthetic significance, the desire to win may never be excluded as one of the determinants of the action. It is for this reason that aesthetic connoisseurs look down their noses at coaches like Notre Dame's Parseghian and Florida State's Peterson. In their calculated decisions to play for ties, they, on one occasion at least, have put the requirement of not losing over the aesthetic ideal of the well-played game.

Lastly, in order to motivate my phenomenological reading of the essence of sporting aesthetics, I have speculated that the declining popularity of baseball in face of the growing interest in football is explicable in aesthetic terms—that the game (or aesthetic product of the one) is inferior in marshalling the aesthetic interest of its viewers.

One point in the foregoing description remains all too sketchy. I refer to the ontological and psychoanalytical commitments in such phrases as "the psychic and moral edification" of the participants in sporting events. For the necessary connections between our existential concept of the body, or consciousness-body, as a "bodily schema" or "bodily image" and the self-creation of the human personality, I can do no better than refer the interested reader to the phenomenological psychoanalytical work of Eugène Minkowski. Two of his central notions, the creative imagination and spontaneity of movement, are contained in articles translated as "Imagination?" and "Spontaneity (. . . spontaneous movement like this!)" found in a recent anthology of readings in existential phenomenology.[3] His point of view on the creation of personality through movement would be necessary for a complete account of aesthetic creation through sensory-motor coordination. We need only keep in mind that any creative artist forms his own personality *qua* artist by transforming his experiences, through significant abstraction, into works of art; and in the arts utilizing human movement as a medium of expression, there is no distinction between the performer and his performance. But a complete account of the communication of aesthetic value through a sporting event was deemed too extravagant a task to be placed upon this author, who chose merely to explain the nature of the aesthetic qualities of a sporting event.

Minkowski's method as well as my own is distinctively phenomenological. His remarks are relevant to an understanding of the way in which the creative locomotor event is performed; mine, to the way in which the sensitive viewer responds to the event as performed. The middle ground, of course, is the event itself. I have only interpreted the rising and falling fortunes of two of our professionalized sports, along with the disgust on the part of some recent football fans at recurring decisions on the part of collegiate coaches to play a game for a tie. Both of these phenomena are meaningful in view of the description given the aesthetic ideal of sporting events, that of the "well-played game."

The beauty of motion referred to as "grace" in the descriptions above is possible at all levels of human motility. For the higher purposes of expressiveness in the dance or of maximal tension in competitive sports it is usually considered of only secondary interest: it represents the exploitation of skill for skill's sake alone. Like the virtuosity of a musical performer, however, that sport technique is the best which is noticed the least.

Give us more coaches who are willing to put their jobs and reputations on the line by going for the well-played game. Let us at least try to go out and win one for the Gipper, who has become in spite of the legend a symbol of the aesthetically dissatisfied sports fan.

NOTES

1. See my "Being in the Body" in the NAPCEW Report *Aesthetics and Human Movement* (Washington, D. C., 1964), pp. 84-103.
2. Cf. its use by Roger Fry in *Transformations* (Garden City, N. Y.: Doubleday Anchor Books, 1956).
3. See Lawrence and O'Connor, eds., *Readings in Existential Phenomenology* (Englewood Cliffs, N. J.: Prentice-Hall, 1967), pp. 75-92, 168-177.

Languages of Sport: Representation

TERENCE J. ROBERTS

That sport "can mean" and on occasion "does have meaning," in a full sense of the term, is not an easy matter for us to accept. When we rely on our common prescientific understanding of the concept of meaning, it is unproblematic that natural language has the capacity "to mean," and, when used appropriately, does indeed "have meaning." We continue to linguistically communicate without any more than our unreflective understanding of the meaning of "meaning" or how it is that language can mean what it does mean when it does mean. Yet, with only our prescientific understanding of meaning and the capacity to mean, an ability often held in reserve for language alone, to say that sport *can* and *does mean* is to jar our sensibilities and to effectively force us to advance beyond our prescientific understanding of the matter.

The impetus and theoretical backdrop of not only the ensuing treatment of the problem, but the very formulation of the problem itself is provided by Nelson Goodman's *Languages of Art.* Through a systematic examination of the symbol systems found in or constituting each, Goodman shows up the common ground of language and art and the source of their capacity to mean.[1] Goodman argues that if we are to achieve a comprehensive grasp of the varieties and functions of symbols, the modes and means of reference, and of their use in and affect on, the operations of the understanding, we must augment our investigations of linguistics with an inten-

sive examination of non-verbal systems. (3:p. xi) This Goodman accomplishes exceedingly well by exposing the nature of many art related non-verbal symbol systems ranging from pictorial representation and expression to musical notation. Employing the same tactic, the present investigation hopes to shed some light on the question of sport's capacities as a bearer of meaning and, consequently, on our understandings of it, by examining the possibilities and ramifications of regarding sport in terms of employed or constitutive symbol systems. Due to demands of time and space, the present paper must restrict its attention to but one mode of reference or symbolism to be found in sport, that of representation as it is found in the sport fake.[2]

It might be wondered why the sport fake merits as much philosophic attention as it is about to receive. Although no one would deny the prevalence of such deceptions in sport and their practical importance to it, their philosophic import is not readily apparent. Yet, wherever and whenever sport fakes are to be found so are symbols: to fake is to employ symbols deceptively; to be faked is to "misread" symbols; to perceive a fake as a fake is to ignore certain symbols while concentrating on others more reliable. Where symbols exist so most often do the attendant meanings that are referred to, stood for or represented by the symbols. Thus, to talk of sport fakes is to talk of symbols is to talk of meaning. If further insight into meaning in or of sport can be gleaned from an examination of the sport fake, then the philosophical relevance of the phenomenon becomes quite apparent.

The question is: Is the sport fake a representation? That is, can the sport fake be viewed as representational in the same or similar way in which some paintings can be said to "represent" that which they are paintings of? Does the same relationship exist between a fake and the "actual" play (which it is deceptively passed off for) as exists between a painting and what it represents? Following a treatment of those questions, the focus shall shift to an examination of some of the implications of viewing the sport fake as representational. By examining the opportunities it provides for artistic-like creativity and the extent or fullness of meaning it can have, the importance of representation in sport to sport's import, meaning and significance shall be more clearly understood.

In paving the way for his own technical theory of representation, Goodman promptly discards three traditional, "simple-minded" accounts: the resemblance, copy and deception theories of representation. Indeed, Goodman's refutations are incisive and perhaps prove fatal to the theories' longevity in the realm of art. Yet, because of a vital difference between the sport fake and the art representation, a difference which mandates the refashioning of the rejected theories into a more consistent, interdependent whole, it will be demonstrated that the sport fake can indeed be understood in terms of them.

The most naive view of representation, so Goodman postulates, is of the opinion that: "'A represents B if and only if A appreciably resembles B' or 'A represents B to the extent that A resembles B'." (3:p.3) Due to the existence of some counterexamples, where resemblance is present in the absence of representation, or the converse of that, Goodman criticizes that resemblance is neither a sufficient nor a necessary condition of representation.[3] Theoretically that may very well be true and is not to be questioned here.[4] Yet, Goodman's injunction is a theoretical one concerning representation in general and, although perhaps quite true, it does not mitigate the fact that for certain practical reasons, resemblance is at least important, if not vital, to a great number of representations. That is, although resemblance may not be a necessary nor a sufficient condition of any representation, because of the practical ways in which they are employed, certain representations are nonetheless somewhat dependent upon it.

Imagine the length of a portrait painter's career if his productions did not resemble his subjects to an "appreciable degree."[5] This is not news to Goodman. Nor does it do much, if any, damage to his position. All that is being asserted here is that, in spite of the fact that resemblance and representation are theoretically independent, not only are they regularly found in association, but, for practical reasons, are often necessarily so conjoined.[6]

A similar case can be made for the performance of effective sport fakes; resemblance between fake and "actual" is a practical necessity. Whether by accident, incompetence or foolishness, the performance of a "fake" which failed to resemble the relevant features of the "actual" play to an "appreciable" degree would prove ineffectual. No matter how often an offensive football squad flawlessly performed their rendition of the "fake" dive play by jumping in unison three times up and down, and no matter how often they patiently explained that such a "fake" was a theoretically legitimate representation of the "actual" dive play, no defensive squad would ever be misled.

One of the great benefits of Goodman's rejection of resemblance is that it handily escapes the sticky problem of determining the degree of resemblance necessary before "representation" can be legitimately employed. What is an "appreciable" degree of resemblance? There are no objective methods of measuring degrees of resemblance, nor any absolute standards to be employed in determining whether resemblance even holds between particular objects. Depending on the criteria employed, a painting can be said to both resemble and not resemble the object it is a painting of. Even a portrait that is generally agreed to be a remarkable likeness of the subject does not likely resemble that person with respect to such criteria as temperature, texture, weight, three-dimensionality and so on. But if these criteria are not important, which are and why? And if these "important ways" objects or events resemble each other can be determined, to what extent must they be satisfied? To calmly assert: "to an appreciable degree" is merely to "question beg" and push the solution one step beyond.

One attempt at providing some such solution is made by the proponents of the "copy theory of representation" who suggest: "To make a faithful picture, come as close as possible to copying the object just as it is." (3:p.6) As Goodman points out, however, such a position is paralyzed by the fact that an object can at any one time be perceived or described in a variety of ways. Thus, ". . . the object before [one] is a man, a swarm of atoms, a complex of cells, a fiddler, a friend, a fool, and much more." (3:p.6) "But," he says, "if all are ways the object is, then none is *the* way the object is. I cannot copy all these at once; and the more nearly I succeeded, the less would the result be a realistic picture." (3:p.6) If all of the ways an object looks cannot be simultaneously copied, then it must be one of them. But which one? Pressed further, the copy theorist might respond: ". . . the object is to be copied as seen under aseptic conditions by the free and innocent eye." (3:p.7) But Goodman, following on the heels of Gombrich, denies the existence of the innocent eye:

> The eye comes always ancient to its work, obsessed by its own past and by old and new associations of the ear, nose, tongue, fingers, heart and brain. It functions not as an instrument self-powered and alone, but as a dutiful member of a complex and capricious organism. Not only how but what it sees is regulated by need and prejudice. (3:pp.7-8)[7]

What is to be copied and to what extent? What is an "appreciable" degree of resemblance? What both the copy and resemblance theories lack is a criterion by which we can determine minimally required degrees of copying and resemblance, by which we can determine the lower limits for what is to be resembled, copied and to what degrees. If the sport fake is to be instructively viewed in terms of either or both the resemblance and copy theories, some effort must be made to uncover a criterion which helps to decide what and to what extent the effective fake copies and/or resembles.

Ironically enough, Goodman supplies the context within which that criterion exists. If, as he suggests, the percipient is so preconditioned to perceive what he perceives, then it would seem that the representative painter, if communicative, cannot go about his work with a total disregard for his audience. He must be somewhat aware of their general perceptual habits, tendencies and abilities to associate representations with the represented. A completely private symbol system would draw no one but himself back from the "representation" to the thing intended to be represented. In this sense, successful (i.e., communicative) pictorial representation presupposes, or shows forth, a unique communion between artist and viewer. To an even greater extent are the por-

trait painters and the performers of sport fakes bound to the perceptual experiences, habits and limitations of their viewers. They literally cannot afford to produce "representations" which draw no one but themselves back to the object intended to be represented. Although the communicative context of percipient dependence within which the criterion operates has been established, the actual criterion has yet to be uncovered and is best shown up through an examination of the deception theory of representation.

The deception theory of representation is of the opinion ". . . that a picture is realistic to the extent that it is a successful illusion, leading the viewer to suppose that it is, or has the characteristics of, what it represents." (3:p.34) Accordingly, to the degree the percipient is led to exhibit responses or have expectations identical or similar to those he normally would have upon the perception of the "actual" object or event is the degree to which the representation is judged successful. But Goodman argues that even effective likenesses in painting, when viewed as bordered by a frame and hanging in the context of a gallery, are incapable of being confused with what is represented. (3:p.35) That is, in the arts, real deception is virtually precluded.

Yet, because of one fundamental difference between art representations and sport fakes, Goodman's criticisms of the deception theory do not mitigate the theory's efficacy for the latter. Representational paintings are usually of objects or events in the world *outside of themselves*, outside of painting or paintings, of a different realm, so to speak. In marked contrast, sport fakes are of events also *in* sport, internal to the sport, and thus of the *same realm*. Put simply, most representational paintings are of such things as apples, landscapes and people and not of other paintings. But for obvious reasons, sport fakes must be fakes of other sport events and to be effective can take no events external to sport to be their objects.

Further, where the representation and the represented are of different realms, the materials which constitute the representation are quite different from those which constitute the represented. That is, it is not chunks of apple, but blobs of paint that plaster the canvas of an apple painting. Conversely, when representation and represented are of the same realm, the materials which constitute each are quite similar. Quite obviously, paintings of paintings, like the paintings they are paintings of, are made of paint. And fake dive plays, like the dive plays they are fakes of, are composed of the same sorts of human movements in certain temporal and spatial relations.

The upshot of these fundamental differences in realms and constitutive materials is, that, unlike the confusion-precluding "gallery" conditions within which representational paintings are viewed, because they are of the same realm and are constituted by the same or similar materials, there are no conditions existing prior to or concurrent with the perception of a fake play which preclude the possibility of confusing it with the "actual" play. Analogous to the sporting case would be a painting of a painting painted on a gallery wall. Although bizarre, such a painting would be of the same realm and constitutive materials as that which it is a painting of. Consequently, and as is the case with the sport fake, no longer would the possibility of confusing the two be precluded. And where confusion can exist, deception can flourish.

In addition, the temporal context within which most representational paintings are viewed virtually eliminates the chance of deception. Seldom, if ever, do any immediately pressing decisions depend on the viewer's determinations as to whether what he sees is representation or "actual" object. His decision is usually an end in itself, made under no temporal restrictions and he is often at his leisure to consider all the relevant details: he can view the representation (or "actual" object) from several angles and distances, examine it under different intensities of light and even consult his colleagues. In short, he can delay his decision until all the evidence is in.

But the athlete must operate in a radically different temporal context. He is not at his leisure. His decision between fake and "actual" is not an end in itself. Effective action, not perception alone, is the end he seeks and his effectiveness depends not merely on his correct perceptions or fakes, but on his appropriate counteractions. Because fakes and what they are fakes of are of a realm where time is crucial, the athlete's perceptions occur within stringent temporal restrictions. In an instant, he must perceive, decide, act. He cannot delay for the arrival of all information and is often forced to act on the scantiest evidence. If he did delay, his determinations between fake plays and "actual" plays would probably be correct, but all effective action would be precluded and he would remain strangely contemplative at mid-field.

Given these temporal exigencies coupled with the identity of realm and constitutive materials, the possibility of deception looms large. Goodman's criticism that deception seldom exists in art is not applicable to sport; deception there is possible and actual. Because the athlete has so little time to determine between two sets of events occurring in identical perceptual contexts, and composed of identical elements, there is every possibility he can be deceived into thinking the "actual" is or is about to occur when it actually is not or will not. That is the very measure of a fake's success.

The resemblance and copy theories of representation have now been supplied with the necessary criterion: deception. The sport fake's reason for being (i.e., deception) cannot be accomplished unless it resembles the "actual" play to an "appreciable" degree. Quite simply, an "appreciable" degree of resemblance is the degree of resemblance necessary to produce an effective deception, that is, where the opponent is led to exhibit the same responses and expectations as he would have upon perceiving the "actual." Thus, the degree of resemblance necessary is ultimately determined through the reactions of one's opponents, through an understanding of their perceptual habits and tendencies. And that is gained primarily by trial and error, by experience. Similarly, with respect to the copy theory of representation, one should copy those aspects of the "actual" the copying of which results in the most effective deception. And again, knowledge of that is to be gained through trial and error.

It can be concluded, then, that despite the resemblance, copy and deception theories' inadequacies as explanations of representation in the arts, they do prove effective in coming to understand the sport fake as representation. Because of the peculiar context within which sport fakes are performed and viewed, deception is a real possibility. The conjoining of the criterion of deception with the resemblance and copy theories thereby renders them immune to Goodman's criticisms; that is to say, as accounts of the sport fake, they can no longer be rejected for the reasons Nelson Goodman gives.

But the case may even be stronger than the above argument would suggest in that the sport fake can perhaps be viewed in terms of Goodman's own highly regarded theory of representation as well. For Goodman, the notion of *denotation* lies at the center of representation, and is the key to understanding it:

The plain fact is that a picture, to represent an object, must be a symbol for it, stand for it, refer to it; and that no degree of resemblance is sufficient to establish the requisite relationship of reference. Nor is resemblance necessary for reference; almost anything may stand for almost anything else. A picture that represents —like a passage that describes—an object refers to and, more particularly, *denotes* it. Denotation is the core of representation and is independent of resemblance. (3:p.5)

Although Goodman nowhere provides an exact account of what "denotation" is or means, it is here assumed that he understands it in no idiosyncratic manner. What *is* idiosyncratic about Goodman's *use* of "denotation," however, is its expanded range of application. What has traditionally been a linguistic concept is now being pressed into pictorial service. The result is that the relation between pictures and what they represent has been assimilated within the reference relation existing between predicates and what they apply to.(3:p.5)

In order for the sport fake to be a representation, in Goodman's sense of the term, it must now be demonstrated that the sport fake not only resembles the "actual" play, but refers to (i.e., denotes) it as well. Once again it is Goodman who supplies the key: by including the pantomime within the denotative realm he supplies all the artillery needed.

> The action of a mime . . . is not usually among the actions it denotes. He does not climb ladders or wash windows but rather portrays, represents, denotes, ladder-climbings and window-washings by what he does. (3:pp.63-64)

By the same token: The action of a quarterback while faking is not usually among the actions it denotes. When faking he does not throw passes or make hand-offs but rather portrays, represents, denotes, pass-throwing and hand-off-making by what he does. While their purposes differ, the observable behavior of the mime and the faking quarterback seem to be of the same form. While the mime aims to portray and the quarterback aims to deceive by his portrayals, both do indeed portray and employ the same sorts of movements to do it. If requested to perform his rendition of a quarterback passing, a mime would attempt to recapture in movement all those motions important to the actual throwing of a pass. But that is precisely what a quarterback endeavors to do when he fakes an "actual" pass.[8] Thus, if it is reasonable to view the mime's actions as denotative and therefore, representational, for the same reasons the quarterback's fake

pass can be said to denote and consequently to represent the "actual" pass.[9]

The argument is technically complete. The sport fake can be viewed as a representation both in terms of the resemblance, copy and deception theories and also in terms of Goodman's denotational theory. That, in itself, is an important accomplishment. But what of sport's capacity as a bearer of meaning? In the early paragraphs it was suggested that the philosophical importance of the sport fake lay in its capacity to provide further insight into meaning in or of sport and consequently, expand our understanding of it. The argument that the sport fake is a legitimate instance of representation must now be related to this larger question of meaning.

Sport Representation: Implications for Creativity and Meaning

Because its reason for being is to deceive, the sport fake, unlike the art representation, can represent no object or event external to the sport of which it is a part. Neither can it represent that which it does represent in a non-resembling fashion. That is, the sport fake is severely restricted both in *what* it represents and the *ways* in which it can represent. Consequently, and as will be outlined below, the sport fake, as compared with its artistic counterpart, allows little room for artistic-like creativity, and, is decidedly shallow in the range and significance of its meaning.

Surely a portion of the creativity involved in the production of representations is tied to the choice of subject: where choice of subject is extremely limited, so creativity is as well. Since it is the case that each and every sport fake, in order to be effective, must be of a particular event from a limited range of events within the sport of which it is a part, choice of subject is very limited. The events which can be the referents of sport representations are numerically few. Painting, on the contrary, has the entire world at its disposal: it is not restricted to a certain set of selected subjects, but can represent virtually anything it wishes. If pictorial representation was somehow restricted to the portrayal of apples, creativity there, as in the production of sport fakes, would be vastly diminished.

But even if painting was confined to the representation of apples, it would still have available to it much opportunity for creativity in the *ways* in which it could portray. One needs only to reflect on the great variety of ways in which single topics (e.g., the Madonna and Child) have been pictorially represented to realize that is so. But the athlete must deceive. He is therefore bound to the ingrained perceptual habits and tendencies of his viewers and thus to the demands of resemblance. Because he must deceive, he must resemble: he must represent in a certain *way* only. Not only is the performer of sport fakes creatively limited in *what* he can represent, but also in the *ways* in which he can represent it.

To reiterate the above point, it can be seen, in general terms, that the painter, as a maker of representations, attempts to communicate some form of knowledge either by pointing out new relationships or by provoking an increased understanding of that which he represents. Goodman expands:

> Representation . . . is apt, effective, illuminating, subtle, intriguing to the extent that the artist . . . grasps fresh and significant relationships and devises means for making them manifest . . . The marking off of new elements or classes, or of familiar ones by labels of new kinds or by new combinations of old labels may provide new insight . . . In sum, effective representation and description require invention. They are creative. (3:pp.32-33)

In sport, however, the intent of the fake is not to intrigue, illuminate or advance any understanding; rather, it is to deceive. Although a "fake" which is significantly novel may provide new insights that inform its observers, because it no longer employs the same signs in the same ways, it would no longer be an effective deception; in fact, it would not deceive at all. The athlete may indeed have fresh and significant insights into the movements he is attempting to fake, but the more he attempts to make those insights manifest, the more he reduces the play's deceptive effectiveness. The production of novel movement representations is the art of the pantomime and dancer, not the athlete.

Perception and the meaning which accompanies it have histories which influence their present operations. Whatever is perceived is, in varying degrees, colored by what has been perceived and understood before. But creation and invention are vehicles leading out of the past; they are the perceptual shuttlebuses between the familiar and the novel. Deception (at least as it occurs in sport), however, can exist only in the past, amongst all that is familiar; any excursion of any depth into novelty, into the unknown, will result in dinosaurian extinction. As such, invention and creation are deception's enemies, ones whose presence precludes its existence. In order for any fake play to work, it first must be of a familiar "actual" play, and second, it must be performed in such a way that the familiarity is clearly felt by those perceiving the fake. Although it may be a representation in the full sense of the term, it cannot, if successful, be perceived as such; it must be *perceived as and mistaken for* the "actual." Any attempts to be creative, that is, any attempts to perform a fake of a non-familiar play, or perform a fake of a familiar play in a non-familiar way are doomed to be deceptive failures. Thus, to an extent unparalleled in the traditional representational arts, the performance of sport representations, if they are to be successful, are bound to their viewers' perceptual pasts and to the demands of resemblance. But the range of possible movements which can effectively satisfy those demands is very limited. Although the athlete has the opportunity to be creative within those strict limits, and perhaps produce a movement which resembles the "actual" to a degree greater than any that have gone before, within those creatively shallow confines of resemblance he must remain.

When it is the case that representation is restricted to the portrayal of a single object in a single way, its ability to advance understanding, either of the world or even of that particular object is severely limited. With its meaning strictly confined to its own realm, not only can the sport representation (i.e, fake) not refer to anything outside of sport, but it cannot even employ aspects extrinsic to itself as aids to understanding that which it does portray. That is, unlike those of art, the representations of sport are unable to draw upon our vast knowledge of the world to supplement our understandings of the meaning of one particular aspect of it. Consequently, in terms of the significance of meaning, sport representation is very shallow. Despite its symbolic nature, despite its being a "language" of sport, denied all access to external knowledge both in what and how it must represent, sport representation can play but an inconsequential role in our further understanding of sport's significant meaning and import.

Notes

1. Briefly characterized, a symbol system ". . . embraces both the symbols and their interpretation, . . ." (3:p.40n). "A symbol system consists of a symbol scheme correlated with a field of reference."(3:p.143) A symbol scheme

". . . consists of characters, usually with modes of combining them to form others. Characters are certain classes of utterances or inscriptions or marks."(3:p.131)

2. Subsequent papers examining additional modes of reference found in or related to sport will concentrate on expression, notation, and sport and the understanding.

3. Goodman's counter-examples to resemblance as a sufficient condition for representation are presented in the following passage:

"An object resembles itself to the maximum degree but rarely represents itself; resemblance, unlike representation, is reflexive. Again, unlike representation, resemblance is symmetric: B is as much like A as A is like B, but while a painting may represent the Duke of Wellington, the Duke doesn't represent the painting. Furthermore, in many cases neither one of a pair of very like objects represents the other: none of the automobiles off an assembly line is a picture of any of the rest; and a man is not normally a representation of another man, even his twin brother." (3:p.4)

His case against resemblance as a necessary condition for representation is not nearly so thorough, however. He merely states: "Nor is resemblance *necessary* for reference; almost anything may stand for almost anything else." (3:p.5)

4. For criticism of Goodman's position on this issue see James W. Mann's "Representation, Relativism and Resemblance." (8:pp.281-87)

5. It has been objected that Goodman wants to argue that resemblance is as much a matter of fiat as representation; if so, the portraiture example is a poor one. Although there is some truth behind that objection, as presently phrased it is too strong and thus misleading. It is better said that resemblance and representation are both conventional, but the former perhaps to a lesser degree. Indeed Goodman suggests that:

". . . we must beware of supposing that similarity (i.e. 'resemblance') constitutes any firm, invariant criterion of realism; for similarity is relative, variable, culture-dependent. And even where, within a single culture, judgements of realism and of resemblance tend to coincide, we cannot safely conclude that the judgements of realism follow upon the judgements of resemblance. Just the reverse may be at least equally true: that we judge the resemblance greater where, as a result of our familiarity with the manner of representation, we judge the realism greater." (4:p.438)

But somehow resemblance has a firmer grasp on our perceptual habits than does representation. It seems more firmly entrenched. As viewers, we seem much more perceptually agreeable to accept radical innovations in representation but not so agreeable and perhaps blind or completely baffled by "resemblance by fiat." Furthermore, one would not think that Goodman would want to argue that effective resemblance, like effective representation, depends upon invention, creativity, the grasping of fresh and significant relationships and the devising of new means for making them manifest. But it may be the case, as Goodman also suggests, that resemblance follows on the heels of representation:

"Representational customs, which govern realism, also tend to generate resemblance. That a picture looks like nature often means only that it looks the way nature is usually painted . . . Resemblance and deceptiveness, far from being constant and independent sources and criteria of representational practice are in some degree products of it." (4:p.39)

Representations repeated over and again entrench themselves, become common, familiar and perhaps even come to resemble what they represent. Representation and resemblance may thereby eventually become one, but once representation takes another of its creative leaps it leaves resemblance behind. Thus, in spite of its probable conventionality, the entrenchment of resemblance in perception makes it an important, if not necessary consideration in the production of some representations (e.g. portraits).

6. Professor Keith Gunderson, in a lecture given at the University of Minnesota, July 7, 1975, nicely pointed out that merely because a feature or characteristic of something is found to be neither a necessary nor a sufficient condition of that thing, philosophers too often automatically discard it as an unimportant, uninteresting ingredient that merits no further discussion. As Gunderson put it, most garbage cans have openings at the top and most automobiles have combustion engines. Although neither necessary nor sufficient conditions, it would be foolish to discard these features as unimportant to our understanding of the great majority of garbage cans and automobiles. The importance and relationship of resemblance to representation may be of the same nature.

7. The notion of the influence of perceptual pasts on current perception pervades the whole of Gombrich's *Art and Illusion*. See especially part three: "The Beholder's Share." (2:pp. 181-290)

8. The quarterback's fake pass would not often be as elaborate or detailed as a mime's pass portrayal, but that is a difference of degree, not of kind. What it points out again, however, is the different temporal restrictions within which the two enterprises operate.

9. Strictly speaking, it is not entirely appropriate to conclude that because the sport fake is de-

notational it is therefore representational. Although necessary, denotation is not a sufficient condition of representation and must be coupled with syntactic density and relative repleteness, two properties which, in a subsequent paper, will be shown to be characteristic of sport.

Bibliography

1. Adams, E. M. "Lewis, Clarence Irving." *Encyclopedia of Philosophy*. Vol. VII.
2. Gombrich, E. H. *Art and Illusion*. Princeton: Princeton University Press, 1969.
3. Goodman, Nelson. *Languages of Art*. New York: The Bobbs-Merrill Co., 1968.
4. ————. "Seven Strictures on Similarity." *Problems and Projects*. New York: The Bobbs-Merrill Co., 1972.
5. Gunderson, Keith. A lecture on aesthetics presented at the University of Minnesota, Minneapolis, July 7, 1975.
6. Kretzman, Norman. "Semantics, History of" *Encyclopedia of Philosophy*. Vol. VII.
7. Langer, Susanne K. *Philosophy in a New Key*. 3rd ed. Cambridge: Harvard University Press, 1957.
8. Manns, James V. "Representation, Relativism and Resemblance." *British Journal of Aesthetics*. (Summer, 1971), 281-87.
9. *Webster's Seventh New Collegiate Dictionary*. Springfield, Mass.: C. & C. V. Merriam Co., 1971.

A Metacritical Aesthetic of Sport

N. GAYLE WULK

One of the potential meanings of sport lies in the aesthetic realm. Sport theorists and aestheticians are now beginning to examine the nature of the sport aesthetic. Such considerations have heuristic value in that they add a dimension of meaning to sport often overlooked. Any discussion which attempts to increase awareness and add to the depth of potential meanings of sport is, it seems, worth pursuing.

A framework is needed, however, to provide boundaries and discipline to an examination of an aesthetic of sport. Such a structure is offered by the systematic aesthetic theory of Beardsley (1958). Beardsley's theory is clearly and completely developed and, unlike many theories, it attempts to take account of the actual practice of critics. It is only one of many ways of examining the nature of art and the aesthetic experience. But Beardsley does, I feel, offer more because he indicates and emphasizes the logical and reasoning processes utilized in critical practices.

Metacritical Aesthetics

In the late 1950's, Monroe Beardsley suggested that aesthetics be conceived of as a philosophy of criticism. His metacritical theory centered on the perceiver/audience as the focus of the valuational process. He saw aesthetics as consisting of principles which clarify and confirm critical statements.

> I take as central the situation in which someone is confronted with a finished work, and is trying to understand it and to decide how good it is (Beardsley, 1958, p. 6).

Beardsley was concerned with practical criticism and he proposed a theory of evaluation based on a "general criterion theory." Critical reasoning about the arts and aesthetic experiences presupposes general principles upon which judgments about particular objects and experiences deductively depend. Beardsley maintained that a distinctive kind of experience can be isolated and described as an aesthetic experience. He defined this experience as the "immediate effect of aesthetic objects" (Beardsley, 1958, p. 559), and proposed five characteristics of the experience.

1. In an aesthetic experience, attention is fixed on heterogeneous yet interrelated parts of an objective phenomenal field. It is composed of some sensory pattern. There is a central focus, as opposed to the looseness of daydreaming, and the aesthetic object controls the experience.

2. The experience is marked with intensity and a concentration of experience. It marshals "the attention for a time into free and unobstructed channels of experience" (Beardsley, 1958, p. 528).

3. The experience is coherent. It "hangs together" with one thing leading to another, with continuity of development and with an overall sense of pattern and coherence. Even if the experience is interrupted, e.g. intermissions, a re-connection is quickly made with what went before and the audience becomes a part of the experience again.

4. The experience is complete in itself. All expectations and impulses which are aroused

are counterbalanced or resolved by other elements within the experience.

> Because of the highly concentrated, or localized, attention characteristic of aesthetic experience, it tends to mark itself out from the general stream of experience, and stand in memory as a single experience (Beardsley, 1958, p. 528).

5. The aesthetic experience is "not real"; in fact, the question of reality never arises. The experience has the capacity to elicit admiration and contemplation with no need for any commitment to practical action.

These five characteristics were condensed by Beardsley into three elements: unity, complexity and intensity:

The characteristics of coherence and completeness comprise the factor of *unity*. Critical comments dealing with form, organization and logic of structure and style are recognized as statements dealing with the unity of an aesthetic experience.

The *intensity* factor is characterized by critical interpretations dealing with the forcefulness, vividness, beauty and vitality of an experience. Comments indicating tragedy, irony, grace, delicacy, tenderness and comedy are descriptive of the intensity of an experience.

The *complexity* factor deals with the range and diversity of elements within the aesthetic experience. Descriptors of the scale, richness and variety, subtlety and imaginativeness of the experience are common critical statements related to this factor.

These are the three aesthetic-designating factors on which judgments about particular aesthetic experiences and works of art depend. Both the work of art and the experience of it involve some degree of unity, complexity and/or intensity. These factors are connected yet independent and aesthetic experiences differ in magnitude as a function of the three variables.

A Metacritical Aesthetic of Sport

The exhibition in sport of the aesthetic factors of unity, complexity and intensity comprises the matrix which defines a metacritical aesthetic of sport. The identification of this matrix describes the features in sport which delineate aesthetic activity and is intended to locate the aesthetic experience or object of sport for the spectator/audience. A discussion of the features of a metacritical aesthetic of sport matrix follows.

Unity. The aesthetic-designating factor of unity is displayed in sport through spatial and temporal boundaries of performance; through technical skill in performance standards concerned with the efficiency and economy of effort; through the display and evaluation of formal design and expressive qualities; and through the twin concepts of harmony and wholeness.

Sport provides unity by being spatially immediate and temporally recurring. Sport contests are definitely organized and "athletic contests, like dramatic tragedy, are divided into time periods of varying lengths" (Keenan, 1972, p. 13). Both sport and art have rules of performance and unique/special ways of using time and space. For instance, Kostelantz (1973) has proposed that the spatial and temporal rhythm of American football has a definite, repeated configuration. The actions of a contest can be traced as the players are seen to form their offensive and defensive huddles; take their positions at the line of scrimmage; execute their various strategies and regroup in their huddles to plan the next action. Kostelantz has labeled these various stages of action "stasis," "purpose," "passionate pursuit," "chaos" and a return to "stasis." Such plotting of the rhythm of a sport shows the formal, coherent patterns which can be identified.

Performance skill is an aspect of unity. Aesthetic response to sport movement is, according to Lowe (1971), derived from two sources: from an empathic response to the action itself or from individual interpretation of the form, technique and composition of the movement itself. Well-executed movements, which display balance, rhythm, economy of effort, smoothness and flow, yield great aesthetic pleasure for the spectator. The total coordination of body and movement parts is fundamental to skill execution and is basic to aesthetic appreciation (Best, 1975).

Form, of bodies moving and interacting, is displayed in all sport performances. Form in sport is perceived as a sense of pattern and is described in both formal and expressive terms. Formal properties such as balance, symmetry and continuity are often linked with the more expressive descriptors such as dynamic, strong and graceful. A real sense of design can be found in sport and Kupfer (1975) even contended that the form of a sport was an essential reason governing the choice of watching or playing one sport rather than another.

Every aspect of a sport contest is an integral

part of the whole. The aesthetic in movement occurs when the actual or empathic feel and the sport goal of the movement are in harmony (Munrow, 1972). Everything is focused on the achievement of the sport goal and useless motions, which do not contribute to the completeness of the movement skills, detract from the unity, wholeness and grace of the sport performance (Browne, 1917).

There is also a unity or wholeness in sport which is found in the context of the opposition necessary for the sport to take place. Kupfer (1975) suggested that in the tensions between opponents and the coordinations among teammates, individual players come together to form a whole. "Concepts such as timing, jelling, flowing, harmonizing, and executing attest to this aesthetic ideal in competitive sport" (p. 88). In terms of the spectator:

> The wholeness and finality possible in competitive sporting events, paradigmatic in the artistic, answers the human desire for completeness and unity, if only in symbol (Kupfer, 1975, pp. 88-89).

Complexity. Complexity in sport is displayed through the range and diversity among the kinds of sport activities available; through the dramatic concepts of reversal and style; through the many "viewpoints" from which sport can be examined; and through the uniqueness, novelty and spontaneity found in sport actions.

The dramatic aspects of sport offer diversity within the experience. Athletic contests often give rise to the dramatic element of reversal, a sudden change of advantage during the contest. Sport is rich in these moments which vividly contrast victory and defeat in a sudden reversal of action.

The concept of personal style of moving also adds drama and complexity to sport performances. Functional perfection, the mastery of bodily movements, allows the performer to move smoothly and fluidly with appropriate rhythms of tension and relaxation. Once this is achieved, then the performer can "give the movement expressive form which is his own creation, and which is meaning-embodied" (Reid, 1970, p. 250). This is what is meant by style. Sport participants display their own assertion of personality in the style quality of their performance. "This individuality asserts itself even, seemingly, at the highest pitch of perfection which characterizes both art and sport" (Maheu, 1963, p. 32).

Another complexity-producing aspect of

sport is created by rules, boundaries and regulations. The rule-imposed confines and precise geometric spatio-temporal boundaries of sport require invention on the part of the participants. Brown and Gaynor (1967) proposed an action theory of creativity which indicated that creativity will occur during athletic action and that it operates in movement like it acts in other processes. They stated that the competitive sport situation is an arena where confusion and chaos are rampant. Invention, improvisation and experimentation by the participants are necessary for adaptation to the ever-changing vista of a sport situation. "Sport instantiates man's capacity to improvise in the midst of structured stress" (Kupfer, 1975, p. 89). Keenan (1972) has suggested that:

> Perhaps it is the ability to cope with the novel immediately and skillfully which provides us [the spectator] with an aesthetic quality in the athletic contest (p. 5).

Intensity. Intensity in sport performances is shown through the power, beauty and formal aesthetic factors displayed by the skilled human form in sport motion; through the dynamic tensions formed by the flow of movement and the rhythmic, force and spatial/temporal inter-relationships of bodies and body parts; through the risk, virtuosity and originality displayed by the participants; through the dynamic tensions produced by the conflict and the opposition of wills to win; and through the dramatic and emotional responses to the action and the uncertainty of outcome.

Sport is perceptually complex and intense. When the focus is on the beauty of the human form in motion, the efficiency, grace, ease of skilled movement, rhythm, tension, flow and suppleness of the sport performance are critically examined. Kovich (1971) suggested that the performer and spectator can share the intensity of the sport experience by becoming sensitive to the movement elements of space, force and time. The feel of freedom in flight; the rhythm of skilled performance; the precarious balance produced by strength, concentration and control all contribute to the shared intensity of sport. As the athlete experiences the movement in relation to a harmony of sensation, the spectator sees the movement in relation to its rhythm, force and space elements.

Risk, originality and virtuosity intensify the aesthetic experience both visually and experientially (Lowe, 1977). Skilled performances heighten the essence of the experience, enabling the spectator to "see" "the poise of balance, the smoothness of rhythm, the power of a leg leaping, the effort of a muscle taut with strain" (Pavlich, 1966, p. 9).

In a discussion of responses to visual form, Arnheim (1951) proposed that visual forms contain directed tensions. His essay repeatedly mentioned the intensity and strong dynamic effect of the aesthetic response to pictures depicting movement as well as the response to movement itself. Sport builds up, sustains, compounds and releases tensions. The conflict produced by opposing wills to win make the game an aesthetic event (Kaelin, 1968). Through conflicts, collisions of interest, climaxes and Dionysian rituals, sport reveals itself as an extremely intense experience for both the performer and the spectator. Aesthetic values related to the intensity of the experience arise from these human interactions.

Intensity in sport is also related to the dramatic and emotional responses to the action and the uncertainty of outcome. Few would deny that sport has the power to excite and, as in art, excitement attracts attention and adds intensity. Sport requires the total involvement of both spectators and participants, thereby encompassing the whole range of human emotions. The drama and doubt over the final outcome provide dramatic tensions and emotional responses to sport display the full spectrum from joy and excitement to sadness and despair (Pavlich, 1966).

Once the features which designate the metacritical aesthetic matrix of sport are defined, there remains one more step. Dickie (1974), whose aesthetic theories were developed from the basic precepts of Beardsley's metacriticism, indicated that the final step in defining aesthetic activity requires that the object or event "has had conferred upon it the status of candidate for appreciation by some person or persons acting on behalf of a certain social institution" (Dickie, 1974, p. 34).

The designation of an art aesthetic is conferred on behalf of an "artworld" (Dickie, 1974; Danto, 1964). The artworld consists of the loosely organized but interrelated core of persons who are necessary for the continuing existence of the art system. The application to sport is apparent. The conferring of aesthetic status on sport is done on behalf of the "sportworld." The minimum core of the sport situation or sportworld is composed of the athletes, coaches, officials and spectators of sport. Other personnel are also important to the sportworld and should be mentioned. This group includes the sport theorists, reporters, critics and his-

torians. The term, "sportworld," refers then to the broad social institution within which sport situations or contests have their place.

Having defined the social institution, the sportworld, it remains to demonstrate how status is conferred by this institution. The status of candidate for appreciation can be acquired if a single person, acting on behalf of the social institution, treats the activity as aesthetic experience. Therefore, a discussion of sport as aesthetic activity would be sufficient to designate it as such. This paper is presented to designate sport as aesthetic activity. The concepts and terminology of metacritical aesthetic theory have been utilized as the framework within which a sport aesthetic has been described. Many other aesthetic viewpoints can be utilized and are ultimately necessary for the complete exploration of the concept.

Discussions of sport aesthetics, once made public, carry a particular kind of responsibility: presenting sport as aesthetic activity always includes the possibility that no one else sees it as such and the person who did the conferring would be seen in a less than favorable light. This has not happened with the sport aesthetic concept, though, for several sport theorists, who can be conceived of as acting on behalf of the sportworld, have designated sport as aesthetic activity (Best, 1975; Browne, 1917; Kaelin, 1968; Keenan, 1972; Kovich, 1971; Kupfer, 1975; Lowe, 1971, 1977; Maheu, 1965; Munrow, 1972; Pavlich, 1966; Reid, 1970).

Most of these theorists, while presenting sport as aesthetic activity, obviously have a theoretical aesthetic framework within which their viewpoints are structured. Some elucidated their aesthetic base and some did not. Such a framework, carefully described to guide and explain the synthesizing processes, is necessary to provide strength to any sport aesthetic theory. Just as art critics are subject to questioning regarding their aesthetic designations and decisions, so too must the sport aesthetic critic/theorists be prepared to explain and defend their positions. All questions and challenges are important and essential in the exploration and development of sport aesthetic theory.

Bibliography

Arnheim, R. Perceptual and aesthetic aspects of the movement response. *Journal of Personality*, 1951, *19*, 265-281.

Beardsley, M. C. *Aesthetics: Problems in the philosophy of criticism*. New York: Harcourt, Brace, 1958.

Best, D. The aesthetic of sport. *Journal of Human Movement Studies*, 1975, *1*, 41-47.

Brown, G. I. and Gaynor, D. Athletic action as creativity. *Journal of Creative Behavior*, 1967, *1*, 155-162.

Browne, G. H. *The esthetics of motion*. New Ulm, Minnesota: Turner, 1917.

Danto, A. The artworld. *The Journal of Philosophy*, 1964, *41*, 571-584.

Dickie, G. *Art and the aesthetic*. Ithaca, New York: Cornell University, 1974.

Kaelin, E. F. The well-played game: Notes toward an aesthetics of sport. *Quest*, 1968, *10*, 16-28.

Keenan, F. W. The athletic contest as a "tragic" form of art. A paper presented at the State University College at Brockport, Brockport, New York, for the Symposium on the Philosophy of Sport, February 12, 1972.

Kostelantz, R. Fanfare for TV football. *Intellectual Digest*, 1973, *3* (12), 53-54.

Kovich, M. Sport as an art form. *Journal of Health, Physical Education and Recreation*, October, 1971, 42.

Kristeller, P. O. The modern system of the arts. In M. Weitz (Ed.), *Problems in aesthetics* (2nd ed.). London: Macmillan, 1970.

Kupfer, J. Purpose and beauty in sport. *Journal of the Philosophy of Sport*, 1975, *2*, 83-90.

Lowe, B. The aesthetics of sport: The statement of a problem. *Quest*, 1971, *16*, 13-17.

Lowe, B. *The beauty of sport: A cross-disciplinary inquiry*. Englewood Cliffs, New Jersey: Prentice-Hall, 1977.

Maheu, R. Sport and culture. *Journal of Health, Physical Education and Recreation*, 1965, *34* (8), 30-32, 49-50, 52-54.

Munrow, A. D. *Physical education: A discussion of principles*. London: Bell and Sons, 1972.

Pavlich, M. The power of sport. *Journal of Arizona Association of Health, Physical Education and Recreation*, 1966, *10* (1), 9-10.

Reid, L. A. Sport, the aesthetic and art. *British Journal of Educational Studies*, 1970, *18* (3), 245-258.

Wulk, N. G. Aesthetics of sport: A metacritical analysis. Unpublished doctoral dissertation, University of North Carolina at Greensboro, 1977.

The Aesthetic in Sport*†

DAVID BEST

INTRODUCTION

There appears to be an increasing interest in looking at various sporting activities from the aesthetic point of view. In this paper I want to examine the relationship between sport and the aesthetic, and to attempt to sketch the logical character of this way of considering physical activities. My method of approach will be to trace out an important logical characteristic of paradigm cases of objects of the aesthetic attitude, namely works of art, and go on to see whether, or to what extent, it is applicable to sport.

THE AESTHETIC: CONCEPT NOT CONTENT

First, it might be asked whether it is possible to consider all sports from the aesthetic point of view, when one takes account of the great and increasingly varied range of such activities. That question, at least, can be answered clearly in the affirmative, for one can look at any object or activity from the aesthetic point of view—cars, houses, mountains, even mathematical proofs and philosophical arguments.

This raises a point about which it is important to be clear at the outset, which is that it is less conducive to error to regard the aesthetic

*From *British Journal of Aesthetics*, 14 (Summer, 1974), 197-213.

†This topic is considered at greater length in Chapter 7 of David Best's recently published book *Philosophy and Human Movement*, (George Allen & Unwin, London: 1978).

as a concept than a content—as a way of perceiving an object or activity rather than a constituent feature of that object or activity. One sometimes hears talk of the aesthetic content of an activity, which gives the misleading impression of the aesthetic as an element or characteristic which could be added or subtracted. Such a misconception is closely related to the pernicious assumption that there must be some common property or set of properties in all those objects which can properly be said to be of aesthetic interest. This sometimes leads to suspicions by the scientifically minded that those who are concerned with the aesthetic must be up to something mistily metaphysical, since the presence of this aesthetic content in an activity or object cannot be empirically verified by scientific procedures. These suspicions are without foundation for despite the dubious metaphysics of much writing on the subject, aesthetic judgements, like any other judgements, are intelligible only if they are ultimately answerable to what is, at least in principle, empirically observable. Yet that is not to say that they are scientifically verifiable, since the scientific is not the only way of considering what is available to sensory perception. A car may be assessed from the point of view of performance—road-holding, acceleration, petrol consumption, etc.—for the accurate testing of which scientific procedures are important. But such procedures would be quite inappropriate for answering questions about whether it were of attractive appearance. Nevertheless, such questions would require answers which referred to observable features

345

of the car. Questions concerning its appearance come under a different aspect; they are answered in a different way.

THE AESTHETIC POINT OF VIEW

It may be true that everything can be considered from the aesthetic aspect, but it is equally true that some activities and objects are more centrally of aesthetic interest than others. Works of art, to take an obvious example, are primarily of aesthetic interest, though even they can be considered from other points of view: a piece of sculpture might be used as a paper-weight, and paintings often are used as an investment. The question now arises as to what it is to look at something from the aesthetic point of view, what it is which marks off this from other ways of looking at objects. One important characteristic which has been the subject of some attention in recent philosophical writings is that the aesthetic is a non-functional or non-purposive concept. To take a central example again, when we are considering a work of art from the aesthetic point of view we are not considering it in relation to some external function or purposes it serves. The work of art cannot be evaluated aesthetically according to its degree of success in achieving some such extrinsic end. By contrast when a painting, for instance, is considered from the point of view of an investment, then it is assessed in relation to an extrinsic end, namely that of maximum appreciation in financial value. Its success is measured against the way in which other investments, say in stocks and shares, increase in monetary value.

This characteristic of the aesthetic immediately raises an insuperable objection to theories which propose an over-simple relation between sport and the aesthetic by identifying them too closely. For example, it is sometimes claimed that sport just *is* an art form (for examples see Anthony, 1968), and sometimes that the aesthetic is the unifying concept or characteristic in all the activities which come under the umbrella of physical education (see Carlisle, 1969). But there are many sports, indeed the great majority, which are like the case of the painting considered as an investment in that there is an identifiable aim or purpose which is of far greater importance than the way it is accomplished. That is, the *manner* of achievement of the primary purpose is of little or no significance as long as it comes within the rules. For example, from the competitive point of view it is far more important

for a football or hockey team *that* a goal is scored than *how* it is scored. In very many sports of this kind the overriding consideration is the achievement of an external end, since that is the mark of success. In such sports the aesthetic is incidental.

Despite the fact that this non-purposive character of the aesthetic is often pointed out, it is also often misunderstood or not fully understood. Such a misunderstanding would be manifested, for instance, in the commonly supposed consequence that therefore there is no purpose or point in art. The misunderstanding arises from the presupposition that an activity can be said to be of some point or value only if it can be assessed in relation to its success in attaining some purpose external to itself towards which it is directed. Now in cases where such an extrinsic end is the primary consideration, evaluation does depend on it. As we saw above, a painting considered solely as an investment would be evaluated entirely according to its degree of success in achieving maximum capital appreciation. Where the attainment of the end is the overriding consideration the means of attaining it is irrelevant. It would not matter, for instance, what sort of painting it were, or even that it were a painting at all, as long as the end were realized. Similarly, if someone wants to improve the petrol consumption of his car by changing the carburetter, considerations about the particular design of the new one, and the materials from which it is made, are unimportant as long as it succeeds in giving maximum mileage per gallon.

The purpose or point of art cannot be specified in this way, however, though the misapprehension we are now considering stems from the mistaken assumption that the point of an activity *must* somehow be identifiable as an end or purpose apart from the activity itself. Yet where art, or more generally the aesthetic, is concerned, the distinction between means and end is inapplicable. Consider, for example, the case of a particular work of art. The question: What is the purpose of that novel? or Why did the novelist write it? can be answered comprehensively only in terms of the novel itself. It might be objected that this is not entirely true, since the purpose of some novels could be given as, for example, exposing certain deleterious social conditions. But such an objection misses the point I am trying to make, for if the purpose is the external one of exposing those social conditions, then it could equally well, or perhaps better, be realized in other ways, such as the publication of a social survey or a political speech. The report of the social survey is evaluated by reference to its purpose, of effectively conveying the information, whereas this would be irrelevant to the *aesthetic* judgement of a novel. To put the same point another way, from the point of view of efficient conveying of information the precise form and style of writing of the report is of no consequence except in so far as it affects the achievement of that purpose. One report could be as good as another, though the style of writing or compilation was different from, or even inferior to, the other. There could not be a parallel situation in art in which, for example, one poem was said to be as good as another though not so well written. This is, of course, an aspect of the well-known problem of form and content in the arts. To put it briefly, there is a peculiarly intimate connection between the form of an object of aesthetic assessment, i.e. the particular medium of expression, and its content, i.e. what is expressed in it. So that in art there cannot be a change of form of expression without a corresponding change in what is expressed. It is important to recognize that this is a logical point. For even if, in fact, one way of writing the report is the clearest and most efficient, this is only a contingent matter since it is always possible that a better method may be devised; but it is not a contingent matter that the best way of expressing the content of *One Day in the Life of Ivan Denisovich* is in the particular form of that novel. So that the question becomes: 'What is the purpose of this particular novel, i.e. of this particular *way* of exposing certain aspects of these social conditions?' The end cannot be specified as 'exposing such and such social conditions,' but only as 'exposing such and such social conditions in this particular way and no other.' And to give a comprehensive account of what is meant by 'in this particular way and no other' one would have to reproduce nothing less than the whole novel. The end cannot even be identified apart from the manner of achieving it, and that is another way of saying that the presupposition encapsulated in the question, of explanation in terms of purposive action directed on to an external end, is inappropriate in the sphere of aesthetics. In short, there is an important sense in which the answer to 'What is the purpose of that novel?' will amount to a rejection of the question.

A further objection, which has important implications for the aesthetic in sport, might be that in that case how can we criticize a work of art if it can be justified only in terms of itself and there is nothing else with which we can compare it? There is a great deal to be said about the misapprehension that to engage in critical reasoning is necessarily to generalize (see Bambrough, 1973). It is sufficient for my argument to recognize that an important part of the activity of critical appreciation of art consists in the giving of reasons why particular features contribute so effectively to, or detract from, *this particular* work of art. The important point, for our purposes, is to see again that the end is inseparable from the means of achieving it, for even when one is suggesting an improvement, that improvement is given in terms of the particular work of art in question. Another way of putting this point is to say that *every* feature of a work of art is relevant to the aesthetic assessment of it, whereas when we are judging something as a means to an end, there are irrelevant features of the means, or equally effective alternative means, of achieving the required end. To say that X is an irrelevant feature is always a criticism of a work of art, whereas this is not true of a functional object.

It is true that the aim or end in a sport cannot be considered in isolation from the set of rules or norms of that particular sport. Scoring a goal in football and hockey is not just a matter of getting the ball between the opponents' posts, but requires conformity to the laws of the game. Such requirements are implicit in the use of terms such as 'scoring a goal.' Nevertheless, in contrast to a work of art, within those limits there are many ways of achieving the end, of scoring a goal, in football and hockey.

THE GAP:
PURPOSIVE AND AESTHETIC SPORTS

At this point we need to direct our attention to the difference between types of sporting activities with respect to the relative importance of the aesthetic. On the one hand there are those sports, which I shall call 'purposive' and which form the great majority, where the aesthetic is relatively unimportant. This category would include football, climbing, athletics, orienteering and squash. In each of these sports the aim, purpose or end can be specified independently of the manner of achieving it as long as it conforms to the limits set by the rules or norms—for example, scoring a goal and climbing the Eiger. Even in such sports as these, of course, certain moves or movements, indeed whole games or performances, can be considered from the aesthetic point of view; but that is a relatively unimportant aspect of the activity. If we were to ask a hockey player, on the eve of an important match: 'Which would you prefer, to score three goals in a clumsy manner, or to miss them all with graceful movements?' there is little doubt what the answer would be, at least in most cases. In sports such as these the aesthetic aspect is subordinate to the main purpose.

On the other hand there is a category of sports in each of which the aim cannot be specified in isolation from the aesthetic, for example trampolining, gymnastics, figure skating and diving. I shall call these the 'aesthetic' sports, since they are similar to the arts in that the purpose cannot be considered apart from the manner of achieving it. There is an intrinsic end, one which cannot be identified independently of the means. In formal gymnastics the end is not simply to get over the box, or to turn a somersault if, for example, one were to do so in a clumsy way and collapse afterwards in an uncontrolled manner. It is not incidental, but central, to these sports *how* one performs the appropriate movements. The end cannot be specified, for instance, as 'getting over the box,' but only in terms of the way in which this end is to be achieved. Indeed a certain degree of aesthetic evaluation is already built in to terms like 'vault' and 'dive.' To vault over a box is not the same as to jump over it or to get over it somehow or other. 'Vault' incorporates certain implicit aesthetic norms. Moreover, although such terms as 'vault' are not used in modern educational gymnastics, the same issue of principle applies. There is greater flexibility in the possibility of answering a particular task in educational, as compared with more formal gymnastics, yet it still matters a great deal how, aesthetically, the task is answered. Clumsy, uncontrolled movements would not be regarded as an adequate way of answering a task, even allowing for the wider choice of movements available for each task in educational gymnastics. Similarly, not any way of dropping into the water would count as a dive. One would have to satisfy at least to some minimal extent the aesthetic requirement built into the meaning of the term for a performance to count as even a bad dive.

In an interesting article on this topic Reid (1970) distinguishes between what I have called purposive and aesthetic sports in the following way: 'Games come at the end of a kind of spectrum. In most games, competition against an opponent (an individual or team) is assumed. In a wide range of athletics, on the other hand—such as hurdling, flat racing, high or long jumping—competition against others, although part of any total picture of athletics, is not absolutely essential to the activity. In any of these sports one can "compete" for long periods only against oneself. At the other end of the spectrum there are gymnastics, diving, skating . . . in which grace, the *manner* in which the activity is carried out, seems to be of central importance.' But it is difficult to understand this suggestion, for it is not clear what is the element or characteristic the degree of which determines the position of various sports on such a spectrum. If the supposed characteristic is competitiveness, then there does not seem to be even a distinction here, let alone a spectrum, for competition in Olympic gymnastics, trampolining, skating and diving can be every bit as keen as it is in Rugby football. Reid appears to be adopting the commonly encountered practice of contrasting the competitive with the aesthetic, but to take a paradigm example there are even competitive music festivals. If on the other hand Reid were thinking of the differences between sports with respect to the relative ineliminability of the aesthetic, then there is a distinction, but hardly a spectrum. As we have seen, there are sports whose purpose can be stated in terms which carry no implications as to the manner of achievement, and there are sports in which the purpose of the activity will inevitably incorporate aesthetic evaluation of the means of achieving it. I can think of only one sport which would qualify for a central position on a spectrum, namely ski jumping, in which points are awarded both for length and for style so that the skier who produces the longest jump does not necessarily win the competition. But one such sport is not enough to provide a spectrum, though this almost total lack of 'mixed' sports is, of course, a contingent matter. One can imagine a game in which, for instance, points are awarded for a goal, and further points are awarded if it was scored in an aesthetically pleasing manner. So that one competitor could 'win' (in our present sense) a high jump, boat race or cricket match, yet lose because the manner of achievement was inferior. Such a situation, in which different sports varied with respect to the relative importance of the aesthetic, *would* give a spectrum. It may be a pity that we do not have more sports of this sort—and perhaps one might take the liberty of commending the idea to physical educationists interested in the aesthetic who may consider devising new sports or modifying old ones. It would provide even greater variety to the growing range of sporting activities, and would specifically cater for the increasing interest in the aesthetic. Nevertheless, at present, to the best of my knowledge there is only one candidate for an intermediate position, and that would seem to be insufficient to uphold the notion of a spectrum.

CLOSING THE GAP

We can now return to the original question concerning the characterization of the aesthetic way of looking at sport. By examining the paradigm cases of sports in which the aesthetic is inseparable from what the performer is trying to achieve we might hope to discover aspects of our way of considering them which can be found to apply even to purposive sports when they are looked at aesthetically.

In figure skating, diving, trampolining and Olympic gymnastics it is of the first importance that there should be no wasted energy, no superfluous movements. Champion gymnasts like Olga Korbutt and Ludmilla Tourischeva not only perform striking physical feats, but do so with such remarkable economy and efficiency of effort that it sometimes looks effortless. There is an intensive concentration of the gymnast's effort so that it is all directed precisely and concisely on to that specific task. Any irrelevant movement or excessive expenditure of energy would detract from the quality of the performance as a whole, just as superfluous or exaggerated words, words which fail to contribute with maximum compression of meaning to the total effect, detract from the quality of a poem as a whole.

However, even in the case of the aesthetic sports there is still, though no doubt to a very limited extent, an externally identifiable aim: for example the requirements set by each particular movement and by the particular group of movements in gymnastics. Now it might be thought that it would be justifiable to regard such stringencies as analogous to, say, the form of a sonnet. That is, it may be thought more appropriate to regard them as setting a framework within which the performer has the opportunity to reveal his expertise in moving gracefully than as an externally identifiable aim. There is certainly something in this notion, but it is significant that there is no analogy in aesthetic sports with poetic licence. The poet may take liberties with the sonnet form without necessarily detracting from the quality of the sonnet, but if the gymnast deviates from the requirements of, say, a vault, however gracefully, then that inevitably detracts from the standard of the performance. Nevertheless the main point for our purposes is that even if in the aesthetic sports the means never quite reaches the ultimate of complete identification with the end which is such an important distinguishing feature of the concept of art, it at least closely approximates to such an identification. The gap between means and end is almost, if not quite, completely closed.

Now I want to suggest that the same consideration applies to our aesthetic appreciation of sports of the purposive kind. However successful a sportsman may be in achieving the principal aim of his particular activity, our *aesthetic* acclaim is reserved for him who achieves it with maximum economy and efficiency of effort. We may admire the remarkable stamina and consistent success of an athlete such as Zatopek, but he was not an aesthetically attractive runner because so much of his movement seemed irrelevant to the ideal of most direct accomplishment of the task. His style was regarded as ungainly because there were extraneous waggles, rolls or jerks which seemed wasteful in that they were not concisely aimed at achieving the most efficient use of his energy.

So to consider the purposive sports from the aesthetic point of view is to reduce the gap between means and end. From a purely purposive point of view any way of winning, within the rules, will do, whereas not *any* way of winning will do as far as aesthetic considerations are concerned. There is a narrower range of possibilities available for the achievement of the end in an aesthetically pleasing way, since the end is no longer simply to win, but to win with the greatest economy and efficiency of effort. Nevertheless the highest aesthetic satisfaction is experienced and given by the sportsman who not only performs with graceful economy but who also *achieves* his purpose. The tennis player who serves a clean ace with impeccable style has, and gives to the spectator, far more aesthetic satisfaction than when he fractionally faults with an equally impeccable style. In the case of the purposive sports there is an objectively specifiable framework, i.e. one which does not require the sort of judgement to assess achievement which is necessary in the aesthetic sports. Maximum aesthetic success still requires the attainment of the end, and the aesthetic in any degree requires direction on to that end; but the number of ways of achieving such success is reduced in comparison with the purely purposive interest of simply accomplishing the end in an externally specifiable sense.

CONTEXT AND AESTHETIC FEELING

This raises two related points. First, movement cannot be considered aesthetically in isolation, but only in the context of a particular action in a particular sport. A graceful sweep of the left arm may be very effective in a dance, but the same movement may look ugly and absurd as part of a service action in tennis or of a bowler's action in cricket, since it detracts from the ideal of total concentration of effort to achieve the specific task. A specific movement is aesthetically satisfying only if in the context of the action as a whole it is seen as forming a unified structure which is regarded as the most economical and efficient method of achieving the required end.

Second, there is a danger of serious misconception arising from a mistaken dependence upon feelings as criteria of aesthetic quality whether in sport or in any other activity, including dance and the other arts. The misconception is to take the feeling of the performer, or spectator, as the ultimate arbiter. But such a feeling is intelligible only if it can be identified by observable phenomena. This is part of what Wittgenstein (1963) meant by saying that an inner process stands in need of outward criteria. It is the observable physical movement which identifies the feeling and not, as is often believed, the inner feeling which suffuses the physical movement with aesthetic quality or meaning. That is, the feeling could not even be understood as a feeling, still less as the specific feeling it is, if it were not experienced in a certain set of empirically recognizable circumstances. We should resist the temptation, commonly encountered in discussion of dance and other forms of movement, to believe that it is how a movement feels which determines its effectiveness, whether aesthetic or purposive. That it feels right is no guarantee that it is right. Inexperienced oarsmen in an 'eight' are often tempted to heave their bodies round violently in an attempt to propel the boat more quickly, because such an action gives a feeling of much greater power. But in fact it will upset the balance of the boat and thus reduce the effectiveness of the rowing of the crew as a whole. The most effective stroke action can best be judged by the coach who is watching the whole performance from the bank, not by the feeling of the individual oarsman or even by that of all the crew. Similarly in tennis and skiing, to

take just two examples, the feeling of an action is often misleading as to its maximum efficiency. A common error in skiing is to lean into the slope and at a certain stage in his progress a learner starts to make turns for the first time which feel very good. Yet however exhilarating the feeling, if he is leaning the wrong way he will be considerably hampered from making further progress because in fact he is not directing his effort in the most effective way. There are innumerable other such examples one could cite, and this of course has important implications for education. If the arbiter of success in physical activities is what the students feel, rather than what they can be observed to do, it is hard to see how such activities can be learned and taught.

It is important, however, not to misunderstand this point by going to the opposite extreme, for I am not saying that we cannot be guided by such feelings or that they are of no value. My point is that they are useful and reliable only to the extent that they are answerable to patterns of behaviour which can be *observed* to be most efficiently directed on to the particular task. This reveals the connection between this and the preceding point, for it is clear that the character and efficiency of a particular movement cannot be considered in isolation from the whole set of related movements of which it forms a part and from the purpose towards which they are, as a whole, directed. Thus the context in which the movement occurs is a factor of an importance which it is impossible to exaggerate, since the feeling could not even be understood, let alone evaluated, if it were not normally experienced as part of an empirically recognizable action.

In this respect I should like to question what is often said about the aesthetic attitude, namely that it is essentially or predominantly contemplative. Reid (*op. cit.*, p. 248), for instance, says: 'In an aesthetic situation we attend to what we perceive in what is sometimes called a "contemplative" way.' Now it may be that a concern with the arts and the aesthetic is largely, or even for the most part, contemplative; but I see no reason to deny, indeed I see good reason to insist, that one can have what are most appropriately called aesthetic *feelings* while actually performing an activity, as long as it is clear that the criterion is answerability to an empirically observable context. A perfect smash in tennis, a well-executed dive, a finely timed stroke in squash, a smoothly accomplished series of movements in gymnastics, an outing in an 'eight' when the whole crew is pulling in unison with unwavering balance, a training run when one's body seems to be completely under one's control, and there are many other examples—for many who engage in sport the feelings derived from such performances are part of the enjoyment of participation in these activities. And 'aesthetic' seems the most appropriate way to characterize such feelings. Reid says (*op. cit.*, p. 252): '. . . a dancer or actor in the full activity of dancing or acting is often, perhaps always, in some degree contemplating the product of his activity' And later (p. 252), of games players: 'There is no time whilst the operation is going on to dwell upon aesthetic qualities. . . . Afterwards, the participant may look back upon his experience contemplatively with perhaps some aesthetic satisfaction.' Again (p. 254), of the aesthetic in cricket: "The batsman may enjoy it too, although at the moment of play he has no time to dwell upon it. But to produce exquisite strokes for contemplation is not part of his dominating motive as he is actually engaged in the game. . . .' Yet the batsman's aesthetic experience is not necessarily dependent upon his having time, at the moment of playing the stroke, to 'dwell upon it,' nor is it limited to a retrospective contemplation of his performance. If he plays a perfectly timed cover drive, with the ball flashing smoothly and apparently effortlessly from the face of his bat to the boundary, the aesthetic satisfaction of the batsman is intrinsic to what he is doing. The aesthetic is not a distinct but perhaps concurrent activity, and it need not depend upon detached or retrospective contemplation. His experience is inseparable from the stroke he is playing, since it is identifiable only by the way in which he is performing. His particular action, in that context, is a criterion of his feeling, and it is quite natural, unexceptionable and perhaps unavoidable, to call such feelings 'aesthetic.' 'Kinaesthetic' or 'tactile' would not tell the whole story by any means, since producing the same physical movement in other circumstances, say in a laboratory, would not produce the same feeling. Indeed it is significant that we tend naturally to employ aesthetic terms to describe the feelings involved in such actions. We say that a stroke felt 'beautiful,' and it was so to the extent that it was efficiently executed in relation to the specific purpose of the action in the sport concerned. Many participants in physical activities have experienced the exquisite feeling of, for instance, performing a dance or gymnastic sequence, of sailing over the bar in a pole vault, and of accomplishing

a fluent series of Christis with skis immaculately parallel. It is difficult to know how to describe these feelings other than as 'aesthetic.' It is certainly the way in which those of us who have taken part in such activities tend spontaneously to refer to them. So, though I do not wish to deny that contemplation is an important part of the aesthetic, I would suggest that it is not exhaustive. It is by no means unusual to experience aesthetic feelings, properly so called, while actually engaged and fully involved in physical activities.

THE AESTHETIC IN THE FUNCTIONAL

This characteristic of the aesthetic in activities which are primarily functional can be seen to apply to the apparently bizarre examples cited earlier of mathematical proofs and philosophical arguments. The proof of a theorem in Euclidean geometry, or a philosophical argument, is aesthetically pleasing when there is a cleanly, sharply and totally directed focus of effort. Any over-elaborate, irrelevant or repetitious section, in either case, would detract from the maximum economy in achieving the conclusion which is a requirement for maximum aesthetic satisfaction. Again the context is crucial. Rhetorical flourishes, however aesthetically impressive in other contexts, as for example a political speech, detract aesthetically from a philosophical argument by fussily blurring the ideal of a clean line of totally focused direction on to the conclusion. The aesthetic satisfaction given by rhetoric in a political speech is related to the latter's different purpose of producing a convincing or winning argument rather than a valid one.

The same characteristic of the aesthetic can be seen to apply, to some extent, to objects which are considered primarily from a functional point of view. For example our aesthetic evaluation of the shape of a car is at least partly related to what we take to be its contribution to optimum efficiency of function— for instance by reducing wind resistance. Of course there are other aspects, such as colour and embellishments, which may contribute to aesthetic effect while being irrelevant to efficiency of function, but even these are unlikely to be highly regarded aesthetically if they actually detract from the achievement of the primary purpose of the car.

The aesthetic pleasure which we derive from sporting events of the purposive kind, such as hurdling and putting the shot, is, then, derived from looking at, or performing, actions which we take to be approaching the ideal of totally concise direction towards the required end of the particular activity. Skiing provides a good example. The stylish skier seems to float, his body automatically accommodating itself, apparently without conscious effort on his part, to the most appropriate and efficient positions for the various types and conditions of terrain. By contrast the skiing in a slalom race often appears ungainly because it seems to be unnecessarily forced. The skier in such an event achieves greater speed, but only by the expenditure of a disproportionate amount of additional effort. Similarly athletes at the end of a distance race often abandon the smooth, economical style with which they have run the greater part of the race. They achieve greater speed but at disproportionate cost, since irrelevant movements appear—the head rolls, the body lurches, etc. In rowing, too, some oarsmen can produce a higher speed with poor style but more, if less effectively produced, power. Even though it is wasteful, the net effective power may still be greater than that of the oarsman who directs his more limited gross power with far more efficiency. It is often said that a good big 'un will beat a good little 'un. It is also true in many sports, unfortunately in my view, that a poor big 'un may well beat a far better little 'un.

Perhaps these considerations do something to explain the heightened aesthetic awareness which is achieved by watching slow-motion films and television replays, since (a) we have more time to appreciate the manner of the performance, and (b) the object of the action, the purpose, in an extrinsic sense, becomes less important. That is, our attention is directed more to the character of the action than to its result. We can see whether and how every detail of every movement in the action as a whole contributes to making it the most efficient and economical way of accomplishing that particular purpose. A smooth, flowing style is more highly regarded aesthetically because it appears to require less effort for the same result than a jerky one. Nevertheless, as we mentioned above, achievement of the purpose is still important. However graceful and superbly directed the movements of a pole-vaulter, our aesthetic pleasure in his performance is marred if he knocks the bar off.

Several questions remain. For example, why do we regard some events as less aesthetically pleasing than others, i.e. where we are not comparing actions within the same context of direction on to a common end but comparing actions in different contexts? For instance, in my view the butterfly stroke in swimming, however well performed, seems less aesthetically pleasing than the crawl. Perhaps this is because it looks less efficient as a way of moving through the water, since there appears to be a disproportionate expenditure of effort in relation to the achievement. A similar example is race walking, which even at its best never seems to me to be an aesthetically pleasing event. Perhaps, again, this is because one feels that the same effort would be more efficiently employed if the walker broke into a run. In each of these cases one is implicitly setting a wider context, seeing the action in terms of a wider purpose, of movement through water and movement over the ground respectively. But what of a sport such as weight lifting, which many regard as providing little or no aesthetic pleasure, though it is hard to discover a wider context, a more economical direction on to a wider or similar end in another activity with which we are implicitly comparing it? Perhaps the explanation lies simply in a general tendency to prefer, from an aesthetic point of view, sports which allow for smooth, flowing movements in the achievement of the primary purpose. Nevertheless, for the devotee, there are no doubt 'beautiful' lifts, so called because they accomplish maximum direction of effort.

ARE THE AESTHETIC SPORTS ART?

In the case of the purposive sports, then, as the actions become more and more directly aimed with maximum economy and efficiency at the required end, they become more and more specific and the gap between means and end is to that extent reduced. That is, increasingly it is less possible to specify the means apart from the end. In these sports the gap will nevertheless never be entirely closed—there cannot be the complete identification of means and end or, more accurately perhaps, the inappropriateness of the distinction between means and end which obtains in the case of art. For even if in fact there is a single most efficient and economical way of achieving a particular end, this is a contingent matter. The evolution of improved high jumping methods is a good example. The scissor jump was once regarded as the most efficient method, but it has been overtaken by the straddle, the Western roll and the Fosbury flop.

But what of the aesthetic sports? Can they justifiably claim to be art forms? I am inclined to give a negative answer, for two reasons.

First, as we have seen, there is good reason to doubt whether the means/end distinction ever quite becomes inappropriate, though it almost reaches that point, even in the aesthetic sports. That is, unlike dance, in these sports there is still an externally specifiable aim even though, for instance, it is very difficult to specify what the gymnast is trying to achieve apart from the way in which he is trying to achieve it. Perhaps this is what some physical educationists are getting at when they say, rather vaguely, that a distinction between gymnastics and dance is that the former is objective while the latter is subjective.

It is the second reason, however, which seems to me the more important one, and this concerns the distinction which seems to be almost universally ignored, or oversimplified and therefore misconceived, between the aesthetic and the artistic. The aesthetic applies, for instance, to sunsets, bird song and mountain ranges, whereas the artistic is limited, at least in its central uses, to artefacts or performances intentionally created by man—*objets trouvés*, if they are accepted as art, would be so in an extended sense. Throughout this paper I have so far followed the common practice of using 'aesthetic' as a broad generic term of which the artistic is a species. My reason for doing so is that the difference between the two terms is of no consequence to my main argument, since their logical character, with respect to the possibility of distinguishing between means and end, is the same. However, when we are discussing the question whether sport can justifiably be regarded as an art form the distinction becomes crucial. This issue seems to me to be a big one, which would take us too far afield to examine in the detail it merits, i.e. in relation to the arts generally; but it will be sufficient here to restrict our attention to the art form most closely related to our present enquiry, namely dance. It seems to me that there are cases where one may appreciate a dance performance aesthetically without appreciating it artistically. Some years ago I went to watch a performance by Ram Gopal, the great Indian classical dancer, and I was quite enthralled by the exhilarating quality of his movements. Yet I did not appreciate, because I could not have understood, his dance artistically, for there is an enormous number of precise meanings given to hand gestures in Indian classical dance, of which I knew none. So it seems clear that my appreciation was of the aesthetic not the artistic.

Reid is prepared to allow that what I call the aesthetic sports may justifiably be called art, but I suggest that he reaches this conclusion as a result of failing sufficiently to recognise the importance to that question of this aspect of the difference between the two concepts. For example, he says (*op. cit.*, p. 249): 'When we are talking about the category of art, as distinct from the category of the aesthetic, we must be firm, I think, in insisting that in art there is someone who has made (or is making) purposefully an artifact, and that in his purpose there is contained as an essential part the idea of producing an object (not necessarily a "thing": it could be a movement or a piece of music) in some medium for aesthetic contemplation.' Again (p. 258): '. . . the movement (of a gymnast, skater, diver), carried out in accordance with the general formula, has aesthetic quality fused into it, transforming it into an art quality. . . .' And again (*loc. cit.*): 'The question is whether the production of aesthetic value is intrinsically part of the purpose of those sports. (If so, on my assumptions, they will be in part, at least, art.)' According to Reid, then, the artistic is that which is intentionally created or performed for its aesthetic value. But I want to suggest that this overlooks the important factor in the distinction between the two concepts which is implicit in my example of Indian dance. In any art form, to put it roughly, there is at least the possibility of a close involvement with life situations—for example, the arts characteristically concern themselves with contemporary moral, social, political and emotional issues. Yet this is not true of the aesthetic, even if the object under consideration has been created for an aesthetic purpose. For example, a wallpaper pattern is normally designed to give aesthetic pleasure but I would not on that account, at least in the great majority of cases, want to call it artistic. To relate this to our present enquiry: it seems to me that even in those sports in which the aesthetic is intrinsic, and which are therefore intentionally performed to give aesthetic satisfaction, we cannot justifiably call them art forms. For in skating, diving, trampolining and gymnastics the performer does not have the possibility of expressing through his particular medium his view of life situations. It is difficult to imagine a gymnast who included in his sequence movements which expressed his view of war, or of love, or of any other such issue. Certainly if he did so it would, unlike art, *detract* to that extent from his performance.

Of course this is inadequate as an examination of the difference between the aesthetic and the artistic, but I think it points to an aspect of that difference which would repay further thought. There are difficult cases, even in the accredited arts, such as 'abstract' paintings and dances, where we are urged not to look for a meaning but simply to enjoy the line, colour, movement, etc., without trying to read anything into it. But it does seem to me that an art form, properly so called, must at least allow for the possibility of the artist's comment, through his art, on life situations and this is not possible in diving, skating, trampolining and gymnastics. Incidentally, if I am right, this may pose problems for those who suggest that these aesthetic sports may provide one method of, perhaps an introduction to, education in the arts, though of course this is not in the least to cast doubt on their aesthetic value. Superb aesthetically, at their best, these sports undoubtedly are; but they are not, in my view, art.

Bibliography

Anthony, W. J., 'Sport and P.E. as a means of aesthetic education,' in *Journal of P.E.*, Vol. 60, No. 179. Published by the P.E. Association, Nottingham Place, London W1, 1968.

Bambrough, J. R., 'To reason is to generalise,' in *The Listener*, Vol. 89, No. 2285, 11 Jan. 1973.

Carlisle, R., 'The concept of physical education,' in *Proceedings of the Philosophy of Education Society of Great Britain*, Vol. 3, Jan. 1969.

Reid, L. A., 'Sport, the aesthetic and art,' in *British Journal of Educational Studies*, Vol. 18, 1970.

Wittgenstein, L., *Philosophical Investigations* (Oxford, 1953).

Purpose and Beauty in Sport*

JOSEPH KUPFER

"Winning isn't the most important thing, it's the only thing." "Success is measured by your record." "Win at all costs." Such ways of talking and taking up sport reflect a pervasive emphasis in our culture almost too well noted. What goes largely unnoticed, however, is that this attitude assumes and fosters the belief that sport, and competitive sport in particular, is inherently purposeful. The purpose of course is to win by out-scoring one's opponent(s). On this view, the play of the sport becomes merely a means to the accomplishment of the distinct, dominant end of winning. The prevalent, unexamined attitude toward competitive sport is based then on the assumption of purposefulness. This assumption is further reflected in the way many respond to the question, "How was the game?" . . . "Great! We won."

Distinguishing between competitive and non-competitive sports is helpful in focusing on this assumption of purposefulness. Competitive sports require for their play opposition, offense and defense, and "scoring." Such aspects are essential, for without them one cannot engage in the sport proper. Noncompetitive sports such as diving, gymnastics, or skating, while staged as "competitions," do not in their nature or form require opposition or scoring for their performance. (Evidence of the externality and "forced" element of competition in such sports is the fact that "judges" are required to make strained translation into numerical notation of their appreciation of the

*From *Journal of the Philosophy of Sport*, II (Sept., 1975), 83-90.

grace or fluidity of the performance. In the genuinely competitive sports, number results naturally or simply from keeping track of scoring play.) Performance in the non-competitive sports serves no end or purpose beyond itself. In these sports "The end cannot be identified apart from the manner of achieving it."[1] The "purpose" of the dive is exhausted by its manner of execution. Because they lack this independently identifiable end or purpose, non-competitive sports are thought by many to be capable of beauty or aesthetic apprehension. The aesthetic appreciation of an object or event requires that we view the object or event "disinterestedly," "as an end in itself," without regard to consequences. Or, as Kant would have it, as a mere representation and not as an existent thing. In contrast, competitive sports are thought incapable of aesthetic viewing because they appear to have ". . . an identifiable aim or purpose which is of far greater importance than the way it is accomplished." (1:p. 199)

It seems as though there is a gap between the fact *that* the purpose is achieved (end) and how it is achieved (means).[2] It might then be concluded that the means-end fusion typifying art (as well as those sports most richly repaying aesthetic apprehension) is lacking in the competitive sports. Such a conclusion, however, would be mistaken because it rests upon the assumption that competitive sport is purposeful. And this assumption is false. As a matter of fact, most people do consider winning more important than the way the game is won, but does this reflect the nature of competitive sport? Is public attitude the criterion conclusive for reflection about the significance of victory or the beauty of sport?

In what follows I shall argue for two related theses: 1) Competitive sport is not determined by an external purpose; 2) Competition affords an added aesthetic dimension lacking in non-competitive sport. Thus I shall argue that competition and the possibility for victory add to, rather than detract from the aesthetic in sport.

I

I should like now to consider several facets of purpose which support the view that scoring in order to win is *not* an external purpose of sport.

The purpose of an activity is the reason or basis for engaging in the activity. Scoring is not the *raison d'être* of competitive sport the way, for example, communication is the reason for the being of a telephone. Scoring or winning is not that in virtue of which competitive sport comes to exist or is engaged in. Scoring or winning, therefore, is not the purpose of competitive sport.

Because purposes are the ground of activities, their reasons for being purposes serve to differentiate activities from one another. That a goal is scored in itself, however, does not differentiate one sport from another or one instance of a particular sport from another. Scoring cannot be, therefore, a (or, *a fortiori*, "the") purpose of sport. Sporting activity is differentiated internally, by what is required to score, by the manner of play whose issue is scoring. The form or structure of the particular sport is the basis for our choosing to watch or play *it* rather than another.

An object or activity may serve some purpose or function external to it. Such is the case with a hammer or the activity of hammering a roof on to the frame of a house. A purpose or end may, on the other hand, be included *within* an activity which activity does not itself serve any purpose or end external to it. Such is the case with "taking tricks" in bridge; achieving perspective in painting a landscape; and singing a harmonic in a barbershop quartet. Such is also the case with scoring or winning in competitive sport. If scoring be a purpose it is not a purpose *of* sport or the play of the game; it is rather a purpose *within* sport or the play. By confounding these two sorts of purpose one is led to the erroneous belief that the play in competitive sport is purposeful in the sense of serving an external purpose or end.[3]

Scoring is not "external" to the play of the game in that it is not an end which could be accomplished by some other means. Scoring is independent of *this* or *that* particular play and so might come to be thought external to playing the game itself. We should not, however, confuse independence from particular plays with externality to the game itself or the play which constitutes the game. In addition to the fact that there can be no scoring without play, scoring and winning are contingently and logically bound to "good" (including the aesthetic sense) play. To score or win as the result of shabby play or luck can by no stretch of the imagination be thought of as achieving the "purpose" of competitive sport. Yet this would be of no matter if winning or scoring were its purpose! Scoring (or winning) is valued as a sign of excellence in play because it helps define excellence: it is part of our concept of good play. Elaboration of this claim will follow presently.

If what I have said above is correct, then scoring is not the "end identifiable apart from the manner of achieving" it most of the sport-watching public takes it to be. Why should we think that scoring cannot be specified apart from the play? In the first place, scoring a goal must be understood in relation to the structure of the sport: scoring serves to define and articulate *overcoming opposition*. It gives definition and form to this overcoming by providing a limit to particular play. In this way it helps define excellence. As the culmination of play scoring helps determine its form and completeness. The scoring aspect of a play is not detachable from it in that the play is partially defined in terms of the success or failure in scoring. It may help here to compare scoring a goal to the termination of a dive: scoring is analogous to "entering the water continuously, smoothly, at a ninety degree angle, without splash." Each is the culmination of excellent performance though each is, as a matter of fact, possible without the preceding excellence. The complete description of the play includes whether or not it issues in scoring. But just as the play cannot be completely specified independent of scoring, neither can scoring be specified or identified independent of the play.

Now, in one sense, of course, scoring can be specified independent of its manner of attainment: "that a goal is scored" can be so specified. What I wish to point out here is that this specification, this counting is an abstraction from how and when the goal is scored. How and when the opposition is overcome is the *scoring* and this is not specified, much less independently specified, by the "score." Scoring is distinct from the score and the score represents different means and manner of scoring indifferently. The "score" is specifiable independent of the manner of scoring since it is number. But the scoring is not itself so identifiable or separable from the play of the game. In short, we should not confuse the independent specifiability of the score (which follows from its numerical nature), with the independent specifiability of scoring. The number which represents the scoring plays of the game is merely an abstraction from the way in which opposition is surmounted or frustrated.

II

The logical claim for the independent specifiability of the purpose of competitive sport typically is accompanied by a valuation. ". . . [the] identifiable aim or purpose [scoring] . . . is of far greater importance than the way it is accomplished." (1:p. 199) This union of the logical and valuational claims is revealing. The issue of value must be introduced in order to demonstrate the significance of the "independent specifiability of scoring." For even if we could identify scoring apart from how the goal is made, unless the score itself be *important* the identifiability of the score would be inconsequential for the aesthetic of sport. The question which now arises is this: why should we think that the end, scoring, is more important than its manner of attainment?

The most obvious way of proceeding is to rely uncritically upon the opinion and valuing of the majority of performers and spectators.

. . . from the competitive point of view it is far more important for a football or hockey team that a goal is scored than *how* it is scored. In very many sports of this [competitive] kind the overriding consideration is the achievement of an external end . . . (1:p.199)

If we were to ask a hockey player, on the eve of an important match: 'Which would you prefer, to score three goals in a clumsy manner, or to miss them all with graceful movements?' there is little doubt what the answer would be, at least in most cases. In sports such as these the aesthetic aspect is subordinate to the main purpose. (1:p.201)

It seems to me that in no sport is the aesthetic subordinate to the "main purpose" since the purpose alluded to is part of the whole game, a reflection of excellence in the play of that game, and the aesthetic concerns the excellence of the whole. There is, however, one standpoint which vitiates my claim: the "professional" point of view through which most of us formulate our considerations. The singular thing to notice about this methodology is that it takes what is "important" or of "overriding consideration" to actual or would-be professionals or partisan spectators as the criterion of what is important in sport. The evaluations of hockey players or interested audiences are our guide in sketching the logic of sport and subsequently its aesthetic. This is symptomatic of our age and philosophy: what is, in fact, believed by the majority becomes the standard by which we judge what is in the nature of things or what is good. I suggest that most people who play or watch competitive sport are as jaded in their appreciation of sport as are art dealers who evaluate art on the basis of market price. We ought not appeal to the priorities of players or typical audiences to determine the place of scoring or winning within the logic of sport. What alternative do we have in examining the logic of sport? In order that an appreciation of the full range of its aesthetic be attained preliminary inquiry into the nature of sport is required.

The concept most basic to our investigation is "play." When we play at anything we act simply for the sake of the enjoyment of the activity. We are not forced by need or external constraint to participate. A man repairing his auto is engaged in activity for the sake of utility, but to the extent that he is playfully repairing the auto he is concerned with the task for its own dimensions, tensions, and resolutions. He enjoys the repair work for its own sake. We speak typically of playing games because games are paradigms of activities in which we participate for no purpose other than the enjoyment of their properties: the strategy and intricacy of chess: the gambling of poker; or the communication and thinking-through-of-the-play demanded in bridge. In *origin* and *ideal* games have no purpose other than the delight taken in their play. To play a game for the monetary or personal gain is to introduce a purpose or basis foreign to the game itself.

Competitive sports are formed as games. Non-competitive sports are essentially physical activities which, as with competitive sports,[4] admit of perfecting. The individual can try to perfect himself in the activity, but the desire to "do one's best" does not detract from or "compete" with the intrinsic value of the activity itself in either sort of sport. The Greeks saw the relationship as complementary: when engaging in an activity fully for its own sake one attempts to bring oneself and the activity to perfection. In this way sport includes man's relation to ideal. My intuition concerning sport, and any activity, is that it and the participant are perfected just when the activity is loved for its own dimensions. But sport, as with any activity or object, including art, may be used as a means to external ends such as making money or satisfying the desire to distinguish oneself.

Playing well, then, is not external to the game, rather, it is the full realization of the activity. Scoring and winning are at once conclusions of play and the "natural" completion of excellent play; they are signs or evidence of such excellence. As argued above, scoring is internal to the play of the game and therefore cannot, save in cases of perversion, "subordinate" the activity itself. A man who has no motive other than to play the game well and enjoy himself in such play would sooner lose a well-played game than win, when playing poorly, through luck or the utter weakness of his opponent. Yet the latter eventualities would not faze the "professional" since his concern *is* with matters extrinsic to the game itself. My point can be made by considering another hypothetical hockey player, one who plays for the sake of the game: would he rather score ten goals through happenstance, or two as a result of splendid execution?[5] The only delight taken in scoring which results from luck or shabbiness of play, and the only pleasure in a lopsided victory is derived from purposes or incentives external to the activity itself. And this brings me to the irony of the empirical methodology noted above.

In an attempt to show that competitive sports are "purposive" (serve an external end) a quasi-empirical appeal to what professional athletes and their audiences would or do value is made. This appeal is persuasive only because we have become inured to the fact that such valuation is itself based on ends extrinsic to sport. The force of reference to the importance of scoring to professional athletes or their audiences stems from the contingent connection between winning in sports and the attainment of "goals" external to the game itself such as financial or social gain. It is ironic that the *contingent* bearing of such extrinsic ends upon sport underlies the attempts to show that in competitive sport the play is *logically* subservient to its "extrinsic end" of scoring (or winning). We should not, then, take current practice or attitude toward competitive sports

as the criterion for locating scoring in the logic of sport.

Having shown that purpose is neither external nor important in the way typically thought, it remains for me to show how competition, the attempt to overcome or thwart opposition, adds to the aesthetic value of sport.

III

The most arresting aesthetic feature of sport *is* the grace of the human form. Economy and efficiency of effort are accomplished in movement which is continuous and fluid: sport provides us distinct balletic values. To their credit, non-competitive sports accentuate these values, but there is more to the aesthetic in sport than simply the individual human body in momentary motion.

Aesthetic values also emerge from human interaction. The activity which constitutes competitive sport involves tension between opponents and (where germane) coordination within the team. A "good" game includes both team cohesiveness and balance between the teams. In such sports the part can be brought to dramatic and athletic completion within the whole in two senses. The athlete realizes his excellence in relation to the team (as the team does collectively in relation to its opposition); the momentary funds and is in turn located within the temporally protracted whole. In the context of the opposition necessary for engaging in such sports, individuals come together to form a whole. As in art proper, the antagonism between part and whole is overcome. The part is brought to full development through its reciprocal relations with the other parts (members). Concepts such as timing, jelling, flowing, harmonizing, and executing attest to this aesthetic ideal in competitive sport. The individual's performance, a delight in itself, is organized and directed in the interdependence called forth by the demands of competition. The team as a whole, moreover, is pushed and pressed to its limit by the performance of the opposition: each "brings out" the best in the other. This mutual enhancement through opposition surely adds an aesthetic quality lacking in the non-competitive sports, especially since it dramatically unfolds over time.

Temporally extended opposition is the significant aesthetic addition competition provides. The aesthetic objects such opposition offers range in scope and duration. We delight in a movement, play, rally or drive, a sub-unit of the game such as inning, (golf) hole, or quarter, as well as a game, series of games, or an entire season. The game itself no doubt is the most typical as well as accessible object of appreciation. Movements and plays, rallies and drives combine to create crucial foci of tension amidst stretches of relative respite. The game is the wider dramatic context for momentary movement: the body moves to the rhythm and tempo of a whole.

Repetitions, balance, pace, variations, crescendoes and decrescendoes conspire to flavor a game with a rhythm and correlative mood or atmosphere. Some games are tense, stingy encounters in which defense dominates and scores are hard earned as if squeezed from a resistant world. Others are sprawling, brawly affairs, scoring barrages threatening to last forever. "Taut," "brisk," "sprawling," "smooth," "torpid," "electric," and "jerky" are but some aesthetically meaningful characterizations of whole games. It is appropriate, moreover, to speak of games in the "expressive" or "emotive" idiom typical in description of art works: games may be "grim," "breezy," "jovial," "solemn," "lively" and so on. As with works of art, games can fail to fill out into discernible wholes possessed of strong aesthetic qualities. Some games never seem to find a rhythm and in others dramatic tension is all but dissipated in early scoring or lackadaisical play; the latter mars the beauty of a game by destroying the rhythmic element dependent upon the crispness of execution.

The resolution of contest in victory and defeat is the way in which competitive sporting episodes are completed-in-themselves. When aesthetically rich, the game builds to a consummation. The see-saw scoring, the delicate balance between offenses and defenses, the entire rhythm of the game is fulfilled in the ending which is, in addition to a terminus, a climax. The strengths and weaknesses of the opponents exhibited throughout reach their final reckoning in the outcome which is in doubt until the last possible moment.[6] The conclusion seems to put all the duels and scores, plays and tensions in their "proper place." Thus do we retrospectively hold the entire game before us looking for omens and "turning points," portents of what seems at the conclusion to have been inevitable.

In this way, competitive sports exhibit just those real-life features lacking in the non-competitive sports: strains, oppositions, pivotal situations, denouements, inclusive rhythms, consummations are real. This stuff of drama is foreign to the form of non-competitive sports. The wholeness and finality possible in competitive sporting events, paradigmatic in the artistic, answer the human desire for completeness and unity, if only in symbol. The interdependence of team members contesting the opposition yields tensions and resolutions which echo those arising from the circumstances in which real people are situated. Within the confines imposed by the rules, which define the play of the game, and the spatio-temporal boundaries, often precise and geometrically exact, the resolution of these tensions requires invention in the exercise of the athlete's talents. Sport instantiates man's capacity to improvise in the midst of structured stress. It emphasizes and crystallizes the element of venture—that summons to new openings within the world's limits, so often unrecognized or unheeded in our everyday lives.

NOTES

1. Unless otherwise noted, all references are to David Best's "The Aesthetic in Sport." (1) Because he so clearly articulates it, I shall take Best to represent philosophically this popular assumption concerning the purposefulness of competitive sports.
2. Paul Ziff (4) seems to view performance in some sports, including the competitive, as "counting," i.e., important, only with regard to scoring. He maintains that form matters (as a "grading factor") *only* in the class of sports which turn out to be of the non-competitive sort. He writes that ". . . if one manages somehow to sink the ball expeditiously enough one may end up a champion." (4:p.101) He is obviously viewing sporting events only with a concern for their outcome, for he continues: "It is not looks but points that win a tennis match." (4:p. 104) My question for Ziff is: But is it points that make a tennis match good or worth watching?
3. The question of purposefulness is clarified by the Kantian distinction between purpose and purposivity. Art is purposive but not purposeful. This means that it displays those properties such as we find in objects which exist in order to serve an external purpose, but it does not in fact serve any such purpose. The unity of art works does not derive from something external to themselves, i.e., (a function), as does say a telephone or car. Although a work of art does not exist in order to serve some external end, it may contain within itself aims or purposes, as for example literary works in which the narrator or characters act or speak in order to attain some end. The purely purposive then may include purposes within it without as a whole being subservient to an extrinsic purpose or end. Sport is like art in being purposive but without external purpose. We engage in the activity or its viewing for its own sake.

4. It is interesting that many of these activities, such as diving, jumping, running, skating, and swimming, and even gymnastics originally met a practical need. Unlike most competitive sports, one swam, dove or vaulted in order to attain a real goal in a practical context, yet these turn out to be the paradigms of non-purposeful sports.

5. The case of the professional athlete includes the following objection to my thesis: one can play ungracefully and score, or gracefully and fail to score. My response is simply that as a function of human anatomy the very *best* plays and players (those who score most and in the most crucial situations) are graceful. Economy and efficiency in effort are always an asset in one's play. To be sure there have been fine athletes who lacked in grace of form but their achievements were not made *because* of awkwardness. Even Ziff (4) seems willing to concede this "natural" relationship.

6. For a more detailed account of cooperation inherent in competition and the role of suspense in sport see Warren Fraleigh's "On Weiss on Records and on the Significance of Athletic Records" (2), and E. F. Kaelin's "The Well-Played Game: Notes Toward an Aesthetics of Sport." (3)

Bibliography

1. Best, David. "The Aesthetic in Sport," *British Journal of Aesthetics*, Vol. 14, No. 3 (Summer, 1974), 197-213.
2. Fraleigh, Warren. "On Weiss on Records and on the Significance of Athletic Records," *Philosophic Exchange*, Vol. 1, No. 3 (Summer, 1972), 105-111.
3. Kaelin, E. F. "The Well-Played Game: Notes Toward an Aesthetics of Sport," *Quest*, No. 10 (May, 1968), 16-28.
4. Ziff, Paul. "A Fine Forehand," *Journal of the Philosophy of Sport*, Vol. 1 (September, 1974), 92-109.

BIBLIOGRAPHY TO SPORTS AND AESTHETICS

Aldrich, Virgil C. "Art and the Human Form." *Journal of Aesthetics and Art Criticism,* 29 (Spring, 1971), 295-302.

Anthony, D. W. J. "Sport and Physical Education as a Means of Aesthetic Education." *Physical Education,* 60 (March, 1968), 1-6.

Aspin, David N. "Sport and the Concept of 'the Aesthetic'." *Readings in the Aesthetics of Sport.* Edited by H. T. A. Whiting and Don W. Masterson. London: Lepus Books, 1974.

Baumbach, Jonathan. "The Aesthetics of Basketball." *Esquire,* LXXIII, no. 1, January, 1970, 140-146.

Best, David. *Expression in Movement and the Arts.* London: Lepus Books, 1974.

Bouet, M. Contribution à l'esthetique du sport. *Revaed' Esthetique,* 1, 180-194 (1948).

————. "The Phenomenology of Aesthetics of Sport." *Sport in the Modern World—Chances and Problems.* Edited by Ommo Grupe, Dietrich Kurz and Johannes Tiepel. New York: Springer-Verlag, 1973.

Brown, George S. and Donald Gayner. "Athletic Action as Creativity." *Journal of Creative Behavior,* 1 no. 2, 1967, 155-162.

Brown, Joe. "Movement and Figurative Sculpture." *Quest,* XXIII (Jan., 1975), 84-87.

Brown, Margaret C. "Sculpture and Physical Education." *Physical Educator,* I (October, 1940), 3-4.

Carlisle, Robert. "Physical Education and Aesthetics." *Readings in the Aesthetics of Sport.* Edited by H. T. A. Whiting and Don W. Masterson. London: Lepus Books, 1974.

Cheney, Gay. "Kine-Aesthetics." Proceedings of the NCPEAM/NA PECW National Conference, Orlando, Florida, Jan. 6-9, 1977.

Dubois, P. E. "The Aesthetic of Sport and the Athlete." *The Physical Educator,* 31, no. 4, 1974, 198-201.

Dufrenne, M.: La Philosophie du Sport. Education Physique et Sport 1, 4-6, (1950).

Edgell, C. H. *Sport in American Art.* Boston: Museum of Fine Arts, 1944.

Elliott, R. K. "Aesthetics and Sport." *Readings in the Aesthetics of Sport.* Edited by H. T. A. Whiting and Don W. Masterson. London: Lepus Books, 1974.

Fetters, Jan L. "The Body Aesthetic: A Symbolic Experience." Proceedings of the NCPEAM/NA PECW National Conference, Orlando, Florida, Jan. 6-9, 1977.

Frayssinet, P.: Le sport parmi les beaux-arts, 1968.

Friesen, Joana. "Laban's Effort/Shape Theories as Aesthetic Material." Proceedings of the NC PEAM/NAPECW National Conference, Orlando, Florida, Jan. 6-9, 1977.

Gablewitz, E. "Aesthetic Problems in Physical Education and Sport." *Bulletin of the Federation International d'Education Physique,* No. 3, 1965.

Gaskin, Geoffrey and Masterson, D. W. "The Work of Art in Sport." *Journal of the Philosophy of Sport,* 1 (September, 1974), 36-66.

Groos, Karl. *The Play of Man.* New York: D. Appleton and Company, 1901.

Hein, Hilde. "Play as an Aesthetic Concept." *Journal of Aesthetics,* 27 (Fall, 1968), 67-71. [Reprinted in *Humanitas,* V (Spring, 1969), 21-28.]

————. "Performances as an Aesthetic Category." *Journal of Aesthetics and Art Criticism,* 28 (Spring, 1970), 381-386.

Hohler, V. "The Beauty of Motion." *Readings in the Aesthetics of Sport.* Edited by H. T. A. Whiting and Don W. Masterson. London: Lepus Books, 1974.

Hohne, E. "Coubertin on the Place of Art in Modern Olympism." *Bulletin of the National Olympic Committee of the German Democratic Republic,* 14, n. 4, 1969. 31-40.

Holme, B. "Sport as a Challenge to Artists." *Design,* 61, January 1960, 125-127.

James, C. L. R. "The Relationship Between Popular Sport and Fine Art." *Readings in the Aesthetics of Sport.* Edited by H. T. A. Whiting and Don W. Masterson, London: Lepus Books, 1974.

Jokl, Ernst. "Sport and Culture" in *Medical Sociology and Cultural Anthropology of Sport and Physical Education.* Illinois: Charles C Thomas, 1964.

Kaelin, E. F. "The Well-Played Game: Notes Toward an Aesthetics of Sport." *Quest,* X (May, 1968), 16-28.

Kapreliam, Mary Haberkorn. *"A Comparison of Two Aesthetic Theories as They Apply to Modern Dance."* Unpublished Ed.D. dissertation, University of Wisconsin, 1969.

Keenan, Francis W. "The Athletic Contest as a 'Tragic' Form of Art." *The Philosophy of Sport: A Collection of Original Essays.* Edited by Robert G. Osterhoudt. Illinois: Charles C Thomas, 1973.

Keller, Hans. "Sport and Art—The Concept of Mastery." *Readings in the Aesthetics of Sport.* Edited by H. T. A. Whiting and Don W. Masterson. London: Lepus Books, 1974.

Kent, Norman. "Art in Sports." *American Artist,* 32 (March, 1968), 45-47, 55.

Kleinman, Seymour. "Effort/Shape: Heightening Aesthetic Awareness of the Self and the Other." Proceedings of the NCPEAM/NAPECW National Conference, Orlando, Florida, Jan. 6-9, 1977.

————. "Movement Notation Systems: An Introduction to Benesh Movement Notation, Labanotation and Eshkol—Wachman Movement Notation." *Quest,* XXIII (Jan., 1975), 33-56.

Kovich, Maureen. "Sport as an Art Form" *Journal of Health, Physical Education, and Recreation,* 42 (October, 1971), 42.

Kuntz, Paul G. "Aesthetics Applies to Sports As

Well As to the Arts." *Journal of the Philosophy of Sport,* I (September, 1974), 6-35.

———. "Paul Weiss on Sports as Performing Arts." *International Philosophic Quarterly,* 17 (June, 1977), 147-165.

———. "The Aesthetics of Sport." *The Philosophy of Sport: A Collection of Original Essays.* Edited by Robert G. Osterhoudt. Illinois: Charles C Thomas, 1973.

Kupfer, Joseph. "Purpose and Beauty in Sport." *Journal of the Philosophy of Sport,* II (September, 1975), 83-90.

Lowe, Benjamin. "The Aesthetics of Sport: The Statement of a Problem" *Quest,* XVI (June, 1971), 13-17.

———. *The Beauty of Sport: A Cross-Disciplinary Inquiry.* Englewood Cliffs, New Jersey: Prentice-Hall, Inc., 1977.

———. "The Representation of Sports in Painting in the United States: 1865-1965." Unpublished Masters' thesis, University of Wisconsin, 1968.

Maheu, Rene. "Sport and Culture." *Journal of Health, Physical Education, and Recreation,* 34 (October, 1963), 30-32, 49-50, 52-54.

Masterson, Don W. "Sport and Modern Painting." *Readings in the Aesthetics of Sport.* Edited by H. T. A. Whiting and Don W. Masterson. London: Lepus Books, 1974.

Metzi, E. "Art in Sports." *American Artist,* 26 (November, 1962), 30-37.

"The Poetry of Football." The Arts of Sport and Recreation. Edited by Derek Stanford. London: Thomas Nelson and Sons, 1967. (Reprinted from *The Times,* October 23, 1962).

Mitchell, Robert Thomas. "A Conceptual Analysis of Art as Experience and Its Implications for Sport and Physical Education." Unpublished Ed.D. dissertation, University of Northern Colorado, 1974.

Nasmark, H. "Aesthetics and Sport." *Bulletin of the International Federation d'Education Physique,* No. 1, 1963.

Osterhoudt, Robert G. "An Hegelian Interpretation of Art, Sport, and Athletics." *The Philosophy of Sport: A Collection of Original Essays.* Edited by Robert G. Osterhoudt. Illinois: Charles C Thomas, 1973.

Perry, R. Hinton. "The Relations of Athletics to Art." *Outing,* 49, (1902), 456-63.

Pouret, H. "Is Sport an Art?" *Report of the Tenth Session of the International Olympic Academy,* 129-133, Athens, 1970.

Rau, Catherine. "Psychological Notes on the Theory of Art as Play." *Journal of Aesthetics and Art Criticism,* 8 (June, 1950), 229-238.

Reid, Louis A. "Sport, The Aesthetic and Art." *British Journal of Educational Studies,* 18 (Oct., 1970), 245-258.

Roberts, Terence J. "Sport and the Sense of Beauty." *Journal of the Philosophy of Sport,* II (September, 1975), 91-101.

———. "Languages of Sport." Unpublished Ph.D. dissertation, University of Minnesota, 1976.

Schiller, Friedrich von. *Essays and Letters.* Volume VIII. Translated by A. Lodge, E. B. Eastwick and A. J. W. Morrison. London: The Anthological Society, 1882.

Seward, George. "Play as Art." *Journal of Philosophy.* XLI (March, 1944), 178-184.

Smith, Hope M. "Movement and Aesthetics." *Introduction to Human Movement.* Edited by Hope M. Smith. Massachusetts: Addison-Welsey, 1968.

Spencer, Herbert. "Aesthetic Sentiments." *Background Readings for Physical Education.* Edited by Ann Paterson and Edmond C. Hallberg. New York: Holt, Rinehart and Winston, 1965.

Studer, Ginny L. "Movement Aesthetics Summary." Proceedings of the NCPEAM/NA PECW National Conference, Orlando, Florida, Jan. 6-9, 1977.

Sweeney, James Johnson. "Contemporary Art: The Generative Role of Play." *Review of Politics,* 21 (April, 1959), 389-401.

Thomas, Carolyn E. "Toward an Experiential Sport Aesthetic." *Journal of the Philosophy of Sport,* 1 (September, 1974), 67-91.

Toynbee, Lawrence. "Artists and Sport." *New Society,* 6 (November 8, 1962), 28.

Whiting, H. R. A., Masterson D. W. *Readings in the Aesthetics of Sport.* London: Lepus Books, 1974.

Ziff, Paul. "A Fine Forehand." *Journal of the Philosophy of Sport,* 1 (September, 1974), 92-109.